NEUROBIOLOGY

SECOND EDITION

NEUROBIOLOGY

SECOND EDITION

Molecules, Cells, and Systems

Gary G. Matthews

Department of Neurobiology and Behavior
State University of New York at Stony Brook

b

Editorial Offices:
Commerce Place, 350 Main Street, Malden, Massachusetts 02148, USA
Osney Mead, Oxford OX2 0EL, England
25 John Street, London WC1N 2BL, England
23 Ainslie Place, Edinburgh EH3 6AJ, Scotland
54 University Street, Carlton, Victoria 3053, Australia
Other Editorial Offices:
Blackwell Wissenschafts-Verlag GmbH, Kurfürstendamm 57, 10707 Berlin, Germany
Blackwell Science KK, MG Kodenmacho Building, 7-10 Kodenmacho Nihombashi, Chuo-ku, Tokyo 104, Japan

Distributors:
USA

Blackwell Science, Inc.
Commerce Place
350 Main Street
Malden, Massachusetts 02148
(Telephone orders: 800-215-1000 or 781-388-8250; fax orders: 781-388-8270)

Canada

Login Brothers Book Company
324 Saulteaux Crescent
Winnipeg, Manitoba R3J 3T2
(Telephone orders: 204-837-2987)

Australia

Blackwell Science Pty, Ltd.
54 University Street
Carlton, Victoria 3053
(Telephone orders: 03-9347-0300; fax orders: 03-9349-3016)

Outside North America and Australia
Blackwell Science, Ltd.
c/o Marston Book Services, Ltd.
P.O. Box 269
Abingdon
Oxon OX14 4YN
England
(Telephone orders: 44-01235-465500; fax orders: 44-01235-465555)

Acquisitions: Nancy Whilton
Development: Jill Connor
Production: Irene Herlihy
Manufacturing: Lisa Flanagan
Marketing Manager: Carla Daves
Cover and text design by Meral Dabcovich, VisPer
Illustrations by Electronic Illustrators Group
Typeset by Northeastern Graphic Services

Printed and bound by Courier Companies/Kendallville

Printed in the United States of America
00 01 02 03 5 4 3 2 1

The Blackwell Science logo is a trade mark of Blackwell Science Ltd., registered at the United Kingdom Trade Marks Registry

Library of Congress Cataloging-in-Pbulication Data

Matthews, Gary G., 1949–
    Neurobiology : molecules, cells, and systems / Gary G. Matthews — 2nd ed.
      p. ; cm.
    Includes bibliographical references and index.
    ISBN 0-632-04496-9
    1. Neurobiology. I. Title.
    [DNLM: 1. Nervous System Physiology.   2. Neurobiology. WL 102 M439n 2001]
  QP355.2 .M38 2001
  573.8—dc21

                                        00-063014

To Karen and David

PART II: CELLULAR ASPECTS OF NEUROBIOLOGY   37

Chapter 3   **39**   ORIGIN OF MEMBRANE POTENTIAL

Chapter 4   **66**   MECHANISM OF NERVE ACTION POTENTIAL

Chapter 5   **92**   SYNAPTIC TRANSMISSION AT THE NEUROMUSCULAR JUNCTION

Chapter 6   **114**   SYNAPTIC TRANSMISSION IN THE CENTRAL NERVOUS SYSTEM

PART III: MOTOR CONTROL SYSTEMS   137

Chapter 8   164   SPINAL CORD MOTOR MECHANISMS

Chapter 9   188   BRAIN MOTOR MECHANISMS

Chapter 15   318   THE VISUAL SYSTEM: RETINA

Chapter 16   352   THE VISUAL SYSTEM: HIGHER VISUAL PROCESSING

Chapter 17   379   HEARING AND OTHER VIBRATION SENSES

Chapter 18   402   CHEMICAL SENSES

PART V: NEURONAL PLASTICITY AND HIGHER CORTICAL FUNCTION 427

Chapter 19 430 NEURAL DEVELOPMENT

Chapter 20   465   SYNAPTIC PLASTICITY

Chapter 21   496   LANGUAGE AND COGNITION

CHANGES IN THE SECOND EDITION

The second edition of *Neurobiology: Molecules, Cells, and Systems* incorporates numerous additions and improvements. For students, several new learning tools have been introduced. The Essential Background section at the beginning of each chapter lists the assumed background information for that chapter, with references to specific chapters when the material is covered in this book. Key Points have been interspersed throughout the text, framed as questions that will be answered in each section. Review questions have been added at the end of each chapter to focus attention on the main points covered in the chapter. Practice midterm and final exams are provided at the book's web site, which is accessible through *www.blackwellscience.com*. In addition, an extensive study guide, *Introduction to Neuroscience*, is available as part of the Blackwell Science 11th Hour series. This study guide includes numerous sample exam questions, with answers, to ensure mastery of the material covered in *Neurobiology: Molecules, Cells, and Systems*. Finally, each chapter includes at least one Internet Assignment, in which students are asked to use the worldwide web to investigate a topic related to the material covered in the chapter. Links relevant to each Internet Assignment are available at the book's web site.

New topics added to the second edition include a chapter devoted to the roles of the hypothalamus, including a description of recent advances in understanding the molecular basis of circadian rhythms. A chapter on language and cognition in the human brain has also been added. Two new Advanced Topics have been included for students and instructors who wish to cover cellular aspects of neurobiology in a more quantitatively rigorous way. One advanced topic discusses ion channel kinetics, and the other describes the passive electrical characteristics of cell membranes.

The most obvious change from the first edition is the artwork, which has been completely redrawn to exploit the book's new four-color format. Each illustration was designed to illuminate a particular principle, and I have always tried to integrate the drawings into the text discussion of each topic. The goal has been to make the figures accessible and readily comprehensible to beginning students of neurobiology, as well as visually attractive. In addition, animations of selected illustrations are available at the book's web site, as indicated by special icons next to the relevant figures.

HOW THIS BOOK APPROACHES THE FIELD OF NEUROBIOLOGY

Although the second edition incorporates many changes, the general approach to the field of neurobiology has not changed from the first edition. Neurobiology is a diverse field. Although *Neurobiology: Molecules, Cells, and Systems* provides broad exposure to this field, I have not attempted to cover all aspects of neuroscience. Instead of an encyclopedic survey, I have selected a subset of topics within neurobiology that illustrate the fundamentals of nervous system function. Within each selected topic, I have chosen specific examples that lend themselves to explanations at the levels of molecules, cells, and neural systems. The intention is to provide a framework for further learning, which individual instructors and students can supplement with additional subject matter. Toward this end, suggested readings for each chapter are included at the book's web site, an approach that will help ensure that the readings are up-to-date.

I thank the instructors and students who used the first edition of the book in their courses and took the time to provide suggestions for improvements in the second edition. Special thanks go to the reviewers of the second edition: Vijaya Kumari, University of California-Davis; Kate Susman, Vassar College; Larry Cahill, University of California-Irvine; Indira Raman, Northwestern University; Janice Naegele, Wesleyan University. They made numerous improvements in the presentation and focused my attention on omissions they considered vital. Even though I was unable to add everything they asked for (without expanding the book to encyclopedic length), it was very useful to obtain their expert perspective.

The most important acknowledgment is to my wife Karen, whose support, good humor, and tolerance made it possible for me to complete this second edition in my "spare time" away from the lab.

GGM

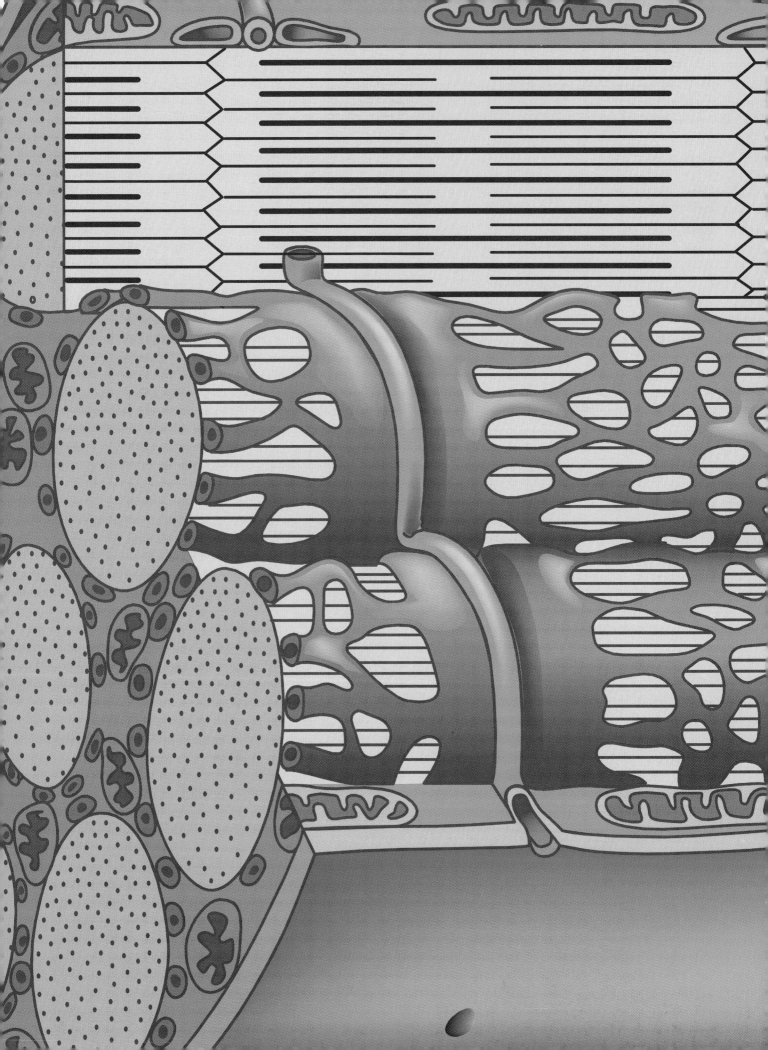

INTRODUCTION TO NEUROBIOLOGY

The goal of the first two chapters is to provide an overview of the function and organization of the nervous system. This will give you a framework for learning more about the details of neurobiology in subsequent parts of the book. Chapter 1 examines some of the different scientific approaches used to study the nervous system. Neurobiology represents a cross section of its parent science, biology, and many different styles of scientific analysis, ranging from studies of intact organisms to fundamentals of gene expression, are employed in neurobiology. Chapter 2 then introduces the overall structural organization of the mammalian central nervous system, which is examined from a developmental perspective, both phylogenetically and embryologically. In both phylogenetic and embryological development, neural organization proceeds from simpler to more complex forms, and study of the simpler forms enables a better understanding of the more complex forms. After this two-chapter introduction to neurobiology and neural organization, we will move on to learn about the specific details of neuronal communication in Part II.

A PREVIEW OF NEUROBIOLOGY

The nervous system is the master control system whose task is to coordinate the other organ systems that make up the organism. To understand how the nervous system carries out this task, students of neurobiology must master a wide variety of facts about the anatomy, cell biology, and biochemistry of the nervous system. This rapidly increasing body of information forms the foundation necessary to appreciate how the nervous system works.

As a student learning about neurobiology, you should also become

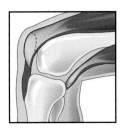

familiar with the scientific approaches neurobiologists use to gather new information about the nervous system. Although our knowledge of the nervous system is impressive, the amount we do not know is also vast. Understanding the scientific tools neurobiologists use in the course of their research will help you keep pace with new advances in the understanding of the brain. For that reason, this introductory chapter examines some of the different approaches neurobiologists use to study the nervous system. In the process, you will also begin to see how the nervous system is organized and what kinds of cellular events underlie its functioning.

This preview also introduces some important terms and principles that are explored in more detail in subsequent chapters. Although a brief explanation of each new concept is included here, you should concentrate at this point on the broader picture and should not be concerned if you find yourself asking questions and wanting a more detailed description of the previewed material. Indeed, one purpose of this chapter is to pique your interest in digging deeper into the material. With this goal in mind, the specific chapters that describe the material in more detail are explicitly referenced at the relevant points.

NEUROBIOLOGY IS A MULTIDISCIPLINARY FIELD

As a scientific discipline, neurobiology differs from most other specialties within the realm of biological science. Molecular biology, for example, is a field organized around a particular set of techniques and methods—a particular way of asking and answering scientific questions. A molecular biologist who works on yeast cells would have a good understanding of the work of her fellow molecular biologist who works on mammalian cells in the lab next door. The details of their respective research systems may differ, but both scientists share a common language and common approaches to their work. The same cannot be said of neurobiology, however. A neurobiologist may be trained as a biochemist, a physiologist, an anatomist, a behaviorist, or a molecular biologist. The common thread that unites neurobiologists of all scientific persuasions is that they all work on the nervous system—the most complex and mysterious of organ systems. Given the many scientific approaches that can be taken to the study of the nervous system, students studying neurobiology (and research neurobiologists, too) face the difficult task of mastering a wide range of information about nerve cells and how they interact.

Like other organs in the body, the nervous system is made up of cells, including the nerve cells themselves, called **neurons**, and their supporting and sustaining cells, called **glial cells**. Much of neurobiology focuses on understanding how the cells of the nervous system are specialized to carry out the transmission and processing of information. Because of the importance of the basic electrical and chemical properties of neurons, the first major subdivision of this book (Part II), beginning with Chapter 3, is devoted to these cellular aspects of neurobiology.

The next two major subdivisions (Parts III and IV) describe neuronal circuits that mediate two of the important functions of the nervous system: formulating a motor response that makes sense for the organism in a particular context (motor systems, Part III), and gathering information about the environment (sensory systems, Part IV). Proper processing of both motor and sensory information depends on the characteristics of the individual neurons as well as the specificity of connections among the numerous cells that make up the nervous system. Knowing the source of a nerve cell's inputs and the location of its outputs is crucial in understanding the cell's role in neural information processing. For this reason, neuroanatomy is an important aspect of neurobiology, and for each neural system described in this textbook, we will consider how that system is organized anatomically.

Finally, in Part V, we will consider how connections among neurons are established during embryonic development and modified on the basis of experience in the adult. Part V also presents information about unique functions of the human brain: language and cognition.

THE PATELLAR REFLEX: AN EXAMPLE OF NERVOUS SYSTEM FUNCTION

What are the afferent and efferent pathways involved in the patellar stretch reflex?

To make this discussion of the various scientific approaches in neurobiology more concrete, it is useful to consider a simple example that can be examined from different viewpoints. The simple behavior we will analyze is perhaps the best-known example of a neural reflex—the knee-jerk reflex, which is more properly called the **patellar stretch reflex**. You can easily demonstrate this reflex on yourself, as shown in Figure 1.1. While seated, cross one leg over the other and relax your thigh muscles. Find the patellar tendon (the soft spot between the knee cap and the lower leg bone) and give it a sharp tap with the side of your open hand. If you are successful, the tap to the patellar tendon will be followed by extension of the lower leg, seemingly acting on its own. If you rest your free hand on the front of the thigh, you can feel the twitch of the quadriceps muscle that causes the involuntary extension of the knee joint and the upward jerk of the lower leg.

Figure 1.2 diagrams the neural circuitry underlying the patellar reflex. Tapping the patellar tendon pulls down on the knee cap (patella), which in turn stretches the quadriceps muscle. Then the nervous system comes into play. Specialized nerve cells (**sensory neurons**) sense the stretch of the muscle and send a signal to the nervous system that the muscle length has increased. This signal is received by other neurons, called **motor neurons**, located within the spinal cord (see Fig. 1.2). The motor neurons command the quadriceps muscle to contract, which produces the reflexive extension of the knee joint.

This simple reflex loop embodies many of the general properties that characterize the operation of the nervous system. A sensory stimulus (muscle stretch) is detected, the signal is transmitted rapidly over a long distance (to and from the spinal cord), and the information is focally and specifically directed to the appropriate target neurons (the quadriceps motor neurons). The sensory pathway, which carries information into the nervous system, is called the **afferent pathway**, and the motor output constitutes the **efferent pathway**. Much of the nervous system is devoted to processing afferent sensory information and then making the proper connections with efferent pathways to ensure that an appropriate response occurs.

Figure 1.1.

A demonstration of the patellar reflex. The goal is to passively stretch the relaxed quadriceps muscle at the front of the thigh by tapping sharply on the tendon attached to the bottom of the knee cap. Take a seat in such a way that the thigh is approximately horizontal, the foot is off the floor, and the muscles of the leg are relaxed. Next, deliver a sharp tap to the patellar tendon. You can use a rubber reflex hammer or the side of your open hand or the ends of your bunched fingers. If you are successful, the lower leg will jerk upward (hence, the name knee-jerk reflex). You can also feel and see the reflexive contraction of the quadriceps muscle

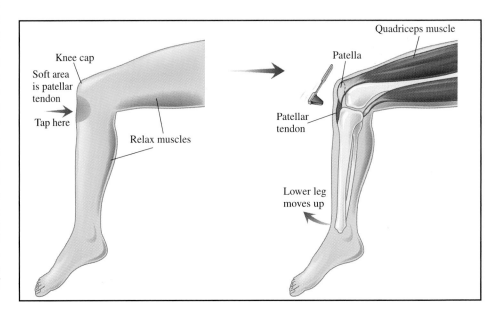

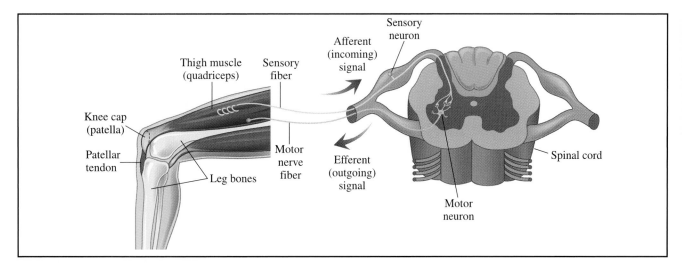

Figure 1.2.

A schematic representation of the patellar reflex. The sensory neuron is activated by stretching the thigh muscle. The incoming (afferent) signal is carried to the spinal cord along the nerve fiber of the sensory neuron. In the spinal cord, the sensory neuron activates motor neurons, which in turn send outgoing (efferent) signals along the nerve back to the thigh muscle, causing it to contract.

Anatomy of the Patellar Reflex

The diagram in Figure 1.2 requires knowledge of where the neurons in the loop are located and where they project—that is, we must be aware of the relevant neuroanatomy. The cell bodies of the sensory neurons in the patellar reflex are located just outside the spinal column in the **dorsal root ganglion**. Each vertebral segment has two dorsal root ganglia, one on each side of the spinal cord. This arrangement is illustrated in Figure 1.3A. Each dorsal root ganglion in the chain of ganglia paralleling the spinal column provides the sensory innervation for a particular region of the body. The ganglia contain the cell bodies of many different kinds of sensory neurons. In addition to those carrying sensory signals from muscles, there are sensory neurons that signal information about touch, pressure, pain, temperature, and so on.

In the patellar reflex, each sensory cell that innervates the quadriceps muscle gives rise to a single thin nerve fiber (the fibers projecting from the cell body of a neuron are collectively called **processes**, or **neurites**). This fiber exits the dorsal root ganglion and bifurcates, sending one long branch through the nerve supplying the quadriceps muscle and another branch via the **dorsal root** into the spinal cord. Once inside the spinal cord, the sensory nerve fiber branches profusely (see Fig. 1.3B) and makes contact with numerous spinal cord neurons.

Among the neurons receiving connections from the sensory neuron in the spinal cord are the motor neurons that control the quadriceps muscle. The cell bodies of these motor neurons are located in the ventral part of the spinal cord. A group of motor neurons that control a particular muscle is shown in Figure 1.3B, and the structure of a single motor neuron is illustrated in Figure 1.3C. The long, thin output process of each motor neuron, called the **axon**, groups together with other motor axons and exits the spinal cord in the **ventral root**. Outside the spinal cord, the ventral root joins with the peripheral nerve fibers of the sensory neurons in the dorsal root ganglion to form the **spinal nerve**. Thus, the spinal nerve exiting each vertebral segment along the spinal column carries a mixture of both afferent sensory fibers and efferent motor fibers.

Where are dorsal root ganglia located and what neurons do they contain?

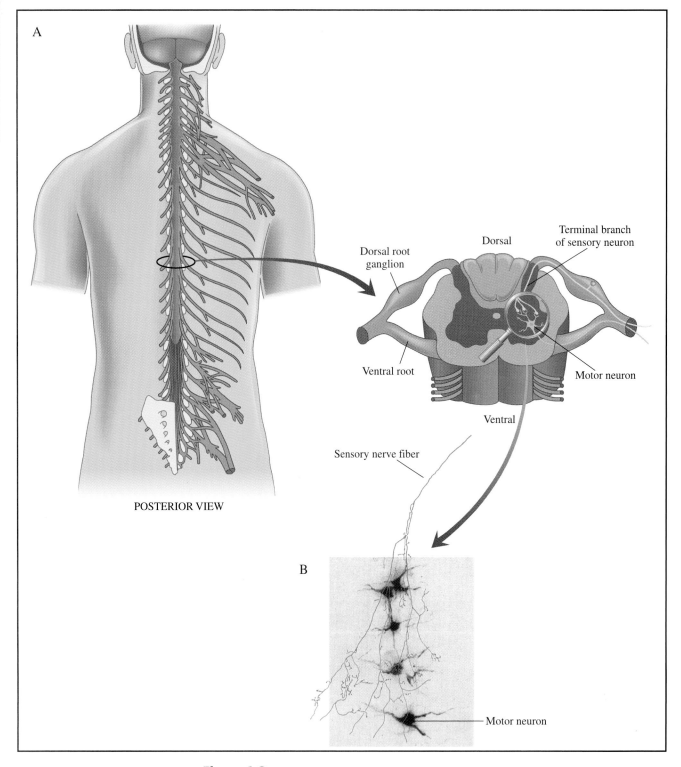

A

POSTERIOR VIEW

Dorsal root
ganglion

Dorsal

Terminal branch
of sensory neuron

Ventral root

Motor neuron

Ventral

Sensory nerve fiber

B

Motor neuron

Figure 1.3.

The organization of sensory and motor neurons in the spinal cord. **A**. At each vertebra in the spinal column, a pair of spinal nerves exits, one on each side of the body. At the spinal cord, the nerve splits into dorsal and ventral branches (called roots). Sensory nerve fibers are found in the dorsal root, and motor nerve fibers are located in the ventral root. **B**. In the spinal cord, incoming sensory nerve fibers branch profusely and make contact with motor neurons. **C**. The drawing shows a single motor neuron, which has many elaborately branching dendrites (white) that receive synapses from other neurons, including sensory neurons. The cell body of the motor neuron (blue) gives rise to a single output fiber, the axon (red), that extends through the spinal nerve to the muscle. **B** and **C**: based on drawings and a photo provided by W. Collins and L. Mendell of the State University of New York at Stony Brook.

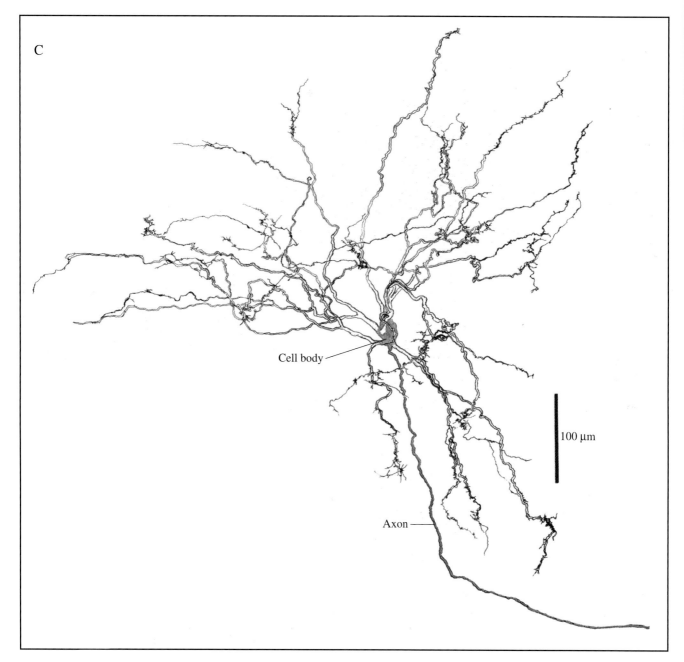

C

Cell body

Axon

100 µm

Figure 1.3.

(continued)

In the patellar reflex, the neuroanatomy is relatively simple. However, the anatomy of neural pathways often is not so straightforward in the mammalian brain, with its tangle of interconnections among neurons in neighboring and distant parts of the brain. Chapter 2 provides an overview of brain organization, to lay the groundwork for understanding the general relationship among brain regions.

Cellular Signals Involved in the Patellar Reflex

For the nervous system to carry out its mission, signals must be sent and received among neurons. Even a simple reflex arc like the patellar reflex involves several different signals, which are summarized in Figure 1.4. The stretch of the quadriceps muscle is sensed by the sensory neurons, which produce a signal that propagates

Figure 1.4.

A block diagram of the sequence of events in the stretch reflex.

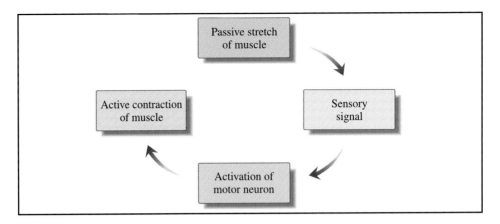

from the muscle to the central nervous system along the long, thin sensory nerve fibers. In the spinal cord, the sensory signal is then transmitted to the motor neurons controlling the quadriceps muscle. The point of contact—where signals are transmitted from one neuron to another—is called a **synapse**. The synaptic contact from sensory neurons activates the motor neurons, which generate a message that is sent back along the nerve supplying the quadriceps muscle, where the motor axons make synaptic contact with their target cells, the muscle cells of the quadriceps muscle. This synapse between a motor neuron and a muscle cell is called the **neuromuscular junction**.

The nervous system relies on two fundamental types of signals, electrical signals and chemical signals, both of which are found in the patellar reflex. First, we will consider the electrical signal generated in the sensory nerve fibers in response to muscle stretch and in the motor axons to command reflexive contraction of the muscle. This signal, called the **action potential**, is one of the fundamental electrical signals of the nervous system. Then, we will examine the chemical transmission of information from one cell to another at the two synapses in the reflex: the connection between the sensory and motor neurons in the spinal cord, and the neuromuscular junction between the motor neurons and the muscle cells. The transmission of information at these synapses involves the release of a chemical messenger, a **neurotransmitter**, which then produces an electrical change in the target cell. Chapters 5 and 6 discuss synaptic transmission in detail.

The Action Potential

What is the long-distance electrical signal of the nervous system?

The nervous system must transmit information rapidly over long distances. Consider, for example, the distance from an elephant's toe to its spinal cord or from a giraffe's brain to the end of its spinal cord. To satisfy this requirement for speed, neurons produce active electrical signals that travel rapidly along the long, thin fibers that make up the transmission paths. Like all other cells, neurons have an electric field (that is, an electrical **voltage**) across their membranes that arises from the inside of the cell being more negative than the outside. The origin of this membrane voltage, which is called the **membrane potential**, is described in Chapter 4. Although the transmembrane voltage is small—typically less than a tenth of a volt—it is central to the functioning of the nervous system. Information is transmitted and processed by neurons by means of changes in the membrane potential.

To observe the electrical signal that carries the message along the sensory nerve fiber in the patellar reflex, we must measure the membrane potential of the sensory neuron by placing an ultrafine voltage-sensing probe, called an **intracellular microelectrode**, inside the sensory nerve fiber. Figure 1.5 illustrates this kind of experiment. A voltmeter is connected to measure the voltage difference between the

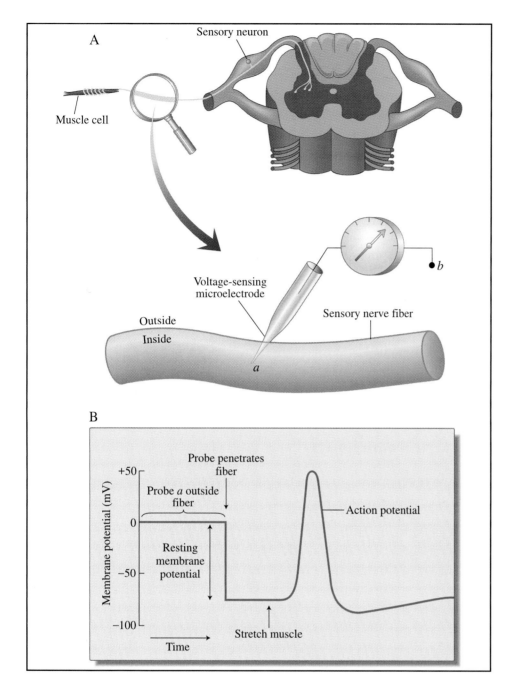

Figure 1.5.

Recording the action potential in the nerve fiber of the sensory neuron in the patellar stretch reflex. **A**. A diagram of the recording configuration. A tiny microelectrode is inserted into the sensory nerve fiber, and a voltmeter is connected to measure the voltage difference (*E*) between the inside (*a*) and the outside (*b*) of the nerve fiber. **B**. When the microelectrode penetrates the fiber, the resting membrane potential of the nerve fiber is measured. When the sensory neuron is activated by stretching the muscle, an action potential occurs and is recorded as a rapid shift in the recorded membrane potential of the sensory nerve fiber.

tip of the intracellular microelectrode (point *a* in the figure) and a reference point in the extracellular space (point *b*). When the microelectrode is located outside the sensory neuron, both points *a* and *b* lie in the extracellular space, and the voltmeter records no voltage difference (see Fig. 1.5B). When the tip of the probe is inserted inside the sensory neuron, however, the voltmeter measures an electrical potential between points *a* and *b*, representing the voltage difference between the inside and the outside of the neuron—that is, the membrane potential of the neuron. As shown in Figure 1.5B, the inside of the sensory nerve fiber is negative with respect to the outside by about 70 thousandths of a volt (1 millivolt, abbreviated mV, equals 1 thousandth of a volt). Because the potential outside the cell is defined as zero and the inside is negative with respect to the outside, the membrane potential is approximately −70 mV.

As long as the sensory neuron is not stimulated by stretching the muscle, the membrane potential remains constant at this resting value. For this reason, the unstimulated membrane potential is known as the **resting potential** of the cell. When the muscle is stretched, however, the membrane potential of the sensory neuron undergoes a dramatic change, as shown in Figure 1.5B. After a delay that depends on the distance of the recording site from the muscle, the membrane potential suddenly moves in the positive direction and transiently reverses sign for a brief period, during which the inside of the cell becomes positive with respect to the outside. The membrane potential then rapidly returns to its usual negative level. This transient jump in membrane potential is the **action potential**—the long-distance signal used to carry information in the nervous system.

If we record the membrane potential at various points along the length of the sensory nerve fiber, we would find that the action potential travels progressively from the sensory endings in the muscle all the way to the synaptic endings of the sensory neuron in the spinal cord. The speed at which it moves is not very fast compared with the speed of electricity in a wire, but it is still quite fast for a biological process. For the stretch-sensitive sensory neurons involved in the patellar reflex, for example, the action potential travels at a velocity of 50 to 100 m/sec along the nerve fiber. Thus, the signal reaches the spinal cord in approximately 10 to 20 thousandths of a second (10–20 msec). A similar action potential occurs in the axon of the motor neuron when the contraction command is sent from the spinal cord to the quadriceps muscle in the return loop of the patellar reflex. A major focus for Part II of this book, beginning with Chapter 3, is to understand the electrical and chemical principles that underlie the action potential.

Synaptic Transmission

How do neurons communicate at synapses?

When the action potential reaches the end of the neuron, the signal must be transmitted to the next cell in the loop. In the patellar reflex, signals are relayed from one cell to another at two locations: the synapse between the sensory neuron and the motor neuron in the spinal cord, and the synapse between the motor neuron and the muscle cells in the quadriceps muscle. There are two general classes of synapses: **electrical synapses** and **chemical synapses**. In both types, specialized membrane structures are formed at the point where the input cell (called the **presynaptic cell**) comes into contact with the receiving cell (called the **postsynaptic cell**). In the patellar reflex, both the synapse between the sensory neuron and the motor neuron and the synapse between the motor neuron and the muscle cells are chemical synapses.

The sequence of events during transmission at a chemical synapse is summarized in Figure 1.6. In this type of synaptic transmission, an action potential in the presynaptic cell causes it to release a chemical substance, called a **neurotransmitter**, that diffuses through the extracellular space at the point of synaptic contact and changes the membrane potential of the postsynaptic target cell. Recall from Figure 1.5B that the membrane potential of the neuron becomes less negative during an action potential—indeed, the inside of the cell actually becomes positive with respect to the outside for a brief time at the peak of the action potential. Reduced negativity of the membrane potential of a cell is called **depolarization** (because the membrane is then less **electrically polarized**). The depolarization of the presynaptic cell during the action potential stimulates release of the chemical neurotransmitter by a process of exocytosis, which is triggered by calcium ions that enter the presynaptic cell at the synapse during the action potential.

Transmission is simpler at an electrical synapse, where the change in membrane voltage during the action potential in the presynaptic cell spreads directly to the postsynaptic cell. Understanding the mechanisms of synaptic transmission is another major focus of Part II, beginning in Chapter 5.

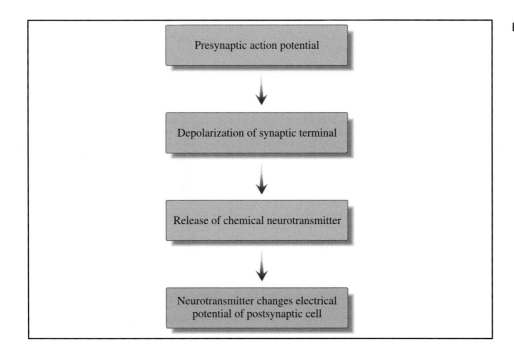

Figure 1.6.

A block diagram of the sequence of events involved in the release of chemical neurotransmitter from the synaptic terminal.

Molecular View of the Patellar Reflex

To this point, we have examined the patellar reflex from an exclusively cellular viewpoint—both in terms of the anatomy and in terms of the physiological signals—without paying much attention to subcellular mechanisms that give rise to the cellular events. Like all other cells, neurons are complex assemblies of molecular components. An important aspect of neurobiology is understanding how the properties of these molecular components contribute to the function of the nervous system. In the patellar reflex, for example, many different molecules are responsible for the various aspects of signal transmission. As an example of how molecular components determine neural function, we will focus on the transmission of information at the synapse between the motor neurons and the muscle cells at the neuromuscular junction.

As described in Figure 1.6, an action potential arriving at a synaptic terminal causes release of a chemical neurotransmitter, which in turn alters the electrical behavior of the postsynaptic cell. At any synaptic junction in the nervous system, identification of the chemical neurotransmitter released at that synapse is an important piece of information. Indeed, a great deal of neurobiological research is devoted to specifying which neurotransmitters are released at which synapses in a neuronal circuit, because this information helps explain how the circuit works. At the neuromuscular junction, the neurotransmitter released from the synaptic terminals of the motor neurons is a simple organic molecule, **acetylcholine**, whose chemical structure is shown in Figure 1.7. Acetylcholine, abbreviated **ACh**, is manufactured in the synaptic terminal by the chemical combination of acetate and choline, a reaction that is catalyzed by an enzyme called **choline acetyltransferase (ChAT)** (see Fig. 1.7).

The presence of the synthetic enzyme for a particular neurotransmitter within a neuron is evidence that the neuron uses that neurotransmitter at its synaptic release sites. Thus, staining neural tissue to reveal the synthetic enzyme ChAT can be used to establish which neurons in a circuit are likely to release ACh as a neurotransmitter. The presence of ChAT inside a neuron can be detected with antibodies directed against the enzyme, using a procedure called **immunocytochemistry**. Neurons that contain ChAT are called **cholinergic neurons**. An

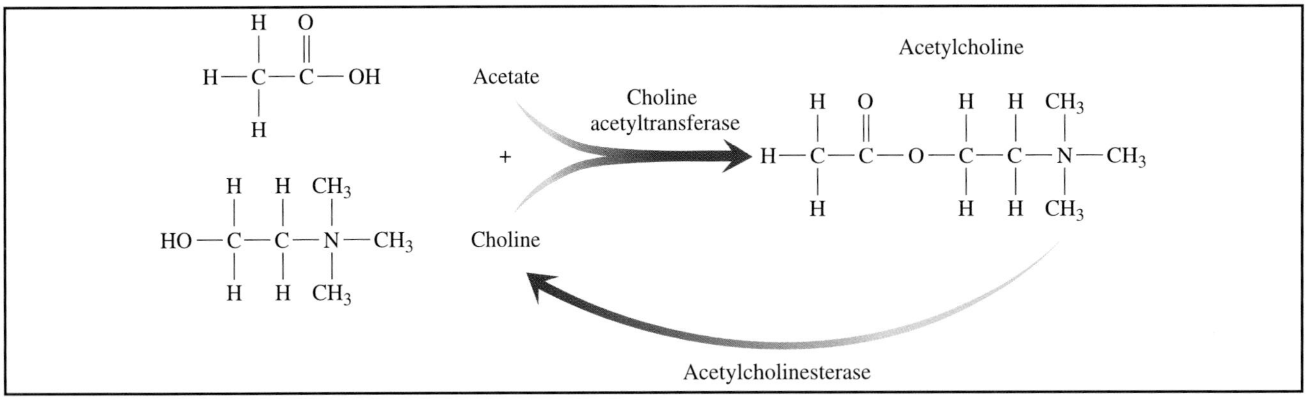

Figure 1.7.

Acetylcholine is a well-studied neurotransmitter in the nervous system. It is released from the synaptic terminals of the motor neurons at the neuromuscular junction. Acetylcholine is synthesized by the enzyme choline acetyltransferase from the precursors choline and acetate. After finishing its job, acetylcholine is inactivated by being spit into choline and acetate by the enzyme acetylcholinesterase.

How are neurotransmitter molecules inactivated after they are released at a synapse?

example of cholinergic neurons labeled with an antibody against ChAT is shown in Figure 1.8.

After a chemical neurotransmitter has been released from the synaptic terminal, its action must be terminated in some way. Otherwise, the continued presence of the transmitter in the extracellular space would continually activate the postsynaptic cell. The action of a neurotransmitter can be terminated in either of two ways:

- The transmitter molecules are removed from the extracellular space by uptake into surrounding glial cells and neurons (including the presynaptic terminal that originally released the transmitter), as the neurotransmitter diffuses away from its site of release.
- The neurotransmitter molecules are chemically degraded into inactive substances.

At the neuromuscular junction, the latter mechanism is used to inactivate ACh released from the synaptic terminals of the motor neurons. The extracellular space between the motor nerve terminals and the postsynaptic muscle cell contains an enzyme that destroys ACh (see Fig. 1.7). Because this destructive enzyme works by cleaving the ester bond between acetate and choline, it is called **acetylcholinesterase** (abbreviated AChase). Just as the synthetic enzyme ChAT can be used as a marker for synapses at which ACh is the neurotransmitter, AChase in the extracellular space at a synaptic junction also can be used to detect cholinergic synapses. For example, AChase staining at the neuromuscular junction marks the postsynaptic muscle cell at the precise location of the nerve terminal (Fig. 1.9).

The goal of synaptic transmission is modification of the electrical properties of the postsynaptic cell by the neurotransmitter released from the presynaptic cell. For this action to occur, the postsynaptic cell must detect the presence of the neurotransmitter in the extracellular space and respond appropriately. Detection of the neurotransmitter is accomplished by specialized postsynaptic **neurotransmitter receptors**—transmembrane protein molecules inserted into the postsynaptic membrane at the point where the presynaptic cell makes contact. The extracellular portion of the receptor molecule contains a binding pocket into which a molecule of neurotransmitter fits precisely. When the binding site is occupied, the receptor protein is activated, triggering a postsynaptic response.

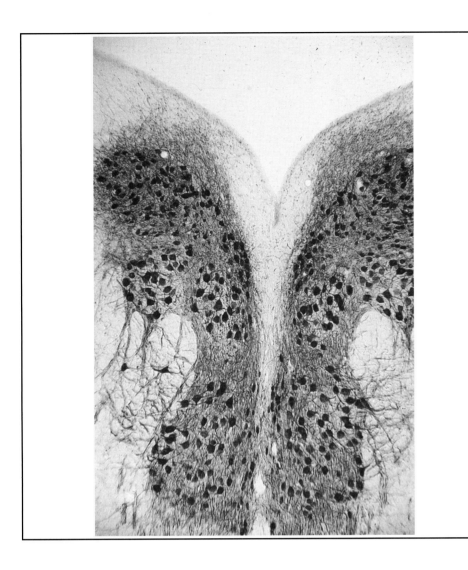

Figure 1.8.

Choline acetyltransferase (ChAT) can be used as a marker to define which neurons in the nervous system are likely to use acetylcholine as a neurotransmitter. The neurons shown here are motor neurons in the oculomotor nucleus, which controls the eye muscles. ChAT has been labeled by incubating a tissue sample with an antibody directed against the enzyme. Photo courtesy of J.T. Erichsen of the University of Wales.

Because the binding site will accept only a particular neurotransmitter substance, many different types of postsynaptic receptor molecules are found in the nervous system, providing specific detectors for the many different types of neurotransmitters. At the neuromuscular junction, for example, the postsynaptic membrane of the muscle cell contains large numbers of **ACh receptors** that detect the ACh released from the terminals of motor neurons. The ACh receptors are formed from the aggregation of five protein subunits, as shown in Figure 1.10A. At

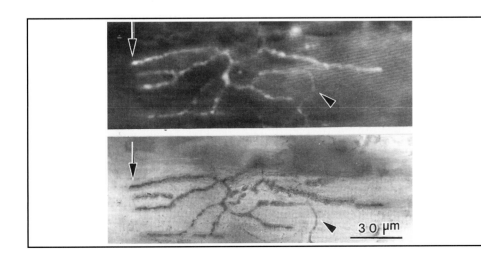

Figure 1.9.

The degradative enzyme for acetylcholine, acetylcholinesterase (AChase), is found at the neuromuscular junction. The nerve terminal is labeled in the *upper picture* and the pattern of AChase is shown in the *lower picture*. Note that AChase precisely mirrors the innervation provided by the nerve terminal. Reproduced by permission from Chen L, Ko C-P. Extension of synaptic extracellular matrix during nerve terminal sprouting in living frog neuromuscular junctions. J Neurosci 1994; 14:796–808.

Figure 1.10.

The acetylcholine (ACh) receptor molecule mediates the postsynaptic response to the neurotransmitter ACh. **A.** Diagram of the structure of ACh receptor molecules. The protein is a transmembrane ion channel, formed from the combination of five subunits: two alpha subunits, and one subunit each of beta, gamma, and delta. When two molecules of ACh bind to the receptor (one to each alpha subunit), the ion channel opens and allows ions to traverse the membrane. **B.** The location of ACh receptors at the neuromuscular junction (nmj). The receptors have been labeled with a toxin from snake venom, alpha-bungarotoxin (α-βgtx), which binds to the ACh binding sites of the receptor. **B:** reproduced by permission from Chen L, Ko C-P. Extension of synaptic extracellular matrix during nerve terminal sprouting in living frog neuromuscular junctions. J Neurosci 1994; 14:796–808.

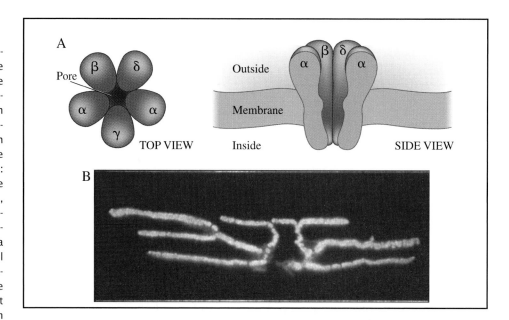

the center of the cluster is a pore that forms a small hole extending across the plasma membrane. When no ACh is bound to the receptor, the pore remains closed. When ACh binds, the pore opens, allowing positively charged ions from the external fluid to flow into the muscle cell (described in detail in Chapter 5).

Membrane proteins that allow ions to move across the membrane are called **ion channels** (see Chapters 3 and 4). Thus, the ACh receptor forms an **ACh-activated ion channel** in the muscle membrane. The influx of positive charge through the channel makes the membrane potential of the muscle cell less negative in the presence of ACh. Thus, ACh depolarizes the muscle cell, and as discussed in Chapter 4, depolarization triggers an action potential in the muscle cell. The action potential itself also is produced by ion channels, which open in response to depolarization and allow positively charged sodium ions to enter the cell. This influx of positive charge, carried by sodium ions, accounts for the rapid movement of the membrane potential in the positive direction during the initial portion of the action potential (see Fig. 1.5B). Because the sodium channels that generate the action potential of neurons and muscle cells open in response to depolarization, these ion channels are called **voltage-sensitive sodium channels**. Their properties are discussed in detail in Chapter 4.

The presence of ACh receptors at a synapse can be used as a marker for synapses that use ACh as a neurotransmitter. Figure 1.10B shows the localization of ACh receptors at the neuromuscular junction, as revealed by a toxin from snake venom that binds tightly to the receptor site where ACh normally interacts with the receptor molecule.

The Neurons of the Patellar Reflex Are Part of Larger Neural Systems

Let's return to the demonstration of the patellar reflex. Once again, cross one leg over the other and prepare to tap the patellar tendon to elicit the reflex. This time, however, command the muscles of your thigh to tense up and lock the knee joint in the flexed position. Now, when you tap the patellar tendon, no reflexive contraction of the quadriceps muscle occurs. You have just demonstrated in a simple way that the neurons of the patellar reflex are subject to control by other parts of the nervous system. This comes as no surprise: voluntary override of spinal cord reflexes is a common part of our daily experience. From the neurobiological point of view, specifying the neural circuitry involved in voluntary control of motor function is a difficult and uncompleted task. In **systems neurobiology**, the goal is not to understand the functional role of a single neuron in the nervous system (although analysis of the behavior of individual neurons plays an important part in systems neurobiology), but rather to understand how groups of neurons are organized into larger neural circuits. The interactions among these neural circuits underlie the ability of the brain to carry out complex motor and sensory functions. We will now examine some of the larger neural circuits that make use of the neurons of the patellar reflex.

In Figure 1.2, we saw that the patellar reflex is the simplest kind of neuronal circuit, consisting of two neurons—the stretch-sensitive sensory neuron and the motor neuron—connected by a single synapse. The motor neurons of a particular muscle (the quadriceps muscle in our example) are part of many other spinal circuits as well. Motor neurons are the only output from the nervous system to muscles; therefore, any task that involves a particular muscle must be coordinated by neural circuits that converge onto the motor neurons supplying that muscle. In the quadriceps muscle, the motor neurons are acted on by neural circuits involved in locomotion, circuits involved in postural control and balance, and all other circuits that involve the knee joint.

Neural circuits that influence the motor neurons are commonly made up of other kinds of neurons within the spinal cord itself, as shown schematically in Figure 1.11. The other spinal neurons include various kinds of **interneurons**, which are neurons that receive inputs only from other neurons and make outputs only to other neurons. In contrast, sensory neurons receive inputs from an external stimulus (for example, muscle stretch), and motor neurons send outputs to non-neuronal targets (for example, muscle cells). In the central nervous system, interneurons make up the majority of the neural circuitry.

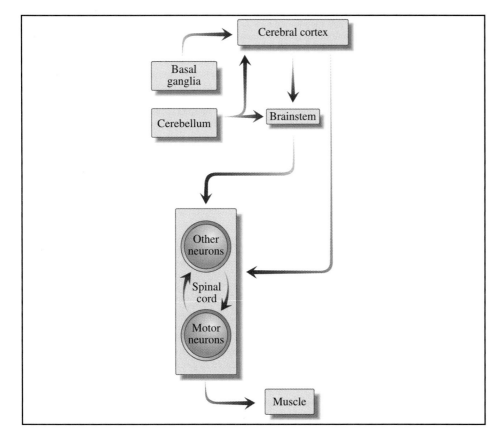

Figure 1.11.

A block diagram of the motor control system, showing brain and spinal cord regions involved in formulating and executing motor commands. The diagram has been simplified by removing the sensory pathways providing inputs to many of the systems. In addition, the diagram does not include subdivisions of the cerebral cortex, basal ganglia, and brainstem motor regions.

Note also that motor neurons send outputs not only to the muscle but also to spinal interneurons. Such feedback from a neuron to the cells from which it receives inputs is a common feature of neuronal circuits in the nervous system.

The neural circuits of the spinal cord coordinate various kinds of reflexive movements, in which a stimulus is closely coupled to a fixed motor output, without the requirement for conscious control or voluntary initiation of the movement. But what about voluntary control of movement, such as you demonstrated when you prevented reflexive contraction of the quadriceps muscle by purposefully locking the knee joint before tapping the patellar tendon? Some of the brain circuitry that regulates the function of spinal motor neurons in this way is illustrated in Figure 1.11. The organizational scheme is rather elaborate, and multiple parts of the brain contribute to voluntary motor control (more detailed information about this circuitry is given in Chapter 9). Commands for voluntary control of movement originate in the motor regions of the **cerebral cortex**. The cerebral cortex is a major part of the brain in mammals, and it forms the highly wrinkled outer surface that most of us envision when we think of the human brain (see Chapter 2). The cerebral cortex sends signals directly to the spinal cord, as well as to brainstem motor nuclei (see Chapter 2 for a description of the anatomical organization of the brain). The brainstem nuclei also send outputs to the spinal circuits. Movement commands from the cortex and brainstem are modulated by brain regions called the **cerebellum** and the **basal ganglia** (see Chapter 9).

The information shown in Figure 1.11 stems from both anatomical studies and physiological studies. Together, such information allows systems neurobiologists to deduce how the parts interact to plan a movement, program its execution, and modify the movement on the basis of sensory feedback. Similar kinds of circuits could be diagrammed for the analysis of sensory information, as described in Part IV (Chapters 13–18).

MOLECULAR BIOLOGICAL AND GENETIC APPROACHES TO THE NERVOUS SYSTEM

As with other fields of biology, recent advances in molecular biological techniques allow manipulations of the nervous system at the molecular level in precise and specific ways. Also, genetics has long been a valuable tool for analyzing complex biological systems and establishing the functional role of a protein. In the nervous system, genetics has played an important role in unraveling the molecular basis of neural function. Traditionally, the genetics approach has relied on naturally occurring or experimentally created mutations that affect a gene important for the biological system of interest. In the case of the nervous system, such mutations are often detected by their effect on some aspect of behavior. More recently, new techniques have been developed that allow targeted disruption of a particular gene.

Genetic and Transgenic Approaches

Genetic analysis is based on information about the organization of genes on the individual chromosomes, using various genetic markers that provide a map of chromosomal organization. Certain organisms have become the standard choices for genetic analysis. Common organisms for genetic analysis are the mouse (*Mus musculus*) among mammals, zebrafish (*Danio rerio*) among cold-blooded vertebrates, and the fruit fly (*Drosophila melanogaster*) among invertebrates.

Mutations in a gene often eliminate the production of a useful protein and so interfere with the cellular function carried out by that protein. Thus, analysis of the defect manifested by animals or humans bearing a mutated gene can provide clues about the functional role of the protein encoded by the gene. Mutations may arise spontaneously, from naturally occurring errors in DNA replication, or they may be induced experimentally by exposing animals to radiation or to chemicals that promote mutation.

In the case of genes that affect the nervous system, mutations are often detected by their effect on the behavior of the affected individuals. For instance, mutations that affect the signaling mechanisms used in the patellar reflex would be expected to produce defects in movement. An example is a mutant strain of mice called *med* that develop progressive paralysis. The mutated gene in *med* mice encodes a voltage-sensitive sodium channel, which is necessary for the generation of action potentials in motor axons controlling the muscles. Other mutations that produce paralysis affect other proteins of the motor signaling system. In zebrafish, a paralyzed mutant has been identified in which the mutation prevents production of one of the protein subunits making up the ACh receptor at the neuromuscular junction (see Fig. 1.10A). Without the ACh receptor, the muscle fails to respond to Ach released from the motor neurons, and the muscles no longer contract when commanded to do so by the nervous system.

In humans, an inherited neurological disease called congenital end-plate acetylcholinesterase deficiency is characterized by prolonged synaptic responses at the neuromuscular junction, so that muscle cells trigger multiple action potentials when the motor neuron is activated. As the name of the disease implies, the mutated gene prevents production of functional AChase enzyme molecules, which are responsible for inactivating the ACh released by the motor neuron (see Figs. 1.7 and 1.9). Thus, ACh persists for an abnormally long time at the neuromuscular junction, causing prolonged postsynaptic depolarization of the muscle cell.

Although mutations that occur randomly (whether spontaneously or induced by mutagenesis) have been valuable in establishing the function of proteins encoded by single genes, new techniques that allow precisely targeted disruption of single genes promise to be even more valuable. This ability to insert novel genes allows the production of **transgenic animals**, most commonly mice, in which DNA is introduced artificially into the natural genetic material of the animal. The inserted gene may either add a new gene (for example, from a different organism) or replace the natural gene. If the natural gene is replaced by a nonfunctional version, the result is a loss of the protein encoded by the gene. This type of transgenic mouse is called a **knockout** mouse, because the protein encoded by the gene is eliminated, or "knocked out."

Functional Expression of Genes and Mutagenesis

Gene knockouts in transgenic animals provide information about physiological function. However, after a gene has been identified and sequenced, detailed information about the physiological function of the encoded protein often requires that the protein be studied in ways that are not possible in the intact nervous system. For this reason, experimenters have developed a number of techniques for expressing a neural protein in simpler systems that are more experimentally approachable. This expression of a protein where it is not normally found is called **heterologous expression**.

To accomplish the expression of a protein, the **messenger RNA (mRNA)** for the protein can be injected into a cell, whose protein translation machinery then synthesizes the protein. Frog oocytes (immature eggs) are commonly used for this purpose because the cells are large and have abundant protein synthesis machinery.

Another method of heterologous expression is to incorporate DNA that codes for the protein into cultured cells, in which transcription of the DNA into mRNA is driven by a viral promoter merged to the target DNA. The process of incorporating the alien DNA into host cells is called **transfection**, and the transfection may be either temporary (transient transfection) or permanent (stable transfection). In some cases, specially engineered viruses have been used to introduce DNA into cells, taking advantage of the infection mechanisms that allow viruses to invade host cells.

A common use of heterologous expression is to make the link between a particular neuronal characteristic and a particular gene expressed in the neuron. However, introduction of engineered DNA also offers the possibility of linking a particular part of a protein molecule to a particular aspect of the function of the protein. The DNA encoding the protein can be altered experimentally to change the amino acid sequence, before the DNA is transfected into cells or transcribed into mRNA to be injected into oocytes. In this way, selected mutations can be introduced into the resulting protein to see how the function of the protein is altered. This procedure is called **site-directed mutagenesis**. It has been used extensively to determine which amino acids in ion channels are important in the functioning of the channel. For example, site-directed mutagenesis, followed by heterologous expression in frog oocytes, was used to establish that positively charged amino acids in a particular part of the molecule are responsible for the voltage sensitivity of the voltage-sensitive sodium channels that underlie the action potential. The amino acid residues that determine which ions can move through the pore of an ion channel also have been studied using site-directed mutagenesis. In the ACh-gated ion channel of the neuromuscular junction, negatively charged amino acids associated with the pore of the channel (see Fig. 1.10A) account for the fact that the open channel allows positively charged ions to move through the pore, but not negatively charged ions. This selectivity accounts for the fact that the muscle cell depolarizes when the ACh-gated channels open.

SUMMARY AND PREVIEW

In this overview, we have used a simple neural circuit—the patellar stretch reflex—to examine some specific examples of questions neurobiologists ask about how the nervous system works. Even for a very simple neural circuit, understanding the circuit requires many pieces of information about the cellular events in the circuit, the molecules responsible for the cellular events, and how the simple circuit fits in with larger neural systems. Although the approaches we have considered are diverse, they barely scratch the surface of the scientific questions that fall within the province of neurobiology.

For example, we have ignored important questions concerning how the nervous system reaches the adult form during the course of development: How does the motor neuron become a motor neuron, rather than some other kind of neuron? How does the sensory neuron from the quadriceps muscle recognize and make synaptic contact with the motor neurons from the same muscle? How do the axons of the sensory and motor neurons find their way over long distances from the spinal cord to the target muscle?

From the molecular point of view, there are also many questions we have not touched on: How does a gene encoding a particular protein become activated in one neuron but not in another, or in neurons but not in glial cells? How are the resulting proteins targeted to the appropriate parts of the cell, especially when the parts of the cell may be more than 1 m apart?

Most of the higher parts of the brain—particularly the cerebral cortex—are not directly concerned with either motor commands or sensory analysis per se, but rather with the integration of sensory and motor information. How do these integrating systems account for cognition, the ability to plan and think? How does the nervous system modify itself and the way it controls the actions of the organism on the basis of past experience? How does the nervous system store and recall the information about those past experiences?

In this book, we will at least touch on many of these questions. We will not have answers to all of them—especially those about complex neural systems—because many aspects of nervous system function remain unsolved mysteries. Instead, this book is intended to introduce ideas, concepts, and facts about neurons and the nervous system and to provide a framework for learning more. Students and instructors alike are invited to expand on the information contained here as their interests direct.

In Part II, we consider in detail the cellular signals discussed in this overview: the electrical and chemical signals of neuronal communication. In Part III, we turn our attention to the motor systems that regulate and control reflex action. Part IV discusses how sensory systems are organized to collect and analyze information about the environment. Finally, Part V considers plasticity in the nervous system, both in terms of development and in terms of learning and memory.

1. Describe three ways to identify a synapse that uses acetylcholine as its neurotransmitter.
2. Draw the waveform of the action potential of a nerve fiber.
3. What is the difference between a chemical synapse and an electrical synapse?
4. List the sequence of events between the arrival of an action potential in the presynaptic cell and the change in membrane potential of the postsynaptic cell at the neuromuscular junction.
5. Describe the synthesis and degradation of the neurotransmitter acetylcholine.
6. Define the following: transgenic animal, heterologous expression, site-directed mutagenesis.
7. List four brain regions involved in motor control.

INTERNET ASSIGNMENT   CHAPTER 1

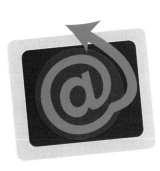

Human diseases that affect motor neurons and the neuromuscular junction—the motor components of the patellar reflex—produce potentially devastating symptoms in patients afflicted by the disease. Three such diseases are myasthenia gravis, myasthenic syndrome, and amyotrophic lateral sclerosis. What aspect of the reflex loop is affected in each of these human diseases? What molecular component is affected in each case? Pick one of the three diseases and write a 150-word report on the scientific history of how the molecular target was identified. You will find PubMed particularly useful in researching your report.

ORGANIZATION OF NERVOUS SYSTEMS

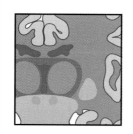

The nervous system is a complicated structure, with elaborate interconnections and communication networks whose complexity makes mastering the detailed neuroanatomy of advanced nervous systems a difficult task. Although the anatomical organization of each specific neural system is presented in the chapter devoted to that system, this chapter establishes some general principles of neural organization. The structure of a mammalian brain can be more readily discerned if we examine simpler nervous systems and look for evolutionary trends in how nervous systems are organized. Similarly, it is also useful to look at the development of the mammalian brain during embryogenesis, as the nervous system progresses from a simple to a complex form during maturation of the organism. By looking at simpler embryonic structures, we can more easily see the interrelationships among parts of adult nervous systems, where distinctions are not so readily apparent. In both viewpoints—evolutionary and developmental—we will utilize simpler forms to illustrate the organization that underlies more intricate forms.

EVOLUTION OF NERVOUS SYSTEMS

Some themes underlying the organization of nervous systems can be appreciated by examining simpler nervous systems and in particular, by examining evolutionary trends in the relationship between body form and style of living on the one hand and nervous system organization on the other. We will see that the basic plan of mammalian nervous systems (including our own) emerges as the outcome of four evolutionary trends in neural organization:

What are the four important trends in the evolution of neural organization?

- Evolution from radial symmetry to bilateral symmetry
- Evolution from general to specialized function of individual neurons
- Cephalization
- Hierarchical organization

Before exploring some specific examples of these trends, we will spend some time considering the origin of neurons as cells specialized for communication.

Electrical Signaling Predates the Emergence of Neurons

It makes sense to talk about a "nervous system" (or any organ system for that matter) only in multicellular animals. Nevertheless, even single-cell organisms exhibit some of the electrical mechanisms usually associated with neurons. For example, Figure 2.1 shows that a protozoan, the paramecium, produces action potentials similar to those of nerve cells, except that the action potential results from an influx of calcium ions rather than sodium ions as in typical nerve action potentials (see Chapter 5). Like neuronal action potentials, the action potential in the paramecium also serves a coordinating function: it regulates the direction of ciliary beating and thus the cell's movement. Mutant paramecia that lack the ion channels underlying the calcium action potential are unable to reverse the direction of ciliary beating and thus cannot swim backward when they encounter noxious environmental stimuli. Because these mutants can only swim forward, they are called "pawn" mutants, after the chess piece that can only move forward. Thus, some of the basic molecular machinery for electrical signaling—one of the hallmarks of nervous system function—predates the origin of the first neuron. This suggests that neural signaling arose by evolutionary modification of preexisting signaling mechanisms found in unicellular organisms.

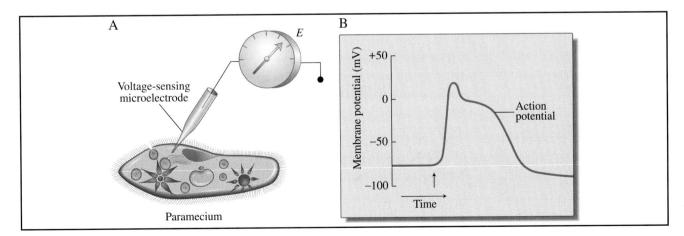

Figure 2.1.

The single-cell protozoan paramecium produces action potentials similar to nerve action potentials. **A.** A diagram of the recording system for measuring the electrical response of paramecium. **B.** An electrical stimulus (at the *vertical arrow*) evokes an action potential.

Preneuronal signaling systems also occur in multicellular animals that lack nervous systems. The cnidarian obelia (genus *Obelia*), for example, forms colonies of polyps sharing a common digestive system. Although there is no nervous system per se, electrical signals spread from one end of the colony to the other along the epithelial cells lining the interior of the digestive cavity. As in the paramecium, the signal takes the form of a calcium action potential.

Early Nervous Systems

Other cnidarians, such as *Hydra*, have the first true nervous system. As shown in Figure 2.2A, this simple nervous system is organized into a **nerve net** in which action potentials propagate from neuron to neuron equally well in all directions. In such a system, no particular neuron could be said to *control* the activity of another, and there is no specialization of function in any one part of the net compared with another. The neurons of the nerve net establish a rapid conduction path for the spread of action potentials throughout the animal, similar to the epithelial conduction system of obelia. With its network of neurons connected via rapidly conducting axons, however, the nerve net provides more rapid spread of signals in a more defined directional pattern than can be attained by electrical signals spreading nonspecifically throughout the epithelial sheet in obelia.

Free-swimming animals require well-coordinated movements to locomote effectively and thus require a nervous system to coordinate their movement. Cnidarians such as jellyfish, for example, swim by rhythmic contractions of the bell and have well-developed nerve nets to ensure the proper coordination of contraction. Interestingly, the free-swimming, reproductive medusae of obelia have a nerve net, although the sessile adult animal does not. Thus, the evolutionary emergence of neurons may coincide with the origination of contractile tissues used for locomotion in animals.

Nerve nets like that of hydra are commonly found in animals whose bodies show **radial symmetry**. In such animals, no particular body part is more likely than another to encounter food or predators. If the animal is mobile, any part of the organism is as likely as any other to lead the way during locomotion. This body symmetry is also seen in echinoderms, such as the starfish shown in Figure 2.2B, in which a set of identical arms radiates from a central core. However, the starfish nervous system provides an early evolutionary example of the selective organization of the neurons into something other than a diffuse network. Each of the starfish's arms is innervated by a neural connective that radiates from a ring of nerve fibers surrounding the mouth at the center of the animal. As nervous systems became more complex during evolution, the trend continued toward more centralized organization, with central clumps of neurons giving rise to nerve fibers that radiate outward to innervate the body. Contrast this radial structure with the more diffuse organization found in the nerve net of hydra, in which neurons are distributed evenly throughout the network (see Fig. 2.2A).

Bilateral Symmetry and the Emergence of Centralized Nervous Systems

The trend toward centralized organization of the nervous system is most strongly apparent in animals whose bodies have **bilateral symmetry**. Compare the nervous system of a segmented annelid, the leech (Fig. 2.2C), with the more diffuse systems of hydra and starfish. The cell bodies of leech neurons are gathered in centrally located **ganglia**, one in each body segment. The nerves that innervate the muscles and skin of each segment radiate out from these central ganglia, and the

What neural organization is typical of animals with radial symmetry and bilateral symmetry?

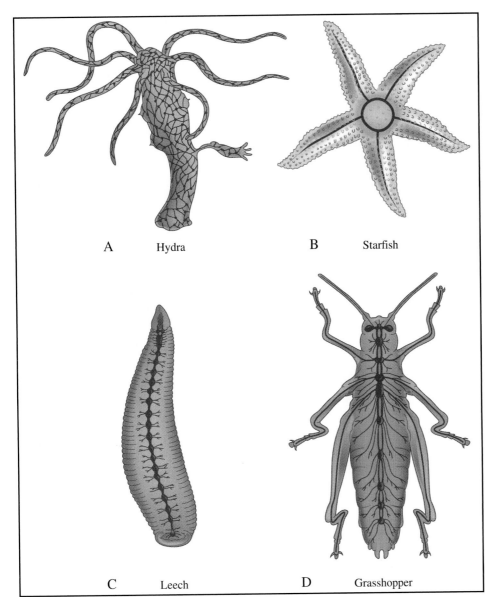

Figure 2.2.

Different organizational schemes of invertebrate nervous systems. **A.** The simplest nervous system consists of a diffuse nerve net, like that found in hydra. **B.** The nervous system of the starfish is organized into a central ring, with nerve fibers radiating out to supply each arm. **C.** The leech has a body with bilateral symmetry, rather than radial symmetry like in the starfish. Correspondingly, the nervous system is arranged longitudinally. The cell bodies of neurons are located in central ganglia along the midline, with nerves radiating out to supply each body segment. In addition, large nerve trunks connect the ganglia into a chain. **D.** Insect nervous systems illustrate the evolutionary trend toward cephalization, with the ganglia at the head end of the animal growing in size and importance and fusing to form a true brain.

A Hydra

B Starfish

C Leech

D Grasshopper

ganglia of successive segments are connected via nerve fibers running longitudinally in a **central nerve trunk**. Thus, annelids exhibit a true central nervous system.

In addition, leech neurons show greater specialization of function than do neurons of nerve nets. Specific sensory neurons in the ganglia carry sensory information in from the environment, whereas other neurons—motor neurons—control the body muscles. Still other neurons are neither sensory nor motor neurons but instead are integrative **interneurons**, which are interposed between sensory and motor neurons. Thus, centralization of neural organization and bilateral symmetry are associated with less generalized and more specific information-processing functions for individual neurons. This specialization of neuronal function becomes more pronounced as organisms and their nervous systems become more complex.

Another trend associated with bilateral symmetry is the trend toward **cephalization**, which refers to the increasing size and importance of the ganglia at the head end of the animal. In most cases, animals with bilateral symmetry locomote in the direction parallel to the long axis of the body. As a result, the leading end (head) of the animal usually comes into contact with food or other environmental stimuli first. The neurons in the ganglia at the head have increased importance, favoring evolutionary development of larger and more elaborate cephalic ganglia. Among invertebrates, insects have perhaps the most complex nervous systems and also the most developed cephalic ganglia (Fig. 2.2D; note that some mollusks, such as the octopus, also have well-developed cephalic ganglia).

As the segmental ganglia at the leading end of the animal grew in size and complexity over evolutionary time, the individual ganglia fused into a single mass that could properly be called a brain. The mammalian brain may not show obvious external signs of it, but it too is organized into clumps of nerve cells separated by interconnecting nerve fiber tracts, much like the segmentally organized leech nervous system. There are in fact many different clusters of neurons within the mammalian brain (called **nuclei** or **ganglia**) that receive inputs from and send outputs to other clusters. Thus, the more primitive organization of the central nervous system into chains of interconnected ganglia is actually retained—albeit in much more intricate form—in the structure of mammalian brains.

A corollary of the trend toward cephalization is the increased importance of cephalic regions of the nervous system in controlling other parts of the nervous system. In more primitive nervous systems, each segmental ganglion coordinates the behavior of a particular body segment; although information is passed along from one ganglion to another, the ganglia are more or less equal partners in controlling behavior of the organism as a whole. However, with the appearance of cephalic ganglia and brains, **hierarchical organization** of the nervous system begins to emerge, with the ganglia in the head taking primary responsibility for initiation of action and overall integration of sensory and motor information into behavior. The segmental ganglia in the rest of the body remain responsible for controlling local actions of individual body segments and integrating those actions into the overall behavior of the animal. Vertebrate nervous systems exhibit this trend most strongly, and the central nervous system is subdivided into the **brain**—the overseer and initiator of behavior—and the **spinal cord**, which coordinates reflex actions and provides circuitry for carrying out the commands descending from higher control centers in the brain.

Subdivisions of the Vertebrate Brain

What are the three major subdivisions of the vertebrate brain?

In vertebrate animals, the brain is subdivided into three main regions, as shown in Figure 2.3: the **hindbrain**, the **midbrain**, and the **forebrain**. In keeping with the general scheme of hierarchical organization, the hindbrain tends to pass information to and receive controlling signals from the midbrain, which in turn is controlled by the forebrain. Of course, there are important exceptions to this hierarchical scheme, as we will see when we discuss specific sensory and motor systems, but it is still useful to think about the organization of the brain in this hierarchical manner.

Figure 2.3.

The basic organizational scheme of the vertebrate central nervous system. The two major divisions are the spinal cord and brain. The brain is further subdivided into the forebrain, midbrain, and hindbrain. Together, the hindbrain and the midbrain are called the brainstem.

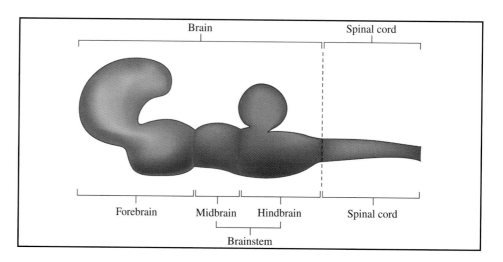

The hindbrain (also called the **rhombencephalon**) is concerned primarily with coordination of body movement and with automatic body functions, such as respiration and cardiovascular function. The midbrain (also called the **mesencephalon**) contains additional motor coordination centers; it also receives and processes sensory information before distributing it to the forebrain for further processing. Collectively, the midbrain and hindbrain are referred to as the **brainstem**. The forebrain (also called the **prosencephalon**) integrates sensory information of various kinds and formulates motor commands that are executed by other parts of the central nervous system.

The vertebrate central nervous system also exhibits the evolutionary trends toward cephalization, specialization of neural function, and hierarchical organization, which we discussed earlier for invertebrate nervous systems. In primitive vertebrates, such as fish, amphibians, and reptiles, the forebrain is a relatively minor part of the brain (see Fig. 2.4). In these animals, the midbrain carries out many of the functions of the forebrain in more complex brains. For example, in animals

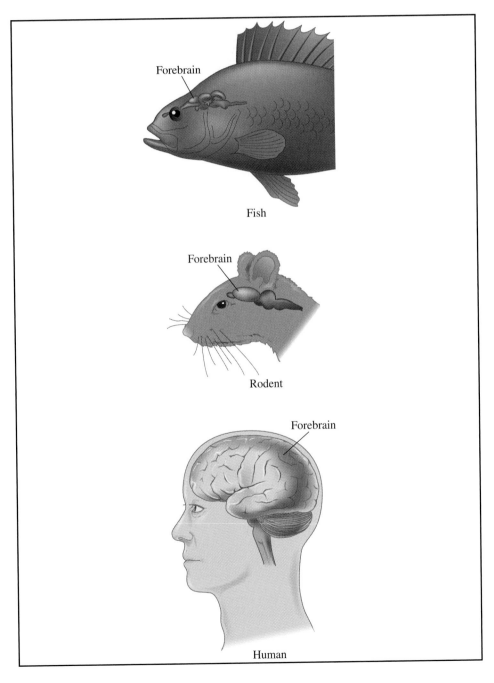

Fish

Rodent

Human

Figure 2.4.

The relative proportions of the brain accounted for by the forebrain in a fish, a rodent, and a primate.

with primitive forebrains, visual information processing occurs in the optic tectum, which is part of the midbrain. In mammals, the corresponding parts of the midbrain serve lower-level visual functions, such as the control of eye movements, while sophisticated visual processing is carried out in the forebrain.

In mammals, increasing importance of the forebrain is associated with increased proportional size of one of the major subdivisions of the forebrain, the **cerebrum** (see Fig. 2.4). The **cerebral cortex**—the outer layer of the cerebrum containing most of the neurons—balloons out to occupy a larger surface area, enveloping the more posterior midbrain and hindbrain structures. Thus, when we look at the exterior surface of a mammalian brain, our view is dominated by the cerebral cortex. In mammals more complex than rodents (see Fig. 2.4), the surface area of the cortex becomes so large that it must form infoldings, or **convolutions**, to fit within the space available for the brain inside the skull. The cerebral cortex is involved in processing of sensory information, formation of perceptions, planning and initiation of movements, and associative learning. Therefore, increased surface area of the cortex—and thus increased numbers of cortical neurons—is correlated with increased complexity and flexibility of behavior.

The forebrain, midbrain, and hindbrain are further subdivided into numerous parts, each with its own specialized functions. Although we will consider each of these subdivisions in detail in later chapters, it is worth mentioning some of them now to give an overall view of the structure of vertebrate brains.

The hindbrain has three principal subdivisions (Fig. 2.5): the **medulla oblongata**, the **cerebellum**, and the **pons**. The medulla oblongata sits at the junction between the brain and the spinal cord and contains neurons that help control many visceral functions, such as breathing, swallowing, and digestion. The pons is located at the junction between the hindbrain and the midbrain. Neurons in the pons also participate in the regulation of respiration. The cerebellum receives a wide variety of sensory information, as well as signals from motor control areas in the forebrain. Based on that sensory and motor information, the cerebellum modifies motor commands to ensure accurate and smooth motor performance. In addition, much of the space in the hindbrain is occupied by tracts of axons carrying information to and from the spinal cord.

In the midbrain, two important subdivisions are the **inferior colliculus** and the **superior colliculus**, which form protrusions on the dorsal surface of the midbrain (see Fig. 2.5). The inferior colliculus is an important relay and processing station in the auditory system, while the superior colliculus is involved in processing visual information. Other parts of the midbrain make up a portion of the **reticular formation**, which controls the level of arousal and contains neurons that play direct and indirect roles in a variety of motor and sensory systems.

What are the diencephalon and the telencephalon?

Figure 2.5 also shows that the forebrain is divided into the **diencephalon** and the **telencephalon**. The diencephalon is composed of the **thalamus** and **hypothalamus**, while the telencephalon consists of the **cerebrum** and the **basal ganglia**. The thalamus is a sensory relay station that distributes sensory information from the various sensory modalities to the appropriate parts of the cerebral cortex for more elaborate processing. The hypothalamus contains a number of nuclei concerned with homeostasis (for example, hunger, thirst, and thermoregulation), the control of sexual behavior, or the regulation of emotion. The basal ganglia help control body movement.

DEVELOPMENT OF THE NERVOUS SYSTEM

With its complicated organization and large forebrain, the mammalian brain represents perhaps the most fully developed example of the evolutionary trends to-

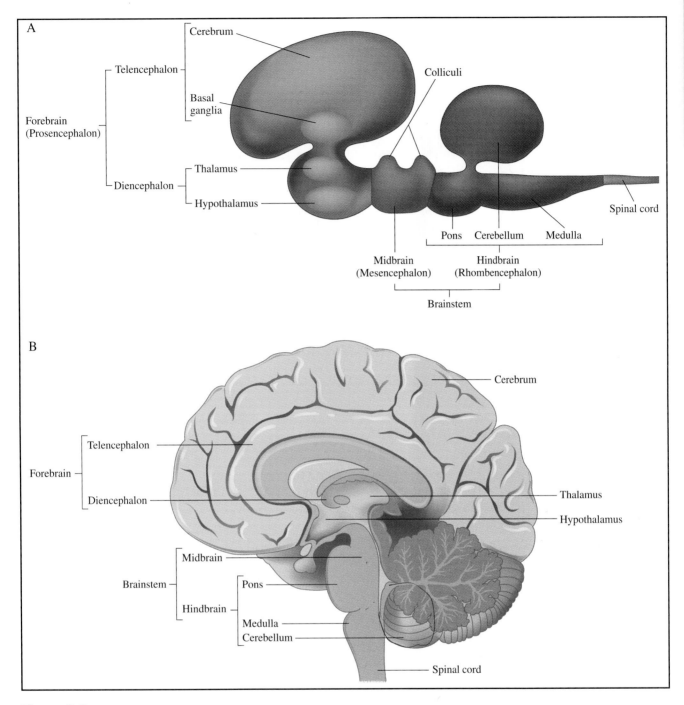

Figure 2.5.

The overall structural organization of the mammalian brain. **A**. The major subdivisions of a prototypical mammalian brain are illustrated schematically in this diagram, in which the brain regions are stretched out linearly to indicate their relative positions. **B**. A human brain sliced longitudinally along the midline reveals the locations of the regions shown schematically in A.

ward cephalization and hierarchical organization. The divisions among the various regions of this complex structure may seem rather arbitrary, however. Why do we divide the brain into three major subdivisions (forebrain, midbrain, and hindbrain)? How are the dividing lines between the three divisions set? Why is the forebrain subdivided into the telencephalon and diencephalon?

From an evolutionary perspective, we have seen that the brains of simpler organisms can give clues about the major divisions of more complex brains. Now, we will examine the developmental sequence during embryogenesis of the mammalian brain to obtain a different perspective on the structural organization of the adult form. In considering this developmental sequence from simple to complex, we will obtain some answers to our questions about the brain's seemingly arbitrary divisions.

Early Neural Development

What is the difference between the neural plate and the neural crest?

During embryonic development, the mammalian nervous system moves through several stages of increasing complexity, culminating in the adult form. The mammalian central nervous system begins as a specialized part of the ectoderm called the **neural plate**, which is located along the dorsal midline of the early-stage embryo (see Fig. 2.6A). Flanking the neural plate on each side are the cells of the **neural crest**, which give rise to the peripheral nervous system, including the dorsal root ganglia. As the cells of the neural plate proliferate, they form an indentation along the midline called the **neural groove**, with the cells of the neural crest forming the top (or crest—hence the name) of each side of the groove (see Fig. 2.6B). As the indentation deepens, the lips of the groove come closer together and finally fuse. At this point, the neural groove becomes a sealed tubular structure, called the **neural tube**, which is separated from the overlying ectoderm (see Fig. 2.6C). The cells of the neural crest lie between the neural tube and the ectoderm at this stage.

IN THE CLINIC

BOX 1

Because the nervous system plays such an important role in the body, damage to the nervous system as a result of disease or accident produces a wide variety of clinically significant symptoms. The nature of the symptoms can give valuable clues about where in the nervous system the damage has occurred. In fact, before the advent of noninvasive imaging techniques, such as computed tomography and magnetic resonance imaging, neurological symptoms were the primary means of determining the locus of damage to the nervous system and guiding possible surgical intervention. A simple example is the loss of sensation and motor control that results when a peripheral nerve is cut: only the part of the body that is innervated by the damaged nerve is affected. The mapping between particular nerves and particular body regions is well established, and the locus of the affected region precisely establishes which nerve or nerve branch is damaged.

In the central nervous system, the situation is often less simple, because the anatomical arrangements are complex and because the damage produced by a stroke or a tumor rarely respects anatomical boundaries between brain regions, producing a spectrum of different symptoms. Nevertheless, neurologists are able to distinguish among a variety of different syndromes that result from specific neurological damage. For example, damage to the cerebellum might produce disorders of balance or gait or might disrupt the ability to make fine movements, depending on the part of the cerebellum that sustains damage. In the cerebral cortex, certain regions are dedicated to the processing of specific types of sensory information, and lesions in those regions disrupt perception of the corresponding sensory modality. Damage to the brainstem is often fatal because the neural circuits in the brainstem are fundamentally important to vital functions like respiration and because both ascending nerve fibers from the spinal cord and descending nerve fibers from the midbrain and forebrain pass through the brainstem.

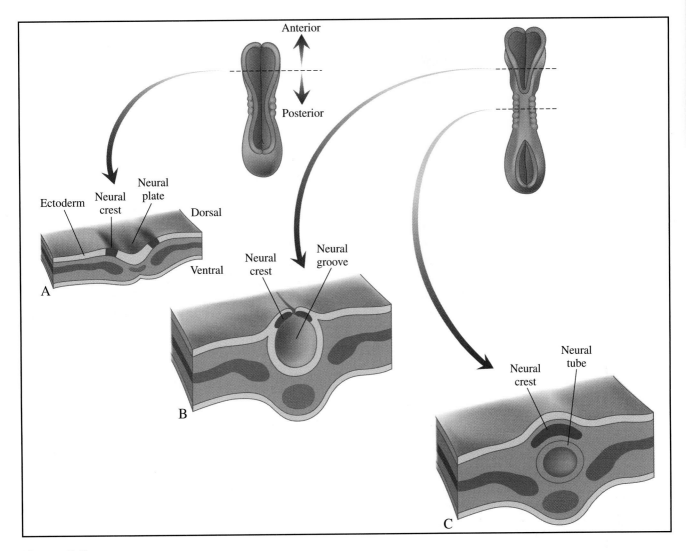

Figure 2.6.

Early differentiation of the nervous system in a vertebrate embryo. **A.** The nervous system begins as undifferentiated ectodermal cells along the dorsal midline, called the neural plate. At this stage, the cells that will form the neural crest lie along each side of the neural plate. **B.** At a later stage, the neural plate invaginates to form the neural groove, with the neural crest running along the lips of the groove. **C.** Later, the neural groove pinches off to form the neural tube, as the two opposing parts of the neural crest fuse and separate from the ectoderm.

The cells lining the neural tube proliferate and differentiate into the neurons and glial cells that make up the brain and spinal cord. At the anterior end of the neural tube, which is destined to form the brain, cells proliferate more rapidly than at the posterior end, which will become the spinal cord. Thus, the anterior end begins to bulge out, forming three protrusions separated by constrictions, as shown in Figure 2.7A. These protrusions, called **vesicles**, have familiar names: the forebrain, the midbrain, and the hindbrain. The part of the neural tube posterior to the three vesicles is the spinal cord. It should now be clear why the adult brain is divided into three major parts, not two or five or ten: three is the number of protobrain protrusions that form early in the development of the central nervous system.

As development proceeds, the lateral portions of the forebrain vesicle begin to balloon out into structures that will become the two hemispheres of the cerebrum (see Fig. 2.7B). Thus, the subdivision of the forebrain into the telencephalon and diencephalon also has an origin in the embryonic development of this part of the

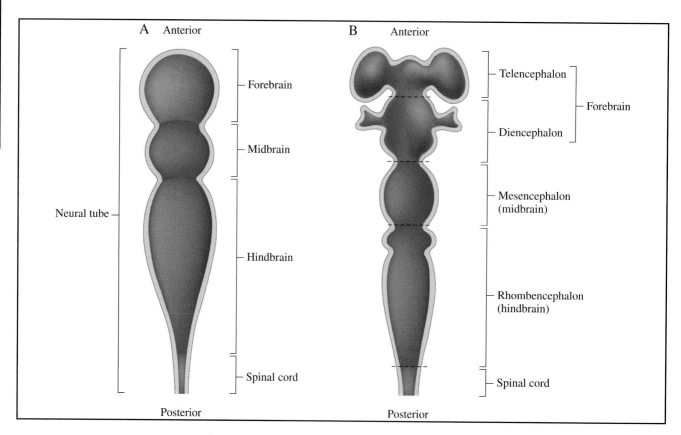

Figure 2.7.

Development of the brain at the anterior end of the neural tube. **A**. At an early stage of development, the anterior neural tube expands into three vesicles: the hindbrain, midbrain, and forebrain. **B**. As development proceeds, the hindbrain and forebrain vesicles subdivide further.

brain: the large protrusions form the telencephalon, while the part left behind forms the diencephalon. A similar subdivision of the hindbrain into its component parts—including the pons, cerebellum, and medulla—begins at these embryonic stages as well. The assignment of a particular structure in the adult brain to the forebrain, midbrain, or hindbrain is determined by which of the primordial brain vesicles gave rise to the structure.

As the telencephalon grows, it folds back on itself, overlapping and enveloping the midbrain and parts of the hindbrain, as illustrated in Figure 2.8. In animals with large cortical regions, such as primates, the growing telencephalon turns back on itself once again, forming a shape somewhat like a ram's horn (see Fig. 2.8). Because of the intricate folding and overlapping, the hierarchical structure of the adult brain may be hard to appreciate without considering the developmental sequence. For example, a cross section of the human brain taken approximately through the middle of the brain (Fig. 2.9) would include structures from the telencephalon, the diencephalon, and the midbrain. The divisions among the parts may be hard to discern in such a cross section. If we keep in mind the embryonic sequence, however, the complicated adult shape is easier to envision.

The Vertebrate Nervous System Is a Fluid-Filled Tube

The brain and spinal cord form from the neural tube, a hollow structure formed when the neural groove pinches off from the ectoderm of the embryo. The hollow

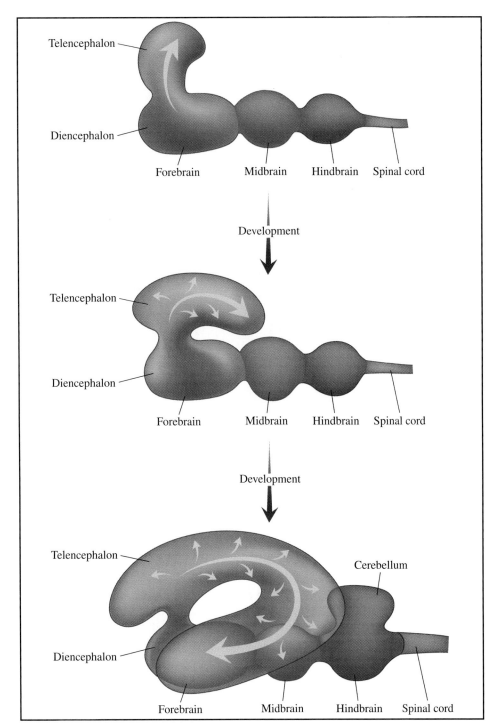

Figure 2.8.

Development of the telencephalon. As the cerebral cortex expands, it extends in the posterior direction to overlie the midbrain and hindbrain. In animals with a larger cortex, the growing telencephalon curls around into a shape similar to that of a ram's horn and virtually completely surrounds the midbrain structures and the diencephalon.

core of the tube persists in adulthood and is called the **spinal canal** in the spinal cord and the **cerebral ventricles** in the brain. The hollow core is filled with fluid called the **cerebrospinal fluid** (abbreviated **CSF**). The ventricles and spinal canal form a continuous, uninterrupted fluid compartment at the core of the central nervous system, extending from the caudal end of the spinal cord to the hemispheres of the cerebral cortex. By tracing this continuous core, we can follow the linear path from the spinal cord to the hindbrain to the midbrain to the forebrain, even though the route has numerous bends and turns introduced during differentiation of the embryonic structure into the adult form.

Figure 2.10 shows the shape of the cerebral ventricles in the adult human brain. This shape reflects the embryonic growth and proliferation of the various parts of

How are the ventricles of the brain organized?

Figure 2.9.

A human brain is sliced perpendicular to the midline to reveal the brain structures in cross section. The slice cuts through forebrain and midbrain structures.

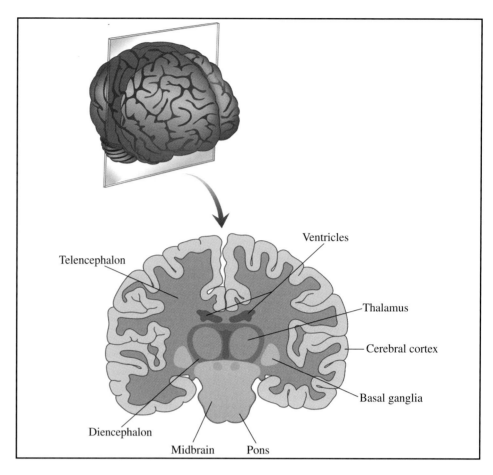

Telencephalon

Ventricles

Thalamus

Cerebral cortex

Basal ganglia

Diencephalon

Midbrain   Pons

IN THE CLINIC

During the early stages of embryonic development, the embryo is especially sensitive to both environmental and genetic factors, which can interfere with the normal sequence of development. Because the nervous system begins to form at these early stages, malformation of the nervous system is a common outcome of exposure to infection or environmental toxins during early embryogenesis or of a genetic abnormality. The severity of the effect depends on exactly when during development the problem arises and which part of the developing nervous system is affected. Particularly severe defects arise from failure of the neural tube to close properly (neural tube defects). If the anterior part of the neural tube fails to fuse, the anterior vesicles that give rise to the brain are malformed, producing anencephaly (absence of the brain). This is obviously a devastating defect. If the failure to fuse properly occurs in more posterior parts of the neural tube, the resulting defect is spina bifida. In spina bifida, neuronal communication within the spinal cord is disrupted at all positions more posterior than the site of the defect, producing varying degrees of paralysis. Defects can also arise at later stages of neural development, after the formation of the neural tube. For example, the anterior part of the forebrain may fail to form two paired telencephalic protrusions, resulting in a single telencephalon (holoprosencephaly) rather than the normal pair of cerebral hemispheres. Severe mental retardation is the outcome of this developmental anomaly.

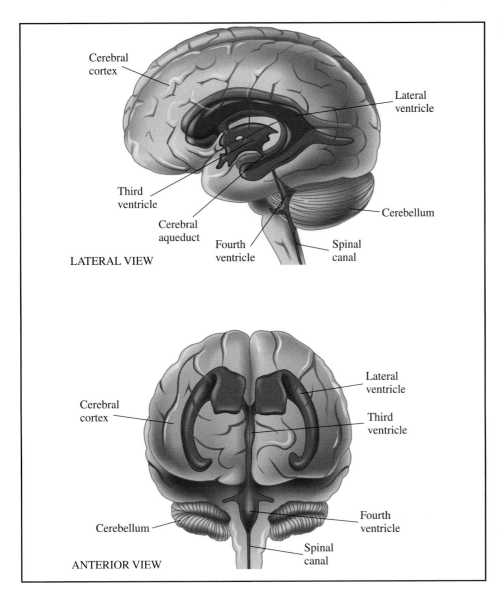

Figure 2.10.

The organization of ventricles in the human brain. The developmental expansion of the telencephalon is reflected in the shape of the lateral ventricles. In addition, the continuity of the ventricles from the spinal canal to the tips of the lateral ventricles demonstrates that the underlying form of the brain is a contorted tube.

the brain. As it enters the brain, the spinal canal expands to form the **fourth ventricle** at the core of the hindbrain. Through the midbrain, the ventricle narrows again to form a structure called the **cerebral aqueduct**. In the diencephalon, the aqueduct opens dorsally and ventrally to form the tall, thin **third ventricle**. As the telencephalon balloons out from the diencephalon during development, the ventricle expands laterally to form the two **lateral ventricles**, one in each hemisphere of the cerebrum. When the telencephalon grows posteriorly and then ventrally and anteriorly, the lateral ventricles follow suit. Thus, the adult lateral ventricles clearly show the shape of a ram's horn resulting from this direction of expansion during development (see Fig. 2.10).

FUNCTIONAL NEUROANATOMY

We have now examined the overall structure of vertebrate—especially mammalian—nervous systems, both in terms of evolutionary trends and as the result of embryonic development from simpler structures. We have discussed the subdivision of the brain into gross structural parts, which provides a framework of nomenclature and a conceptual reference point for more detailed discussions of brain organization that follow in subsequent chapters. The remainder of the discussion of brain anatomy in this book emphasizes **functional neuroanatomy**, in which boundaries are drawn in the nervous system based on considering which nuclei and pathways carry out related functions. In discussing functionally defined neural systems, we will find that forebrain, midbrain, and hindbrain structures might all participate in different aspects of a single neural system. For this reason, the anatomical organization of each neural system will be discussed in the context of the physiological description of that system.

SUMMARY

The overall structure of the mammalian central nervous system can be better appreciated by examining the evolutionary origin and embryonic development of the nervous system. Neurons probably arose during evolution to provide rapid and reliable control of motor structures and rapid distribution of sensory information. Electrical signaling is found in single-cell animals and thus predates the development of nervous systems. The simplest nervous systems are nerve nets like those found in hydra, in which electrical signals can propagate from neuron to neuron in any direction throughout the network. The advent of animals with bilateral symmetry (for example, worms), rather than radial symmetry (for example, starfish), was associated with the clustering of neurons into ganglia along a centralized nerve cord. As nervous systems became more complex, the ganglia at the front end (the head) of the animal became larger and more important in the control of the rest of the nervous system, a process called cephalization. The dominance of the head ganglia in controlling the rest of the nervous system is an example of the evolutionary trend toward hierarchical organization of the nervous system.

The organization of the vertebrate nervous system can be more easily comprehended by examining the relatively simple structure of the nervous system during embryonic development. The nervous system develops from a fluid-filled tube, called the neural tube, which is formed from the neural plate of the early embryo. As development proceeds, the anterior part of the neural tube forms three protrusions, or vesicles, that give rise to the three parts of the vertebrate brain: the hindbrain, the midbrain, and the forebrain. The lateral portions of the forebrain vesicle balloon out to form the two hemispheres of the cerebrum and the cerebral cortex, which spreads out to envelop most of the midbrain and hindbrain in mammalian nervous systems. The developmental history of a mammalian brain can also be appreciated by examining the three-dimensional structure of the fluid-filled center of the nervous system, the cerebral ventricles and the spinal canal.

The forebrain, midbrain, and hindbrain can be subdivided into numerous subregions, based on anatomical connections and on the functional roles of the subregions. In the hindbrain, three major subdivisions are the medulla oblongata, the cerebellum, and the pons. In the midbrain, three important subregions are the superior colliculus, the inferior colliculus, and the reticular formation. The two main subdivisions of the forebrain are the diencephalon and the telencephalon, which includes the cerebral cortex.

1. Describe the role of the calcium action potential in the paramecium.
2. Provide definitions for the following terms: cephalization, hierarchical organization, nerve net, segmental ganglion.
3. List the three principal subdivisions of the hindbrain.
4. Name the two subdivisions of the diencephalon.
5. Describe the formation of the neural tube and neural crest from the neural plate.
6. Define the following: cerebral aqueduct, cerebrospinal fluid, lateral ventricle, fourth ventricle.
7. Name the major subdivision of the brain to which each of the following belongs: cerebellum, thalamus, basal ganglia, medulla oblongata, cerebral cortex, hypothalamus, pons.

INTERNET ASSIGNMENT   CHAPTER 2

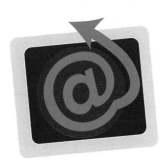

1 The process of gastrulation is an important transition from a single cell layer to three layers in vertebrate embryos. Search the Internet to find videos or animated movies that illustrate the three-dimensional movement of cells during gastrulation. Note that some search sites (for example, altavista.com) allow you to specify that the search results should be restricted to videos and movies.

2 A variety of neuroanatomical information is available on the Internet. For instance, "atlases" of brain sections have been published on the Internet. Locate sources that provide atlases of primate and rodent brains and use these resources to become familiar with the overall structure of these brains. You may find a list of neuroanatomical information sources at neuroguide.com or in the neurosciences section of about.com. The Digital Anatomist is another particularly useful site, maintained by the University of Washington.

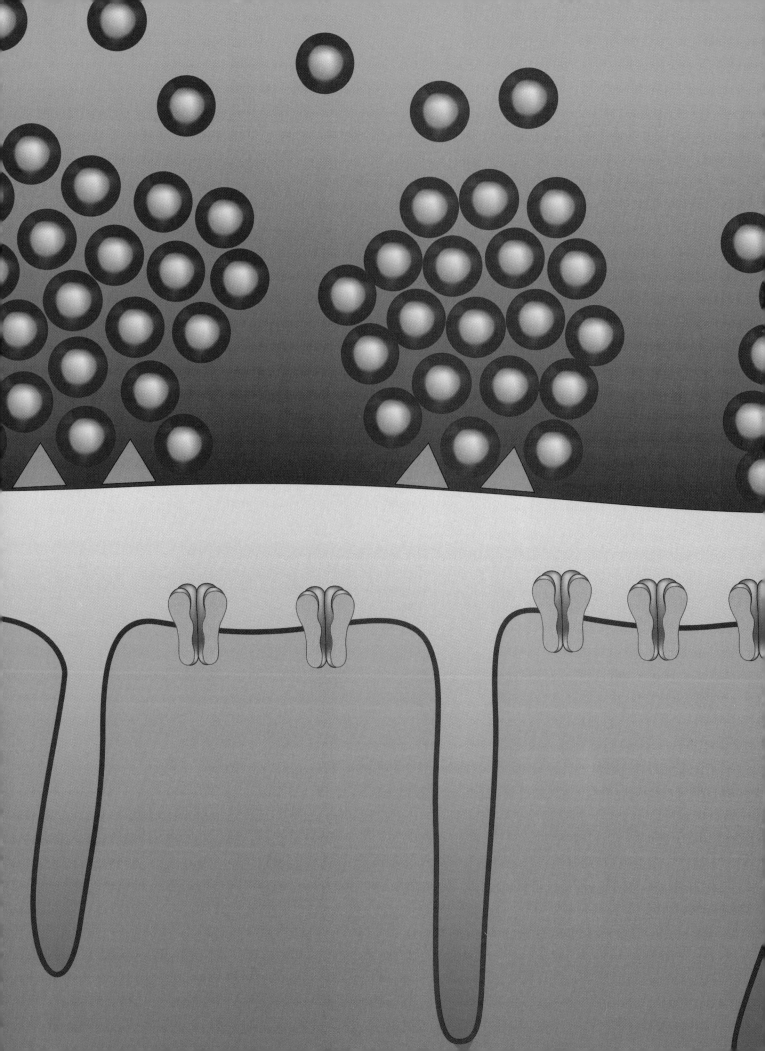

CELLULAR ASPECTS OF NEUROBIOLOGY

In this section of the book, we will examine the fundamental properties of communication in the nervous system. The nervous system employs electrical communication, and we cannot understand its functioning without a firm understanding of how electrical signals are generated and transmitted in nerve cells. The patellar reflex, which we considered in Chapter 1, provides the organizational framework for this part of the book because this simple reflex exemplifies the basic electrical signals underlying information transmission in the nervous system. In the patellar reflex, information must be transmitted over a long distance along the axons of the sensory and motor neurons in the nerve connecting the spinal cord and the muscle. The electrical signal that transmits the information is the action potential. To study the cellular mechanisms of the action potential, we must first understand the physical and chemical principles that govern the generation of the electrical membrane potential in cells. Then, we will apply the principles that govern the membrane potential to comprehend how neurons actively modulate the membrane potential to produce the long-distance signal of the nervous system, the action potential. Finally, we will turn our attention to communication among neurons, and examine mechanisms of synaptic transmission.

Chapter 3 describes osmotic and electrical equilibrium and the nonequilibrium steady-state membrane potential of cells.

A series of model systems are used to illustrate the important principles underlying the electrical membrane potential of cells. Each model system is tailored to illustrate a particular principle, and as we proceed, the models become progressively more complex and more realistic. By working through these models, even students who lack a quantitative background in physics and chemistry will be able to reach an understanding of the principles governing the electrical behavior of cells. In Chapter 4, we will use these principles to examine the membrane mechanisms of the action potential. Chapter 5 considers synaptic transmission from motor neurons to muscle cells at the neuromuscular junction, and Chapter 6 discusses neuron-to-neuron synaptic transmission in the spinal cord.

In Part III, beginning in Chapter 7, we then move on from this cellular viewpoint to see how the patellar reflex fits in with the overall scheme of motor control systems, both in the spinal cord and in the brain.

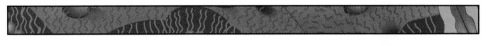

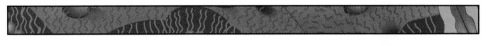

ORIGIN OF MEMBRANE POTENTIAL

ESSENTIAL BACKGROUND

Osmolarity and diffusion

Dissociation of salts in solution

Logarithms (base 10 and base e)

ATP as a cellular energy source

Electrical voltage and electrical current

DNA, genes, and protein production

In the nervous system, changes in the membrane potential are central to the generation and processing of signals. To understand how cells can change their membrane potential, we must first understand the basic physical and chemical principles that govern the electrical behavior of cells. By working through a series of simplified models, we will see that the membrane potential is an essential feature of the mechanisms cells use to maintain differences in the composition of the **intracellular fluid** (ICF) and the **extracellular fluid** (ECF). The membrane potential arises from a differential distribution of charged substances (**ions**) in the ICF and ECF and from differential permeability of the plasma membrane to different ions. We will begin by examining the compositions of fluids inside and outside cells, and then consider the maintenance of osmotic balance, the principles of ionic equilibrium, and the membrane mechanisms for sustaining a nonequilibrium ionic steady state.

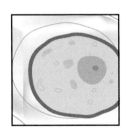

COMPOSITION OF BODY FLUIDS

If we were to dissociate an organism into its component molecules and sort them by type, we would find that special biological molecules—proteins, DNA, RNA, and so on—constitute only about 0.25% of the total. Most of the molecules in the body are far more ordinary. In fact, the most common molecule is water, which makes up about 75% of the weight of a human body, excluding nonessential body fat. Because water is a comparatively light molecule, 75% of the body weight translates into a huge number of water molecules, accounting for about 99% of all molecules in the body. Excluding water and the special biological molecules, the remainder consists of simple inorganic substances, such as sodium, potassium, and chloride ions. We concern ourselves with these mundane molecules because cells could not exist and life would not be possible if cells did not possess mechanisms to control the distribution of water and ions across their membranes. In the course of examining these control mechanisms, we will uncover the physical principles underlying the origin of the membrane potential and the electrical signals that transmit information in the nervous system.

Intracellular and Extracellular Fluids

The water in the body can be divided into two compartments: the ICF and the ECF. The wall separating the intracellular and extracellular compartments is the outer cell membrane, also called the **plasma membrane** of the cell. Both the ECF and ICF compartments can be further divided into subcompartments, but for our purposes it will suffice to treat both of them as single, uniform compartments.

What substances are dissolved in the ICF and ECF?

Although organic and inorganic substances are dissolved in both intracellular and extracellular water, the compositions of the two compartments differ. Table 3.1 lists simplified compositions of ECF and ICF for a typical mammalian cell. The simplification arises because the table includes only the substances that are important in governing the basic osmotic and electrical properties of cells. A variety of other inorganic and organic solutes are found in both ECF and ICF, and many of them have important physiological roles in other contexts. For our examination of the membrane potential, however, they can be safely ignored.

The principal **cation** (positively charged ion) outside the cell is sodium, although the ECF also contains a small amount of potassium. Inside cells, the situation is reversed. In the ICF, the potassium concentration is high, and the sodium concentration is low. Negatively charged chloride ions, which are present at high concentration in the ECF, are relatively scarce in the ICF. The major **anion** (negatively charged ion) inside cells is actually a class of molecules that bear a net negative charge. These intracellular anions (abbreviated $A^{1.2-}$) represent a diverse group of molecules, including proteins, charged amino acids, and inorganic ions such as sulfate and phosphate. Some of these substances carry a single negative charge, while others have a charge of -2, -3, or more. Taken as a group, the average charge per molecule is approximately -1.2. The presence of this class of anions outside cells can be ignored for our discussion of membrane potential, and we will assume that chloride is the sole extracellular anion.

The concentration of water on the two sides of the membrane must also be considered (see Table 3.1). It may seem odd to speak of the "concentration" of the solvent in ECF and ICF. However, the concentration of water inside and outside the cell must be the same. Otherwise, water will move across the membrane and cell volume will change.

Another important consideration is the permeability of the membrane to each substance. The plasma membrane is permeable to water, potassium, and chloride

	Internal Concentration (mM)	External Concentration (mM)	Can It Cross Plasma Membrane?
K^+	125	5	Y
Na^+	12	120	N*
Cl^-	5	125	Y
$A^{1,2-}$	108	0	N
H_2O	55,000	55,000	Y

Membrane Potential = −60 to −100 mV

Table 3.1

Simplified compositions of intracellular and extracellular fluids for a typical mammalian cell

*As we will see later, this "no" is not as simple as it seems to be at first.

but is effectively impermeable to sodium (however, sodium permeability is discussed in detail later). Of course, if the membrane is to do its job properly, it must keep the organic anions inside the cell; otherwise all of a cell's essential biochemical machinery would simply diffuse away into the ECF. Thus, the membrane is impermeable to $A^{1,2-}$.

Finally, the inside of the cell is more negative than the outside, producing a transmembrane voltage difference. The typical value of the membrane potential (abbreviated E_m) is −60 to −100 mV, as shown in Table 3.1.

The Structure of the Plasma Membrane

The control mechanisms responsible for the differences between the ICF and ECF shown in Table 3.1 reside within the barrier between the intracellular and extracellular compartments, the plasma membrane. C. Ernest Overton made the first systematic observations of the kinds of molecules that would cross the plasma membrane, in the early part of the twentieth century. He found that in general, substances that are highly soluble in lipids enter cells more easily than do substances that are less soluble in lipids. Lipids are molecules that are not soluble in water or other polar solvents but are soluble in oil or other nonpolar solvents. Thus, Overton suggested that the plasma membrane consists of lipids and that substances can cross the membrane by dissolving in the membrane lipid.

Lipid solubility cannot account for the membrane permeability of all substances, however. Electrically charged substances, like potassium and chloride ions, are almost totally insoluble in lipids yet they manage to cross the plasma membrane. To account for these exceptions, Overton suggested that the lipid membrane is shot through with tiny holes or pores that allow highly water-soluble (hydrophilic) substances, such as ions, to cross the membrane. Only hydrophilic substances that are small enough to fit through these small aqueous pores can cross the membrane. Larger molecules like proteins and amino acids cannot fit through the pores and thus cannot cross the membrane without the help of special transport mechanisms.

The plasma membrane is a **lipid bilayer membrane**, with the lipid molecules arranged in a layer only two molecules thick. This bilayer arrangement makes sense considering the type of lipid molecules found in the plasma membrane. The membrane lipids are largely phospholipids, which are molecules that have both a hydrophilic region and a hydrophobic region. When spread out in a sheet with water on each side, phospholipids form a bimolecular sandwich, with the hydrophilic parts on the outside toward the water and the hydrophobic parts in the middle,

What is the molecular composition of the plasma membrane?

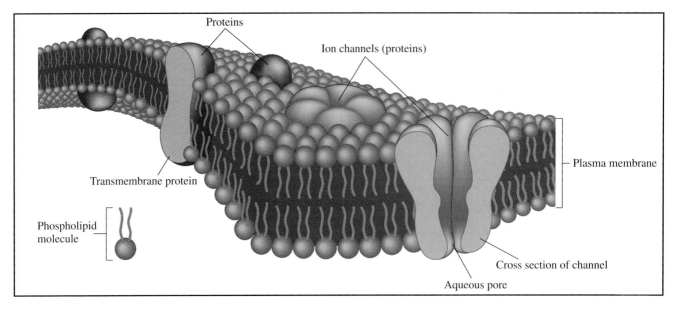

Figure 3.1.

A schematic diagram of a section of the plasma membrane. The backbone of the membrane is a sheet of lipid molecules two molecules thick. Inserted into this sheet are various types of protein molecules. Some protein molecules extend all the way across the sheet, from the inner to the outer face. These transmembrane proteins sometimes form aqueous pores or channels through which small hydrophilic molecules, such as ions, can cross the membrane. The diagram shows two such channels; one is cut in cross section to reveal the interior of the pore.

pointed toward each other. The bilayer structure of the plasma membrane is illustrated in Figure 3.1.

Figure 3.1 also shows that the membrane contains protein molecules, as well as lipid molecules. Some proteins are attached to the inner or outer surface of the cell membrane, and others penetrate all the way through the membrane. Some of the transmembrane proteins form the aqueous pores, or channels, that allow ions and other small hydrophilic molecules to cross the membrane. Although lipids form the backbone of the membrane, proteins are an important part of the picture. By weight, lipids account for only about one-third of the membrane material; most of the remainder is protein. As we will see later, the proteins are important in controlling the movement of substances, particularly ions, across the cell membrane.

The importance of membrane proteins for life can be appreciated by considering how much of the entire genome of a simple organism is devoted to genes encoding membrane proteins. The genome of the microbe *Mycoplasma genitalium* is one of the smallest of any nonviral organism and thus represents the minimum set of genes required for independent, cellular life. The genomic DNA of *M. genitalium* has been completely sequenced, revealing a total of 482 individual genes. Of this total, 140 genes (approximately 30%) encode membrane proteins. Thus, *M. genitalium* expends a large fraction of its total available DNA to provide membrane proteins that reside at the interface between the microbe and its external environment.

Membrane proteins can be observed directly using freeze-fracture electron microscopy, a technique illustrated in Figure 3.2. A thin sliver of tissue is shaved from a sample frozen in liquid nitrogen. The line of fracture between the sliver and the sample sometimes runs between the two layers of the membrane bilayer, leaving holes where protein molecules remain behind and protrusions where membrane proteins come along with the shaved sliver. Figure 3.3 shows a freeze-fracture sample viewed through the electron microscope. The membrane proteins appear as small bumps in the otherwise smooth surface of the plasma membrane, like grains of sand sprinkled on a freshly painted surface.

MAINTENANCE OF CELL VOLUME

At an early stage of evolution, the advent of a cell membrane solved the problem of how to keep biological molecules together to form a coherent organism. This

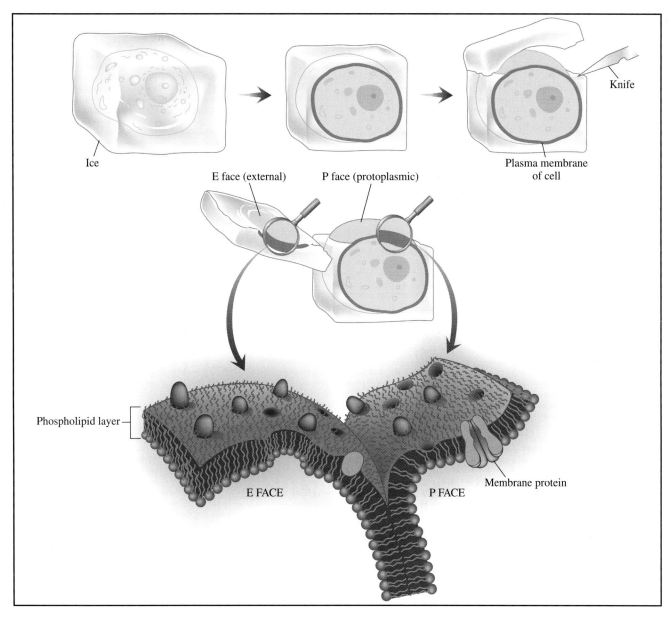

Figure 3.2.

The freeze-fracture procedure for electron microscopy. When a fracture line runs between the two lipid layers of the plasma membrane, some membrane proteins stay with one monolayer, others with the other layer. When examined with the electron microscope, the remaining proteins appear as protruding bumps in the surface.

was the origin of cellular life. While solving one problem, the cell membrane brought a new one: the need to achieve osmotic balance. To see how this problem arises, we must examine the factors that govern the movement of water.

Molarity, Molality, and Diffusion of Water

Examine Figure 3.4, which illustrates the change in water concentration when a solute is added to pure water. When sugar is added to a container of water, the dissolved sugar molecules take up some space that was formerly occupied by water molecules, increasing the volume of the solution. The total number of water molecules is the same before and after the sugar is dissolved, but the water is distributed throughout a larger volume in the sugar-water solution. Because the concentration

Figure 3.3.

A fractured membrane surface containing protein molecules, as viewed through the electron microscope. The protein molecules are the small bumps scattered about on the planar surface of the membrane. Reproduced with permission from C.-P. Ko. Regeneration of the active zone at the frog neuromuscular junction. J. Cell Biol. 1984;98:1685–1695 by copyright permission of the Rockefeller University Press.

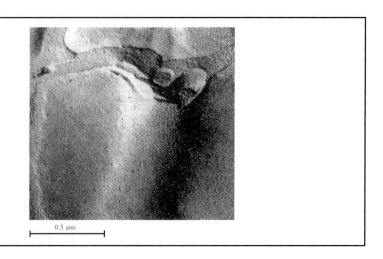

0.5 μm

How do we determine the concentration of water in a solution?

of a substance is defined as the number of molecules of that substance per unit volume of solution, the concentration of water in the sugar solution is lower than it was in pure water.

To compare the concentration of water in solutions containing different concentrations of dissolved substances, we will use the concept of **osmolarity**. A solution containing 1 mole of dissolved solute particles per liter (a 1 molar, or 1 M, solution) has an osmolarity of 1 osmolar (1 Osm), and a 1 millimolar (1 mM) solution has an osmolarity of 1 milliosmolar (1 mOsm). *The higher the osmolarity of a solution, the lower the concentration of water.* For practical purposes in biological solutions, the identity of the dissolved particle does not greatly influence the resulting osmolarity; that is, the concentration of water is effectively the same in a solution of 0.1 Osm glucose, 0.1 Osm sucrose, or 0.1 Osm urea. To be strictly correct in discussing the concentration of water in various solutions, we would have to compare the molality, rather than the molarity, of the solutions. **Molality** is defined as moles of solute per kilogram of solvent. As a result, it takes into account the fact that larger solutes displace more water per mole of solute than do smaller solutes. That is, a liter of solution containing 1 mole of a large molecule, such as a protein, would contain less water (and thus fewer kilograms of solvent) than would a liter of solution containing 1 mole of a small molecule, such as urea. The molality of the protein solution would be greater than the molality of the urea solution, even though both solutions have the same molarity (that is, 1 M). For our purposes, however, it is adequate to treat molarity and osmolarity as equivalent to molality and osmolality.

The osmolarity of a solution also takes into account how many dissolved particles result from each molecule of the dissolved substance. Molecules of glucose, sucrose, and urea do not dissociate in solution, and so a solution containing 0.1 mole

Figure 3.4.

The effect of adding a solute on the volume of a solution. When sugar molecules (*red circles*) are dissolved in a liter of water, the resulting solution occupies a volume greater than a liter because the sugar molecules take up some space formerly occupied by water molecules (*clear circles*). As a result, the concentration of water (number of molecules of water per unit volume) is lower in the sugar-water solution.

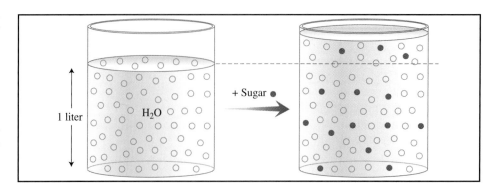

of glucose has an osmolarity of 0.1 Osm. Sodium chloride (NaCl), however, produces two dissolved particles—a sodium and a chloride ion—from each molecule of dissolved salt. Thus, a 0.1 M NaCl solution is a 0.2 Osm solution. To be strictly correct, we must take into account interactions among the ions in a solution, making the effective osmolarity less than expected if all dissolved particles behave independently. For dilute solutions like those usually encountered in biology, ionic interactions are weak and can be safely ignored. Thus, for practical purposes we will assume that all dissolved particles independently determine the total osmolarity of a solution. Consequently, each of the following solutions would have the same total osmolarity (300 mOsm):

- 300 mM glucose
- 150 mM NaCl
- 100 mM NaCl + 100 mM glucose
- 75 mM NaCl + 75 mM potassium chloride

When solutions of different osmolarity are placed in contact through a water-permeable barrier, water diffuses across the barrier according to its concentration gradient (that is, from the lower to the higher osmolar solution). Movement of water down its concentration gradient is called **osmosis**. Consider the example shown in Figure 3.5A, which shows a container divided into two equal compartments filled with glucose solutions. The barrier dividing the container is made of an elastic material, allowing it to stretch freely. If the barrier allows both water and glucose to cross, water will move from side 1 to side 2, down its concentration gradient, and glucose will move from side 2 to side 1. The movement of water and glucose will continue until their concentrations on the two sides of the barrier are equal. Thus, side 1 gains glucose and loses water, and side 2 loses glucose and gains water until the glucose concentration on both sides is 150 mM. No net change occurs in the volume of solution on either side of the barrier at equilibrium, as shown in Figure 3.5B.

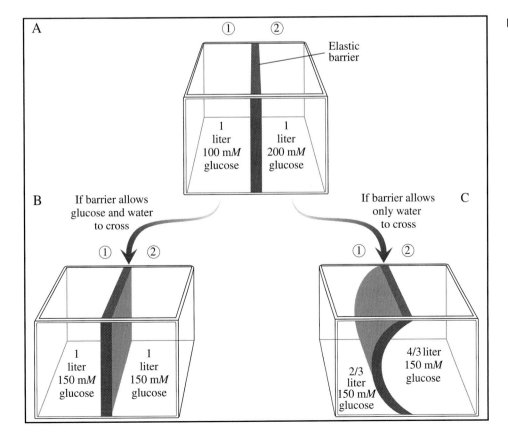

Figure 3.5.

The effect of properties of the barrier separating two different glucose solutions on final volumes of the solutions. **A.** The starting conditions. **B.** If the barrier allows both glucose and water to cross, the volumes of the two solutions do not change when equilibrium is reached. **C.** If the barrier allows only water to cross, osmolarities of the two solutions are the same at equilibrium, but the final volumes differ.

If the barrier in Figure 3.5A allows water but not glucose to cross, the outcome is quite different, however. Water will move down its concentration gradient from side 1 to side 2, but the loss of water will not be offset by a gain of glucose. As water leaves side 1 and accumulates on side 2, the volume of side 2 increases and the volume of side 1 decreases. The accumulating water exerts pressure on the elastic barrier, causing it to expand to the left to accommodate the volume changes (see Fig. 3.5C). Because of the volume changes, the osmolarity of side 1 increases and the osmolarity of side 2 decreases. This process will continue until the osmolarities of the two sides are equal at 150 mOsm. To prevent these volume changes, we would have to exert pressure against the elastic barrier to keep it from stretching. This pressure would be equal and opposite to the pressure moving water down its concentration gradient and would provide a measure of the osmotic pressure gradient across the barrier.

Osmotic Balance and Cell Volume

Consider now the osmotic effect of biological molecules trapped inside the cell by the plasma membrane. If the ECF and ICF have the same composition except for the internal organic molecules, the cell faces an imbalance of water on the two sides of the membrane. This is shown schematically in Figure 3.6. The solutes that are common to the ICF and ECF are grouped together and symbolized by S. The extra solute inside the cell—that is, the organic molecules (symbolized by P, for protein)—reduce the concentration of water inside the cell compared to the outside. Put another way, the total osmolarity is greater inside the cell than outside. There are two solutes inside, S and P, and only one outside. Consequently, water will continue to enter until the osmolarity on the two sides of the membrane is the same. If external volume is infinitely large relative to the volume of the cell (as would occur for a single-cell organism floating in the sea, for instance), internal osmolarity could equal external osmolarity only if the internal concentration of organic solutes is zero, which would require infinite cell volume. Real cell membranes are not infinitely elastic, however. Water will enter the cell, causing it to swell until the membrane ruptures and the cell bursts.

If a substance is at diffusion equilibrium across a cell membrane, there is no net movement of that substance across the membrane. For any solute, S, that can cross the cell membrane, diffusion equilibrium will be reached when

$$[S]_i = [S]_o \qquad (3.1)$$

Figure 3.6.

A simple model cell containing protein molecules (P). The extracellular fluid is a solution of solute (S) in water. Both water and the solute can cross the cell membrane, but the protein molecules cannot.

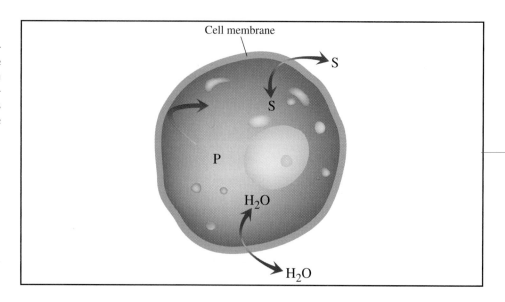

The square brackets indicate the concentration of a substance, and the subscripts i and o refer to the inside and outside of the cell, respectively. For water to be at equilibrium, total osmolarity inside the cell must equal total osmolarity outside the cell, which can be stated in equation form as

$$[S]_i + [P]_i = [S]_o \qquad (3.2)$$

For the cell shown in Figure 3.6, diffusion equilibrium will be reached only when the concentrations of all substances that can cross the membrane (in this case, S and water) are equal inside and outside the cell. This situation requires that equations 3.1 and 3.2 must be true simultaneously, which can occur only if $[P]_i$ is zero.

Answers to the Problem of Osmotic Balance

Four basic strategies are used in different cell types to solve the problem of osmotic balance.

- Make the cell membrane impermeable to water.
- Build a cell wall around the plasma membrane to physically prevent the cell from swelling.
- Actively extrude the accumulating intracellular water.
- Make the cell membrane impermeable to selected extracellular solutes to balance the impermeant internal solutes.

Although the membranes of some epithelial cells and protozoa have low water permeability, water moves relatively freely across most biological membranes, and so the first strategy is not commonly observed in practice. The strategy of building a cell wall is commonly encountered and is used by bacteria and plants. The third strategy is employed by protozoa such as paramecia, which live in very dilute pond water containing few extracellular solutes. We will focus on the fourth strategy, which is the mechanism found in animal cells.

To see how preventing an extracellular solute from crossing the membrane allows animal cells to achieve osmotic balance, let us consider some examples using a simplified model of an animal cell whose membrane is permeable to water. Suppose that the model cell contains only one solute: nonpermeating protein molecules, P, dissolved in water at a concentration of 0.25 M. We place the model cell in various ECFs and observe what happens to its volume in each case. Assume that the initial volume of the cell is one billionth of a liter (1 nanoliter, or 1 nl) and that the volume of the ECF is infinite. An infinite external volume means that the concentration of extracellular solutes does not change, even if water and solutes move across the cell membrane.

In the first example, shown in Figure 3.7A, the cell is placed in a 0.25 M solution of sucrose, which does not cross cell membranes. In this situation, only water can cross the cell membrane. For water to be at equilibrium, the internal osmolarity must equal the external osmolarity, or

$$[P]_i = [\text{sucrose}]_o \qquad (3.3)$$

Because the internal and external osmolarities are both 0.25 Osm, this condition is met. No net diffusion of water occurs, and cell volume does not change.

In the example shown in Figure 3.7B, the cell is placed in 0.125 M sucrose. Again, only water can cross the membrane, and equation 3.3 must be satisfied to achieve equilibrium. In 0.125 M sucrose, the internal osmolarity is greater than the external osmolarity, and water will enter the cell until the internal osmolarity falls to 0.125 M. This will happen when the cell volume doubles to 2 nl.

What strategy is used by animal cells to maintain constant cell volume?

What determines whether a particular ECF causes cell volume to change?

47

Figure 3.7.

The effect of the composition of the extracellular fluid (ECF) on the volume of a simple model cell containing impermeant protein molecules (P). **A.** The ECF contains an impermeant solute (sucrose), and the osmolarity is the same as that inside the cell. **B.** The ECF contains an impermeant solute, and the osmolarity is lower than that inside the cell. **C.** The ECF contains a permeant solute (urea), and external and internal osmolarities are equal. **D.** The ECF contains a mixture of permeant and impermeant solutes.

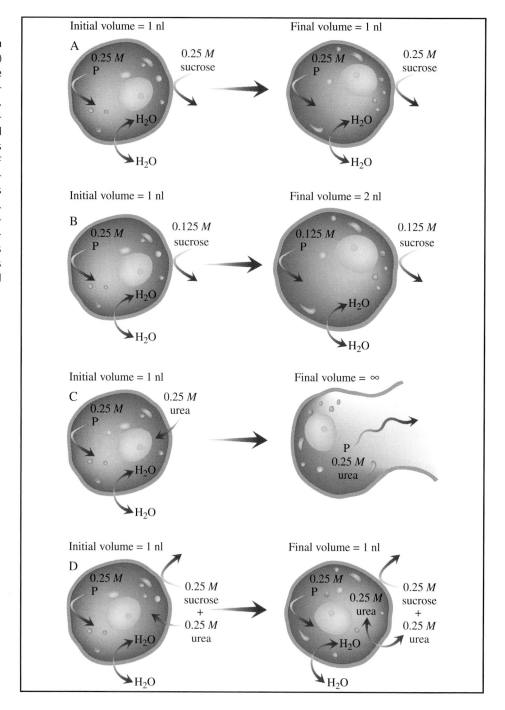

We see from these two examples that water is at equilibrium if the concentration of impermeant extracellular solute is the same as the concentration of impermeant internal solute. To see that the external solute must not be able to cross the cell membrane, consider the example shown in Figure 3.7C. The model cell is placed in 0.25 M urea, rather than sucrose. Unlike sucrose, urea can cross the cell membrane, and so we must take into account both urea and water in determining diffusion equilibrium. In equation form, equilibrium will be reached when the following relations hold:

$$[\text{urea}]_i = [\text{urea}]_o \qquad (3.4)$$

$$[\text{urea}]_i + [P]_i = [\text{urea}]_o \qquad (3.5)$$

Because the external volume is infinite, $[urea]_o$ will be 0.25 M at equilibrium. According to equation 3.4, $[urea]_i$ must also be 0.25 M. Thus, equations 3.4 and 3.5 can be satisfied simultaneously only if $[P]_i$ is zero at equilibrium. The equilibrium volume must be infinite, and the cell will swell until it bursts. Thus, an extracellular solute that can cross the cell membrane cannot help a cell achieve osmotic balance.

In the example shown in Figure 3.7D, the model cell is placed in mixture of 0.25 M urea and 0.25 M sucrose. The equilibrium for urea is once again governed by equation 3.4, and water will be at equilibrium when

$$[urea]_i + [P]_i = [urea]_o + [sucrose]_o \qquad (3.6)$$

Both equations 3.4 and 3.6 will be satisfied when $[P]_i = 0.25\ M$, which is the initial condition. Therefore, in this example, the cell volume at equilibrium will be equal to the initial volume, 1 nl. Even if some extracellular solutes are permeant, the cell can maintain its volume, provided sufficient impermeant solute is present in the ECF to balance impermeant solute in the ICF. Table 3.1 shows that sodium ions are the impermeant extracellular solute responsible for osmotic balance in animal cells.

In all the examples of osmotic equilibrium given here, we arrived at the answer by using just one rule: *For each permeating substance (including water), the inside concentration must equal the outside concentration at equilibrium.*

Tonicity

In the examples given in Figure 3.7, 0.25 M sucrose and 0.25 M urea had the same osmolarity (0.25 Osm) but produced dramatically different effects on cell volume. In 0.25 M sucrose, cell volume did not change; in 0.25 M urea, the cell exploded.

To account for the differing biological effects of solutions of the same osmolarity, we will introduce the concept of **tonicity**. An **isotonic** solution has no final effect on cell volume, a **hypotonic** solution causes cells to swell at equilibrium, and a **hypertonic** solution causes cells to shrink at equilibrium. Thus, the 0.25 M sucrose solution was isotonic, whereas the 0.25 M urea solution was hypotonic. Note that an isotonic solution must have the same osmolarity as the fluid inside the cell. However, having the same osmolarity as the ICF does not guarantee that an external fluid is isotonic.

MEMBRANE POTENTIAL: IONIC EQUILIBRIUM

Until now, we have considered only the diffusion of uncharged particles. However, Table 3.1 shows that the solutes of both ICF and ECF are electrically charged. We will now examine how cells can achieve equilibrium when both diffusional and electrical forces must be considered.

To illustrate the important principles that apply to ionic equilibrium, we will work through a series of model cells of increasing complexity and increasing similarity to real animal cells. At the culmination, we will arrive at a model cell that is at equilibrium and has ICF and ECF with the compositions shown in Table 3.1.

Diffusion Potential

The first example we will consider is the diffusion potential, which arises when two or more ions are diffusing down a concentration gradient from one location to another. Consider the situation illustrated in Figure 3.8, in which a rigid container is divided into two compartments by a porous barrier. The left compartment contains a 0.1 M NaCl solution, and the right compartment contains a 1.0 M NaCl solution.

Figure 3.8.

A schematic diagram of an apparatus for measuring the diffusion potential. A voltmeter measures the electrical voltage difference across the barrier separating the two salt solutions.

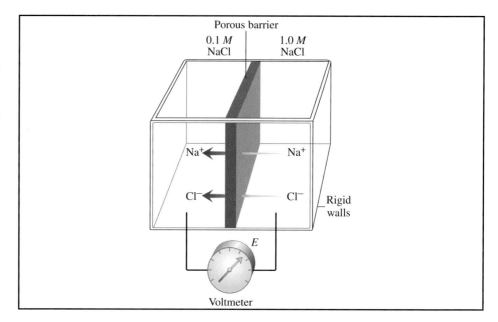

The porous barrier allows Na^+, Cl^-, and water to pass through, but the rigid walls prevent the compartment volume from changing. Thus, water cannot move, and osmotic factors can be neglected. Both Na^+ and Cl^- will move down their concentration gradients from right to left until their concentrations are equal in both compartments. In aqueous solution, Na^+ and Cl^- do not move at the same rate; Cl^- is more mobile and accumulates on the left side more quickly than does Na^+.

Because Cl^- moves faster, an excess of negative charges builds up in the left compartment, and a voltmeter connected across the barrier would record a voltage difference, E. This voltage difference is the diffusion potential. Because the negativity on the left repels Cl^- and attracts Na^+, the electrical potential across the barrier retards Cl^- movement and speeds Na^+ movement. The diffusion potential continues to build up until the voltage exactly counteracts the greater mobility of Cl^-, and the two ions cross the barrier at the same rate.

Equilibrium Potential: The Nernst Equation

What conditions apply to the equilibrium of a charged substance across the plasma membrane?

The diffusion potential is not an equilibrium state but rather a transient voltage that occurs only when net diffusion of ions across the barrier takes place. Equilibrium would be achieved in Figure 3.8 only when the concentrations of Na^+ and Cl^- are the same in both compartments, at which point no net diffusion occurs and no voltage is present across the barrier. However, a small modification of our model, shown in Figure 3.9, will produce a steady voltage across the barrier at equilibrium. In this model, the barrier between the two compartments is selectively permeable to Cl^-, and Na^+ cannot cross. Once again, the box has rigid walls so that water movement can be neglected.

The new situation is similar to that of the diffusion potential, except that the "mobility" of Na^+ is effectively reduced to zero by the permeability characteristics of the barrier. Chloride ions move down their concentration gradient from compartment 1 to compartment 2, but no positive charges accompany them and excess negativity quickly builds up in compartment 2. The electrical gradient across the barrier drives Cl^- out of compartment 2. Negativity stops building up in compartment 2 when the voltage gradient driving Cl^- out of compartment 2 exactly balances the concentration gradient driving Cl^- into compartment 2. At that point, no net movement of Cl^- occurs and chloride is at equilibrium. When the concen-

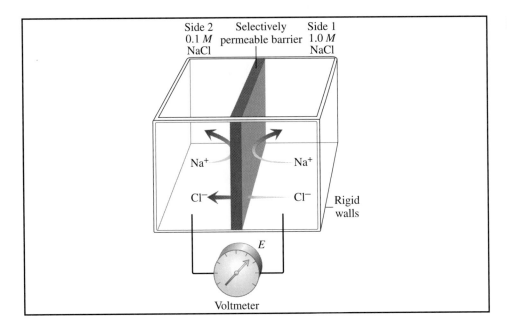

Figure 3.9.

A schematic diagram of an apparatus for measuring the equilibrium, or Nernst, potential for a permeant ion. At equilibrium, a steady electrical potential (the equilibrium potential) is measured across the selectively permeable barrier separating the two salt solutions.

tration and electrical gradients are in exact balance, a chloride ion moves from side 1 to side 2 down its concentration gradient for every chloride ion that moves from side 2 to side 1 down its electrical gradient.

The measured value of the voltage across the barrier at equilibrium in Figure 3.9 is provided by the **Nernst equation**:

What equation is used to calculate the equilibrated value of membrane potential for a permeant ion?

$$E_{Cl} = \frac{RT}{ZF} \ln\left(\frac{[Cl^-]_1}{[Cl^-]_2}\right) \quad\quad (3.7)$$

In the Nernst equation, E_{Cl} is the voltage difference between sides 1 and 2 at equilibrium, R is the gas constant, T is the absolute temperature, Z is the valence of the ion in question (-1 for chloride), F is Faraday's constant, ln is the symbol for the natural, or base e, logarithm, and $[Cl^-]_1$ and $[Cl^-]_2$ are the chloride concentrations in compartments 1 and 2.

The value of electrical potential calculated from equation 3.7 is called the **equilibrium potential**, or **Nernst potential**, for the ion in question. The equilibrium potential specifies the amount of voltage required to exactly balance a given concentration gradient. In Figure 3.9, the permeant ion is chloride, and the electrical potential, E_{Cl}, across the barrier is called the chloride equilibrium potential. If the barrier allowed Na^+ to cross rather than Cl^-, the Nernst equation would again be used to calculate the sodium equilibrium potential, E_{Na}, but $[Na^+]_1$ and $[Na^+]_2$ would be used instead of $[Cl^-]$, and the valence, Z, would be $+1$ instead of -1. The Nernst equation applies only to one ion at a time and only to ions that can cross the barrier. A derivation of equation 3.7 is given in Advanced Topic 1: The Nernst and Goldman Equations.

A simplified form of the Nernst equation is commonly used in biology:

$$E_{Cl} = \frac{58 \text{ mV}}{Z} \log\left(\frac{[Cl^-]_1}{[Cl^-]_2}\right) \quad\quad (3.8)$$

The constant, 58 mV, arises from evaluating (RT/F) at standard room temperature (20°C), converting from natural to base 10 logarithms, and expressing the result in millivolts (mV). Using equation 3.8, we calculate that E_{Cl} in Figure 3.9

would be -58 mV. That is, in crossing the barrier from side 1 to side 2, a voltage change of 58 mV would be encountered, with side 2 being negative.

The Principle of Electrical Neutrality

In calculating $E_{Cl} = -58$ mV in Figure 3.9, we used the initial concentrations of 1.0 M and 0.1 M for $[Cl^-]_1$ and $[Cl^-]_2$, even though some chloride ions moved from compartment 1 to 2 to produce the electrical potential. It is legitimate to use the starting concentrations because only a very small number of charges are needed to generate the voltage required to counteract even a large concentration gradient.

This fact leads to an important concept, called the **principle of electrical neutrality**. It states that *under biological conditions, the bulk concentration of cations within any compartment must equal the bulk concentration of anions in that compartment.* This principle is an acceptable approximation because the number of charges necessary to reach transmembrane potentials of the magnitude encountered in biology is insignificant compared with the total number of cations and anions in the ICF and ECF.

Incorporating Osmotic Balance

Animal cells are not enclosed in a box with rigid walls, and thus we must consider osmotic balance to make our models more realistic. An example of how equilibrium can be reached when the rigid walls are removed is shown in Figure 3.10A. In this model, the cell contains 50 mM Na^+ and 100 mM P, an uncharged impermeant protein. What concentrations of the other intracellular and extracellular solutes are required for the model cell to be at equilibrium? The principle of electrical neutrality tells us that for practical purposes, the concentrations of cations and anions within any compartment are equal. Thus, because P is assumed to have no charge, $[Cl^-]_i = [Na^+]_i = 50$ mM. For osmotic balance, the external osmolarity must equal the internal osmolarity (200 mOsm), and the principle of electrical neutrality requires that $[Na^+]_o = [Cl^-]_o$. These requirements can be satisfied if $[Na^+]_o = [Cl^-]_o = 100$ mM. Thus, the model cell can be at equilibrium if the concentrations of intracellular and extracellular solutes are as shown in Figure 3.10B. The electrical potential across the membrane of the model cell (the membrane potential, E_m) would be given by the Nernst equation for chloride:

$$E_m = E_{Cl} = -58 \text{ mV} \log\left(\frac{[Cl^-]_o}{[Cl^-]_i}\right) = -17.5 \text{ mV}$$

Donnan Equilibrium

How can two permeant ions simultaneously achieve equilibrium across the cell membrane?

The model shown in Figure 3.10B is not very realistic as yet. In real cells, the principal internal cation is K^+, not Na^+. Also, the ECF contains some potassium, and the cell membrane is permeable to both K^+ and Cl^-. With two permeant ions, the electrical potential across the cell membrane must exactly balance the concentration gradients for both K^+ and Cl^- if equilibrium is to be reached. This equilibrium condition will be satisfied only when the equilibrium potentials for Cl^- and K^+ are equal. In equation form, this condition can be written as follows:

$$E_K = 58 \text{ mV} \log\left(\frac{[K^+]_o}{[K^+]_i}\right) = E_{Cl} = -58 \text{ mV} \log\left(\frac{[Cl^-]_o}{[Cl^-]_i}\right)$$

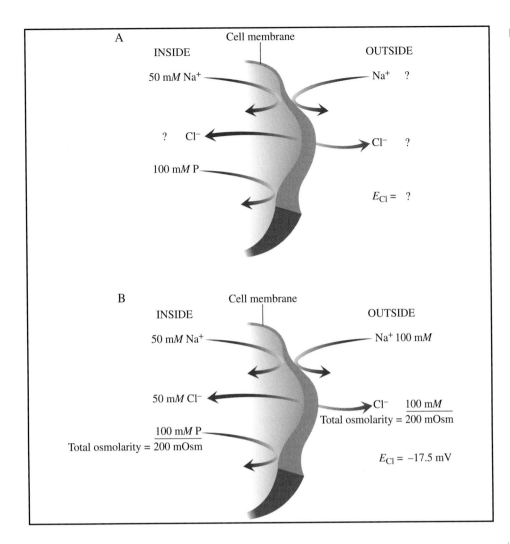

Figure 3.10.

A model cell in which both osmotic and electrical factors must be considered at equilibrium. **A.** The starting conditions, with initial values of some parameters provided. **B.** The values of all parameters required for the cell to be at equilibrium.

The minus sign on the far right arises from the fact that the valence of chloride is −1. Canceling 58 mV from this equation leaves the following:

$$\log \left([K^+]_o/[K^+]_i\right) = -\log \left([Cl^-]_o/[Cl^-]_i\right) \tag{3.9}$$

The minus sign on the right side can be moved inside the parentheses of the logarithm to yield $\log \left([Cl^-]_i/[Cl^-]_o\right)$. Thus, equilibrium will be reached when

$$\left([K^+]_o/[K^+]_i\right) = \left([Cl^-]_i/[Cl^-]_o\right) \tag{3.10}$$

This equilibrium condition, which is called the **Donnan** (or **Gibbs-Donnan**) **equilibrium**, specifies the conditions that must be met if two permeant ions are simultaneously to be at equilibrium. Equation 3.10 is usually written in a slightly rearranged form as the product of concentrations:

$$[K^+]_o[Cl^-]_o = [K^+]_i[Cl^-]_i \tag{3.11}$$

For a Donnan equilibrium to hold, *the product of the concentrations of the permeant ions outside the cell must be equal to the product of the concentrations of those two ions inside the cell.*

Figure 3.11A shows an example of Donnan equilibrium for a model cell containing K^+, Cl^-, and P, placed in ECF containing Na^+, K^+, and Cl^-. What concentrations of these substances would be required for the model to be at equilibrium, assuming that $[Na^+]_o$ is 120 mM and $[K^+]_o$ is 5 mM? From the principle of electrical neutrality, $[Cl^-]_o$ must be 125 mM. Because P is uncharged, the principle of electrical neutrality requires that $[K^+]_i = [Cl^-]_i$. Because two ions—K^+ and Cl^-—can cross the membrane, the defining relation for a Donnan equilibrium shown in equation

Figure 3.11.

An example of a model cell at Donnan equilibrium. The cell membrane is permeable to both potassium and chloride. **A.** The starting conditions, with initial values of some parameters provided. **B.** The values of all parameters required for the cell to be at equilibrium.

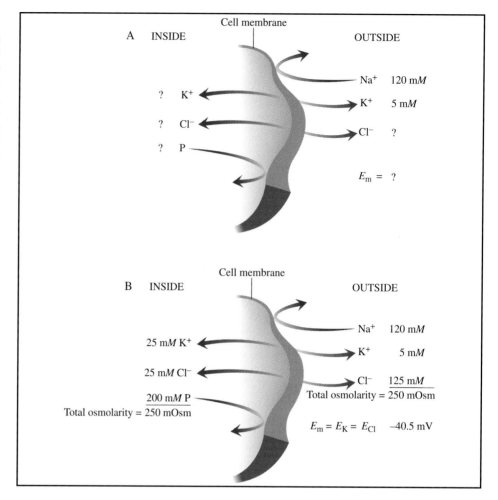

3.11 must be obeyed. Thus, at equilibrium, $[K^+]_i[Cl^-]_i$ must equal $[K^+]_o[Cl^-]_o$, which is 5×125, or 625 mM^2. Because $[K^+]_i = [Cl^-]_i$, the Donnan condition reduces to $[K^+]_i^2 = 625$ mM^2, and $[K^+]_i$ and $[Cl^-]_i$ must be 25 mM. For osmotic balance, the internal osmolarity must equal the external osmolarity, which is 250 mOsm. Thus, $[P]_i$ must be 200 mM for the model cell to be at equilibrium. The membrane potential of the model can be calculated from the Nernst equation for either potassium or chloride. For $[K^+]_o = 5$ mM and $[K^+]_i = 25$ mM, $E_K = -40.5$ mV. Figure 3.11B summarizes the equilibrated values of the parameters for this model cell.

A Model Cell That Looks Like a Real Animal Cell

The model in Figure 3.11B still lacks many features of real animal cells. For instance, the internal organic molecules are electrically charged, which must be considered in the balance between cations and anions required by the principle of electrical neutrality. In addition, the ICF contains some Na$^+$. Adding these complications leads to a model that includes all the constituents shown in Table 3.1. What concentrations of these constituents in the ECF and ICF would be required to construct an equilibrated model? Figure 3.12A shows the assumed starting conditions for our model: $[K^+]_o = 5$ mM, $[Na^+]_o = 120$ mM, $[Cl^-]_i = 5$ mM, and $[A^{1.2-}]_i = 108$ mM. (We could actually calculate the concentration of A from the other parameters, but for mathematical simplicity, we will assume that it is known initially.) Because Cl$^-$ is the sole external anion, the principle of electrical neutrality requires that $[Cl^-]_o$ be 125 mM. Because both K$^+$ and Cl$^-$ can cross the membrane, the condition

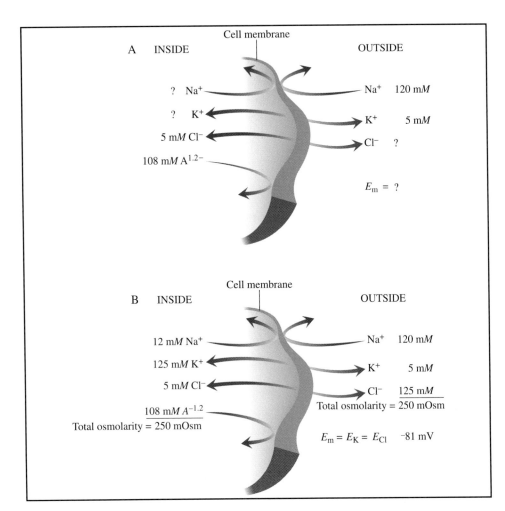

Figure 3.12.

A model cell that is at both electrical and osmotic equilibrium. The compositions of the extracellular and intracellular fluid for the equilibrated model cell are the same as for a typical mammalian cell (see Table 3.1). **A**. The starting conditions, with initial values of some parameters provided. **B**. The values of all parameters required for the cell to be at equilibrium.

for Donnan equilibrium (equation 3.11) must be satisfied, which requires that $[K^+]_i$ = 125 mM. The equilibrated value of $[Na^+]_i$ can then be obtained from the requirement for osmotic balance: $[Na^+]_i$ must be 12 mM if internal and external osmolarities are to be equal. From the Nernst equation for either Cl^- or K^+, the membrane potential at equilibrium can be determined to be approximately −81 mV.

The equilibrium values for this model cell are shown in Figure 3.12B. Note that the concentrations of all intracellular and extracellular solutes in the model cell are the same as real mammalian cells (see Table 3.1). This similarity implies that the real cell is also at equilibrium and is able to maintain the ionic gradients and membrane potential without expending metabolic energy. From this viewpoint, the animal cell seems to be a beautiful example of efficiency, in harmony with its electrochemical environment. In reality, however, the model cell is not an accurate representation of the situation in real animal cells. Real cells are not at equilibrium and must expend metabolic energy to maintain the status quo.

The Sodium Pump

Unlike the model in Figure 3.12B, real cell membranes are permeable to sodium, which would be catastrophic for the model cell. If sodium can cross the membrane, then all extracellular solutes can cross the membrane. A cell placed in ECF containing only permeant solutes swells and bursts. To achieve osmotic balance, the cell membrane must exclude an extracellular solute to balance impermeant organic solutes inside the cell. Sodium ions played that role for the model cell.

What is the role of the sodium-potassium pump in osmotic balance and maintenance of ion gradients, and how does the pump operate?

How can the permeability of the plasma membrane to sodium be reconciled with the requirement for osmotic balance? The experiments that first demonstrated that sodium crosses the membrane suggested an answer to this question. In these experiments, red blood cells were incubated in ECF containing radioactive sodium ions. When the cells were removed from the radioactive medium and washed thoroughly, they remained radioactive, indicating that the cells had taken up some of the radioactive sodium. This showed that the plasma membrane is permeable to sodium. The important clue, however, was that cells lost their radioactive sodium when incubated in normal ECF, and the rate of loss of radioactive sodium slowed dramatically when the cells were cooled. This observation indicated that a source of energy was being tapped to actively "pump" sodium out of the cell against its concentration and electrical gradients. The energy to drive active pumping of sodium out of the cell is derived from the high-energy phosphate compound adenosine triphosphate (ATP).

Active extrusion of sodium prevents sodium from accumulating intracellularly as it leaks in down its concentration and electrical gradients. The result is that sodium behaves osmotically as though it cannot cross the membrane. Metabolic inhibitors, such as cyanide or dinitrophenol, prevent the pumping of sodium out of the cell and cause cells to gain sodium and swell. Similarly, other manipulations that reduce the rate of ATP production, such as cooling, lead to sodium accumulation and increased cell volume.

The molecular mechanism of the sodium pump has been identified. The sodium pump is a membrane protein that binds sodium ions and ATP at the intracellular face of the membrane. The protein is an ATPase that cleaves ATP and uses the released energy to translocate the bound sodium to the extracellular face of the membrane, where it is released into the ECF. Potassium ions in the ECF then bind to the pump, a step required to return the protein to the configuration in which it can again bind ATP and sodium at the inner surface of the membrane. Potassium bound on the outside is released again on the inside. In this manner, the protein molecule acts as a shuttle that carries Na^+ out across the membrane and releases it in the ECF, then carries K^+ in across the membrane and releases it in the ICF. Because the pump molecule splits ATP and binds both sodium and potassium ions, biochemists refer to this membrane-associated enzyme as a Na^+-K^+ ATPase.

MEMBRANE POTENTIAL: IONIC STEADY STATE

Equilibrium Potentials for Sodium, Potassium, and Chloride

If the permeability of the cell membrane to Na^+ is not zero, then sodium must contribute to the membrane potential of the cell, even though the sodium pump removes any sodium that leaks into the cell. The electrical contribution of Na^+ must be considered because the electrical force per particle is much stronger than the concentrational force per particle. Even a tiny trickle of sodium that causes a negligible change in internal concentration produces a large change in membrane potential. Because the sodium pump responds only to changes in the bulk concentration of sodium inside the cell, it cannot prevent the tiny changes in internal sodium that accompany even large changes in membrane potential.

The sodium equilibrium potential is very different from the potassium and chloride equilibrium potentials. Given the ion concentrations from Table 3.1, E_K and $E_{Cl} = -80$ mV, but $E_{Na} = +58$ mV. The membrane potential, E_m, cannot simultaneously equal -80 mV and $+58$ mV, and its actual value will fall somewhere between these two extremes. There will be a struggle between Na^+ on the one hand, tending to make $E_m = +58$ mV, and K^+ and Cl^- on the other, tending to make $E_m = -80$ mV.

Two factors determine the actual value of E_m: (1) ion concentrations, which determine the equilibrium potentials for the ions; and (2) relative ion permeabilities, which determine the relative importance of a particular ion in governing E_m. Before expressing these relations quantitatively, it will be useful to consider the mechanism of ionic permeability in more detail.

Ion Channels in the Plasma Membrane

The permeability of a membrane to a particular ion is a measure of the ease with which that ion can cross the membrane. Ions must cross the membrane through aqueous pores or channels. The permeability of a membrane to a particular ion is governed by the total number of channels that allow that ion to cross and by the ease with which the ion can pass through a single channel. Not all membrane channels allow all ions to cross with equal ease. Some channels allow only cations to enter, while others pass only anions. Other channels are even more selective, allowing only K^+ through but not Na^+, or vice versa. Thus, the permeability of cell membranes to different ions can vary substantially, depending on the properties of the ion channels available in the membrane.

What governs the permeability of a membrane to an ion?

Membrane Potential and Ionic Permeability

To see how the membrane potential depends on the relative permeabilities of the competing ions, consider a cell whose membrane is more permeable to K^+ than Na^+, shown in Figure 3.13A. Initially, we hold the membrane potential at E_K, -80 mV. What happens when we stop holding E_m at E_K and allow it to seek its own level? To answer this question, we must examine the factors that govern net movement of an ion across the membrane in response to changes in E_m, illustrated in Figure 3.13B for K^+. If $E_m = E_K$, the electrical force driving K^+ into the cell balances the concentrational force driving K^+ out of the cell, and the net movement of K^+ is zero. This balance is destroyed, however, if E_m is not equal to E_K.

When E_m is more positive than E_K (time a in Fig. 3.13B), the electrical force moving K^+ into the cell is weaker than the concentration gradient moving K^+ out of the cell, resulting in net movement of K^+ out of the cell. At time b, we suddenly make E_m more negative than E_K. Now the electrical force is stronger than the concentrational force, producing a net movement of K^+ into the cell. Note that in each case, the ion moves across the membrane in such a way as to force the membrane potential toward the equilibrium potential for the ion. The amount of permeability of the membrane to potassium determines how much potassium movement occurs per millivolt of disparity between the actual value of membrane potential and the equilibrium potential.

In Figure 3.13A, the membrane is permeable to sodium as well as potassium. With an equilibrium potential of $+58$ mV, sodium will enter the cell, bringing positive charge into the cell. When we stop holding E_m at E_K, Na^+ influx moves E_m in the positive direction, toward E_{Na}. As E_m moves toward E_{Na}, however, it becomes more positive than E_K, and K^+ moves out of the cell in response. Thus, a struggle ensues between K^+ efflux, which drives E_m toward E_K, and Na^+ influx, which forces E_m toward E_{Na}. Because K^+ permeability is much higher than Na^+ permeability, potassium efflux is large for a small difference between E_m and E_K, whereas sodium re-

Figure 3.13.

Movement of ions is determined by the difference between the membrane potential and the equilibrium potential. **A.** The resting membrane potential of a cell that is more permeable to potassium than to sodium. At the *upward arrow*, an apparatus that artificially holds the membrane potential (E_m) at the equilibrium potential for potassium (E_K) is abruptly switched off, and the membrane potential is allowed to seek its own resting level. **B.** The effect of changes in membrane potential on the movement of potassium ions across the plasma membrane. When the membrane potential is manipulated (*upper trace*), potassium ions move across the membrane (*lower trace*) in a direction governed by the difference between E_m and E_K.

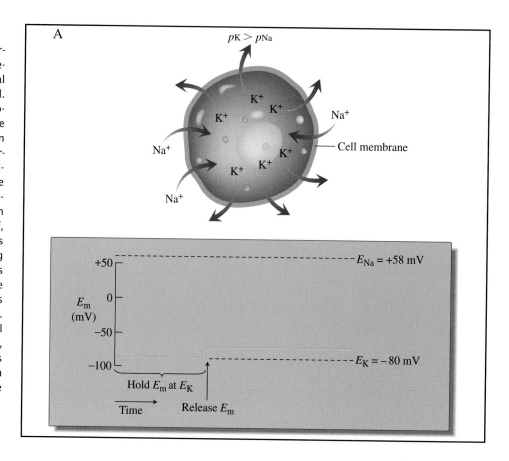

quires a larger difference between E_m and E_{Na} to attain the same level of influx. In this situation, the balance between the movement of Na^+ into the cell and the exit of K^+ from the cell is struck relatively close to E_K.

Figure 3.14 shows a different situation. In this case, sodium permeability is much greater than the potassium permeability. We begin with $E_m = E_K = -80$ mV and then allow E_m to seek its own value. Sodium, with $E_{Na} = +58$ mV, enters the cell down its electrical and concentration gradients and depolarizes the cell. The low potassium permeability in this instance prevents potassium from moving out as readily as sodium can move in, and sodium influx will not be balanced as readily by potassium efflux. Thus, E_m will reach a steady value closer to E_{Na} than to E_K.

The point of the last two examples is that E_m is governed by the relative permeabilities of the permeant ions. *If a cell membrane is highly permeable to an ion, that ion can respond readily to deviations away from its equilibrium potential, and E_m will tend to be near that equilibrium potential.*

The Goldman Equation

The equation that gives the quantitative relation between E_m on the one hand and ion concentrations and permeabilities on the other is the **Goldman equation**, which is also called the **constant-field equation**. For a cell that is permeable to K^+, Na^+, and Cl^-, the Goldman equation is the following

What equation is used to calculate the resting membrane potential of a cell whose plasma membrane is permeable to more than one type of ion?

$$E_m = \frac{RT}{F} \ln\left(\frac{p_K[K^+]_o + p_{Na}[Na^+]_o + p_{Cl}[Cl^-]_i}{p_K[K^+]_i + p_{Na}[Na^+]_i + p_{Cl}[Cl^-]_o}\right) \quad (3.12)$$

This equation is similar to the Nernst equation, except that it simultaneously takes into account the contributions of all permeant ions. A derivation of the

B

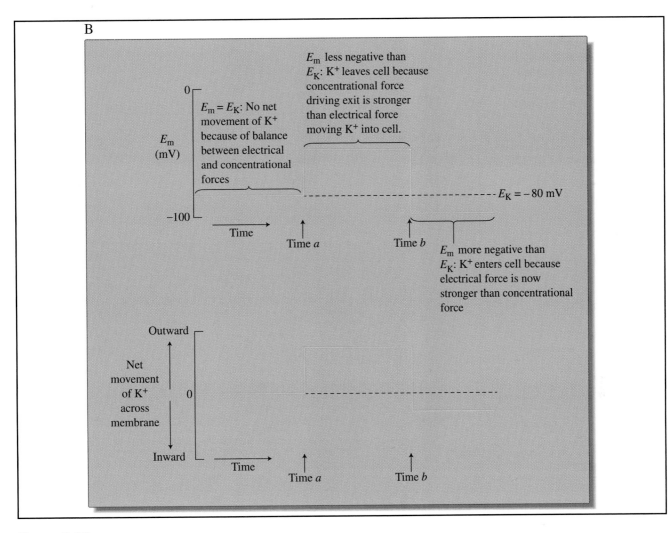

$E_m = E_K$: No net movement of K^+ because of balance between electrical and concentrational forces

E_m less negative than E_K: K^+ leaves cell because concentrational force driving exit is stronger than electrical force moving K^+ into cell.

$E_K = -80$ mV

E_m more negative than E_K: K^+ enters cell because electrical force is now stronger than concentrational force

Figure 3.13.

(continued)

Goldman equation is provided in Advanced Topic 1: The Nernst and Goldman Equations.

In the Goldman equation, the concentration of each ion is scaled according to its permeability, p. Thus, if the cell is highly permeable to potassium, the potassium term dominates, and E_m will be close to E_K. If p_{Na} and p_{Cl} are zero, the Goldman equation reduces to the Nernst equation for potassium, and E_m would be exactly equal to E_K, as expected if potassium is the only permeant ion.

Because it is easier to measure relative ion permeability than absolute permeability, the Goldman equation is often written in a slightly different form:

$$E_m = 58 \text{ mV} \log\left(\frac{[K^+]_o + b[Na^+]_o + c[Cl^-]_i}{[K^+]_i + b[Na^+]_i + c[Cl^-]_o}\right) \quad (3.13)$$

In this case, permeabilities are expressed relative to potassium permeability. Thus, $b = p_{Na}/p_K$, and $c = p_{Cl}/p_K$. We have also evaluated RT/F at room temperature, converted from base e to base 10 logarithm, and expressed the result in millivolts.

For most nerve cells, the Goldman equation can be simplified even further by dropping the chloride term. This approximation is valid because the contribution

Figure 3.14.

The resting membrane potential of a cell that is more permeable to sodium than to potassium. An apparatus holding the membrane potential (E_m) at the equilibrium potential for potassium (E_K) is abruptly turned off at the *upward arrow*.

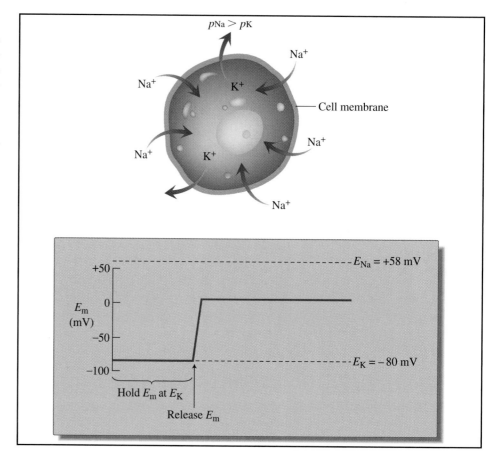

of chloride to the resting membrane potential is insignificant in most nerve cells. In this case, the Goldman equation becomes

$$E_m = 58 \text{ mV} \log\left(\frac{[K^+]_o + b[Na^+]_o}{[K^+]_i + b[Na^+]_i}\right) \qquad (3.14)$$

In nerve cells, the ratio of sodium to potassium permeability, b, is commonly approximately 0.02, although it may vary somewhat from one cell to another. That is, p_K is roughly 50 times higher than p_{Na}. According to equation 3.14, $E_m \approx -71$ mV for a cell with $[K^+]_i = 125$ mM, $[K^+]_o = 5$ mM, $[Na^+]_i = 12$ mM, $[Na^+]_o = 120$ mM, and $b = 0.02$.

Ionic Steady State

The membrane potential of the cell takes on a steady-state value that reflects a fine balance between competing influences. Neither sodium nor potassium is in equilibrium at the steady-state membrane potential. Sodium ions are continually leaking into the cell, and potassium ions are continually leaking out. If this leakage continued, the concentration gradients for sodium and potassium would eventually run down and the membrane potential would decline to zero as the ionic gradients collapsed.

To prevent the intracellular accumulation of sodium and loss of potassium, the cell must expend energy to restore the ionic gradients. This is another important role for the sodium pump. Metabolic energy stored in ATP is used to pump out the sodium that leaks in and to regain the potassium that was lost. In this way, the cell's "batteries" are recharged using metabolic energy. Viewed in this light, the steady-state membrane potential represents chemical energy that has been converted into a different form and stored in the ionic gradients across the cell membrane.

The Chloride Pump

Given the internal and external concentrations shown in Table 3.1, the chloride equilibrium potential is approximately −80 mV, but the resting membrane potential is about −71 mV. Under these conditions, chloride flows steadily into the cell. Eventually, this influx would raise the internal chloride concentration to the point where the chloride equilibrium potential reached −71 mV, equal to the resting membrane potential. At that point, the concentration gradient for chloride would be reduced sufficiently to come into balance with the resting membrane potential. From the Nernst equation, internal chloride concentration would have to rise to 7.5 mM to establish this new equilibrium state.

In some cells, internal chloride does indeed rise to a new equilibrium governed by the resting membrane potential. (The cell also gains the same amount of potassium; because the cell contains so much potassium, a change of a few millimolar in potassium concentration alters the potassium equilibrium potential very little, however.) In other cells, internal chloride remains out of equilibrium with the resting membrane potential, just as the sodium and potassium equilibrium potentials remain different from E_m. The only way this nonequilibrium condition can be

BOX 1

IN THE CLINIC

The resting membrane potential of cells depends on both the ionic permeability of the plasma membrane and the ionic gradients across the membrane. In certain pathological conditions, reduction in those ionic gradients—and the resulting reduction in membrane potential—can have life-threatening consequences. This is especially true for victims of heart attacks. When the delivery of oxygen to the body's organs is interrupted by a reduction in blood flow (ischemia), metabolic activity and the production of ATP decrease. ATP is required to fuel the sodium-potassium pump of the plasma membrane and thus to maintain the sodium and potassium gradients between the ECF and ICF. Thus, one consequence of ischemia can be the loss of intracellular potassium and a corresponding increase in extracellular potassium (hyperkalemia). From the Nernst equation, a doubling of external potassium from 5 mM to 10 mM would cause a shift in the potassium equilibrium potential from about −80 mV to about −63 mV, for example. Because the resting, steady-state membrane potential of cells is near the potassium equilibrium potential, there will be an approximately comparable reduction in the membrane potential of the cells in the body. The reduction in membrane potential is particularly important for the cardiac-muscle cells, which depend on electrical mechanisms for proper coordination of contractions to pump the blood through the circulatory system. During a heart attack, then, a vicious cycle can arise in which reduced blood flow leads to hyperkalemia, which in turn interferes further with cardiac function. This cycle can culminate in complete cessation of electrical activity of the heart. The importance of extracellular potassium concentration for the heart is exploited with lethal intent by the criminal justice systems of some states in the United States, which use potassium injections to execute condemned prisoners.

maintained is by expending energy to keep the internal chloride constant—that is, there must be a chloride pump similar to the sodium-potassium pump. In most cells, the chloride pump moves chloride ions out of the cell, keeping the chloride equilibrium potential more negative than the resting membrane potential. In a few cases, however, an inwardly directed chloride pump has been discovered. The chloride pump is an ATPase in some instances, using hydrolysis of ATP to drive chloride movement. In other cases, the pump uses energy stored in gradients of other ions to drive the movement of chloride.

Electrical Current and the Movement of Ions Across Membranes

An electrical current is the movement of charge through space. The movement of ions through space—such as from the outside of a cell to the inside of a cell—constitutes an electrical current, just as the movement of electrons through a wire constitutes an electrical current. At the steady-state membrane potential, a steady influx of sodium ions balances a steady efflux of potassium ions. Thus, a steady electrical current carried by sodium ions flows across the membrane in one direction, and a second current, carried by potassium ions, flows across the membrane in the opposite direction. By convention, the transfer of positive charge from the outside to the inside of the membrane is called an *inward* membrane current, whereas the transfer of positive charge from the inside to the outside is an *outward* current. The influx of sodium therefore represents an inward current, and the potassium efflux is an outward membrane current.

In the steady state, the sodium current, i_{Na}, is equal and opposite to the potassium current i_K. In equation form, this can be written as follows:

$$i_K + i_{Na} = 0 \qquad (3.15)$$

If the sum of i_{Na} and i_K were not zero, there would be a net flow of current across the membrane, producing a net transfer of charge into or out of the cell and altering the membrane potential. Equation 3.15, then, is a requirement for the steady-state condition. In cells with an appreciable flow of chloride ions across the membrane, the steady-state equation must be expanded to include chloride current, i_{Cl}:

$$i_K + i_{Na} + i_{Cl} = 0 \qquad (3.16)$$

Factors Affecting Ionic Current Across a Cell Membrane

The difference between the equilibrium potential for an ion and the actual membrane potential is one important factor governing the amount of current that is carried across the membrane by the ion. If $E_m = E_K$, there is no net movement of potassium across the membrane and $i_K = 0$. If $E_m \neq E_K$, the imbalance between electrical and concentrational forces drives a net movement of potassium across the membrane. The larger the difference between E_m and E_K, the larger the net potassium flux. Thus, i_K depends on $E_m - E_K$. This difference is called the **driving force** for membrane current carried by an ion.

The permeability of the membrane to an ion is also an important determinant of the amount of membrane current carried by that ion. If the permeability is high, the ionic current for a particular amount of driving force is higher than if the permeability were low. Because resting p_K is much greater than p_{Na}, the potassium current resulting from a 10-mV difference between E_m and E_K will be much larger than the sodium current resulting from a 10-mV difference between E_m and E_{Na}. This difference in the amount of current per millivolt of driving force explains why the steady-state membrane potential lies closer to E_K than to E_{Na}: to satisfy equation 3.15, the driving force for sodium entry $(E_m - E_{Na})$ must be much greater than the driving force for potassium exit $(E_m - E_K)$.

Membrane Conductance

What scaling factor relates electrical driving force to ionic current?

To place the discussion of membrane current on more quantitative ground, it will be necessary to introduce the concept of **membrane conductance**. The conductance of a membrane to an ion is an index of the ability of that ion to carry current across the membrane. The higher the conductance, the greater the ionic current for a given driving force. Conductance is analogous to the reciprocal of the resistance of an electrical circuit to current flow. The higher the resistance of a circuit, the lower the amount of current that flows in response to a particular voltage. This behavior of electrical circuits is summarized by Ohm's law: $i = V/R$. In this relation, i is the current flowing through a resistor, R, in the presence of a voltage gradient, V. The equivalent form for the flow of potassium current across a membrane is

$$i_K = g_K(E_m - E_K) \tag{3.17}$$

where g_K is the conductance of the membrane to potassium ions. The unit of electrical conductance is the siemen, abbreviated S; a voltage of 1 V will drive 1 ampere of current (1 A) through a conductance of 1 S.

Similar equations can be written for sodium and chloride:

$$i_{Na} = g_{Na}(E_m - E_{Na}) \tag{3.18}$$

$$i_{Cl} = g_{Cl}(E_m - E_{Cl}) \tag{3.19}$$

For the usual values of E_m (−71 mV), E_K (−80 mV), and E_{Na} (+58 mV), the potassium current is a positive number and the sodium current is a negative number, as required by the fact that the two currents flow in opposite directions across the membrane. By convention in neurophysiology, an outward membrane current (such as i_K, at the steady-state E_m) is positive and an inward current (such as i_{Na}, at the steady-state E_m) is negative.

Behavior of Single Ion Channels

Equations 3.17 through 3.19 show that the ionic current across a membrane is equal to the product of the electrical driving force and the membrane conductance for each ion. Similar considerations apply to the ionic current flowing through a single open ion channel. For a potassium channel, for example, the single-channel current, i_S, is given by

$$i_S = g_S(E_m - E_K) \tag{3.20}$$

where g_S is the **single-channel conductance** for the potassium channel. Analogous equations can be written for single sodium and chloride channels.

We have treated ion channels as simple open pores or holes that allow ions to cross the membrane. Ion channels exhibit more complex behavior, however. The protein molecule that forms the channel can take on two conformations: one in which the pore is open and ions are free to move through it, and one in which the pore is closed and ion movement is blocked. (Actually, channels frequently show more than two functional states, but for our purposes, we can treat channels as being either open or closed.) Channels behave as though access to the pore is controlled by a "gate" that can be open or closed; for this reason, we refer to the opening and closing of the channel as **channel gating**.

How large is the current flowing through a single open channel? Although there is considerable variation in single-channel conductance among different kinds of ion channels, a single-channel conductance of approximately 20 pS might be considered typical (pS is the abbreviation for picosiemens, or 10^{-12} S). If the conductance is 20 pS and the driving force is 50 mV, then equation 3.20 indicates that the single-channel current would be 10^{-12} A (or 1 pA, which corresponds to approximately 6 million monovalent ions per second). Although this is a small current indeed, a measurement technique called the patch clamp allows direct measurement of the electrical current flowing through a single open ion channel.

What is the relationship between the total conductance of the cell membrane to an ion (equations 3.17, 3.18, and 3.19) and the single-channel conductance? If a cell membrane contains only one type of potassium channel with single-channel conductance g_S, then the total membrane conductance to potassium would be given by

$$g_K = Ng_SP_o \tag{3.21}$$

where N is the number of potassium channels in the entire cell membrane and P_o is the average proportion of time that an individual channel is open. If the individual channels are always closed, then P_o is zero and g_K is also zero. Conversely, if individual channels are always open, then P_o is 1 and g_K will be the sum of all individual single-channel conductances (i.e., $N \times g_S$).

SUMMARY

To survive, cells must maintain proper osmotic balance between the ICF and ECF. Animal cells achieve osmotic balance by excluding an extracellular solute to compensate for the osmotic effect of impermeant biological molecules trapped within the cell. The compensating extracellular solute is sodium, which is actively pumped out of the cell by use of metabolic energy.

The movement of charged substances across the plasma membrane is governed not only by the concentration gradient across the membrane, but also by the electrical potential across the membrane. Equilibrium for an ion is reached when the electrical gradient exactly balances the concentration gradient. The Nernst equation expresses this equilibrium condition quantitatively, allowing us to calculate the equilibrium potential for an ion. The equilibrium potential is the value of membrane potential that will exactly balance a given concentration gradient.

The cell membrane is permeable to both sodium and potassium, and these ions have very different equilibrium potentials. The resting membrane potential of a cell therefore will lie somewhere between the sodium and potassium equilibrium potentials, at the membrane voltage where sodium influx is exactly balanced by potassium efflux. This balance point depends on the relative membrane permeabilities to sodium and potassium. In most cells p_K is much higher than p_{Na} and the balance is struck close to E_K. The Goldman equation quantitatively expresses the relation between membrane potential on the one hand and ion concentrations and permeabilities on the other.

Because the steady-state membrane potential lies between the equilibrium potentials for sodium and potassium, sodium is continually moving into the cell and potassium is continually moving out. The concentration gradients are restored by the sodium-potassium pump, which uses energy from hydrolysis of ATP to expel sodium and take up potassium. The steady fluxes of potassium and sodium ions constitute electrical currents across the cell membrane, and at the steady-state membrane potential, these currents cancel each other so that the net membrane current is zero.

1. A cell containing 0.25 M impermeant solute is placed in an infinite volume of an extracellular solution containing 0.5 M sucrose and no other solute. What would you predict the equilibrium cell volume to be?

2. For the example shown in Figure 3.7D, draw a graph showing the cell volume as a function of time after the cell is placed in the external solution. Explain the time course you have drawn.

3. Calculate the equilibrium potential for potassium if intracellular and extracellular potassium concentrations are equal.

4. Suppose a cell is permeable to potassium ions, the internal potassium concentration equals 100 mM, and the external potassium concentration equals 10 mM. If the membrane potential of the cell is set to -80 mV, in which direction will potassium ions move across the membrane?

5. Describe the factors that determine the value of the resting membrane potential in a neuron.

6. Why is the resting membrane potential of a neuron closer to the potassium equilibrium potential than to the sodium equilibrium potential?

7. What would happen to the resting membrane potential of a neuron if both sodium and potassium permeabilities were doubled?

8. Write the Goldman equation and define each of the parameters in the equation.

INTERNET ASSIGNMENT   CHAPTER 3

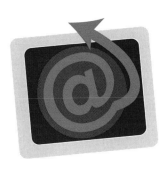

1 Table 3.1 is a simplified representation of the ionic composition of the ECF. Find a source that lists a more complete ionic composition of mammalian ECF. What is the largest single difference in ions between Table 3.1 and the actual composition of the ECF? In what way is the table simplified with regard to this substance?

2 The Nernst equation figures prominently in this chapter. Research the biographical history of Walther Hermann Nernst, the chemist who derived the equation.

3 The sodium pump (or sodium-potassium ATPase) plays an important role in the maintenance of water balance and ionic gradients. What is known about the molecular structure of this membrane protein? Search the Internet for images that illustrate the sodium pump and its action.

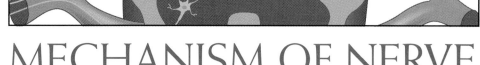

MECHANISM OF NERVE ACTION POTENTIAL

The nervous system must transmit information rapidly over long distances. To satisfy this requirement, neurons actively generate an electrical signal—the **action potential**—that travels rapidly along the long, thin fibers that connect each neuron with its targets. The action potential propagates from one end of a nerve fiber to the other at speeds as high as 100 m/sec. Cells that generate action potentials in response to stimuli are called **excitable cells**, and exam

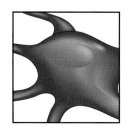

ples include muscle cells and endocrine cells, in addition to neurons. In this chapter, we will see that simple modifications of the scheme for the origin of the membrane potential presented in Chapter 3 can explain how neurons generate active electrical signals that allow the nervous system to achieve its goal of rapid signal transmission.

To set the stage for our discussion of the generation and transmission of signals in the nervous system, we will return to the patellar reflex, the knee-jerk reflex described in Chapter 1. Figure 4.1 summarizes the neural circuit for this reflex. Stretch-sensitive sensory neurons are activated when the quadriceps muscle is

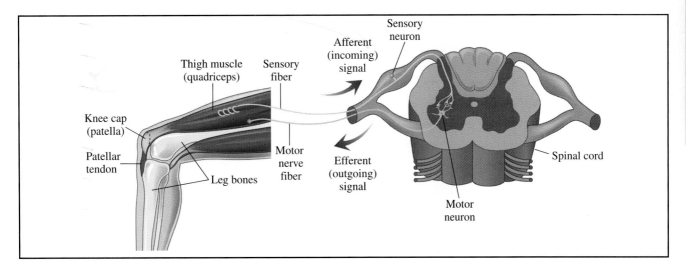

Figure 4.1.

A schematic representation of the patellar reflex. The sensory neuron is activated by stretching the thigh muscle and subsequently activates motor neurons in the spinal cord. Activity in the motor neuron causes the thigh muscle to contract.

passively stretched. The message that the muscle has been stretched travels along the axon of the sensory neuron to the spinal cord, where the message is passed along to motor neurons that send axons back to the quadriceps muscle. Activity in the motor neurons causes the muscle to contract, which opposes the passive stretch.

Neurons are structurally complex cells, with long fibrous extensions (called **processes**) that are specialized to receive and transmit information. This complexity can be appreciated by examining the structure of a motor neuron, which is shown schematically in Figure 4.2A. The cell body, or **soma**, of the motor neuron—where the nucleus resides—is only a small part of the cell. In the motor neurons involved in the patellar reflex, the soma is typically only about 20 to 30 μm in diameter. The soma gives rise to numerous branching processes called **dendrites**, which might spread out for several millimeters within the spinal cord. The dendrites receive signals from other neurons, including the stretch-sensitive sensory neurons, and funnel those signals to the soma. The soma also gives rise to a thin fiber, the **axon**, that transmits activity to other neurons, or in the case of motor neurons, to muscle cells. In many neurons, the axon also branches profusely and carries signals to many targets in the nervous system.

As shown in Figure 4.2B, the sensory neuron of the patellar reflex is structurally simpler than the motor neuron. Its soma, which is located just outside the spinal cord in the **dorsal root ganglion**, gives rise to only a single process. This process bifurcates to form the axon that carries the signal activated by stretching the muscle from the muscle into the spinal cord.

THE ACTION POTENTIAL

Ion Permeability and Membrane Potential

In Chapter 3, we learned that membrane potential is governed by the relative membrane permeability to sodium and potassium, as specified by the Goldman equation. If sodium permeability is greater than potassium permeability, the membrane potential will be closer to the equilibrium potential for sodium (E_{Na}) than to the equilibrium potential for potassium (E_K). Conversely, if potassium permeability is greater than sodium permeability, the membrane potential will be closer to E_K.

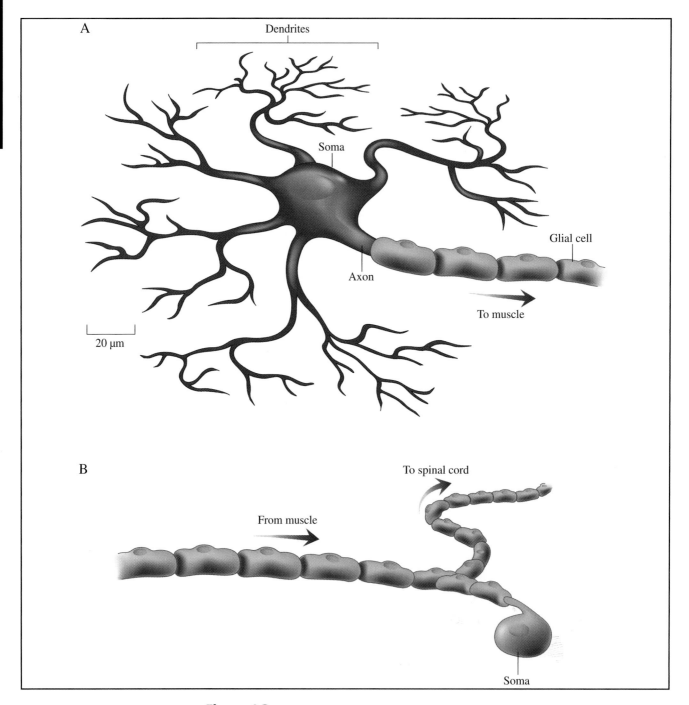

Figure 4.2.

Structures of single neurons involved in the patellar reflex. **A**. A motor neuron within spinal cord. **B**. A sensory neuron just outside spinal cord.

Until now, ionic permeability has been treated as a fixed characteristic of the cell membrane. However, the ionic permeability of the plasma membrane of excitable cells can vary. Specifically, a transient, dramatic change in relative sodium and potassium permeability underlies the action potential.

Measuring the Long-Distance Signal in Neurons

What does an action potential look like?

The change in membrane potential during an action potential can be measured as shown in Figure 4.3. An ultrafine probe (a **microelectrode**) is placed inside the

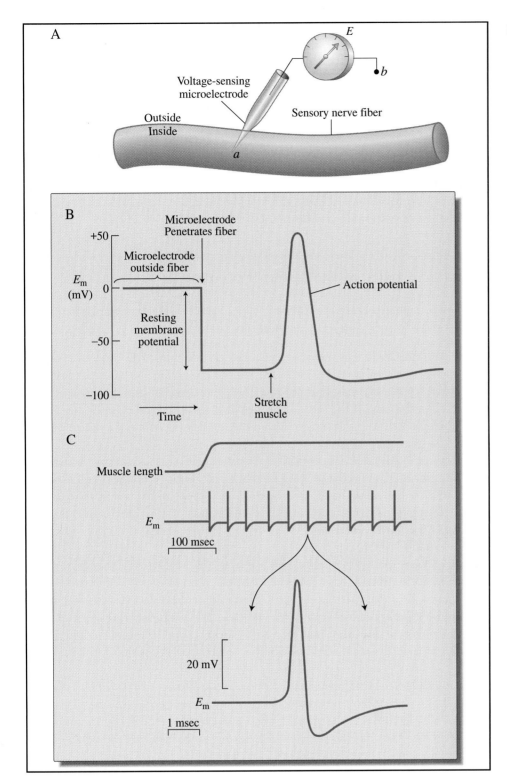

Figure 4.3.

An example of an action potential in a neuron. **A.** An experimental arrangement for recording the membrane potential of a nerve fiber. **B.** The resting membrane potential and an action potential recorded via a voltage-sensing probe inside the sensory neuron of the patellar reflex. **C.** A series of action potentials in a single stretch-receptor sensory fiber during stretch of the muscle. The *lower trace* shows a single action potential on an expanded time scale to illustrate its waveform in more detail.

sensory axon in the patellar reflex to measure the electrical membrane potential of the sensory neuron. A voltmeter is connected to measure the voltage difference between point *a*, at the tip of the microelectrode, and point *b*, a reference point in the extracellular fluid (ECF). As shown in Figure 4.3B, when the probe is outside the sensory axon, both the probe and the reference point are in the ECF, and the voltmeter records no voltage difference. When the microelectrode is inserted into the sensory fiber, however, the voltmeter records the voltage difference between the inside and outside of the neuron, the membrane potential. As expected from the discussion in Chapter 3, the membrane potential of the sensory fiber is approximately −70 mV.

When the muscle is stretched (see Fig. 4.3B), the membrane potential of the sensory neuron undergoes a dramatic series of changes. After a small delay, the voltage across the membrane suddenly moves in a positive direction (a **depolarization**) and actually reverses sign, so that the inside of the cell is positive with respect to the outside for a brief time. When the potential returns toward its resting value, it transiently becomes more negative than its normal resting value. This rapid sequence of changes in membrane potential is an action potential. If the stretch is sufficiently strong, it might elicit a series of several action potentials, each with the same shape and amplitude, as illustrated in Figure 4.3C.

Characteristics of the Action Potential

The action potential has several important characteristics that can be explained in terms of the underlying ionic permeability changes:

1. *Action potentials are triggered by depolarization.* The stimulus that initiates an action potential in a neuron is reduction in the membrane voltage—that is, depolarization. Normally, depolarization is produced by some external stimulus, such as muscle stretch in the case of the sensory neuron in the patellar reflex, or by the action of another neuron, as in transmission from the sensory neuron to the motor neuron in the patellar reflex.

2. *A threshold level of depolarization must be reached to trigger an action potential.* A small depolarization from the normal resting membrane potential will not produce an action potential. Typically, the membrane must be depolarized by about 10 to 20 mV in order to trigger an action potential. If a neuron has a resting membrane potential of about –70 mV, the membrane potential must be reduced to −60 to −50 mV to trigger an action potential.

3. *Action potentials are "all-or-none" events.* Once a stimulus is strong enough to reach threshold, the amplitude of the action potential is independent of the strength of the stimulus. The event either goes to completion (if the depolarization exceeds threshold) or doesn't occur at all (if the depolarization is below threshold). In this manner, triggering an action potential is like firing a gun: the speed of the bullet leaving the barrel is independent of whether the trigger was pulled softly or forcefully.

4. *An action potential propagates without decrement throughout a neuron, but at a relatively slow speed.* If we recorded simultaneously from a sensory fiber in the patellar reflex near the muscle and near the spinal cord, we would find that the action potential at the two locations has the same amplitude and form. Thus, as the signal travels from the muscle—where it originated—to the spinal cord, its amplitude remains unchanged. However, there would be a significant delay of about 0.1 sec between the appearance of the action potential near the muscle and its arrival at the spinal cord. The conduction speed of an action potential in a typical mammalian nerve fiber is about 10 to 20 m/sec, although speeds as high as 100 m/sec have been observed.

5. *At the peak of the action potential, the membrane potential reverses sign, becoming positive inside the cell.* As shown in Figure 4.3, the membrane potential during an action potential transiently overshoots zero, and the inside of the cell becomes positive with respect to the outside for a brief time. This phase is called the **overshoot** of the action potential. As the membrane potential returns toward the normal resting membrane potential at the end of the action potential, it transiently becomes

more negative than normal. This phase is called the **undershoot** of the action potential.

6. After a neuron fires an action potential, there is a brief period, called the absolute refractory period, during which it is impossible to make the neuron fire another action potential. The absolute refractory period varies a bit from one neuron to another, but usually lasts about 1 ms. The refractory period limits the maximum firing rate of a neuron to about 1000 action potentials per second.

We will now consider how all of these characteristics of the action potential are explained in terms of changes in the ionic permeability of the cell membrane and the resulting movement of ions.

INITIATION AND PROPAGATION OF ACTION POTENTIALS

What stimulus triggers an action potential?

Figure 4.4 shows an arrangement for studying some of the fundamental properties of action potentials. A long section of a single axon is removed, and intracellular electrodes are placed inside the fiber at two locations, *a* and *b*, 10 cm apart. The probe at point *a* can pass positive or negative charges into the fiber and record the resulting change in membrane potential. The probe at point *b* records the membrane potential at that location. The effect of injecting negative charges at a constant rate at point *a* is shown in Figure 4.4B. The extra negative charges make the interior of the fiber more negative, and the membrane potential increases; that is, the membrane becomes **hyperpolarized**. In contrast, the membrane voltage at point *b* does not change, because the plasma membrane is leaky to charge. In other words, the membrane is not a very good electrical insulator. In Chapter 3, we learned that ion channels in the plasma membrane provide a path for electrical current to flow across the membrane. Thus, charges injected at point *a* do not travel very far down the fiber before leaking out across the plasma membrane. There is no change in membrane potential at location *b* because all of the charges leak out before reaching that location. When we stop injecting negative charges at *a*, all the injected charges leak out of the cell, and the membrane potential at location *a* returns to its normal resting value. See Advanced Topic 2: Electrical Properties of Cells for a quantitative description of the response of cells to injection of electrical charge.

The effect of injecting positive charges into the axon is shown in Figure 4.4C. If the number of positive charges injected is small, the effect is simply the reverse of the effect of injecting negative charges. That is, the membrane depolarizes while the charges are injected, but the effect does not reach location *b*. When charge injection ceases, the extra positive charges leak out of the fiber, and membrane voltage returns to normal. As shown in Figure 4.4D, a larger positive current produces a larger depolarization. If the depolarization is sufficiently large, an all-or-none action potential, like that recorded when the muscle was stretched (see Fig. 4.3), is triggered at point *a*, and the probe at point *b* now records a replica of the action potential at point *a*, except that a time delay separates the occurrence of the action potential at *a* and its arrival at *b*.

These experiments show that action potentials are triggered by depolarization, not by hyperpolarization (characteristic 1 in the list given earlier); the depolarization must be large enough to exceed threshold (characteristic 2); and the action potential travels without decrement along the nerve fiber (characteristic 4). Now we will discuss the ionic properties of the neuron membrane that explain these characteristics.

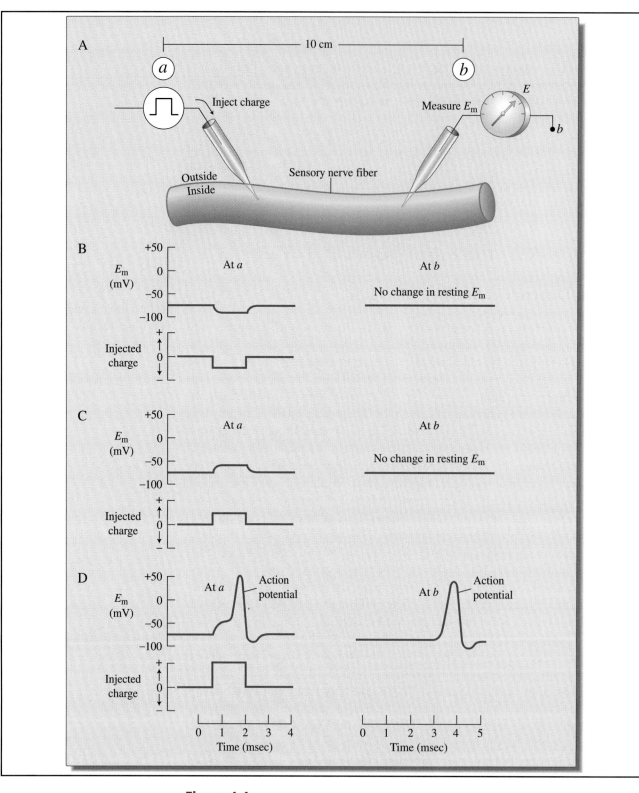

Figure 4.4.

The generation and propagation of an action potential in a nerve fiber. **A.** Apparatus for recording electrical activity of a segment of a sensory nerve fiber. The probes at points *a* and *b* allow recording of the membrane potential, and the probe at *a* also allows injection of electrical current into the fiber. **B.** Injecting negative charges at *a* causes hyperpolarization at *a*. All injected charges leak out across the membrane before reaching *b*, and no change in membrane potential is recorded at *b*. **C.** Injection of a small amount of positive charge produces a depolarization at *a* that does not reach *b*. **D.** If a stronger depolarization is induced at *a*, an action potential is generated. The action potential propagates without decrement along the fiber and is recorded at full amplitude at *b*.

CHANGES IN RELATIVE SODIUM PERMEABILITY DURING AN ACTION POTENTIAL

The key to understanding the origin of the action potential lies in the Goldman equation (see Chapter 3). Recall that the resting membrane potential will be somewhere between E_K and E_{Na}, and that the ratio of sodium to potassium permeability, p_{Na}/p_K, determines the exact balance point. The resting value of p_{Na}/p_K is approximately 0.02, and the resting membrane potential is relatively close to E_K. However, if sodium permeability increased a thousandfold (Fig. 4.5), leaving potassium permeability unchanged, p_{Na}/p_K would increase to 20. From the Goldman equation, we calculate that the membrane potential would shift from -70 mV to $+50$ mV, near E_{Na}. If p_{Na}/p_K then returns to 0.02, the membrane potential would move back to its usual value near E_K. This sequence of permeability changes in fact underlies the action potential.

Voltage-Dependent Sodium Channels

Recall that ions must cross the membrane through transmembrane protein molecules called ion channels. The changes in sodium and potassium permeability during an action potential are produced by special ion channels whose ability to conduct ions across the membrane is determined by the membrane potential. The increase in sodium permeability during the depolarizing phase of the action potential is produced by **voltage-dependent sodium channels**. These sodium channels are closed as long as the membrane potential is near its normal negative resting level, and open upon depolarization. The increase in sodium permeability upon depolarization causes an increased flux of positively charged sodium ions into the cell, which leads to greater depolarization and hence to the opening of still more voltage-dependent sodium channels (Fig. 4.6). Thus, the response to depolarization is inherently explosive, or **regenerative**, producing a large increase in sodium permeability and driving the membrane potential near the sodium equilibrium po-

What changes in membrane permeability account for the action potential?

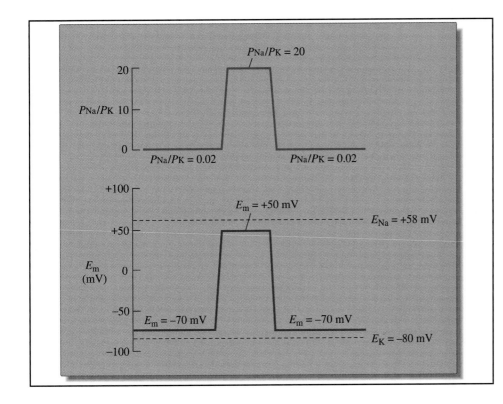

Figure 4.5.

The relationship between relative sodium permeability and membrane potential. When the ratio of sodium to potassium permeability (*upper trace*) changes, the position of the membrane potential (E_m) relative to potassium equilibrium potential (E_K) and sodium equilibrium potential (E_{Na}) is altered accordingly.

Figure 4.6.

The explosive cycle leading to the depolarizing phase of an action potential.

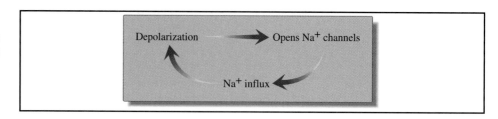

tential. This regenerative response explains the all-or-none behavior of the nerve action potential—once triggered, the process tends to run to completion.

At this point, it may seem that any depolarization that opens sodium channels, no matter how small, would trigger an action potential. However, according to characteristic 2 above, an action potential occurs only when a depolarization exceeds the threshold potential for triggering an action potential. We will now consider the factors that lead to the requirement for a threshold level of depolarization to stimulate an action potential. In considering the effect of a depolarization, we must take into account the total current that flows across the membrane in response to depolarization, not just the current carried by sodium ions. At the resting membrane potential, potassium permeability is very much greater than sodium permeability; therefore, the flow of K^+ out of the cell can readily counteract the influx of Na^+, even if sodium permeability increases moderately. Thus, for a moderate depolarization, potassium efflux will exceed sodium influx, and the explosive cycle underlying the action potential will not occur.

To initiate the explosive process, a depolarization must produce a net inward membrane current, which will in turn produce further depolarization. A depolarization that produces an action potential must be sufficiently large to open sufficient sodium channels to overcome the efflux of potassium resulting from the depolarization. The **threshold potential** will be reached at that value of the membrane potential where the influx of Na^+ exactly balances the efflux of K^+; any further depolarization will allow Na^+ influx to dominate, producing an explosive action potential.

One factor that determines the amount of depolarization required to reach threshold is the density of voltage-sensitive sodium channels in the plasma membrane. If voltage-sensitive sodium channels are densely packed in the membrane, opening only a small fraction of them will produce a sizable inward sodium current. The threshold depolarization would be smaller than if the channels were sparse. Often, the density of voltage-sensitive sodium channels is highest at the **initial segment**, where a neuron's axon leaves the cell body. Thus, the initial segment often has the lowest threshold for generation of an action potential.

Another important factor in determining the threshold is the strength of the connection between depolarization and sodium channel opening. In some cases, sodium channels have "hair triggers," and only a small depolarization is required to open large numbers of channels. The threshold would then be close to the resting membrane potential. In other neurons, larger depolarizations are necessary to open appreciable numbers of sodium channels, and the threshold is further from the resting membrane potential.

Repolarization

Two factors cause the membrane potential to return to rest again following the regenerative depolarization during an action potential:

- The increase in sodium permeability during depolarization is transient.
- Potassium permeability also increases in response to depolarization.

Sodium channels open for only a short time upon depolarization, and the channels close again within a millisecond or two after depolarization. The sodium channel behaves as though the flow of sodium ions is controlled by two independent gates, as summarized in Figure 4.7. One gate, called the **m gate or activation gate**, remains closed when the membrane potential is equal to or more negative than the usual resting potential. This gate thus prevents Na$^+$ from entering the channel at the resting potential. The other gate, called the **h gate or inactivation gate**, is open at the usual resting membrane potential. Both gates respond to depolarization but with different speeds and in opposite directions. The m gate opens rapidly in response to depolarization; the h gate closes in response to depolarization but does so slowly. Rapid opening of the m gate produces the explosive upstroke of the action potential, whereas delayed closing of the h gate returns sodium permeability to its

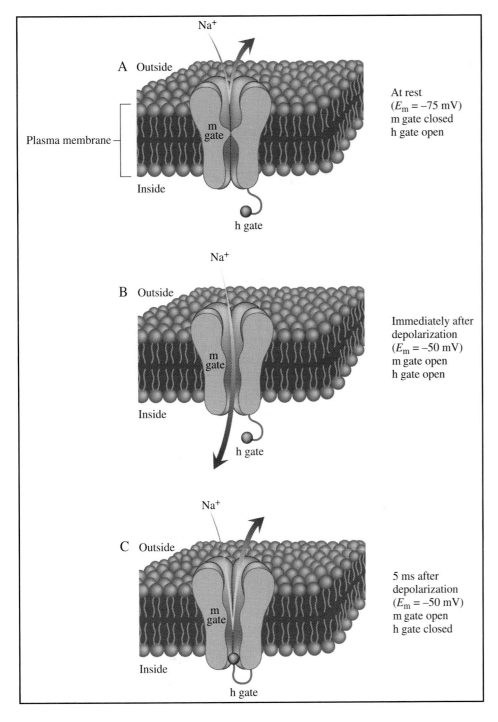

Figure 4.7.

A schematic representation of the behavior of a single voltage-sensitive sodium channel in the plasma membrane of a neuron. **A.** The state of the channel at the normal resting membrane potential. **B.** Upon depolarization, the m gate opens rapidly and sodium ions are free to move through the channel. **C.** After a brief delay, the h gate closes, returning the channel to a nonconducting state.

Na$^+$

A   Outside

At rest
($E_m = -75$ mV)
m gate closed
h gate open

Plasma membrane

m gate

Inside

h gate

Na$^+$

B   Outside

Immediately after depolarization
($E_m = -50$ mV)
m gate open
h gate open

m gate

Inside

h gate

Na$^+$

C   Outside

5 ms after depolarization
($E_m = -50$ mV)
m gate open
h gate closed

m gate

Inside

h gate

resting level. As shown in Figure 4.5, returning sodium permeability to its resting level would alone be sufficient to bring the membrane potential back to rest.

In addition to the voltage-sensitive sodium channels, neurons also possess voltage-dependent potassium channels, whose response to depolarization is summarized in Figure 4.8. The gates of the potassium channels (called **n gates**) are closed at the normal resting membrane potential and open slowly upon depolarization, allowing potassium ions to move through the channel when the membrane potential becomes more positive. The delayed opening of these voltage-dependent potassium channels causes a delayed increase in potassium permeability, which is the other factor responsible for the repolarizing phase of the action potential. Unlike the sodium channel, the potassium channel has no second gate that closes upon depolarization. Instead, the channel remains open as long as the depolarization is maintained and closes only when membrane potential returns to its normal resting value.

The repolarizing phase of the action potential is produced by a simultaneous decline of sodium permeability to its resting level and increase of potassium perme-

Figure 4.8.

The behavior of a single voltage-sensitive potassium channel in the plasma membrane of a neuron. **A.** At the normal resting membrane potential, the channel is closed. **B.** Immediately after a depolarization, the channel remains closed. **C.** After a delay, the n gate opens, allowing potassium ions to cross the membrane through the channel. The channel remains open as long as depolarization is maintained.

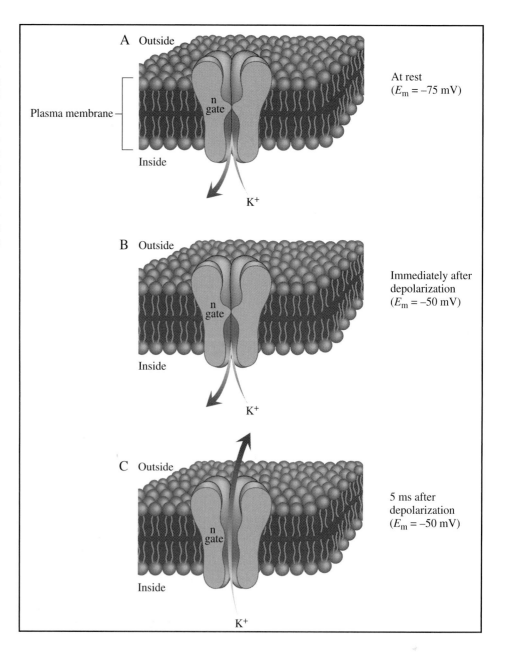

ability to a higher-than-normal level. During this time, p_{Na}/p_K is actually *smaller* than its usual resting value. This smaller ratio explains the undershoot at the end of an action potential, when the membrane potential approaches nearer to E_K. Membrane potential returns to rest as the slow n gates respond to the repolarization by closing and returning potassium permeability to its normal value.

Figure 4.9 summarizes the behavior of the voltage-dependent sodium and potassium channels during an action potential, and characteristics of the various gates

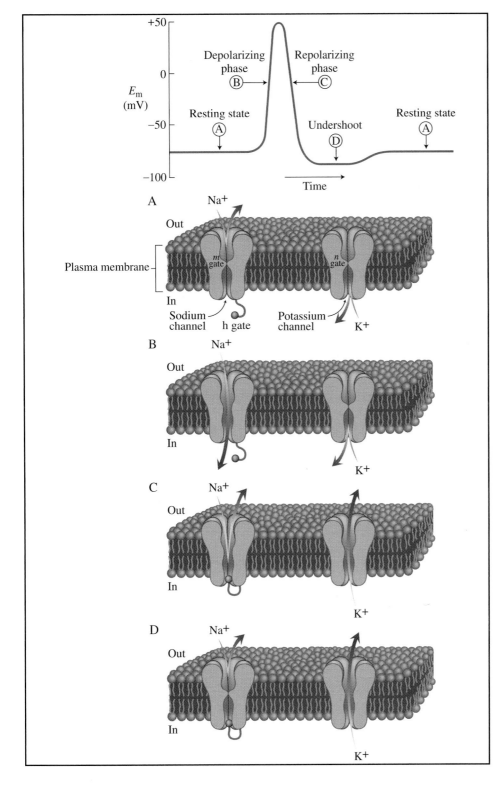

Figure 4.9.

The states of voltage-sensitive sodium and potassium channels at various times during an action potential in a neuron. **A**. At rest, neither channel is in a conducting state. **B**. During the depolarizing phase of the action potential, the sodium channels open, but the potassium channels have not yet responded to the depolarization. **C**. During the repolarizing phase, sodium permeability begins to return to its resting level as h gates respond to the preceding depolarizing phase. At the same time, potassium channels respond to the depolarization by opening. **D**. During the undershoot, sodium permeability returns to its usual low level; potassium permeability, however, remains elevated because n gates respond slowly to the repolarization of the membrane. The resting state of the membrane is restored after h gates and n gates return to their resting configurations.

Table 4.1

Summary of Responses of Voltage-Sensitive Sodium and Potassium Channels to Depolarization

Type of Channel	Gate	Response to Depolarization	Speed of Response
Sodium	m gate	Opens	Fast
Sodium	h gate	Closes	Slow
Potassium	n gate	Opens	Slow

are summarized in Table 4.1. Note that the sodium channel h gates remain closed for a period after repolarization. During this period, called the refractory period, the neuron cannot fire another action potential, even if it receives another depolarizing stimulus. The refractory period arises because the channels will not conduct sodium ions while the h gates are closed, even if the m gates open again in response to depolarization.

THE MECHANISM OF ACTION POTENTIAL PROPAGATION

How do action potentials propagate along nerve fibers?

To transmit information over long distances, the action potential must propagate rapidly from one end of an axon to the other. The stimulus for triggering an action potential is depolarization, and the action potential itself is a large depolar-

BOX 1

IN THE CLINIC

Action potentials are the signals that transmit information along the long, thin fibers that connect neurons with each other or with their sensory or motor targets in the body. If the conduction of action potentials is prevented in a nerve fiber, then the information normally conveyed by that neuron is blocked. Blockade of action potentials is frequently used in medicine to produce local anesthesia. Many local anesthetics act by blocking voltage-dependent sodium channels, which are required for the generation of action potentials. Commonly used local anesthetics that act in this manner are procaine, lidocaine, and tetracaine. Interestingly, the first local anesthetic of this type to be described and used clinically was cocaine, a drug better known for its other pharmacological actions on the central nervous system and for its addictive properties. Injection of a local anesthetic near a peripheral nerve blocks action potentials in all sensory and motor nerve fibers within the nerve, producing loss of all sensation and motor paralysis in the area of the body supplied by that nerve.

Naturally occurring biological toxins are also known to block the sodium channels of nerve membranes. Tetrodotoxin is a potent sodium channel blocker made by puffer fish. Saxitoxin, another sodium channel blocker, is produced by marine dinoflagellates and is responsible for paralytic shellfish poisoning in humans who eat shellfish that have ingested the poisonous dinoflagellates ("red tide" organisms).

ization, greatly in excess of the threshold. Thus, once an action potential occurs at one end of a neuron, the strong depolarization will bring the neighboring region of the cell above threshold, setting up a regenerative depolarization in that region. The action potential in the neighboring region in turn will bring the next region above threshold, and so on. Therefore, action potential is a self-propagating wave of depolarization sweeping along the nerve fiber. At each successive location along the axon, the action potential is recreated by the precisely timed opening and closing of sodium and potassium channels at that location. This behavior is analogous to that of a lighted fuse, in which the heat generated in one segment of the fuse ignites the neighboring segment.

Figure 4.10 shows the spatial profile of depolarization as an action potential propagates along an axon. At the peak of the action potential (point 1 in Fig. 4.10A), an inward flow of sodium ions moves the membrane potential near E_{Na}. This region of axon therefore will be depolarized with respect to more distant parts of the axon, such as points 2 and 3. This difference in electrical potential drives positive charges along the inside of the axon, producing depolarization of neighboring regions of the axon, where the action potential has not yet reached. The depolarization produced by an action potential decays with distance, because the membrane is a leaky insulator (recall Fig. 4.4). Figure 4.10B illustrates the profile of the membrane potential along the axon at the instant the action potential at point 1 reaches its peak. Note that there is a region of axon over which the depolarization is above threshold for generating an action potential in that

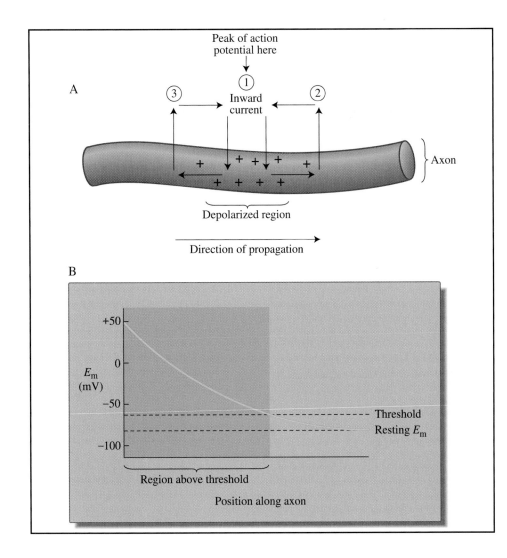

Figure 4.10.

The decay of depolarization with distance from the peak of the action potential at a particular instant during propagation of the action potential from left to right along the axon. **A.** A diagram of the flow of electrical current around a portion of an axon that is undergoing an action potential. **B.** The membrane potential gradually decays from +50 mV, at the location of the action potential, to the normal resting membrane potential. The large depolarization produced by the action potential raises the membrane potential of neighboring regions of the axon above the threshold potential.

part of the membrane. At the next instant, then, this region that is above threshold will generate its own action potential. This process will continue as the action potential sweeps along the axon, bringing each successive segment of axon above threshold.

The depolarization produced by an action potential at a particular location will depolarize the axon in both directions. Thus, current flows from point 1 to both point 2 and point 3 in Figure 4.10A. Nevertheless, the action potential in an axon propagates in only one direction, because the region just traversed by the action potential (e.g., point 3) is in the refractory period and is thus incapable of responding to depolarization. If an action potential is artificially stimulated in the middle of a nerve fiber, that action potential will propagate in both directions along the fiber. The normal direction of propagation in an axon—the direction taken by normal action potentials—is called the **orthodromic** direction; an abnormal action potential propagating in the opposite direction is called an **antidromic** action potential. For example, in the sensory neuron of the patellar reflex, the orthodromic direction is from the muscle to the spinal cord, whereas for the motor neuron, the orthodromic direction is from the spinal cord to the muscle.

Factors Affecting the Speed of Action Potential Propagation

Action potentials propagate at greatly different speeds in different axons, with velocities ranging from 0.1 to 100 m/sec. The propagation velocity is determined by the diameter of the axon and by whether the axon is covered by an insulating myelin sheath. As Figure 4.10B shows, depolarization falls off with distance along the axon from a region where the action potential is occurring. If depolarization falls off less steeply with distance, the length of axon brought above threshold by an action potential will be larger, an action potential at a particular location will set up a new action potential at a greater distance down the axon, and propagation speed will be greater. Thus, the rate at which depolarization decreases with distance determines propagation speed.

The decline of voltage with distance in turn depends on the relative resistance to current flow of the plasma membrane and the intracellular path down the axon. At each point along the axon, positive charges moving away from a depolarized region (see Fig. 4.10A) either continue down the interior of the fiber or cross the membrane. The portion of current taking each path depends on the relative resistances of the two paths. If the resistance of the membrane is high or if the resistance down the inside of the axon is low, the path down the axon is favored. In this situation, depolarization resulting from an action potential reaches farther along the axon, and propagation speed increases.

Thus, two strategies can be employed to increase the speed of action potential propagation: (1) increase the electrical resistance of the plasma membrane to current flow, and (2) decrease the resistance of the longitudinal path down the inside of the fiber. Both strategies have been adopted in nature. Among invertebrate animals, fast-conducting axons have a large diameter. A larger axon offers a greater cross-sectional area to the internal flow of current, which reduces resistance by providing many parallel paths for current to continue down the interior of the axon. For the same reason, electric power companies use large-diameter copper wires for the cables leaving a power-generating station; these cables must carry massive currents and thus must have low resistance to current flow to avoid burning up. Some invertebrate axons, with diameters up to 1 mm, represent the neuronal equivalent of these power cables. These giant axons are the fastest-conducting nerve fibers of the invertebrate world.

Vertebrate animals also have axons of widely varying diameter, ranging from less than 1 μm to 50 μm. However, even the largest mammalian axons do not begin to rival the size of the giant axons of invertebrates. Nevertheless, the fastest-conducting vertebrate axons are actually faster than the giant invertebrate axons, owing to evolution of a method for increasing the membrane resistance to current, as well as increasing internal diameter. Fast-conducting vertebrate axons are wrapped with extra layers of insulating cell membrane, as shown in Figure 4.11. To reach the exterior, electrical current must flow not only through the resistance of the axon membrane, but also through the cascaded resistance of the tightly wrapped layers of extra membrane. The cell that provides the spiral of insulating membrane surrounding the axon is a type of **glial cell**, a non-neuronal supporting cell of the nervous system that provides a sustaining mesh in which the neurons are embedded. In peripheral nerves, the insulating glial cells are

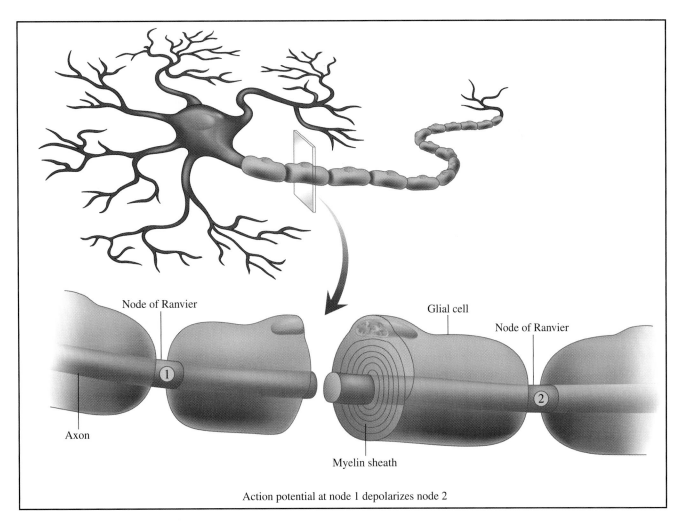

Node of Ranvier

Glial cell

Node of Ranvier

Axon

Myelin sheath

Action potential at node 1 depolarizes node 2

Figure 4.11.

The propagation of an action potential along a myelinated nerve fiber. A cross section of a myelinated axon shows the spiral wrapping of the glial cell membrane around the axon. The depolarization produced by an action potential at one node of Ranvier spreads along the interior of the fiber because the insulating myelin prevents the leakage of current across the plasma membrane. This spread of depolarization ensures that the next node of Ranvier along the axon triggers an action potential, and the action potential jumps progressively from one node to the next along the myelinated axon.

Schwann cells, and in the central nervous system, oligodendrocytes form the insulating cover of axons.

The insulating sheath around the axon is called myelin. By increasing the resistance of the path across the membrane, the myelin sheath forces a larger portion of the current flowing as the result of voltage change to move down the interior of the fiber. Thus, the spatial spread of a depolarization increases along the axon, and action potentials propagate more rapidly. In order to set up a new action potential at a distant point along the axon, however, external sodium ions must have access to the axon membrane to flow in through open sodium channels. To provide that access, the myelin sheath is interrupted at regular intervals, at nodes of Ranvier (see Fig. 4.11). The depolarization resulting from an action potential at one node of Ranvier spreads along the interior of the fiber to the next node, where it sets up a new action potential. The action potential leaps along the axon, jumping from one node to the next. This form of action potential conduction is called saltatory conduction, and it greatly speeds action potential propagation.

MOLECULAR PROPERTIES OF VOLTAGE-SENSITIVE SODIUM CHANNELS

By what molecular mechanism does membrane potential influence the opening of voltage-dependent sodium channels?

Ion channels are proteins, and like all proteins, the sequence of amino acids making up a particular ion channel is encoded by a particular gene. Thus, it is possible to study ion channels by applying techniques of molecular biology to isolate and analyze the corresponding gene. This has been done for an increasing variety of ion channels, including the voltage-sensitive sodium channel that underlies the action potential.

The sodium channel is a large protein, containing approximately 2000 amino acid residues. A model of how the protein folds up into a three-dimensional structure has been developed, as summarized in Figure 4.12. The protein consists of four distinct domains, each having six separate transmembrane segments, labeled S1 through S6. Within a domain, then, the protein threads its way through the membrane six times. The amino acid sequence of each transmembrane segment within a domain is similar to the corresponding segment in other domains. Thus, the overall structure of the channel can be thought of as a series of six transmembrane segments, repeated four times.

The four domains aggregate in a circular pattern as shown in Figure 4.12B to form the pore of the channel. The lining of the pore determines the permeation properties of the channel and makes it selective for sodium ions. Interestingly, the lining is actually made up of the external-loop connecting segments S5 and S6 within each of the four domains, shown in red in Figure 4.12A. To form the transmembrane pore, the external loop must fold down into the pore in the manner shown in Figure 4.12C.

Part of the large protein that comprises the sodium channel detects changes in the membrane potential and thus imparts voltage sensitivity. Evidence shows that the voltage sensor is segment S4 (see Fig. 4.12A). Segment S4 contains many positively charged arginine and lysine residues, which provide sensitivity to the electric field across the membrane. To test the idea that the charges in S4 are the voltage sensors, artificial sodium channels were constructed by altering the encoding DNA to replace one or more of the arginines or lysines in S4 with a neutral or negatively charged amino acid. These altered channels were less sensitive to depolarization than normal channels, as expected if the charges in S4 detect depolarization and trigger channel opening.

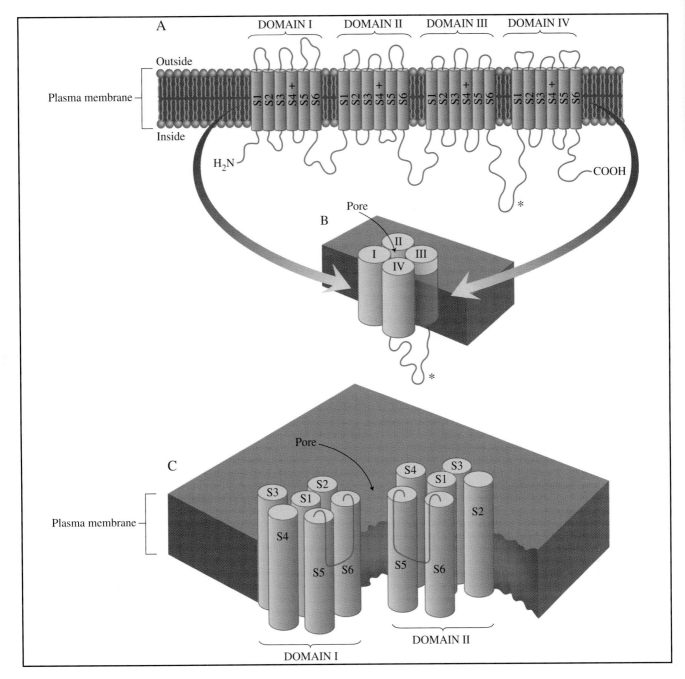

Figure 4.12.

The molecular structure of the voltage-sensitive sodium channel. **A.** The molecule consists of four domains of similar makeup, labeled with Roman numerals. Each domain has six transmembrane segments (S1–S6). The highly positively charged segment S4 is indicated in each domain by a *plus sign* (+). The linkage between domains III and IV, indicated by an *asterisk* (*), is involved in inactivation gating. **B.** The domains are shown in a linear arrangement in **A**, but in reality, the domains likely form a circular arrangement with the pore at the center. **C.** The extracellular loop shown in *green* may fold in as indicated to line the entry to the pore. This region controls the ionic selectivity of the channel.

Experimentally altered channels have identified the sodium inactivation gate, the h gate. If the part of the protein connecting domains III and IV (marked with an *asterisk* in Fig. 4.12A, B) is deleted or altered, inactivation is greatly impaired, though activation remains normal.

MOLECULAR PROPERTIES OF VOLTAGE-DEPENDENT POTASSIUM CHANNELS

The DNA encoding voltage-activated potassium channels has also been analyzed to reveal the sequence of amino acids making up those proteins. It is interesting that potassium channels are structurally related to voltage-sensitive sodium channels (and to voltage-sensitive calcium channels). For example, segment S4 of potassium channels imparts voltage sensitivity. Thus, voltage-activated channels of various kinds represent a family of proteins encoded by related genes that probably arose during the course of evolution from a single ancestral gene. Potassium channel genes, however, encode proteins that are much smaller than sodium channels, corresponding to a single one of the four domains present in the voltage-activated sodium channel. Functional potassium channels are formed by aggregation of four of these individual protein subunits, so that the whole channel is arranged similarly to the sodium channel (see Fig. 4.12B). In sodium channels, however, the four domains are combined together into one large, continuous protein molecule, whereas in potassium channels each domain consists of a separate protein subunit.

CALCIUM-DEPENDENT ACTION POTENTIALS

How do calcium ions contribute to action potentials in some neurons?

In the discussion of the evolution of the nervous system in Chapter 2, we learned about action potentials in single-cell paramecium and in multicellular obelia. In these organisms, the depolarizing upstroke of the action potential is caused by an influx of positively charged calcium ions, rather than sodium ions. In the case of calcium action potentials, calcium channels that open upon depolarization underlie the depolarizing phase of the action potential, just as sodium channels produce depolarization in the conventional nerve action potential.

Voltage-dependent calcium channels are found in most neurons. In some neurons, they contribute significantly to the action potential. Figure 4.13 compares typical waveforms of action potentials with and without a contribution from calcium channels. Often, the depolarization produced by calcium influx is slower and more sustained than the spike-like action potential generated by sodium and potassium channels alone. Because voltage-activated calcium channels commonly inactivate more slowly than voltage-activated sodium channels, they produce a more sustained influx of positive charges and thus a more prolonged depolarization. In neurons with a calcium component, the action potential shows a rapid upstroke caused by the opening of sodium channels, followed by a longer-duration plateau produced by voltage-dependent calcium channels.

The influx of calcium ions through voltage-dependent calcium channels has functional consequences beyond its contribution to the action potential. This calcium influx triggers a variety of internal cellular events. For example, an increase in intracellular calcium concentration stimulates the release of neurotransmitter molecules from the presynaptic terminal during synaptic transmission.

A rise in internal calcium concentration also activates other kinds of ion channels. In addition to the potassium channels opened by depolarization, neurons fre-

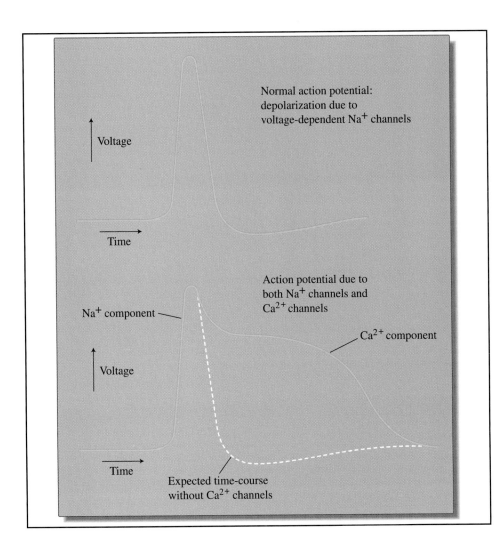

Normal action potential: depolarization due to voltage-dependent Na$^+$ channels

Voltage

Time

Na$^+$ component

Action potential due to both Na$^+$ channels and Ca^{2+} channels

Ca^{2+} component

Voltage

Time

Expected time-course without Ca^{2+} channels

Figure 4.13.

A comparison between action potentials in neurons without a contribution from voltage-dependent calcium channels (*top*) and in neurons with a calcium component (*bottom*). The rising phase of the action potential on the bottom is produced by depolarization-activated sodium channels, and the *dashed white line* shows the expected time course of the action potential in the absence of calcium channels. The *yellow line* shows the plateau depolarization caused by the opening of voltage-sensitive calcium channels.

quently possess potassium channels that open when internal calcium concentration increases. The activation scheme for calcium-activated potassium channels is summarized in Figure 4.14. Calcium-activated potassium channels contribute to action potential repolarization in neurons whose action potential included a calcium component. Increased potassium permeability accounts in part for the repolarizing phase of the action potential and produces the hyperpolarizing undershoot after repolarization. The increase in potassium permeability can be accomplished with either voltage-activated potassium channels or calcium-activated potassium channels.

An important functional difference between voltage-activated and calcium-activated potassium channels is the amount of time the channels remain open after the membrane potential has returned to its negative level at the end of the action potential. The action potential undershoot occurs because voltage-dependent potassium channels remain open for a period, making the ratio p_{Na}/p_K smaller than usual and driving the membrane potential nearer E_K. The undershoot ends as the voltage-dependent potassium channels close in response to repolarization, which takes a few milliseconds. In contrast, calcium-activated potassium channels remain open as long as the intracellular calcium concentration remains elevated after the action potential, which can be hundreds of times longer than the undershoot produced by voltage-dependent potassium channels (Fig. 4.15). This longer-lasting hyperpolarization is called the **afterhyperpolarization**, to distinguish it from the undershoot. The afterhyperpolarization requires both significant calcium influx during the action potential and significant numbers of

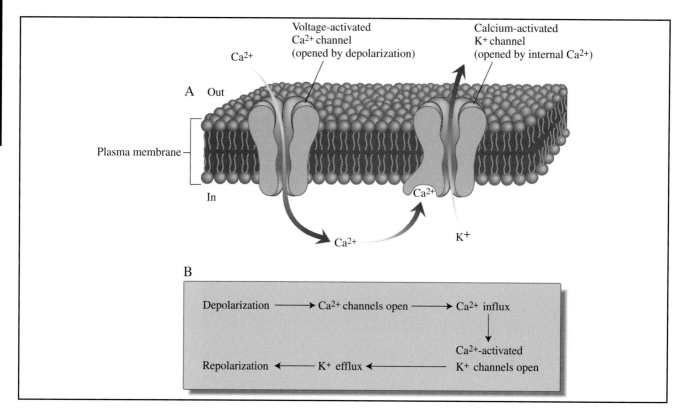

Figure 4.14.

Activation of potassium channels by internal calcium ions. **A.** Upon depolarization, voltage-dependent calcium channels open and calcium ions enter the cell from the extracellular fluid (ECF). The calcium ions then bind to and open calcium-activated potassium channels, which allow potassium ions to exit from the cell. **B.** A summary of the sequence of events leading to the activation of calcium-activated potassium channels.

calcium-activated potassium channels. Neurons that have only a small amount of calcium influx during a single action potential may exhibit afterhyperpolarization only after a rapid burst of action potentials. The internal calcium contributed by each action potential may accumulate to reach the level necessary to open calcium-activated potassium channels. The afterhyperpolarization helps determine the temporal patterning of action potentials, because the long period of increased potassium permeability makes it more difficult for the neuron to continue to fire action potentials. In neurons that require a burst of several action potentials to initiate the afterhyperpolarization, calcium-activated potassium channels help terminate the burst. We will encounter such a mechanism for regulating burst duration, for example, when we discuss neuronal circuits controlling locomotion in Chapter 10.

VOLTAGE-CLAMP ANALYSIS OF THE ACTION POTENTIAL

How can the voltage-dependent changes in ion permeability be tracked using the voltage clamp technique?

During an action potential, sodium and potassium permeability changes as a function of both voltage and time. To study these permeability changes quantitatively, experimenters use a technique called voltage clamp, in which membrane voltage is held constant ("clamped") by a voltage-clamp apparatus that injects

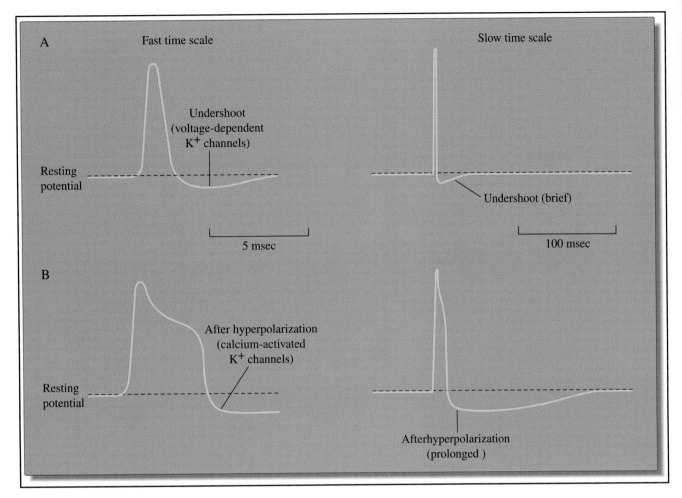

A Fast time scale   Slow time scale

Undershoot
(voltage-dependent
K⁺ channels)

Resting
potential

Undershoot (brief)

5 msec   100 msec

B

After hyperpolarization
(calcium-activated
K⁺ channels)

Resting
potential

Afterhyperpolarization
(prolonged)

Figure 4.15.

The time course of the undershoot compared with the time course of the afterhyperpolarization produced by calcium-activated potassium channels. **A.** The action potential of a
neuron with only voltage-dependent sodium and potassium channels. **B.** The action potential of a neuron with voltage-dependent calcium channels and calcium-activated potassium
channels in addition to the usual voltage-dependent sodium and potassium channels. The
left traces in both **A** and **B** show the action potential on a fast time scale (milliseconds),
while the *right traces* show the same action potentials on a slower time scale (hundreds of
milliseconds).

enough current at any given time into the recorded cell to prevent the membrane
potential from changing. Changes in the injected current can then be measured
and used as an index of the underlying changes in ionic permeability as a function
of time, at the fixed voltage level.

Figure 4.16 shows the response of a neuron to depolarization applied while the
membrane potential is clamped. In this example, the membrane potential is first
clamped at the resting potential (–70 mV) and then stepped to a depolarized level
of –20 mV. The current injected by the voltage-clamp apparatus to maintain the
membrane potential at –20 mV varies over time, as voltage-dependent channels
respond to the depolarization. Voltage-dependent sodium channels open in response to the depolarization, and sodium begins to flow into the neuron. Without
voltage clamp, a regenerative depolarization would be triggered, driving the membrane potential to +50 mV (near E_{Na}). To counter this depolarizing influence and
maintain the voltage at –20 mV, the voltage-clamp apparatus must inject a

Figure 4.16.

A diagram of the current injected by a voltage-clamp amplifier into a neuron in response to a depolarizing voltage step.

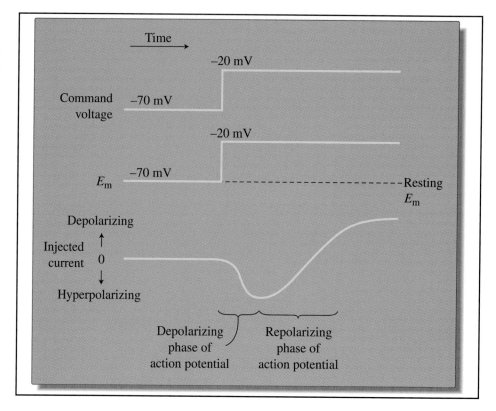

hyperpolarizing (negative) current during the depolarizing phase of the action potential, as shown in Figure 4.16.

With time, however, sodium permeability declines as inactivation gates (h gates) close, and potassium permeability rises as voltage-dependent potassium channels open in response to the depolarization to -20 mV. If not for the voltage clamp, these changes in permeability would drive the membrane potential to near E_K, producing the repolarizing phase of the action potential and the undershoot. To maintain the membrane potential at -20 mV, the voltage clamp must now pass a depolarizing current. Because the voltage-sensitive potassium channels do not inactivate, this depolarizing current persists as long as the membrane potential is held at -20 mV.

To separate the sodium and potassium currents, specific drugs are used to selectively block either the sodium or the potassium channels. Sodium channels are commonly blocked using the biological toxins tetrodotoxin or saxitoxin, which interact with specific sites in the pore of the channel and plug it to prevent sodium influx. Figure 4.17 shows that tetrodotoxin eliminates the early component of hyperpolarizing current injected by the voltage clamp, as expected if sodium influx is eliminated. Without sodium influx, the voltage dependence and time course of the potassium channels can be readily studied in isolation.

Blockers of potassium channels include tetraethylammonium (TEA), which is a large cation that enters the potassium channel pore and blocks it. When potassium channels are blocked, the delayed positive current is eliminated in response to a depolarizing stimulus (see Fig. 4.17). This procedure allows the sodium permeability change to be studied in isolation, revealing the activation and inactivation phases produced by the opening of m gates and closing of h gates, respectively. For a quantitative description of the sodium and potassium permeability changes based on voltage-clamp experiments, see Advanced Topic 3: Analysis of Ion Channel Gating.

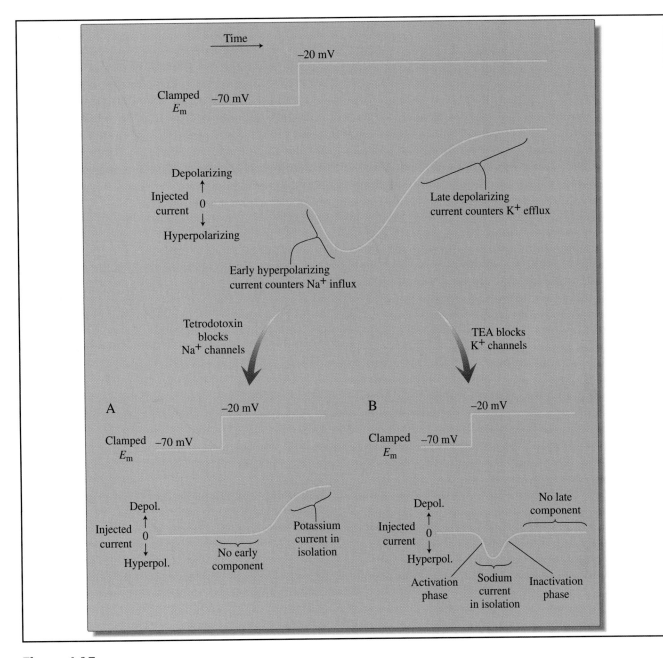

Figure 4.17.

The use of specific channel blockers to separate the ionic current through voltage-dependent sodium and potassium channels. **A**. Tetrodotoxin blocks voltage-dependent sodium channels and selectively eliminates the early, hyperpolarizing component of the voltage-clamp current in response to depolarization. This hyperpolarizing current injected by the voltage-clamp apparatus counters the depolarizing influence of sodium entering the cell, which is absent when sodium channels are blocked. **B**. Tetraethylammonium (TEA) blocks voltage-dependent potassium channels and selectively eliminates the late, depolarizing component of the voltage-clamp current in response to depolarization. This depolarizing current counters the hyperpolarizing influence of potassium efflux, which is absent when potassium channels are blocked.

SUMMARY

The basic long-distance signal of the nervous system is a self-propagating depolarization called the action potential. The action potential arises because of a sequence of voltage-dependent changes in the ionic permeability of the neuron membrane. This voltage-dependent behavior of the membrane is due to gated sodium and potassium channels. The conducting state of the sodium channels is controlled by m gates, which close at the usual resting membrane potential and open rapidly upon depolarization, and by h gates, which open at the usual resting membrane potential and close slowly upon depolarization. The voltage-sensitive potassium channels are controlled by a single type of gate, called the n gate, which closes at the resting membrane potential and opens slowly upon depolarization. In response to depolarization, sodium permeability increases dramatically as m gates open, and membrane potential is driven up near E_{Na}. With a delay, h gates close, restoring sodium permeability to a low level, and n gates open, increasing potassium permeability. As a result, the p_{Na}/p_K ratio falls below its normal resting value, and the membrane potential is driven back to near E_K. The resulting repolarization restores the membrane to its resting state. The gating of voltage-dependent sodium and potassium channels can be studied quantitatively using a technique called voltage clamp, in which membrane voltage is held constant by injecting whatever current is required to prevent the membrane potential from changing, even when channels open and close.

The behavior of the voltage-dependent sodium and potassium channels can explain (1) why depolarization is the stimulus for the generation of an action potential, (2) why action potentials are all-or-none events, (3) how action potentials propagate along nerve fibers, (4) why the membrane potential becomes positive at the peak of the action potential, (5) why the membrane potential is transiently more negative than usual at the end of an action potential, and (6) the existence of a refractory period after a neuron fires an action potential.

Action potentials of some neurons have components contributed by voltage-dependent calcium channels, which open upon depolarization like voltage-dependent sodium channels but specifically allow the influx of calcium ions. The influx of calcium ions through these channels can increase the intracellular concentration of calcium. Calcium-activated potassium channels open when internal calcium concentration is elevated, contributing to the repolarization of the action potential and producing a prolonged period of elevated potassium permeability during which the membrane potential is more negative than the usual resting membrane potential.

REVIEW QUESTIONS

1. Explain why the membrane potential at the peak of the action potential reverses sign, becoming positive inside.

2. What two factors account for returning the membrane potential to its normal level during the repolarizing phase of the action potential?

3. Describe the mechanism underlying the refractory period.

4. Summarize the responses of the gates of the voltage-dependent sodium and potassium channels to depolarization. Include a description of the speed of response of the gates.

5. Diagram the current that would be injected by a voltage-clamp apparatus after a step depolarization from -70 mV to -20 mV. Label the

phases of the current and specify which components correspond to sodium and potassium membrane currents.

6. Diagram the states of the gates controlling the voltage-dependent sodium and potassium channels during the depolarizing phase, repolarizing phase, and undershoot of the action potential.

INTERNET ASSIGNMENT   CHAPTER 4

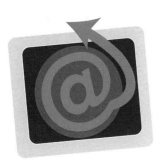

1 As described in Advanced Topic 3, Alan L. Hodgkin and Andrew F. Huxley first described the ionic mechanism of the action potential and developed the gated ion channel model to explain the changes in ion permeability during the action potential. Use the Internet to research the biographies of these important scientists and write a 150-word description of their contributions.

2 Search the Internet to find images of the molecular structure of potassium channels. You will find the following name and reference useful in your research: Roderick MacKinnon of Rockefeller University, *Science* 1998;280:69–77. Use PubMed to look up the reference and related articles.

SYNAPTIC TRANSMISSION AT THE NEUROMUSCULAR JUNCTION

Ion permeability and the basis of the resting membrane potential (Chapter 3)

The Nernst and Goldman equations (Chapter 3)

Voltage-sensitive ion channels (Chapter 4)

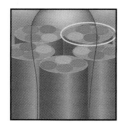

In Chapter 4 we learned about the ionic basis of the action potential, the electrical signal that carries messages long distances along nerve fibers. Using the patellar reflex as an example, we discussed the mechanism that allows the message, "the muscle was stretched," to travel along the membrane of the sensory neuron from the sensory endings in the muscle to the termination of the fiber in the spinal cord. In this chapter we will focus on the mechanism by which activity in the motor neuron is passed along to the cells of the muscle, causing the muscle to contract. Chapter 6 will then consider how action potentials in the sensory neuron influence motor neuron activity.

CHEMICAL AND ELECTRICAL SYNAPSES

The point where activity is transmitted from one nerve cell to another, or from a motor neuron to a muscle cell, is called a **synapse**. The patellar reflex includes two synapses: one between the sensory neuron and the motor neuron in the spinal cord, and another between the motor neuron and the cells of the quadriceps muscle. The two general classes of synapses are electrical synapses and chemical synapses. Both types are characterized by specialized membrane structures at the point where the input cell, called the **presynaptic cell**, comes into contact with the output cell, called the **postsynaptic cell**.

At a chemical synapse, an action potential in the presynaptic cell triggers release of a chemical substance (called a **neurotransmitter**), which diffuses through the extracellular space and changes the membrane potential of the postsynaptic cell. At an electrical synapse, a portion of the presynaptic change in membrane potential (such as the depolarization during an action potential) spreads directly to the postsynaptic cell. Both synapses in the patellar reflex—and indeed most synapses in mammalian nervous systems—are chemical synapses.

At chemical synapses, the membranes of the presynaptic and postsynaptic cells come close to each other but are still separated by a small gap of extracellular space. At an electrical synapse, the presynaptic and postsynaptic membranes touch and the cell interiors are directly interconnected by means of special ion channels called gap junctions, which allow the flow of electrical current from one cell to the other. This chapter focuses on chemical synaptic transmission. Chapter 11 describes in more detail electrical synaptic transmission.

Although the details may differ somewhat, the basic features of the neuromuscular junction apply to all chemical synapses. The neuromuscular junction is a particularly well-studied chemical synapse that provides a convenient model for how chemical synapses work. This chapter discusses the characteristics of the neuromuscular junction. The next chapter then considers some of the differences between the neuromuscular junction and synapses in the central nervous system.

TRANSMISSION AT A CHEMICAL SYNAPSE

Figure 5.1 summarizes the sequence of events during synaptic transmission at the neuromuscular junction. At the end of the axon of the motor neuron is a specialized structure called the **synaptic terminal**. When an action potential arrives in the synaptic terminal, depolarization produced by the action potential induces the release of chemical messenger molecules stored inside the terminal. At the vertebrate neuromuscular junction, the chemical messenger is **acetylcholine (ACh)**, whose chemical structure is shown in Figure 5.2. ACh is released from the synaptic terminal and diffuses across the space separating the presynaptic motor neuron terminal from the postsynaptic muscle cell. ACh depolarizes the muscle cell by altering the ionic permeability of the muscle cell membrane.

What neurotransmitter substance is released from the presynaptic motor nerve terminal at the neuromuscular junction?

Presynaptic Action Potential and Acetylcholine Release

An action potential in the synaptic terminal triggers the release of ACh. Depolarization during the action potential is the necessary stimulus for transmitter release. The coupling between depolarization and release is not direct, however, and is instead mediated by an influx into the synaptic terminal of calcium ions from the extracellular fluid (ECF).

How is presynaptic depolarization linked to the release of neurotransmitter?

Figure 5.1.

The sequence of events during transmission at a chemical synapse.

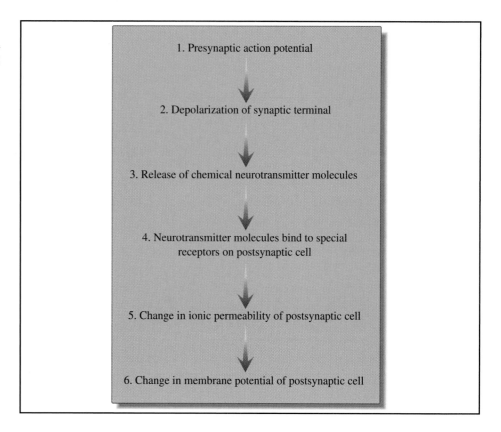

Although calcium is a relatively minor component of the ECF, its presence is required for the release of chemical neurotransmitters. If calcium ions are removed from the ECF, depolarization of the synaptic terminal no longer releases ACh. External calcium is necessary because calcium ions enter the synaptic terminal in response to depolarization and trigger the release of ACh.

Calcium is a divalent cation (Ca^{2+}) that must cross the membrane through ion channels. The membrane of the synaptic terminal contains calcium channels that are closed as long as the membrane potential is near its normal resting level. These channels open upon depolarization and close again when the membrane potential returns to rest. Thus, when an action potential invades the synaptic terminal, the calcium permeability of the membrane increases during the depolarizing phase of the action potential and declines again as membrane potential returns to normal.

The concentration of Ca^{2+} in the ECF is relatively low (approximately 1 mM), but the internal concentration of calcium ions that are free to diffuse across the plasma membrane is about 10,000 times smaller (approximately $10^{-7} M$). From the Nernst equation, we calculate that the equilibrium potential for calcium would be $+116$ mV (remember that $Z = +2$ for calcium). Therefore, both the concentration and the electrical gradients drive Ca^{2+} into the terminal, and calcium will enter the terminal when Ca^{2+} channels open. During a presynaptic action potential,

Figure 5.2.

The chemical structure of acetylcholine (ACh), the chemical neurotransmitter at the neuromuscular junction.

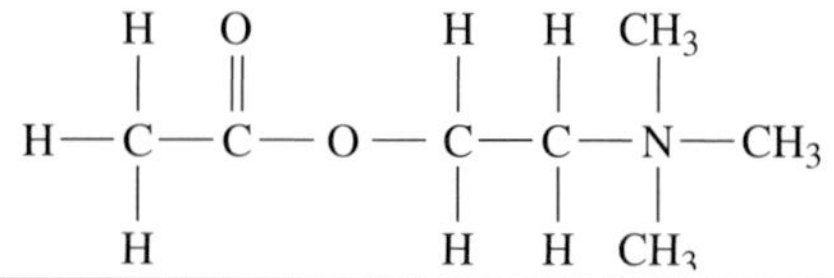

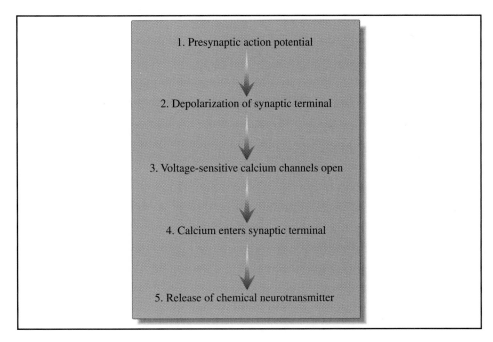

Figure 5.3.

The sequence of events between the arrival of an action potential at a synaptic terminal and the release of a chemical transmitter.

1. Presynaptic action potential

2. Depolarization of synaptic terminal

3. Voltage-sensitive calcium channels open

4. Calcium enters synaptic terminal

5. Release of chemical neurotransmitter

the opening of Ca^{2+} channels allows a spike of calcium to enter the terminal, resulting in the release of neurotransmitter into the extracellular space. Figure 5.3 summarizes this sequence of events.

Effect of Acetylcholine on the Muscle Cell

The goal of synaptic transmission at the neuromuscular junction is contraction of the postsynaptic muscle cell. ACh released from the synaptic terminal accomplishes this goal by depolarizing the muscle cell. Because muscle cells are excitable cells (like neurons), a depolarization that exceeds the threshold level will trigger an all-or-none propagating action potential in the muscle cell. The coupling between the muscle action potential and contraction is described in detail in Chapter 7. Here, we will focus on the mechanism by which ACh depolarizes muscle cells.

The region of muscle membrane where synaptic contact is made is called the **end-plate** region, which is illustrated in Figure 5.4. The end-plate membrane is rich in a transmembrane protein that acts as both an ion channel and a receptor molecule for ACh. Figure 5.4 shows the location of these ACh receptor molecules, which are situated strategically in the muscle cell membrane, just across from the sites of ACh release in the presynaptic terminal. Unlike the voltage-dependent channels discussed in Chapter 4, the ACh receptor channel is little affected by the membrane potential. Instead, the channel opens when it binds ACh. As shown schematically in Figure 5.5, the channel is closed in the absence of ACh. When ACh binds to the receptor, however, the protein undergoes a conformational change, and the channel opens, allowing ions to cross the membrane. Two ACh molecules must bind to the receptor before the channel will open. The ACh-binding site is highly specific, and only ACh or structurally similar compounds can bind to the site and cause the channel to open.

The ACh-activated channel of the muscle end-plate allows both sodium and potassium to cross the membrane equally well. Thus, ACh increases the permeability of the muscle cell to both sodium and potassium by the same amount. Figure 5.6

How does the neurotransmitter substance cause a change in the membrane potential of the postsynaptic cell?

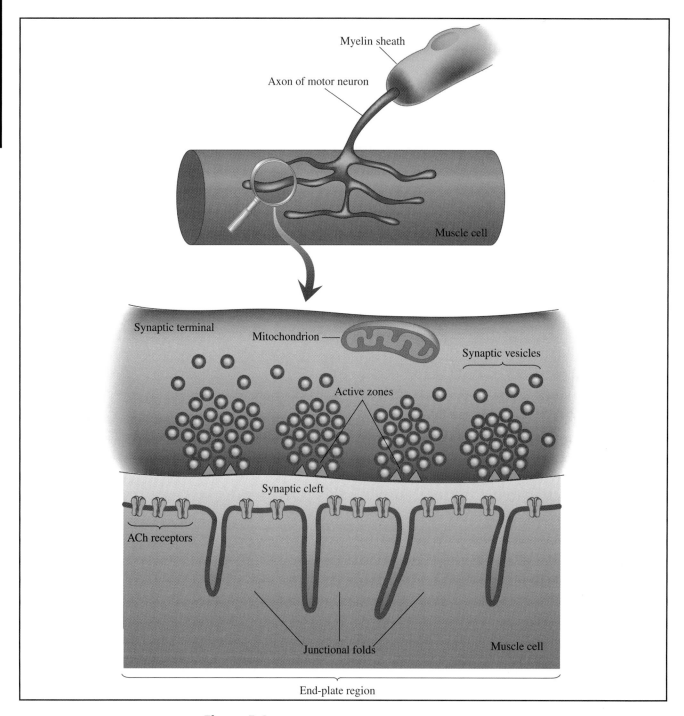

Figure 5.4.

The structure of the motor end-plate, illustrating the major structural features of the presynaptic and postsynaptic elements.

shows how this permeability change depolarizes the muscle cell. According to the Goldman equation (see Chapter 3), the membrane potential depends on the relative sodium and potassium permeabilities of the membrane. If the resting sodium-potassium permeability ratio (p_{Na}/p_K) is 0.02, we calculate that the resting membrane potential would be about −74 mV, assuming typical compositions of the ECF and intercellular fluid (ICF) (see Table 3.1). In the presence of ACh, the sodium and potassium permeabilities increase by equal amounts. For the example

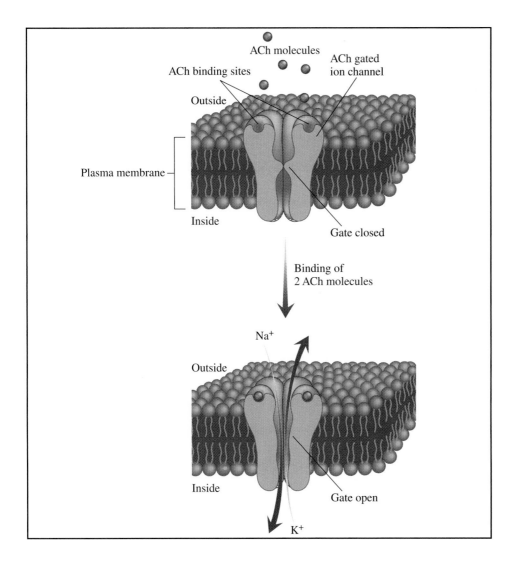

Figure 5.5.

Schematic representation of the behavior of the acetylcholine (ACh)-sensitive channel in the end-plate membrane. The binding of two molecules of ACh to sites on the channel opens the gate, allowing sodium and potassium ions to flow through the channel.

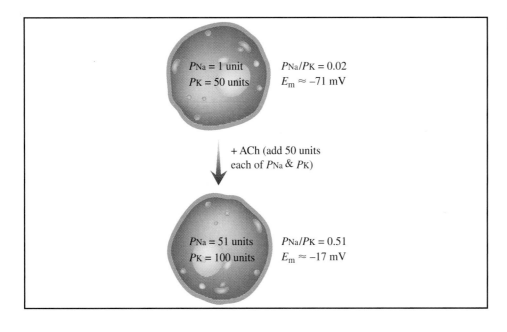

Figure 5.6.

Opening a channel that allows both potassium and sodium to cross the membrane results in a higher value for the ratio of sodium permeability to potassium permeability (p_{Na}/p_K) and causes depolarization.

shown in Figure 5.6, p_{Na}/p_K then becomes 0.51, and the membrane potential depolarizes to about -17 mV.

In a muscle cell, the ACh-activated channels are spatially restricted to the end-plate region, and therefore the permeability increase occurs in only part of the cell membrane. This situation is somewhat more complicated than the example in Figure 5.6, but the qualitative effect of an equal increase in sodium and potassium permeability would be the same. Because the resting sodium permeability is much smaller than the resting potassium permeability, adding the same amount to both will produce a much larger proportional increase in sodium permeability.

NEUROTRANSMITTER RELEASE

Acetylcholine Is Released in Multimolecular Quanta

We will now return to the synaptic terminal for a more detailed examination of the mechanism of neurotransmitter release. ACh is released from the motor nerve terminal in a multimolecular packet, called a **quantum**. Thus, the basic unit of release is not a single molecule of ACh, but the quantum. At the neuromuscular junction, a single quantum of ACh consists of approximately 10,000 molecules. An individual quantum is either released as a whole or not released at all. A "puff" of ACh molecules suddenly appears in the extracellular space as the entire contents of a quantum are expelled during synaptic transmission. A single presynaptic action potential normally causes the release of more than a hundred quanta from the synaptic terminal. Therefore, a strong postsynaptic depolarization during neuromuscular transmission is guaranteed by the sudden appearance of more than a million molecules of ACh in the extracellular space, just across from the ACh receptor molecules of the postsynaptic membrane (see Fig. 5.4).

Statistical analysis of the response of the postsynaptic muscle cell to action potentials in the presynaptic motor neuron gave rise to the idea that ACh is released in multimolecular quanta. This analysis, first carried out by P. Fatt and B. Katz, initiated a series of studies by Katz and coworkers that laid the foundation for our current understanding of chemical neurotransmission. Katz won the Nobel Prize in 1975, in recognition of his contributions. The key experimental trick that revealed the quantal nature of transmitter release was to reduce the extracellular calcium concentration to the point where a single presynaptic action potential released on average only one or two quanta of ACh instead of the usual hundred or more.

Figure 5.7 shows examples of depolarizations recorded in a muscle cell (called **end-plate potentials**) during a series of presynaptic action potentials. Because of the reduced Ca^{2+} concentration in the ECF, the end-plate potentials are much smaller than usual and do not reach the threshold for generating an action potential in the muscle cell. Under these conditions, the size of the depolarization of the muscle cell fluctuates considerably during the series of presynaptic action potentials. Sometimes the response is larger, and other times there is no response at all. Fatt and Katz measured a large number of end-plate potentials and found that the amplitudes clustered around particular values, shown in Figure 5.7B. These clusters were separated by approximately equal amounts of depolarization, and the separation was equal to the size of the smallest observed response. In Figure 5.7, for example, some end-plate potentials were 1 mV in amplitude, others were 2 mV, and still others 3 mV. These values are integral multiples of the smallest ob-

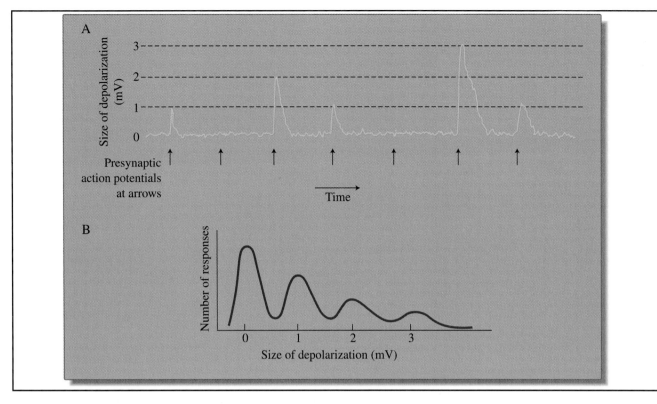

Figure 5.7.

Quantized responses of a muscle cell to action potentials in the presynaptic motor neuron, under conditions in which acetylcholine release is reduced by decreasing external calcium concentration. **A.** Examples of individual postsynaptic responses to presynaptic action potentials, which occur at the times indicated by the *arrows*. **B.** A graph showing the peak response amplitudes recorded in response to a series of several hundred presynaptic action potentials, like those shown in **A**.

served response (1 mV). This statistical behavior shows that the postsynaptic response is quantized in irreducible units of 1 mV. Fatt and Katz correctly surmised that the quantized postsynaptic response arose because presynaptic action potentials release ACh in quantal units corresponding to the amount of ACh required to depolarize the muscle cell by 1 mV. Thus, a presynaptic action potential might release three, two, one, or no quanta, but not one-half or one-and-one-half quanta.

Fatt and Katz also observed occasional small depolarizations of the muscle cell that occurred in the absence of presynaptic action potentials. These spontaneous depolarizations, called **miniature end-plate potentials**, were the same size and shape as the single-quantum response produced by presynaptic action potentials in low-calcium ECF. That is, if the irreducible unit of evoked muscle response was 1 mV, then the spontaneous events also had an amplitude of 1 mV. Therefore, miniature end-plate potentials result from the spontaneous release of single quanta of ACh from the synaptic terminal. Figure 5.8 shows spontaneous miniature end-plate potentials recorded in a muscle cell. Under normal conditions, spontaneous release occurs at a low rate—about one or two quanta per second. Any manipulation that depolarizes the nerve terminal increases the rate of miniature end-plate potentials, however, confirming that they represent spontaneous operation of the process that couples depolarization to quantal ACh release during presynaptic action potentials.

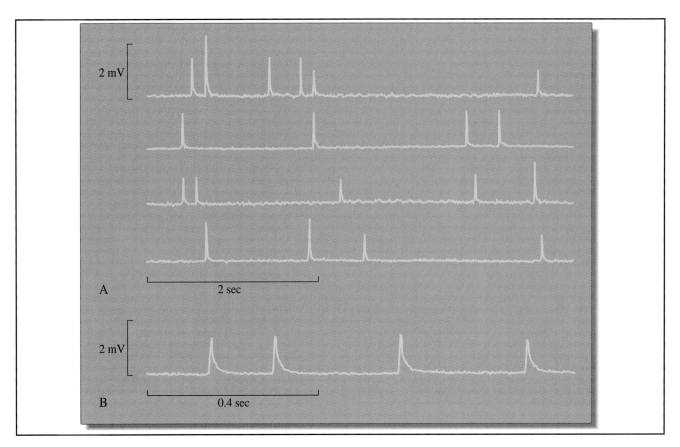

Figure 5.8.

Spontaneous miniature end-plate potentials recorded from the end-plate region of a muscle cell. These randomly occurring, small depolarizations of the muscle cell are generated by spontaneous release of single quanta of acetylcholine from the synaptic terminal of the motor neuron. **A**. Four 5-sec samples of muscle-cell membrane potential (Em), measured via an intracellular microelectrode placed near the end-plate region of the muscle cell. The spontaneous depolarizations occur at a rate of approximately one per second. **B**. Spontaneous miniature end-plate potentials viewed on an expanded time scale to show the shape of the events more clearly.

Synaptic Vesicle Exocytosis Accounts for Quantal Transmitter Release

Molecules of neurotransmitter are released into the synaptic cleft by what mechanism?

To understand the basis of the packaging of ACh in quanta, we must examine the structure of the synaptic terminal, shown in Figure 5.9. The terminal contains a large number of tiny, membrane-bound structures called **synaptic vesicles**, which contain ACh. The vesicles represent the packets of ACh that are released in response to a presynaptic action potential. A quantum of ACh (approximately 10,000 molecules) represents the number of ACh molecules contained in a single vesicle. Because synaptic vesicles are enclosed by a membrane, release of the neurotransmitter into the extracellular space requires the fusion of the vesicle membrane with the plasma membrane of the terminal. In other words, neurotransmitter is released by **exocytosis**.

Synaptic vesicles do not fuse with the plasma membrane indiscriminately. Instead, they fuse only at specialized regions, called **release sites** or **active zones**, that are located just across from the ACh receptor molecules of the postsynaptic muscle cell. Thus, quanta of ACh are released directly into the narrow space, the

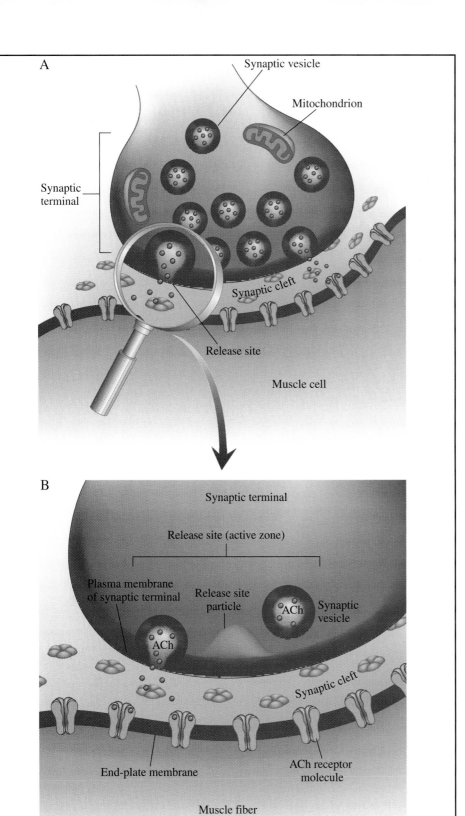

A

Synaptic vesicle

Mitochondrion

Synaptic
terminal

Synaptic cleft

Release site

Muscle cell

B

Synaptic terminal

Release site (active zone)

Plasma membrane
of synaptic terminal

Release site
particle

ACh

Synaptic
vesicle

ACh

Synaptic cleft

End-plate membrane

ACh receptor
molecule

Muscle fiber

Figure 5.9.

A schematic diagram of synaptic vesicles fusing with the plasma membrane to release acetylcholine (ACh) at the neuromuscular junction. **A.** Release occurs at specialized active zones in the presynaptic terminal. **B.** A close-up view of the active zone during release of Ach.

synaptic cleft, separating the presynaptic and postsynaptic cells. Figure 5.10 shows the structure of the active zone observed with freeze-fracture electron microscopy. The active zone of the presynaptic terminal is marked by a double row of large membrane particles, which likely represent membrane proteins (such as calcium channels) that regulate fusion of vesicle membrane with the plasma membrane. A double row of synaptic vesicles is located very near the plasma membrane, lined up along the active zone. These vesicles are available for rapid exocytosis when an action potential arrives in the synaptic terminal.

Evidence for exocytosis as the mechanism of ACh release has been obtained from freeze-fracture experiments. After a muscle and its attached nerve are rapidly frozen while ACh is undergoing release from the synaptic terminals, freeze-fracture electron microscopy reveals synaptic vesicles caught in the act of fusing with the plasma membrane, as shown in Figure 5.10C. The fusing vesicles appear as ice-filled pits or depressions in the presynaptic membrane, lined up along the active zones. Occasionally, fusing vesicles are also observed in terminals that are not stimulated (see Fig. 5.10B). These spontaneously fusing vesicles probably produce miniature end-plate potentials, like those illustrated in Figure 5.8.

Mechanism of Vesicle Fusion

The fusion of the vesicle membrane with the plasma membrane is not a unique feature of synaptic transmission. Many other cellular processes require intracellular vesicles to fuse with the plasma membrane. For instance, plasma membrane proteins are synthesized intracellularly within the Golgi apparatus and are then conveyed to their target sites by transport vesicles, which must then fuse with the plasma membrane to deliver their cargo. Also, secretion of substances to the extracellular space frequently occurs via exocytosis. The molecular mechanism of synaptic vesicle exocytosis shares common features with other forms of exocytosis. However, the requirement for a rapid triggering of exocytosis in response to a Ca^{2+} influx sets synaptic vesicle exocytosis apart from other forms of exocytosis. The delay time between a presynaptic action potential and the first appearance of the postsynaptic response is less than 0.5 msec. Therefore, there is little time for complex, multistage processes to prepare vesicles for membrane fusion. For this reason, vesicles must be placed very near the membrane at the active zone (see Fig. 5.10), ready for fusion when Ca^{2+} enters during an action potential.

Three membrane proteins play a central role in synaptic vesicle fusion: **synaptobrevin**, which is associated with the vesicle membrane; and two plasma membrane proteins, **syntaxin** and **SNAP-25** (synaptosome-associated protein of 25 kilodaltons molecular mass). These proteins bind to each other to form the **core complex**, which brings the vesicle in close proximity to the plasma membrane, as shown in Figure 5.11. Formation of the core complex is required for neurotransmitter release. It is not yet clear, however, whether the core complex is directly involved in fusion or plays a vital role in preparing vesicles for fusion, a process called **priming**. Energy to prime vesicles for fusion is provided by hydrolysis of ATP, which is carried out by an ATPase called **NSF** (N-ethylmaleimide-sensitive factor) that interacts with proteins of the core complex.

In other forms of exocytosis, fusion follows immediately after priming. Primed synaptic vesicles, however, must be prevented from fusing until the influx of Ca^{2+} triggers the process. Therefore, the molecular machinery of fusion requires a brake, which is removed when Ca^{2+} enters during an action potential. This role is carried out by **synaptotagmin**, a protein associated with the synaptic vesicle (see Fig. 5.11). Synaptotagmin includes two binding sites for Ca^{2+} and also interacts with

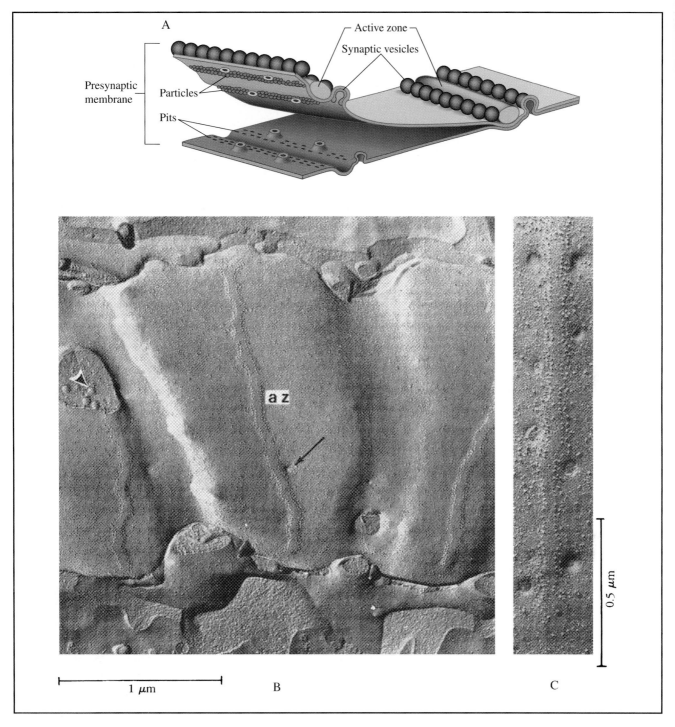

Figure 5.10.

Freeze-fracture electron microscopy reveals the structure of the active zone at the neuromuscular junction. **A.** An illustration of the components of the active zone and the fracture plane shown in the electron micrographs in **B** and **C**. **B.** An unstimulated nerve terminal. Note the double row of particles defining a presynaptic release site or active zone (*az*). The *arrow* points to a synaptic vesicle spontaneously fusing with the presynaptic membrane. Such spontaneous fusions presumably underlie the spontaneous miniature end-plate potentials shown in Figure 5.8. The arrowhead indicates a synaptic vesicle inside the synaptic terminal, revealed at a region where the fracture plane extends through the membrane and into the cytoplasm. **C.** A higher-power view of an active zone of a nerve terminal frozen during release of acetylcholine stimulated by presynaptic action potentials. The depressions arrayed along either side of the active zone represent synaptic vesicles in the process of fusing with the presynaptic membrane. **B** and **C:** Reproduced with permission from C.-P. Ko. Regeneration of the active zone at the frog neuromuscular junction. J. Cell Biol. 1984;98:1685–1695 by copyright permission of the Rockefeller University Press.

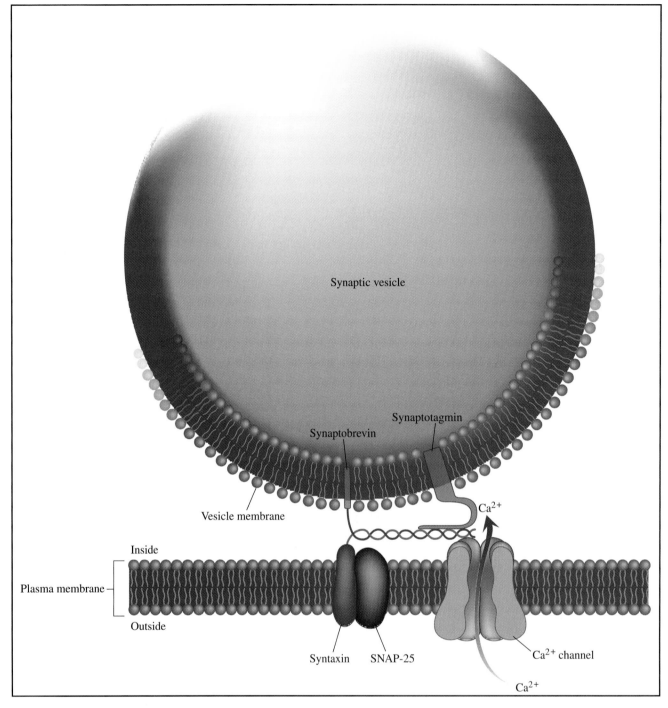

Synaptic vesicle

Synaptotagmin

Synaptobrevin

Vesicle membrane

Ca²⁺

Inside

Plasma membrane

Outside

Syntaxin   SNAP-25

Ca²⁺ channel

Ca²⁺

Figure 5.11.

Proteins of the synaptic vesicle and the plasma membrane. These proteins participate in synaptic vesicle exocytosis at the active zone in the presynaptic terminal.

the proteins of the core complex. This interaction prevents fusion from proceeding until calcium ions bind to synaptotagmin. If the gene for synaptotagmin is knocked out by genetic manipulation, rapid coupling between calcium influx and neurotransmitter release is lost.

The final component of the complex of proteins that regulate calcium-dependent fusion of synaptic vesicles is the calcium channel itself. Voltage-dependent calcium channels of the synaptic terminal directly bind to syntaxin, which is part of the core complex. Thus, the source of the calcium ions that trigger neurotransmitter release is held in close proximity to the calcium sensor molecule (synaptotagmin) and the rest of the fusion machinery.

Recycling of the Vesicle Membrane

When synaptic vesicles fuse with the plasma membrane of the terminal during transmitter release, the surface area of the terminal increases. With continued use, as more and more synaptic vesicles fuse with the terminal membrane, the area of the presynaptic terminal would become larger and larger. However, this expansion does not occur because the vesicle membrane does not remain incorporated into the plasma membrane. Instead, the added membrane is retrieved by endocytosis and recycled to form new synaptic vesicles, as summarized in Figure 5.12.

Retrieval of the vesicle membrane is thought to be carried out by **clathrin-mediated endocytosis**, which leads to the formation of **coated pits** that pinch off to form **coated vesicles**. Coated vesicles get their name because in the electron microscope, they appear to be covered with a fuzzy coat. Clathrin is a protein that forms a lattice in combination with other clathrin molecules and an adapter protein, called **AP-2**. The three-dimensional structure of this lattice is like a dome, which forms a scaffold around the coated vesicle. As the scaffold is constructed by the progressive addition of molecules of adapter protein and clathrin, the membrane attached to the lattice bulges inward to form a coated pit. Then, when the lattice is complete and the pit is ready to pinch off from the plasma membrane, another protein, called **dynamin**, provides the energy to complete the process of endocytosis and separate the coated vesicle from the plasma membrane. Dynamin is a GTPase, which binds and hydrolyzes the high-energy phosphate compound, guanosine triphosphate (GTP). In this regard, GTPases act much like ATPases, such as the sodium pump, except that the released energy is derived from GTP rather than ATP.

The importance of dynamin for endocytosis at the synapse is illustrated nicely by a *Drosophila* mutant called *shibire*, which bears a mutation in the gene encoding dynamin. The mutation causes replacement of an amino acid in the GTPase domain of dynamin, and the mutated protein is thermally unstable. Thus, if the temperature is elevated above approximately 32°C, dynamin unfolds and can no longer function as a GTPase. If temperature is restored to normal levels, dynamin refolds and regains its function. Behaviorally, *shibire* flies are normal at room temperature, but at temperatures above 32°C the flies become paralyzed. Without functional dynamin, synaptic vesicle membrane piles up in the plasma membrane of the synaptic terminal, vesicles cannot be recycled, and neuromuscular transmission fails when the existing pool of synaptic vesicles is exhausted. If the paralyzed flies are returned to room temperature, endocytosis starts again, coated pits are able to pinch off to form coated vesicles, and the flies "wake up" as new synaptic vesicles become available.

The clathrin coat of coated vesicles is disassembled, and the recycling vesicles are thought to fuse with each other inside the synaptic terminal to form an endosome. New synaptic vesicles then bud off from the endosome, as shown in Figure 5.12. To perform its function, the new vesicle must be refilled with neurotransmitter. This task is accomplished by special transporter molecules in the membrane of the synaptic vesicles, which actively accumulate neurotransmitter at high concentration inside the newly formed vesicles. The recycled vesicles are then ready for docking, priming, and a new cycle of exocytosis in response to presynaptic action potentials.

Figure 5.12.

The recycling of vesicle membrane in the presynaptic terminal at the neuromuscular junction. ACh = acetylcholine.

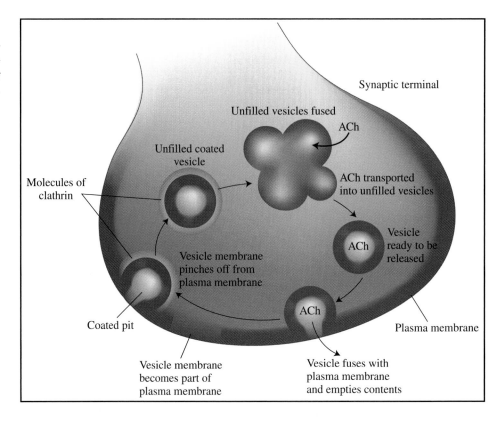

Synaptic terminal

Unfilled vesicles fused

ACh

Unfilled coated vesicle

Molecules of clathrin

ACh transported into unfilled vesicles

Vesicle membrane pinches off from plasma membrane

ACh

Vesicle ready to be released

ACh

Coated pit

ACh

Plasma membrane

Vesicle membrane becomes part of plasma membrane

Vesicle fuses with plasma membrane and empties contents

IN THE CLINIC

BOX 1

The neuromuscular junction is the gateway through which all communication between the nervous system and the skeletal muscles must flow. Because of this central position, the neuromuscular junction is both the target of clinically useful drugs and the root of clinically important diseases. For instance, blockade of neuromuscular transmission is often employed as an adjunct to general anesthesia in surgical operations that require immobility of the patient. Some drugs used for this purpose are derivatives of the naturally occurring poison curare, which occupies the acetylcholine (ACh) binding sites of ACh receptor molecules and prevents ACh itself from binding. Unlike ACh, curare does not cause the channel to open, however, and the result is paralysis of skeletal muscles.

Other drugs that block neuromuscular transmission block the action of acetylcholinesterase, the enzyme that degrades ACh at the neuromuscular junction. At first glance, it may seem that blocking acetylcholinesterase would potentiate the effect of ACh on the postsynaptic cell, not prevent it. However, without degradation, the ACh concentration in the synaptic cleft builds up to a steady level, the postsynaptic muscle cells are chronically depolarized, and subsequent further ACh release can no longer stimulate action potentials in the muscle. Thus, acetylcholinesterase inhibitors also cause muscle paralysis. Some forms of "nerve gas" are also acetylcholinesterase inhibitors.

A disease that involves the neuromuscular junction is myasthenia gravis, which is an autoimmune disease in which the body produces antibodies that attack ACh receptor molecules. These antibodies interfere with the postsynaptic response to ACh and lead to muscle weakness in affected patients. Another autoimmune disease that affects the neuromuscular junction is Lambert-Eaton myasthenic syndrome. In this disease, the antibodies are thought to interfere with the calcium

INACTIVATION OF RELEASED ACETYLCHOLINE

After ACh is released from the synaptic terminal and depolarizes the post-synaptic muscle cell, it must be inactivated somehow to restore the resting state. Inactivation is carried out by the extracellular enzyme acetylcholinesterase, which splits ACh into acetate and choline. Because neither acetate nor choline can bind to and activate the ACh-activated channel, acetylcholinesterase effectively halts the action of ACh.

ACh released from the synaptic terminal has two possible fates. Some of the released ACh molecules bind to ACh-activated channels, causing them to open and depolarizing the postsynaptic muscle cell. Other ACh molecules bind to acetylcholinesterase and are destroyed. ACh bound to the ACh-gated channels remains on the binding site for only about 1 msec. When an ACh molecule comes off the channel, it may bind again to an ACh-activated channel, or it might bind to acetylcholinesterase and be inactivated. With time following release, the concentration of ACh in the cleft rapidly declines until all of it has been split into acetate and choline by acetylcholinesterase.

Choline produced by hydrolysis of ACh in the synaptic cleft is taken back into the synaptic terminal, where it is reassembled into ACh by the enzyme choline acetyltransferase. Thus, both the vesicle membrane (the packaging material of the quantum) and the released neurotransmitter (the contents of the quantum) are effectively recycled in the synaptic terminal.

What is the role of acetylcholinesterase at the neuromuscular junction?

BOX 1

IN THE CLINIC (cont.)

channels of the motor nerve terminal, reducing calcium influx during action potentials and thus reducing the release of ACh from the synaptic terminal.

Many biological toxins also target aspects of neuromuscular transmission. For example, the fish-eating marine snail, *Conus geographicus*, injects its prey with a paralyzing venom containing a number of toxins, including omega-conotoxin GVIA, which blocks the voltage-dependent calcium channels of synaptic terminals. This prevents the release of neurotransmitter at synapses and effectively shuts down all neural communication in the prey. Another example is the poisonous snake, *Bungarus multicinctus*, whose venom includes a toxin (alpha-bungarotoxin) that binds to the postsynaptic ACh receptors that detect the release of the neurotransmitter ACh at the neuromuscular junction. Alpha-bungarotoxin blocks the ACh binding site of the receptor molecule, thus paralyzing the prey animal. The use of alpha-bungarotoxin to label ACh receptor molecules was illustrated in Chapter 1.

Clostridial neurotoxins are produced by bacteria of the genus *Clostridium*, including *Clostridium botulinum*, which causes the lethal form of food poisoning called botulism. Paralysis occurs in botulism because synaptic vesicles no longer fuse with the plasma membrane in response to presynaptic action potentials. Botulinum toxin is a mixture of several different proteins that enter motor nerve terminals and act as proteases. The toxins specifically attack proteins of the core complex necessary for synaptic vesicle docking and fusion at the active zone. Synaptobrevin, syntaxin, and SNAP-25 are all cleaved by different forms of botulinum toxin and are no longer able to drive exocytosis. The loss of neurotransmitter release in botulism provides strong evidence that the core complex plays a vital role in synaptic vesicle exocytosis.

RECORDING THE ELECTRICAL CURRENT FLOWING THROUGH A SINGLE ACETYLCHOLINE-ACTIVATED ION CHANNEL

When an ACh-gated channel opens, the flow of ions through the channel represents an electrical current flowing across the membrane. This minute electrical current through a single open ion channel can be measured directly using a technique called **patch clamp**, which is illustrated in Figure 5.13. A miniature glass pipette is

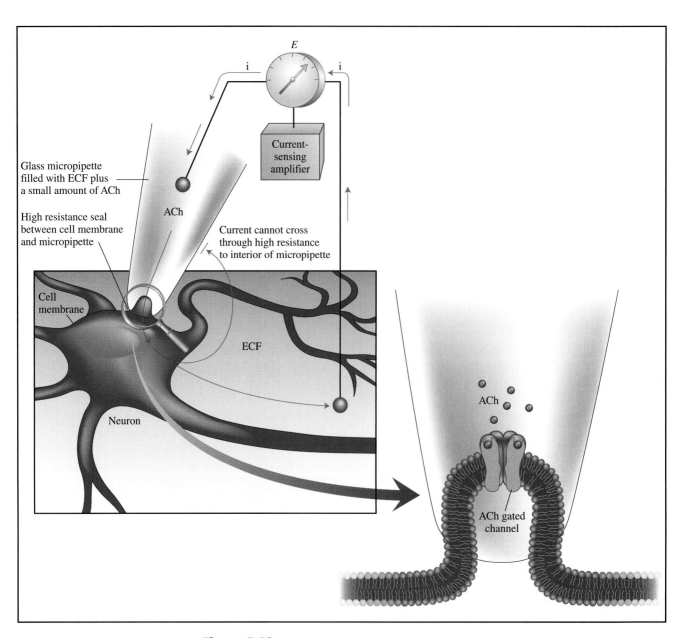

Figure 5.13.

The procedure for recording the current through a single acetylcholine (ACh)-activated channel in a cell membrane. A micropipette with a tip diameter of 1 to 2 mm is placed on the external surface of the membrane. A tight electrical seal is made between the membrane and the glass of the micropipette so that a resistance greater than 10^{10} ohms is imposed in the extracellular path for current flow through the channel. When a channel in the patch of membrane inside the micropipette opens, a current-sensing amplifier connected to the interior of the pipette detects the minute current flow (*red arrows*). ECF = extracellular fluid.

placed in close contact with the postsynaptic membrane so that a tight seal forms between the membrane and the glass. When an ion channel opens in the patch of membrane inside the pipette, the resulting ionic current is recorded by a current-sensing amplifier connected to the interior of the pipette. To detect the tiny current through a single channel, the electrical resistance of the seal between the cell membrane and the glass of the patch pipette must be greater than approximately 10^9 ohms—a very large resistance indeed. Fortunately, seal resistances greater than 10^{10} ohms can be readily obtained.

If a small amount of ACh is included in the solution inside the patch pipette, ACh-gated channels in the patch open when ACh binds. Figure 5.14A shows the expected current when a channel opens. A rapid step of inward current appears as

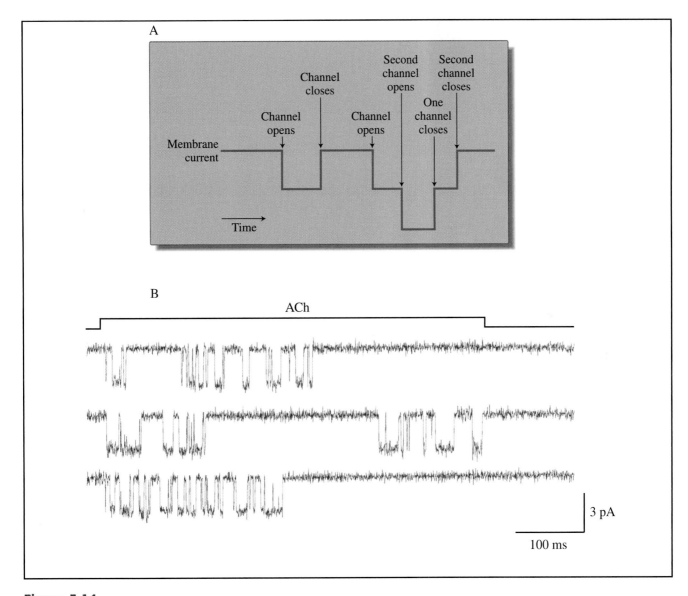

Figure 5.14.

The current through single acetylcholine-activated ion channels. **A.** A schematic diagram of the current expected to flow through a single acetylcholine (ACh)-activated channel if the conducting state of the channel is controlled by a gate that is either completely open or completely closed. When ACh binds, the channel opens and a stepwise pulse of inward current flows through the channel. When ACh unbinds, the channel closes and the current abruptly disappears. **B.** Actual recordings of current flowing through single ACh-activated channels. Part B provided by D. Naranjo and P. Brehm of the State University of New York at Stony Brook.

the channel opens, and the current continues at a constant level as long as the channel is open. The current terminates when ACh unbinds from one of the receptor sites, causing the channel to close. If a second channel opens while the first is still open, the two currents produce a current twice as large as the single-channel current (see Fig. 5.14A).

Actual patch-clamp recordings of currents through single ACh-activated channels are shown in Figure 5.14B. These recordings confirm directly the view of ion permeation and channel gating that we have used to explain the electrical behavior of neurons. Clearly, the gated ion channels carrying electrical current across the plasma membrane are not just figments of the neurophysiologist's imagination.

MOLECULAR PROPERTIES OF THE ACETYLCHOLINE-ACTIVATED CHANNEL

What is the molecular structure of the ACh receptor?

Techniques of molecular biology are being applied with great success to the study of ion channel function, particularly when these techniques are combined with measurements of single-channel behavior using the patch-clamp technique. The ACh-activated channel of the muscle end-plate is an aggregate of five individual protein subunits: two copies of an alpha-subunit, and single beta-, gamma-, and delta-subunits. Each of the four different subunit types is encoded by a separate gene in the muscle cell. The subunits come together as shown in Figure 5.15 to form the ACh-activated channel, with parts of each subunit forming the aqueous pore through which cations cross the membrane. The composition shown in Figure 5.15 represents the ACh-activated channel observed in muscle cells during embryonic development. In adult muscle cells, a different subunit, the epsilon-subunit, replaces the gamma-subunit.

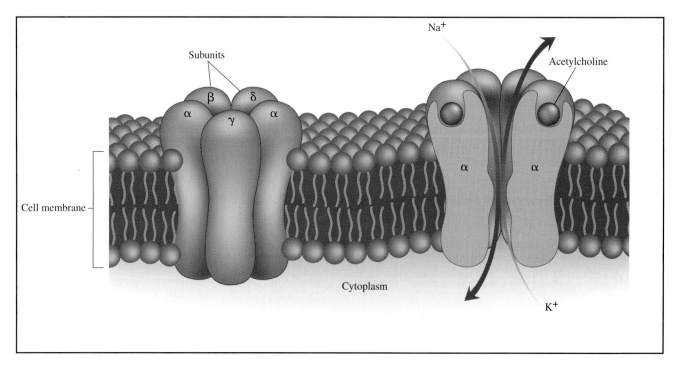

Figure 5.15.

The subunit structure of the acetylcholine-activated channel. The five subunits interact to form the gated ion channel of the end-plate membrane, with the pore at the center.

The genes encoding each of the subunits have been identified and analyzed, and the sequence of amino acids making up the protein has been deduced from the sequence of nucleic acids in the DNA. This sequence of amino acids gives valuable structural information about the ACh-activated channel, shown in Figure 5.16. Each subunit consists of four membrane-spanning segments, M1, M2, M3, and M4. The M2 segments of the five subunits form the lining of the pore at the center of the channel. Amino acids on the outer surface of each alpha-subunit form a binding pocket for ACh, in conjunction with neighboring gamma- or delta-subunits, as shown in Figure 5.16B. Each channel contains two alpha-subunits, and thus two binding sites, accounting neatly for the fact that binding of two ACh molecules is required to open the channel (see Fig. 5.5).

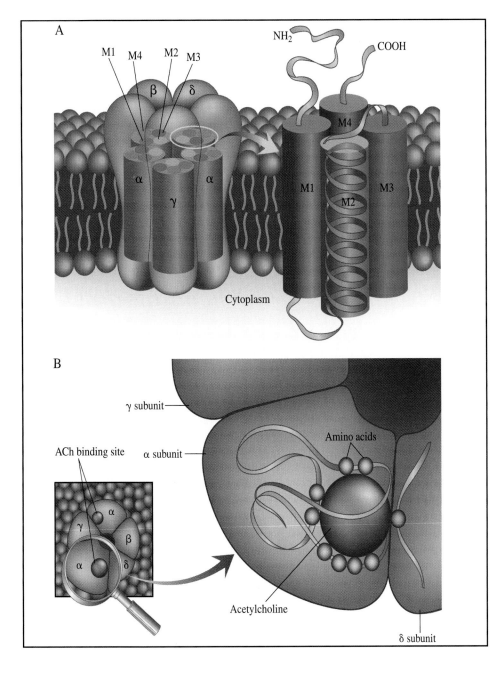

Figure 5.16.

The overall structure of the acetylcholine (ACh)-activated channel. **A**. Each of the five subunits consists of four transmembrane segments. The M2 segments of each subunit form the lining of the pore through which ions move across the membrane. **B**. The two binding sites for ACh are formed predominantly by amino acids of the two alpha-subunits of the channel. In addition, part of the binding site is contributed by the delta-subunit for one binding site and the gamma-subunit for the other.

Figure 5.17.

Summary of the sequence of events during synaptic transmission at the neuromuscular junction.

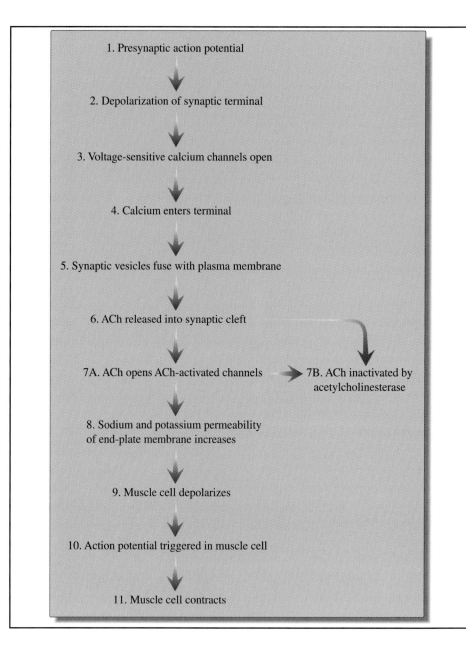

1. Presynaptic action potential

2. Depolarization of synaptic terminal

3. Voltage-sensitive calcium channels open

4. Calcium enters terminal

5. Synaptic vesicles fuse with plasma membrane

6. ACh released into synaptic cleft

7A. ACh opens ACh-activated channels → 7B. ACh inactivated by acetylcholinesterase

8. Sodium and potassium permeability of end-plate membrane increases

9. Muscle cell depolarizes

10. Action potential triggered in muscle cell

11. Muscle cell contracts

SUMMARY

The sequence of events during synaptic transmission at the neuromuscular junction is summarized in Figure 5.17. Calcium channels in the membrane of the synaptic terminal open during the depolarization produced by a presynaptic action potential. Calcium ions enter the terminal through the open channels, triggering synaptic vesicles filled with ACh to fuse with the plasma membrane facing the muscle cell. The released ACh diffuses to the muscle membrane and combines with specific receptor molecules in the postsynaptic muscle membrane. The ACh receptor molecule forms an ion channel that opens when ACh is bound, allowing sodium and potassium ions to cross the membrane. The muscle cell then depolarizes, which triggers an action potential in the muscle cell. The action of ACh is terminated by the enzyme acetylcholinesterase, which splits ACh into acetate and choline.

1. Why does the removal of calcium ions from the extracellular fluid prevent the release of chemical neurotransmitter substances?

2. Describe the experimental evidence for the idea that acetylcholine is released in multimolecular packets, or quanta.

3. List at least four protein molecules thought to be important in the docking and fusion of synaptic vesicles at the active zone, and describe the functional role of each protein.

4. How does opening an ion channel that is equally permeable to sodium and potassium ions cause depolarization of the muscle cell?

5. Draw the structure of the ACh-activated channel at the neuromuscular junction, label its constituent parts, and specify which parts form the binding site for ACh.

6. Briefly define each of the following: synaptic vesicle, synaptic cleft, active zone, clathrin, dynamin.

INTERNET ASSIGNMENT   CHAPTER 5

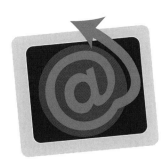

1 Much of what we know about acetylcholine release at the neuromuscular junction stems from work by Bernard Katz and his colleagues. Find information about Bernard Katz and describe his contributions.

2 Vesicle recycling is an important feature of synaptic transmission. Endocytosis of the vesicle membrane after exocytosis occurs by means of a protein called clathrin. Search the Internet for images that illustrate the role that clathrin plays in the vesicle recycling process.

SYNAPTIC TRANSMISSION IN THE CENTRAL NERVOUS SYSTEM

ESSENTIAL BACKGROUND

Ion permeability and the basis of the resting membrane potential (Chapter 3)

The Nernst and Goldman equations (Chapter 3)

Voltage-sensitive ion channels (Chapter 4)

ATP and GTP as sources for the synthesis of cyclic nucleotides

Aspartic acid
(Aspartate)

Chemical synapses between neurons operate according to the same general principles as the synapses between motor neurons and muscle cells discussed in Chapter 5. In the patellar reflex, for example, presynaptic sensory neurons activate postsynaptic motor neurons through a sequence of events similar to those occurring at the neuromuscular junction. However, despite the overall similarity between neuron-to-neuron synapses and neuron-to-muscle synapses, some important differences do exist. This chapter considers some of these differences, as well as the similarities.

EXCITATORY AND INHIBITORY SYNAPSES

At the neuromuscular junction, acetylcholine (ACh) depolarizes the muscle cell, causing it to fire an action potential. Synapses of this type are called **excitatory synapses** because the depolarization produced by the neurotransmitter brings the membrane potential of the postsynaptic cell toward the threshold for firing an action potential, which tends to "excite" the postsynaptic cell. The synapse between the sensory neuron and the quadriceps motor neuron in the patellar reflex is an excitatory synapse. Synapses between neurons are not always excitatory, however. At **inhibitory synapses,** the neurotransmitter tends to prevent the postsynaptic cell from firing an action potential, by keeping the membrane potential of the postsynaptic cell more negative than the threshold potential. Thus, the postsynaptic cell is "inhibited" by the release of the inhibitory neurotransmitter. The fact that not all synapses in the nervous system are excitatory is one major difference between synaptic transmission at the neuromuscular junction and synaptic transmission in the nervous system in general.

We will return to a discussion of inhibitory synapses later in this chapter and will focus now on the properties of excitatory synaptic transmission between neurons in the nervous system.

What is the difference between an excitatory synapse and an inhibitory synapse?

EXCITATORY SYNAPTIC TRANSMISSION BETWEEN NEURONS

The synapse at the neuromuscular junction is unusual in one important aspect: a single action potential in the presynaptic motor neuron produces a sufficiently large depolarization in the postsynaptic muscle cell to trigger a postsynaptic action potential. In such a "one-for-one" synapse, one action potential appears in the output cell for each action potential in the input cell. Most synapses between neurons are not so strong, however. Instead, a single presynaptic action potential usually produces only a small depolarization of the postsynaptic cell. The synapse between a single stretch-receptor sensory neuron and a quadriceps motor neuron is typical of this situation, as illustrated schematically in Figure 6.1.

Temporal and Spatial Summation of Synaptic Potentials

Figure 6.1A shows an experimental arrangement for recording the change in membrane potential of a motor neuron in response to action potentials in a single presynaptic sensory neuron. An intracellular microelectrode is placed inside the postsynaptic motor neuron, and presynaptic action potentials are triggered by electrical stimuli applied to the sensory nerve fiber. Figure 6.1B illustrates responses of the motor neuron to a single action potential in the sensory neuron and to a series of four action potentials. A single presynaptic action potential produces only a small depolarization of the motor neuron, called an **excitatory postsynaptic potential (e.p.s.p.).** A single e.p.s.p. is typically much too small to reach threshold for triggering a postsynaptic action potential.

If a second action potential arrives at the presynaptic terminal before the e.p.s.p. produced by the first action potential has dissipated, the second e.p.s.p. will sum with the first to produce a larger peak postsynaptic depolarization. As shown in Figure 6.1B, the e.p.s.p.'s produced by a rapid series of presynaptic action potentials can add up sufficiently to reach threshold for triggering a postsynaptic action potential. **Temporal summation** of sequential postsynaptic effects of an individual

In what ways do excitatory postsynaptic potentials summate to reach threshold for firing a postsynaptic action potential?

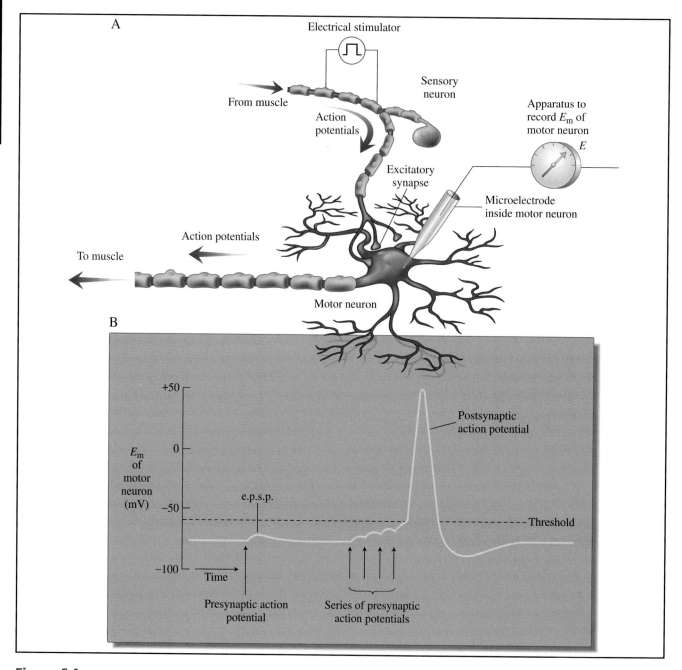

Figure 6.1.

Synaptic transmission at an excitatory synapse between two neurons. **A**. An experimental arrangement for examining transmission between a sensory and a motor neuron in the patellar reflex loop. **B**. Responses of the postsynaptic motor neuron to action potentials in the presynaptic sensory neuron. At the *upward arrows*, action potentials are triggered in the presynaptic neuron by an electrical stimulus.

presynaptic input is an important mechanism that allows even a weak excitatory synaptic input to stimulate an action potential in a postsynaptic cell.

Figure 6.2 shows a recording of an e.p.s.p. in a motor neuron produced by an action potential in a single sensory neuron. In this experiment, an intracellular electrode was placed inside the sensory fiber to record the presynaptic membrane potential and to inject depolarizing current that elicited an action potential in the presynaptic fiber. A second intracellular microelectrode in the motor neuron recorded the change in membrane potential of the postsynaptic cell. Note that the single e.p.s.p. is only about 1 mV in amplitude, which is much smaller than the 10- to 20-mV depolarization required to reach threshold. Thus, summation of e.p.s.p.'s is required to trigger a postsynaptic action potential in the motor neuron.

Temporal summation of e.p.s.p.'s is illustrated in the intracellular recordings shown in Figure 6.3, which were obtained from a motor neuron of the sympathetic

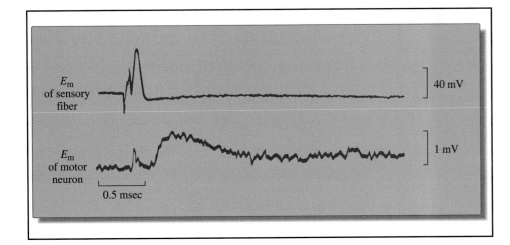

Figure 6.2.

Simultaneous intracellular recordings from a single stretch-sensitive sensory nerve fiber and a motor neuron receiving synaptic input from the sensory fiber. The upper trace shows an action potential triggered in the sensory fiber by passing a depolarizing electrical current through the intracellular electrode. After a brief delay, a small excitatory postsynaptic potential was evoked in the postsynaptic motor neuron (lower trace). Note the different voltage scales for the two traces. Data provided by W. Collins, M. Honig, and L. Mendell, State University of New York at Stony Brook.

nervous system. Each set of traces in the figure consists of superimposed responses to three postsynaptic stimuli. In each case, one stimulus fails to activate the presynaptic input and so produces no postsynaptic response (trace a), one stimulus produces a postsynaptic response that fails to reach threshold (trace b), and one stimulus produces a postsynaptic response that reaches threshold (trace c). Only if the successive e.p.s.p.'s summate sufficiently to reach threshold is an action potential triggered in the postsynaptic cell.

Another way that e.p.s.p.'s can sum to reach threshold is via the simultaneous firing of action potentials by several presynaptic neurons. A single neuron in the

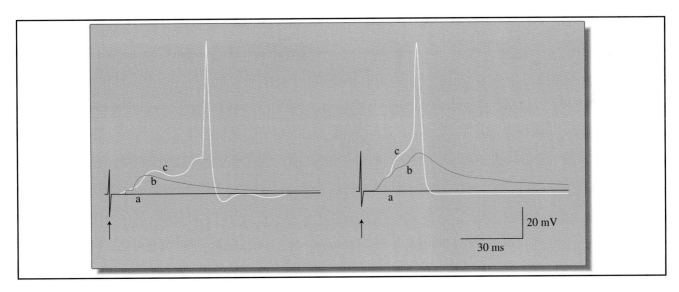

Figure 6.3.

Intracellular recordings of excitatory postsynaptic potentials (e.p.s.p.) in a neuron, showing summation of successive e.p.s.p.'s. Each set of traces shows three superimposed responses. The *arrow* indicates the electrical stimulus that triggered action potentials in the presynaptic neurons making excitatory synaptic contact with the recorded cell. Trace a (*black*) in each set shows a stimulus that failed to trigger the presynaptic input. Trace b (*red*) shows e.p.s.p.'s that failed to sum sufficiently to reach threshold. Trace c (*white*) shows summated e.p.s.p.'s that reached threshold and produced a postsynaptic action potential. In this experiment, the postsynaptic cell is a motor neuron of the sympathetic nervous system. Drawn from data provided by H.-S. Wang and D. McKinnon, State University of New York at Stony Brook.

nervous system commonly receives synaptic inputs from hundreds or even thousands of presynaptic neurons. In the patellar reflex, for example, a single quadriceps motor neuron will receive excitatory synaptic connections from many stretch receptor sensory neurons, shown schematically in Figure 6.4A. An action potential in a single presynaptic cell produces only a small postsynaptic depolarization, as we have seen. If several presynaptic cells fire simultaneously, however, their postsynaptic effects sum together and can reach threshold (see Fig. 6.4B). This **spatial summation** of e.p.s.p.'s occurs when several spatially distinct synaptic inputs are active nearly simultaneously.

In the patellar reflex, both temporal and spatial summation are important in eliciting the reflexive response. To produce reflexive contraction of the quadriceps muscle, a tap to the patellar tendon must stretch the muscle sufficiently to fire a rapid series of action potentials in each of a number of individual sensory neurons. The combination of the temporal summation of the effects of action potentials within the series and the spatial summation of the effects of all of the individual sensory neurons ensures that postsynaptic motor neurons fire action potentials and trigger muscle contraction.

Some Possible Excitatory Neurotransmitters

The chemical neurotransmitter at the neuromuscular junction is ACh, as discussed in Chapter 5. ACh is also used as a neurotransmitter at some neuron-to-neuron synapses. In addition, many other substances act as neurotransmitters at excitatory synapses in the nervous system. The molecular structures of a representative sample of excitatory neurotransmitter substances are shown in Figure 6.5. Many excitatory neurotransmitters are relatively small molecules, often derived from amino acids by simple chemical modifications. Amino acids are more commonly thought of as the basic building blocks for the construction of proteins. In the nervous system, however, amino acids are also often used for cell-to-cell signaling in neurotransmission. For example, glutamate and aspartate are unmodified amino acids, norepinephrine and dopamine are derived from the amino acid tyrosine, and serotonin is derived from tryptamine. Glutamate is thought to be the excitatory transmitter at the synapse between the sensory and motor neurons in the patellar reflex.

Other neurotransmitters are more structurally complex than the small amino acid derivatives. These substances—called **peptide neurotransmitters**, or more simply **neuropeptides**—are formed from a series of individual amino acids linked by peptide bonds, like a small piece of a protein molecule. Indeed, neuropeptides are synthesized by neurons as larger protein precursors, which are then processed proteolytically to release the embedded neuropeptide fragment. An example of a neuropeptide is substance P, whose amino acid sequence is shown in Figure 6.5.

Conductance-Decrease Excitatory Postsynaptic Potentials

In most cases, the mechanism by which an excitatory neurotransmitter produces an e.p.s.p. in the postsynaptic cell is the same as that by which ACh depolarizes the muscle at the neuromuscular junction. That is, the transmitter opens channels in the postsynaptic membrane that are permeable to sodium and potassium ions. The altered balance of sodium and potassium permeability then depolarizes the postsynaptic cell.

Membrane potential is controlled by the ratio of sodium to potassium permeability (p_{Na}/p_K), as described in Chapter 3. Consequently, a depolarization might

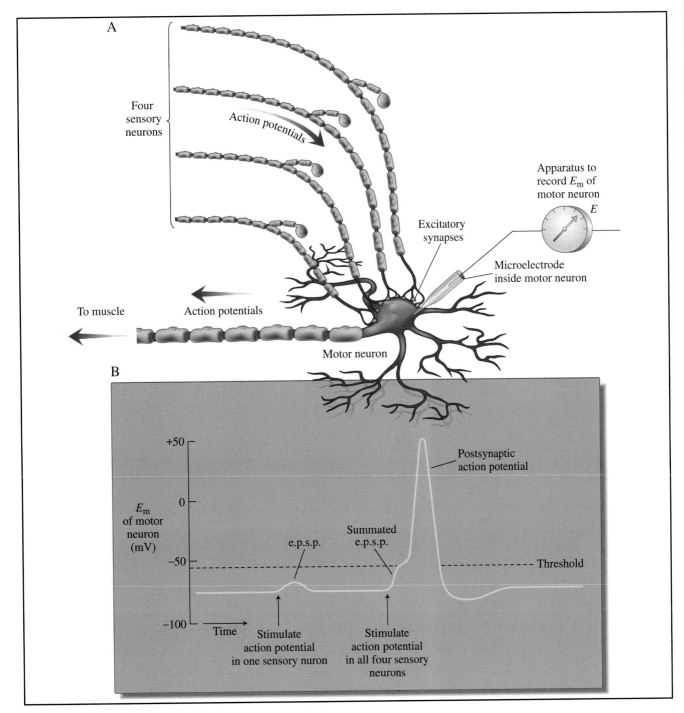

A

Four
sensory
neurons

Action potentials

Excitatory
synapses

Apparatus to
record E_m of
motor neuron

E

Microelectrode
inside motor neuron

To muscle

Action potentials

Motor neuron

B

E_m
of motor
neuron
(mV)

+50

0

−50

−100

e.p.s.p.

Summated
e.p.s.p.

Postsynaptic
action potential

Threshold

Time

Stimulate
action potential
in one sensory nuron

Stimulate
action potential
in all four sensory
neurons

Figure 6.4.

Spatial summation of excitatory inputs to a motor neuron. **A**. A diagram of the neural circuit and the recording configuration. **B**. The change in postsynaptic membrane potential
evoked by an action potential in a single presynaptic sensory neuron (first *arrow*) and by
action potentials in all four presynaptic sensory neurons (second *arrow*).

Figure 6.5.

Structures of some substances used as excitatory neurotransmitters in the nervous system.

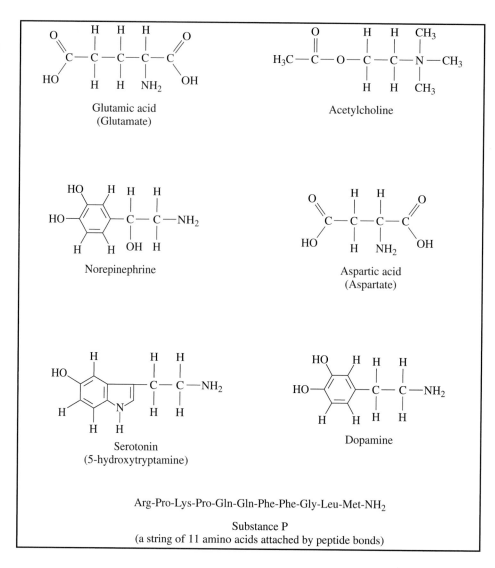

Glutamic acid
(Glutamate)

Acetylcholine

Norepinephrine

Aspartic acid
(Aspartate)

Serotonin
(5-hydroxytryptamine)

Dopamine

Arg-Pro-Lys-Pro-Gln-Gln-Phe-Phe-Gly-Leu-Met-NH$_2$

Substance P
(a string of 11 amino acids attached by peptide bonds)

result from either an increase in sodium permeability or a decrease in potassium permeability. Indeed, at some excitatory synapses, the e.p.s.p. is produced by a reduction in postsynaptic potassium permeability. For instance, ACh produces a long-lasting depolarization of sympathetic ganglion neurons in the frog, caused by a decrease in the potassium permeability of the neuron. ACh closes a type of potassium channel in the neuron membrane, so that outward potassium current declines and the resting inward sodium current exerts a greater influence on the membrane potential.

INHIBITORY SYNAPTIC TRANSMISSION

The Synapse Between Sensory Neurons and Antagonist Motor Neurons in the Patellar Reflex

In the patellar reflex, muscles other than the quadriceps muscle must be taken into account for a more complete description, shown in Figure 6.6. Whereas the quadriceps muscle extends the knee joint, antagonistic muscles at the back of the thigh flex the knee joint. These flexor muscles also have a stretch reflex analogous

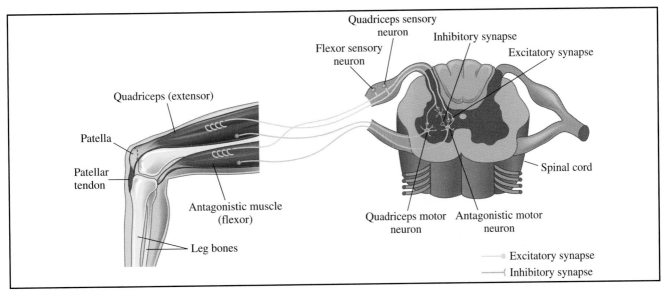

Figure 6.6.

A revised diagram of the circuitry involved in stretch reflexes of thigh muscles.

to that of the quadriceps. That is, stretching the flexor muscle stimulates action potentials in stretch-sensitive sensory neurons, which then make excitatory synaptic connections in the spinal cord with motor neurons of the flexor muscle. When the patellar tendon is tapped, the quadriceps muscle reflexively contracts, causing the knee joint to extend (the "jerk" of the knee-jerk reflex). Extension of the joint stretches the flexor muscles at the back of the thigh, which should then contract because of the action of their own stretch-reflex mechanism. The resulting flexion of the joint should again stretch the quadriceps and elicit reflexive extension, which should elicit another reflexive flexion, and so on. Thus, a single tap to the patellar tendon would send the knee joint into a series of oscillations that would continue until muscle exhaustion sets in.

You might ask, then, why tapping the patellar tendon elicits only a single knee jerk. The answer lies in the neuronal circuitry diagrammed in Figure 6.6. The nerve fibers of the stretch-sensitive sensory neurons from the quadriceps muscle branch profusely when they enter the spinal cord, making synaptic connections with many kinds of neurons in addition to quadriceps motor neurons. As shown in Figure 6.6, the sensory neuron makes an excitatory synaptic contact with interneurons that in turn make inhibitory synaptic contact with motor neurons of the antagonistic muscles. Thus, action potentials in quadriceps sensory neurons not only excite quadriceps motor neurons but also indirectly prevent antagonistic motor neurons from being excited by antagonistic sensory neurons.

Characteristics of Inhibitory Synaptic Transmission

We will now consider some of the properties of postsynaptic responses at an inhibitory synapse and then discuss the underlying mechanisms in the postsynaptic membrane. Figure 6.7 shows schematically an experimental arrangement to examine the inhibition of the antagonistic motor neuron in the patellar reflex. An intracellular microelectrode monitors the membrane potential of the motor neuron, while the inhibitory presynaptic neuron is stimulated electrically to fire action potentials.

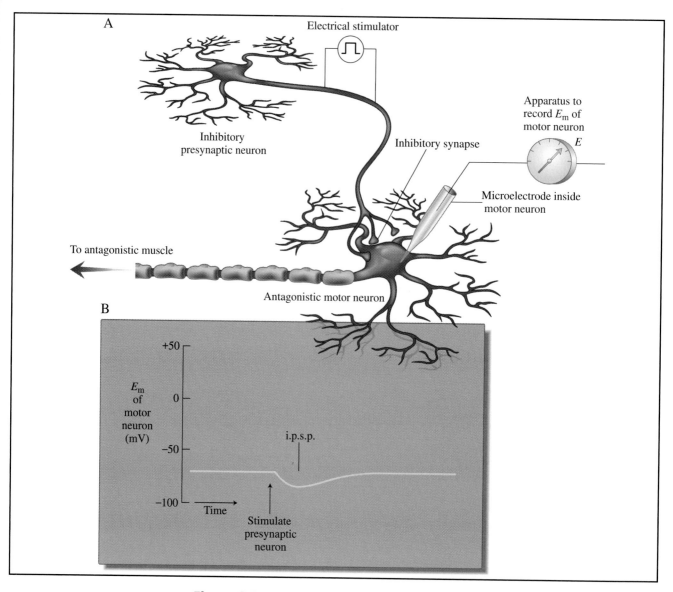

Figure 6.7.

Inhibitory synaptic transmission between two neurons in the circuit shown in Figure 6.6. **A.** A diagram of the neural circuit and the experimental arrangement. **B.** An action potential in the presynaptic neuron releases a neurotransmitter that hyperpolarizes the postsynaptic neuron.

Release of a neurotransmitter at the inhibitory synapse follows the same basic scheme as at other chemical synapses: depolarization produced by the presynaptic action potential stimulates calcium entry through voltage-sensitive calcium channels, inducing synaptic vesicles containing the neurotransmitter to fuse with the membrane and release their contents. However, Figure 6.7B shows that the postsynaptic effect of the neurotransmitter differs from the action of ACh at the neuromuscular junction. An action potential in the presynaptic cell is followed by a transient increase in the postsynaptic membrane potential. When the membrane potential becomes more negative, the cell is said to be **hyperpolarized**. Because hyperpolarization moves the membrane potential away from the threshold for firing an action potential, an excitatory input is less likely to trigger an action potential and the postsynaptic cell is inhibited. The hyperpolarization of the postsynaptic cell caused by the inhibitory neurotransmitter is called an **inhibitory postsynaptic potential (i.p.s.p.)**.

Mechanism of Inhibition in the Postsynaptic Membrane

We have seen repeatedly that changes in membrane potential are produced by changes in ionic permeability of the plasma membrane. The i.p.s.p. is no different in this regard. When the permeability of the membrane to a particular ion increases, the membrane potential tends to move toward the equilibrium potential for that ion.

What changes in postsynaptic permeability could produce an inhibitory postsynaptic potential in a neuron?

To see how a hyperpolarizing response might result from a change in ionic permeability, consider the situation diagrammed in Figure 6.8. If potassium permeability of a cell membrane increases, the membrane potential would move toward E_K, which is approximately −85 mV for a typical mammalian cell (see Chapter 3). In this situation, p_{Na}/p_K would be smaller than usual, and the balance between potassium and sodium would be struck closer to the potassium equilibrium potential (E_K). Note that a similar situation arises during the undershoot at the end of an action potential, when p_{Na}/p_K is transiently smaller than normal. Therefore, an inhibitory transmitter could hyperpolarize the postsynaptic cell by opening potassium channels in the postsynaptic membrane, as shown in Figure 6.8B. When the inhibitory neurotransmitter molecules bind to specific binding sites associated with the channel, the gate controlling movement through the channel opens, and potassium ions can move out of the cell, driving the membrane potential closer to E_K.

At many inhibitory synapses, however, the transmitter-activated postsynaptic channels are not potassium channels. Instead, inhibitory neurotransmitters commonly open postsynaptic chloride channels, as illustrated schematically in Figure 6.9. In many neurons, the chloride equilibrium potential (E_{Cl}), is maintained more negative than the resting membrane potential by chloride pumps in the plasma membrane. An increase in chloride permeability will drive the membrane potential toward E_{Cl} and hyperpolarize the neuron. Thus, opening chloride channels can produce an i.p.s.p. in a postsynaptic cell.

In general, inhibition of a postsynaptic cell results when a neurotransmitter increases permeability to an ion whose equilibrium potential is more negative than the threshold potential for triggering an action potential. If the equilibrium potential for an ion is more negative than threshold, the ion will oppose any attempt to reach threshold as soon as the depolarization exceeds the ion's equilibrium potential. Thus, it is possible that inhibition could occur without any visible change in membrane potential from the resting level. For example, if E_{Cl} is equal to the resting potential, then opening a chloride channel would cause no change in membrane potential. However, if an excitatory input is activated, the size of the resulting e.p.s.p. would be reduced because of the enhanced ability of chloride ions to oppose depolarization.

Some Possible Inhibitory Neurotransmitters

Figure 6.10 shows the structures of some inhibitory neurotransmitters in the central nervous system. Gamma-aminobutyric acid (GABA) and glycine are the most common transmitters at inhibitory synapses. Note that some of the molecules in Figure 6.10 also are excitatory neurotransmitters (see Fig. 6.5). A particular neurotransmitter substance may have an excitatory effect at one synapse but an inhibitory effect at another. Whether a neurotransmitter is excitatory or inhibitory at a particular synapse depends on the type of ion channel it opens in the postsynaptic membrane. If the transmitter-activated channel is a sodium or a sodium-potassium channel (as at the neuromuscular junction), an e.p.s.p. will result and the postsynaptic cell will be excited. If the transmitter-activated channel is a chloride

Figure 6.8.

The mechanism by which increasing potassium permeability produces an inhibitory postsynaptic potential in a postsynaptic neuron. **A.** The membrane potential (E_m) moves toward the potassium equilibrium potential (E_K) when potassium permeability (p_K) increases. **B.** At an inhibitory synapse, neurotransmitter molecules may act by opening potassium channels in the plasma membrane of a postsynaptic neuron. Efflux of potassium ions through the open channel then drives the membrane potential toward E_K. p_{Na}/p_K = sodium-potassium permeability ratio.

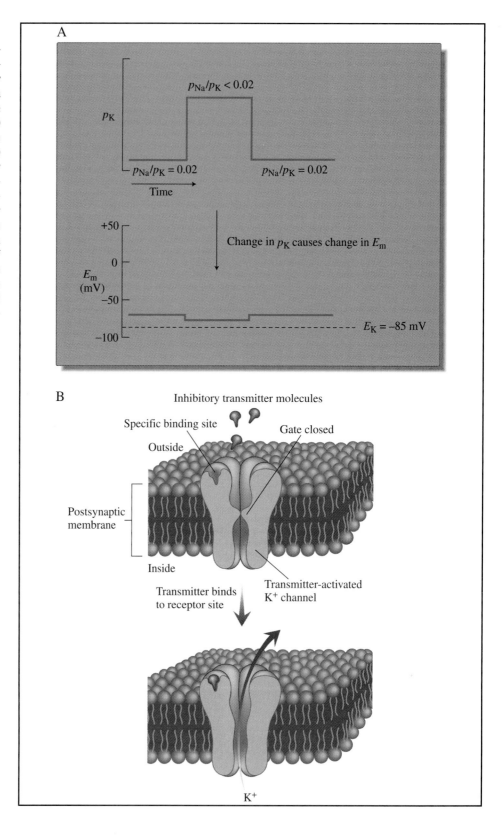

A

p_K

$p_{Na}/p_K < 0.02$

$p_{Na}/p_K = 0.02$

$p_{Na}/p_K = 0.02$

Time

Change in p_K causes change in E_m

E_m (mV)

+50

0

−50

−100

$E_K = -85$ mV

B

Inhibitory transmitter molecules

Specific binding site

Gate closed

Outside

Postsynaptic membrane

Inside

Transmitter-activated K⁺ channel

Transmitter binds to receptor site

K⁺

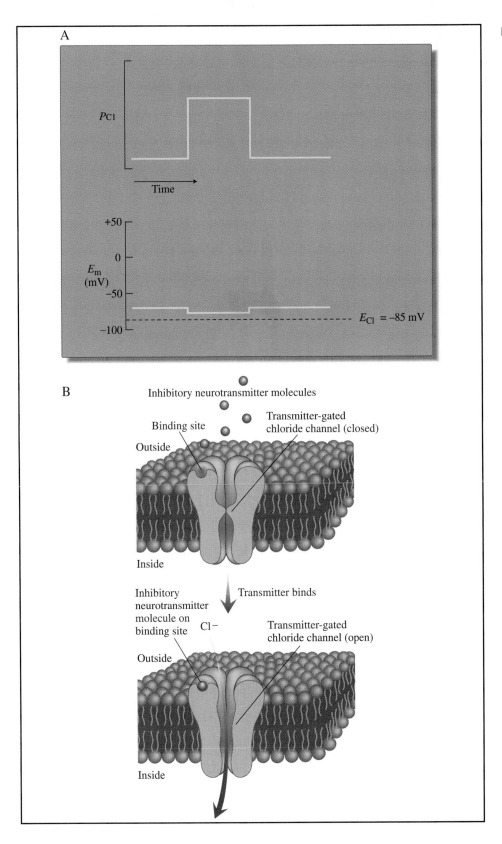

Figure 6.9.

The mechanism by which increasing chloride permeability (P_{Cl}) produces an inhibitory postsynaptic potential in a postsynaptic neuron. **A.** The membrane potential (E_m) moves toward the chloride equilibrium potential (E_{Cl}) when chloride permeability increases. **B.** At an inhibitory synapse, neurotransmitter molecules commonly act by opening chloride channels in the plasma membrane of a postsynaptic neuron. Chloride ions then enter the cell through the open channels to drive the membrane potential toward E_{Cl}.

Figure 6.10.

Structures of some substances that act as inhibitory neurotransmitters in the nervous system.

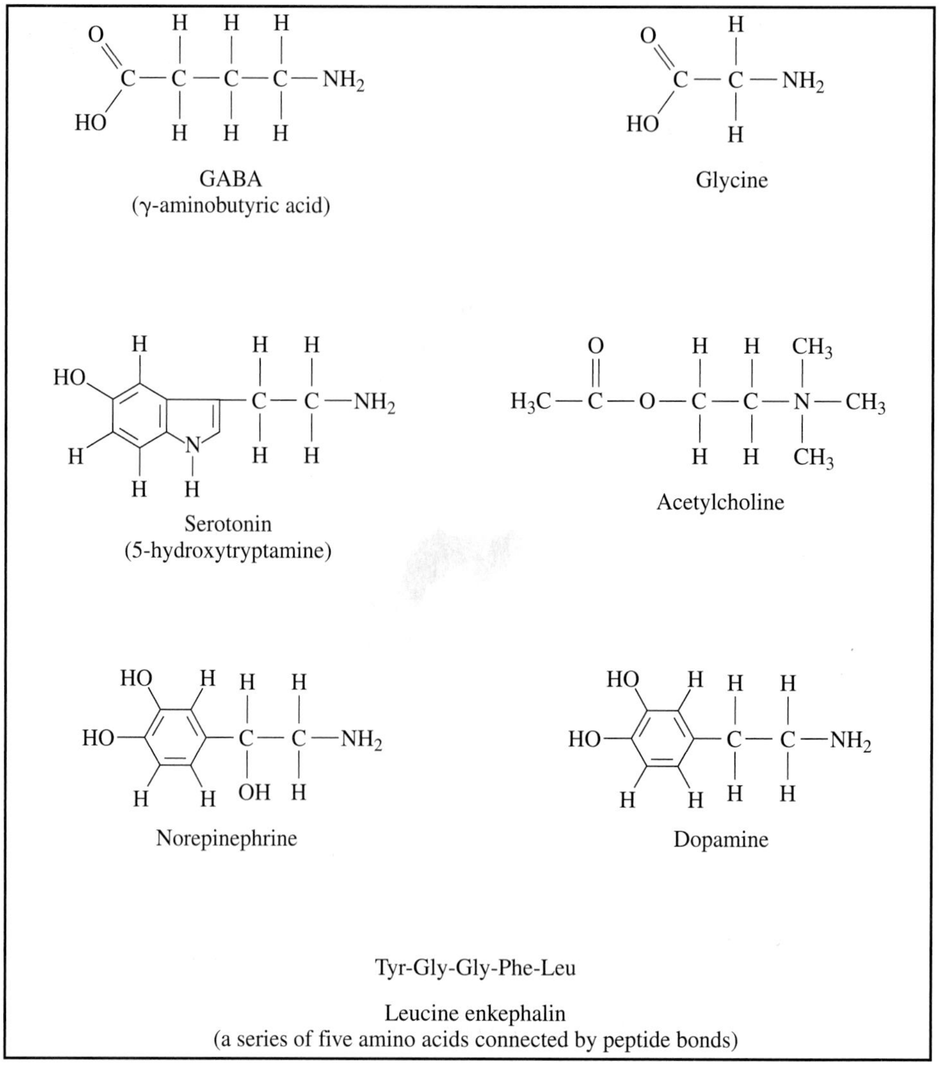

GABA
(γ-aminobutyric acid)

Glycine

Serotonin
(5-hydroxytryptamine)

Acetylcholine

Norepinephrine

Dopamine

Tyr-Gly-Gly-Phe-Leu

Leucine enkephalin
(a series of five amino acids connected by peptide bonds)

or potassium channel, the postsynaptic cell will be inhibited. The same neurotransmitter could even have opposite effects at two different synapses on the same postsynaptic neuron.

THE FAMILY OF NEUROTRANSMITTER-GATED ION CHANNELS

The ACh-gated channel at the neuromuscular junction is formed by the aggregation of several protein subunits (see Chapter 5). The ion channels that underlie excitatory and inhibitory postsynaptic potentials have also been studied at the molecular level. Like the ACh-gated channel, these ion channels are formed by aggregates of individual subunits, with each type of subunit encoded by a specific gene. The amino acid sequences of subunits making up the different neurotransmitter-gated channels are roughly similar. For example, GABA-activated channels are structurally similar to glycine-activated channels and ACh-activated channels; glutamate-activated channels also are related to ACh-activated channels, albeit more distantly. Therefore, the genes encoding the subunits of neurotransmitter-gated ion channels constitute a family of related genes, called the **ligand-gated ion chan-**

nel family. As the name implies, members of the family form ion channels that are opened by the binding of a chemical signal (the ligand) to a specific binding site on the channel.

Of course, there are also important functional differences among the members of this gene family. First, each channel type must be specifically activated by a particular neurotransmitter: a glutamate-activated channel is not activated by GABA, even though glutamate and GABA are structurally quite similar (see Figs. 6.5 and 6.10). (In fact, GABA is formed enzymatically by modification of glutamate.) Thus, the part of the protein that forms the neurotransmitter binding site must be unique for each type of ligand-gated channel. Second, the ion-conducting pore differs among

IN THE CLINIC

BOX 1

Neurotransmitters and their postsynaptic receptors are fundamental for the functioning of the nervous system. Pharmacologists are exploiting the wide variety of different neurotransmitter receptors found at different synapses in the nervous system to devise drugs that selectively target particular aspects of nervous system function. Many drugs that affect the nervous system act by either inhibiting or potentiating the action of natural neurotransmitters. This is especially true of psychoactive drugs, which alter behavior in important ways. An example is the tranquilizer diazepam (Valium), which is a member of a class of psychoactive drugs called benzodiazepines. Drugs of this class act by binding to a special binding site on GABA receptor molecules, the ligand-gated chloride channels opened in postsynaptic cells by the common inhibitory neurotransmitter GABA. When benzodiazepines bind to the GABA receptor, the action of GABA is potentiated, inhibitory postsynaptic potentials are larger and last longer, and the overall level of activity in the nervous system is "calmed down." Because of this potentiation of inhibitory synapses, benzodiazepines are also used as anticonvulsant drugs.

Conversely, drugs that block the action of inhibitory neurotransmitters produce runaway excitation in the nervous system and result in convulsions. An example is strychnine, which has been used for centuries as a poison to control rodents. This poison blocks glycine receptor molecules, the postsynaptic receptors at inhibitory synapses that use the neurotransmitter glycine. In the absence of glycine-mediated inhibitory postsynaptic potentials, the result is uncontrolled and uncoordinated neural excitation and death from convulsions.

Clinically useful drugs can also affect neurotransmitter function without directly interacting with the neurotransmitter receptor molecules. An example is the antidepressant fluoxetine (Prozac). This drug blocks the reuptake of the neurotransmitter serotonin, which is the principal method of terminating the action of serotonin that has been released from synaptic terminals in the brain. At the neuromuscular junction, the action of acetylcholine is terminated when the neurotransmitter is destroyed by the extracellular enzyme acetylcholinesterase. At many synapses in the brain, however, neurotransmitter action is stopped when released neurotransmitter is taken back into the presynaptic terminal by special pump molecules in the membrane of the terminal. Blocking these uptake pumps prolongs the presence of the neurotransmitter and potentiates the postsynaptic effect of the transmitter. Serotonin-releasing neurons are important in the regulation of emotion and mood, but it is not yet clear exactly what role they play or why blocking serotonin uptake improves depression.

members of the ligand-gated ion channel family. Some ligand-gated channels form cation pores (for example, glutamate-gated channels or ACh-gated channels), whereas others form anion pores (for example, glycine-gated or GABA-gated channels). This difference in ionic selectivity reflects underlying differences in how the pore region is constructed. Differences in the pore region determine whether the postsynaptic effect of opening the channel is excitation or inhibition.

INDIRECT ACTIONS OF NEUROTRANSMITTERS

The ligand-gated ion channels provide a direct linkage between neurotransmitter binding and the change in postsynaptic ion permeability. The binding site for neurotransmitter molecules is part of the ion channel protein. In addition, however, postsynaptic effects of neurotransmitters often involve an indirect linkage, in which neurotransmitter binding and the change in ion permeability are carried out by distinct protein molecules. Separation of neurotransmitter binding and the postsynaptic response allows a single neurotransmitter to have diverse effects on a postsynaptic neuron—closing one type of ion channel while opening others, affecting the metabolism of the postsynaptic cell as well as its membrane permeability, or altering gene expression.

The basic scheme for indirect actions of neurotransmitters is shown in Figure 6.11. Neurotransmitter molecules bind to a postsynaptic receptor molecule, as with ligand-gated ion channels. The receptor molecule is not itself an ion channel. Instead, the activated receptor molecule stimulates or inhibits production of an internal substance, called a **second messenger** (the neurotransmitter being the first messenger), that alters the state of the postsynaptic cell. Common second messenger molecules include

- Cyclic adenosine monophosphate (cAMP), which is produced from adenosine triphosphate (ATP) by the enzyme adenylyl cyclase
- Cyclic guanosine monophosphate (cGMP), which is produced from guanosine triphosphate (GTP; the guanine nucleotide equivalent of ATP) by the enzyme guanylyl cyclase

Figure 6.11.

An overview of the indirect linkage of a neurotransmitter to a change in postsynaptic ion permeability, by means of an intracellular second messenger in the postsynaptic cell.

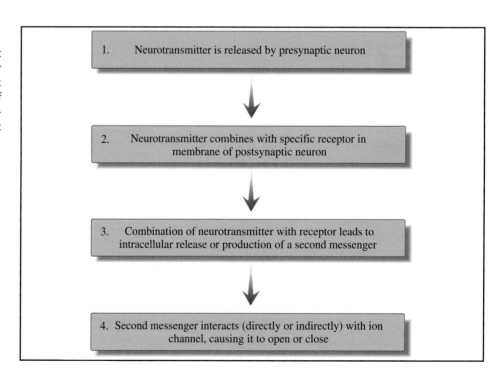

1. Neurotransmitter is released by presynaptic neuron

2. Neurotransmitter combines with specific receptor in membrane of postsynaptic neuron

3. Combination of neurotransmitter with receptor leads to intracellular release or production of a second messenger

4. Second messenger interacts (directly or indirectly) with ion channel, causing it to open or close

- The dual second messengers diacylglycerol and inositol triphosphate, both of which are produced from a particular kind of membrane lipid molecule by the enzyme phospholipase C
- Arachidonic acid, which is produced from membrane lipid molecules by the enzyme phospholipase A

Second messenger substances have a variety of effects in postsynaptic cells. Excitation results if the second messenger promotes opening of sodium channels or closing of potassium channels. Conversely, if the second messenger results in opening of potassium or chloride channels, or closing of sodium channels, then inhibition results.

The second messenger and the target ion channel are linked either directly or indirectly. In some cases, the second messenger molecule directly binds to the ion channel, causing it to open or close. For example, in photoreceptor cells of the retina, cyclic GMP directly opens sodium channels in the plasma membrane. In other instances, the second messenger acts indirectly, by activating an enzyme that then affects the ion channel. For example, cyclic AMP activates an enzyme called cyclic AMP–dependent protein kinase (or protein kinase A). Protein kinase A phosphorylates proteins, by attaching inorganic phosphate to specific amino acids in the protein. Phosphorylation is a common biochemical mechanism by which the function of proteins, including ion channels, is altered. For example, phosphorylation of voltage-activated calcium channels is necessary for normal operation of the channel. Thus, a neurotransmitter might indirectly affect calcium channels in a postsynaptic cell by altering the level of cyclic AMP and hence altering phosphorylation of the channels.

The activated neurotransmitter receptor molecule also is linked indirectly to enzymes that alter second messenger levels. The linkage involves a protein called GTP-binding protein (or G-protein). In its inactive state, guanosine diphosphate (GDP) is bound to the G-protein. The neurotransmitter receptor molecule catalyzes the replacement of GDP by GTP on the G-protein and thus activates the G-protein. The activated G-protein then stimulates the enzyme that produces the second messenger (adenylyl cyclase in the case of cyclic AMP, for example).

What role do G-proteins play in synaptic transmission?

Numerous varieties of G-proteins have been identified, each with specific effects on specific target enzymes. Some G-proteins stimulate the activity of the target enzyme, while others inhibit it. Thus, activation of one type of neurotransmitter receptor molecule might increase the level of a second messenger, whereas activation of a different receptor molecule might decrease the level of the second messenger, depending on the type of G-protein to which the receptor is coupled. In addition to acting via second messengers, activated G-proteins sometimes serve as a messenger that directly activates ion channels.

The indirect actions of neurotransmitters are summarized in Figure 6.12. This sequence can be envisioned as an enzymatic cascade, in which an activated neurotransmitter receptor acts as an enzyme to activate G-protein, which in turn activates an enzyme that produces a second messenger. The second messenger then activates another enzyme that affects ion channel operation. In this sequence, an ion channel might be affected at three different points:

- Activated G-protein might bind to and activate an ion channel.
- The second messenger might directly bind to the channel.
- An enzyme, such as a protein kinase, that depends on the presence of the second messenger might act on the ion channel.

In all cases, the net excitatory or inhibitory effect of the neurotransmitter depends on the type of ion channel affected in the postsynaptic membrane and on whether the ion channel is opened or closed by the indirect action of the neurotransmitter.

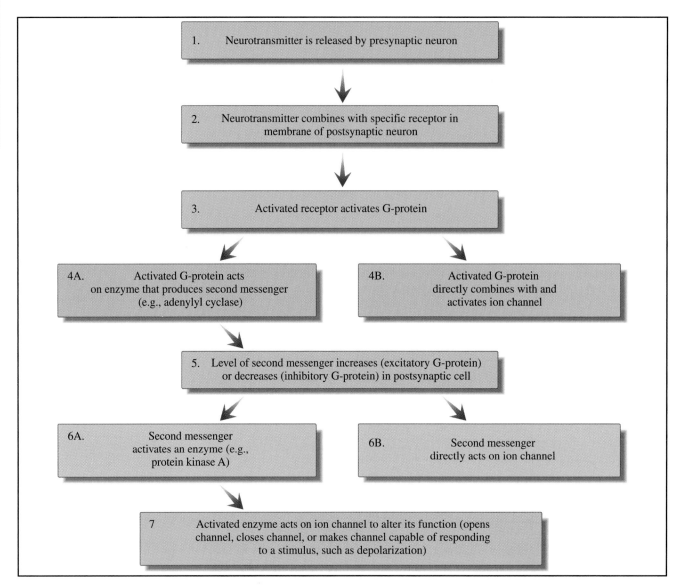

1. Neurotransmitter is released by presynaptic neuron

2. Neurotransmitter combines with specific receptor in membrane of postsynaptic neuron

3. Activated receptor activates G-protein

4A. Activated G-protein acts on enzyme that produces second messenger (e.g., adenylyl cyclase)

4B. Activated G-protein directly combines with and activates ion channel

5. Level of second messenger increases (excitatory G-protein) or decreases (inhibitory G-protein) in postsynaptic cell

6A. Second messenger activates an enzyme (e.g., protein kinase A)

6B. Second messenger directly acts on ion channel

7 Activated enzyme acts on ion channel to alter its function (opens channel, closes channel, or makes channel capable of responding to a stimulus, such as depolarization)

Figure 6.12.

The sequence of events in the indirect action of a neurotransmitter on membrane permeability of a postsynaptic cell. Ion channel activity may be altered when G-proteins, second messengers, or second messenger–dependent enzymes interact with the ion channels.

PRESYNAPTIC INHIBITION AND FACILITATION

What is presynaptic inhibition and how does it differ from conventional postsynaptic inhibition?

Inhibition in the nervous system is sometimes accomplished indirectly by targeting excitatory presynaptic terminals, instead of the postsynaptic cell. This type of inhibition, called **presynaptic inhibition**, is illustrated schematically in Figure 6.13. The inhibitory terminal makes synaptic contact with an excitatory synaptic terminal, which in turn contacts the cell to be inhibited. Inhibition is produced by decreasing the release of excitatory neurotransmitter by the excitatory synaptic terminal. The electron micrograph in Figure 6.13B shows a synaptic arrangement that might give rise to presynaptic inhibition.

Presynaptic inhibition often involves reduced calcium influx into the excitatory terminal during a presynaptic action potential. In some cases, reduced calcium influx during presynaptic inhibition results from a decreased size or duration of the depolarization during the presynaptic action potential, which could be accom-

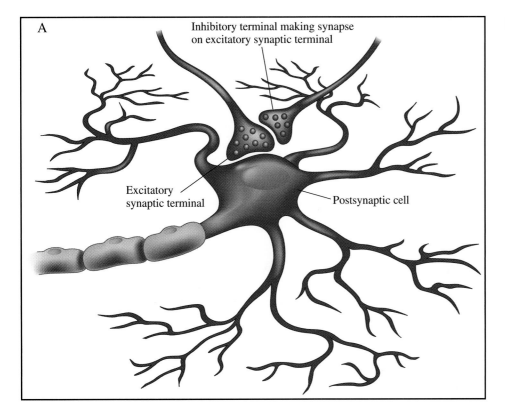

A

Inhibitory terminal making synapse on excitatory synaptic terminal

Excitatory synaptic terminal

Postsynaptic cell

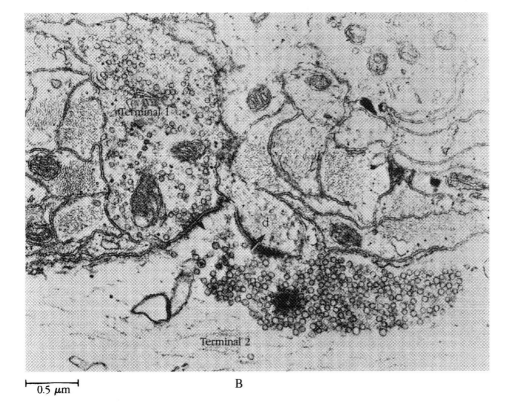

Terminal 1

d

Terminal 2

0.5 μm

B

Figure 6.13.

In presynaptic inhibition, inhibitory synaptic connections are made onto excitatory synaptic terminals. **A.** A schematic diagram of the arrangement for presynaptic inhibition in the nervous system. The inhibitory synaptic terminal makes contact with another synaptic terminal, rather than directly with the postsynaptic cell. **B.** An electron micrograph showing a possible presynaptic inhibitory connection in the nervous system. A synaptic terminal (terminal 1) makes contact with an axon (terminal 2) that in turn makes synaptic contact with a third neuronal process (labeled *d*, for dendrite). The *arrows* show the direction of synaptic transmission from terminal 1 to terminal 2 and from terminal 2 to the dendrite. Note the accumulations of synaptic vesicles in terminals 1 and 2. **B:** Reproduced with permission from W. O. Wickelgren. Physiological and anatomical characteristics of reticulospinal neurons in lamprey. J. Physiol. 1977;270: 89–114.

plished by activating potassium channels in the terminal. Smaller depolarization opens fewer voltage-sensitive calcium channels, and less calcium enters the excitatory terminal. In other cases, presynaptic inhibition involves a reduced opening of voltage-sensitive calcium channels, possibly by decreased phosphorylation of the channels.

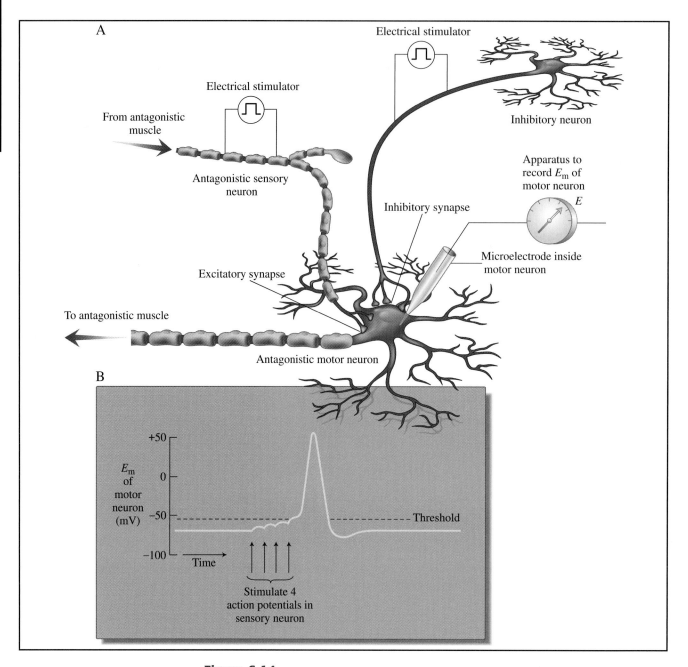

Figure 6.14.

The integration of excitatory and inhibitory synaptic inputs by a postsynaptic neuron. **A**. A schematic diagram of the experimental arrangement for the measurements shown in **B**, **C**, and **D**. **B**. Stimulation of the excitatory presynaptic neuron (the sensory neuron) produces a postsynaptic action potential if temporal summation is sufficient to reach threshold. **C**. Stimulation of the inhibitory presynaptic neuron prevents the excitatory inputs in **B** from reaching threshold. **D**. The inhibitory effect can be overcome by increasing the amount of excitatory stimulation. E_m = membrane potential.

A synapse onto a synapse, such as the arrangement shown in Figure 6.13, might also facilitate rather than inhibit the release of neurotransmitter from the excitatory terminal. Presynaptic facilitation is known to occur, for example, in the nervous system of a sea slug, *Aplysia californica*. The neurotransmitter serotonin increases the effectiveness of an excitatory synaptic connection from presynaptic sensory neurons onto postsynaptic motor neurons in *Aplysia*. Serotonin inhibits (indirectly via a second messenger) voltage-sensitive potassium channels in the

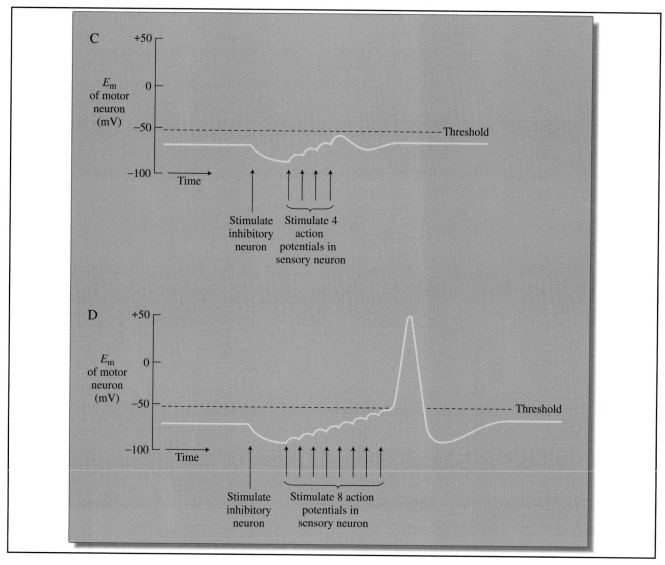

Figure 6.14.

(continued)

presynaptic neuron, slowing the repolarizing phase of the presynaptic action potential. The prolonged depolarization during the action potential increases presynaptic calcium influx and enhances transmitter release.

NEURONAL INTEGRATION

In the nervous system, neurons receive both excitatory and inhibitory synaptic inputs. The decision of a postsynaptic neuron to fire an action potential is determined by only one factor: whether the threshold level of membrane potential has been reached. Reaching threshold is determined at any instant by the sum of all existing excitatory and inhibitory synaptic potentials. This process of summing up, or integrating, synaptic inputs is called **neuronal integration**.

Neuronal integration in the neural circuitry of the patellar reflex is shown in Figure 6.14. When the sensory neuron from the antagonistic muscle fires action potentials, e.p.s.p.'s are produced in the motor neurons that control the antagonist muscle. If there is sufficient temporal summation among the e.p.s.p.'s, an action potential is triggered (see Fig. 6.14B). If the inhibitory neuron is stimulated at the same time, however, the same series of excitatory inputs might be unable to reach threshold (see Fig. 6.14C). As shown in Figure 6.14D, this inhibitory effect can be overcome by increasing the strength of the excitatory input, which could be accomplished by increasing the number of presynaptic action potentials in the sensory neuron (temporal summation) or by increasing the number of sensory neurons activated (spatial summation). The balance between the excitatory and inhibitory inputs dictates whether a postsynaptic action potential is generated.

The information-processing capacity of a single neuron is considerable. A typical neuron receives hundreds or thousands of synapses from hundreds or thousands of other neurons and makes synaptic connections with an equal number of postsynaptic neurons. This capacity is increased still further by the widely varying weights of different synaptic inputs to a cell. Some synapses produce large changes in postsynaptic membrane potential, while others cause only tiny changes. Furthermore, the weight given a particular input might vary with time, as in the case of presynaptic inhibition. A network of some 10^{10} of these sophisticated units, like the human brain, has staggering information-processing ability.

SUMMARY

Chemical synapses between neurons in the nervous system are similar to the synapse at the neuromuscular junction in the following ways:

- Neurotransmitter molecules are stored in the synaptic terminal in membrane-bound synaptic vesicles.
- An influx of external calcium ions into the terminal triggers the release of a neurotransmitter.
- Synaptic vesicles fuse with the plasma membrane of the terminal to release their neurotransmitter content.
- Neurotransmitter molecules combine with specific postsynaptic receptors' molecules and open ion channels in the postsynaptic membrane.

Nervous system synapses differ from the neuromuscular junction in the following ways:

- At most synapses, a single presynaptic action potential produces only a small change in postsynaptic membrane potential. In contrast, a single presynaptic action potential at the neuromuscular junction produces a large depolarization of the muscle cell and triggers a postsynaptic action potential.
- Synapses between neurons can be either excitatory or inhibitory.
- ACh is the neurotransmitter at the neuromuscular junction, but many different neurotransmitter substances (including ACh) are released at synapses in the nervous system.
- A skeletal-muscle cell receives synaptic input from only one neuron—a single motor neuron. A neuron in the nervous system may receive synaptic connections from thousands of different neurons. The output of a neuron depends on the integration of all the inhibitory and excitatory inputs active at a given instant.
- At the neuromuscular junction, ACh directly opens channels by combining with postsynaptic binding sites that are part of the channel protein. In other parts of the nervous system, a neurotransmitter may directly bind to an ion channel or may indirectly affect ion channels via an internal second messenger in the postsynaptic cell.

1. Suppose that the chloride equilibrium potential is equal to the resting potential of a neuron. If a neurotransmitter opens chloride channels, would the neuron be excited or inhibited, or would the neurotransmitter have no effect on the neuron? Explain your answer.

2. How is it possible for a particular neurotransmitter substance (for example, ACh) to have an excitatory effect at one synapse and an inhibitory effect at another synapse?

3. Describe the steps in the linkage between a neurotransmitter receptor molecule and a change in ion permeability of the postsynaptic cell in the case of G-protein–coupled receptors.

4. Would a neuron be excited, inhibited, or unaffected by a neurotransmitter that closes potassium channels in the postsynaptic cell?

5. What is meant by neuronal integration of synaptic potentials? What roles are played by spatial summation and temporal summation in neuronal integration?

6. Describe three different changes in postsynaptic permeability that could in principle produce an inhibitory postsynaptic potential in a neuron.

7. List three second messenger substances and the enzymes that produce them.

8. List at least three ways in which neuron-to-neuron synapses differ from the neuromuscular junction.

INTERNET ASSIGNMENT   CHAPTER 6

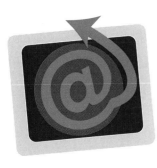

1 Glutamate is the most prevalent excitatory neurotransmitter in the central nervous system. Find information about glutamate receptors, using PubMed. How many different subtypes of glutamate receptors, based on their pharmacological profiles and molecular structure, can you identify?

2 John Eccles was one of the early pioneers in the study of synaptic transmission in the central nervous system. Find information about John Eccles and describe his contributions.

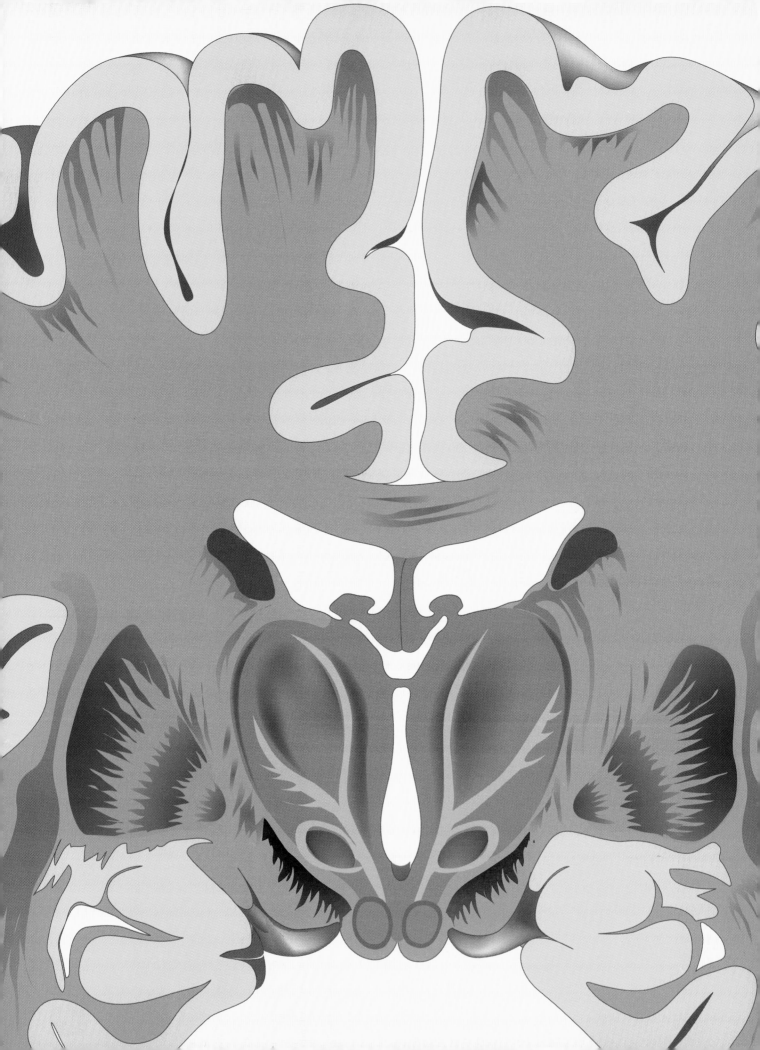

MOTOR CONTROL SYSTEMS

In Part II of this book, we studied in some detail the cellular signals involved in the patellar reflex. We have reached an understanding of the membrane mechanisms that generate the action potential and that allow neurons to communicate at synapses. These fundamental neuronal signals form the basis of the nervous system's ability to transmit and analyze information.

In Part III, we will examine that information-processing ability in somewhat more global terms. Continuing with our analysis of the patellar reflex, we will move beyond the cellular view to consider how the motor control systems of the spinal cord are organized to provide fast, flexible control of the musculoskeletal apparatus, including aspects such as muscle length, joint position, and response to external loads. To understand these control systems, we first must become familiar with the mechanical properties of muscles, which are described in Chapter 7. In Chapter 8, we will consider motor control systems in the spinal cord, and in Chapters 9 and 10, motor systems in the brain. In Chapter 11 we will describe a different type of motor control system—the autonomic nervous system, which controls other motor targets such as the heart. In Chapter 12, we will discuss some of the functions of the hypothalamus, which coordinates high-level functions involving the autonomic nervous system and regulates behaviors related to homeostasis.

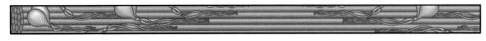

NEURAL CONTROL OF MUSCLE CONTRACTION

ESSENTIAL BACKGROUND

General anatomy of the musculoskeletal system in vertebrates

Ionic permeability and membrane potential (Chapter 3)

Action potential (Chapter 4)

ATP as a cellular energy source

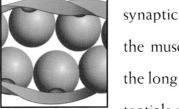

In previous chapters, the patellar reflex served as an example for exploring the cellular signals underlying the function of the nervous system. The final stage of the patellar reflex is contraction of the muscle, which is the subject of this chapter. The arrival of an action potential in the synaptic terminal of the motor neuron stimulates the release of acetylcholine, which depolarizes the postsynaptic muscle cell and initiates an action potential in the muscle cell. The action potential propagates along the long, thin muscle cell in the same way that action potentials propagate along nerve fibers. The muscle action potential triggers contraction of the muscle cell. In this chapter we first will examine the events that link the action potential to activation of the contraction—the process called **excitation-contraction coupling**. Then, we will consider how the nervous system integrates the twitch-like contractions of individual muscle fibers into smooth and graded contractions of the muscle as a whole.

EXCITATION-CONTRACTION COUPLING IN SKELETAL MUSCLE

Types of Muscle Cells

The two general classes of muscle are striated and smooth muscle, both of which are named for the characteristic appearance of the muscle cells when viewed through a microscope. **Striated-muscle cells** (Fig. 7.1) exhibit closely spaced, crosswise stripes (**striations**). **Smooth-muscle cells** have no striations and thus have a smooth appearance. Smooth muscle is found in the gut, blood vessels, uterus, and other locations in which contractions are usually slow and maintained. In contrast, the muscles that move and support the skeletal framework of the body—the **skeletal muscles**—consist of striated-muscle cells. This chapter focuses on the structure and properties of skeletal-muscle cells.

The cells that make up the muscle of the heart are also striated. Because the membranes of cardiac-muscle cells are electrically quite different from those of skeletal-muscle cells, **cardiac muscle** is usually regarded as a distinct class of muscle in its own right. The characteristics of cardiac muscle are discussed in Chapter 11.

Structure of Skeletal Muscle

Figure 7.1 shows the structure of mammalian skeletal muscle at progressively greater magnification. A muscle consists of bundles of individual muscle cells, also called **muscle fibers**. In mammalian muscle, each cell is approximately 50 μm in diameter and is typically as long as the whole muscle. Thus, muscle cells are long, thin fibers similar in shape to neuronal axons. The end-plate region, where synaptic input from the motor neuron is located, is only a few microns in length. Therefore, a rapidly propagating action potential—like that of a nerve cell—is required in skeletal-muscle cells to transmit the depolarization initiated at the end-plate along the entire length of the muscle fiber.

> What is the anatomical organization of single skeletal muscle cells?

Individual muscle cells consist of bundles of still smaller fibers called **myofibrils**, as shown in Figure 7.1. The plasma membrane of a single muscle cell encloses many myofibrils. At the level of the myofibrils, the structural basis of the crosswise striations of skeletal-muscle cells becomes apparent. Myofibrils exhibit a regular, repeating pattern of crosswise light and dark stripes: the A band, I band, and Z line. The I band is a predominantly light region with the dark Z line at its center, while the A band is a darker region separating two successive I bands of the repeating pattern. The A band consists of two darker areas at the outer edges, separated by a lighter region with a faint dark line, the M line, at the center. The basic repeating unit of the striation pattern of a myofibril is the **sarcomere** (see Fig. 7.1), which is defined as extending from one Z line to the next Z line.

Through the electron microscope, a myofibril can be seen to consist of two kinds of longitudinally oriented filaments, called **thick filaments** and **thin filaments**, which are arrayed in parallel groups. Figure 7.1 shows that the parallel thin filaments are connected to each other by perpendicular cross connections at the Z line. Similarly, the thick filaments within a sarcomere are joined together at the M line. The lighter I band corresponds to the region occupied by only thin filaments, while the darker A band corresponds to the spatial extent of the thick filaments. The darker regions at the two edges of the A band correspond to the region where the thick and thin filaments overlap. Small appendages extend to the side from the thick filaments and link to the thin filaments in the region of overlap, forming **cross-bridges** between the thick and thin filaments.

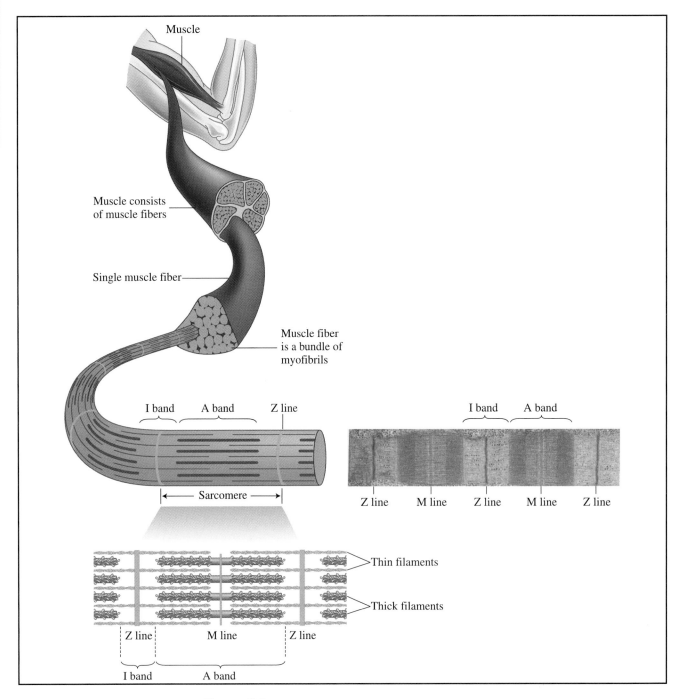

Figure 7.1.

The structure of a skeletal muscle, viewed at increasing magnification. A muscle consists of individual muscle cells (muscle fibers), each of which is a bundle of myofibrils. Each myofibril exhibits a repeating pattern of alternating light and dark bands, which arise from the underlying arrangement of parallel thick and thin filaments. The inset shows the actual appearance of a myofibril viewed through the electron microscope. Electron micrograph provided by B. Walcott of the State University of New York at Stony Brook.

When a muscle cell contracts, each sarcomere shortens in length; that is, the distance from one Z line to the next diminishes. The width of the A band remains constant during contraction, and only the I band shortens. This pattern of changes during contraction is explained by the **sliding filament hypothesis**, which is illustrated in Figure 7.2. Neither the thick filaments nor the thin filaments change in length during a contraction. Instead, shortening occurs because the thick filaments

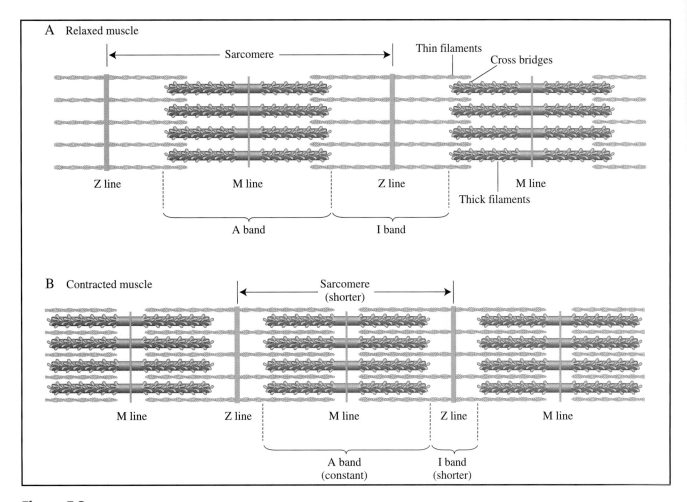

Figure 7.2.

A schematic representation of the relationship among the thick and thin filaments of a myofibril in a relaxed muscle (**A**) and a contracted muscle (**B**). In a contracted muscle, the sarcomere is shorter, because the degree of overlap of thick and thin filaments is greater.

and thin filaments slide past each other, increasing the region of overlap (see Fig. 7.2B). To understand how this sliding occurs, we must examine the molecular makeup of the thick and thin filaments.

Molecular Composition of Filaments

The thick filaments are aggregates of a protein called **myosin**, which consists of a long fibrous "tail" connected to a globular "head" region, as shown schematically in Figure 7.3. The fibrous tails of myosin molecules interact with each other, forming long filaments with the globular heads projecting to the side (Fig. 7.4). These polymers of myosin account for the structure of thick filaments in myofibrils. The aggregated tails form the backbone of the thick filament, and the globular heads form the cross-bridges that connect with adjacent thin filaments.

The thin filaments within a myofibril largely consist of the protein **actin**. Thin filaments also contain two other kinds of protein molecules, **troponin** and **tropomyosin**, whose roles in contraction will be discussed later. Actin is a globular protein that polymerizes to form long chains that form the backbone of the thin filament. Each thin filament consists of two actin chains entwined about each other in a helix, as shown schematically in Figure 7.5. Each actin molecule contains a site that binds the globular head of a myosin molecule. This binding site forms the point of attachment for the cross-bridge on the thin filament.

What protein molecules make up the contractile apparatus of muscle cells?

Figure 7.3.

The overall structure of a single molecule of the thick filament protein, myosin. The flexible fibrous tail is connected to the globular head region via a hinged pivot point. The globular head includes a region that can bind and split a molecule of adenosine triphosphate (ATP).

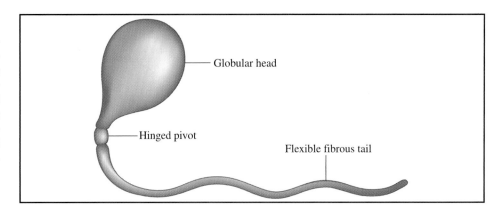

The globular head of myosin acts as an ATPase that binds and hydrolyzes adenosine triphosphate (ATP) into adenosine diphosphate (ADP) and inorganic phosphate (P_i), releasing the stored chemical energy. The energy provided by the ATP is transferred to the myosin molecule, which is transformed into an "energized" state. This sequence can be summarized as follows:

$$\text{Myosin} + \text{ATP} \rightarrow \text{Myosin} \cdot \text{ATP} \rightarrow \text{Energized Myosin} \cdot \text{ADP} + P_i$$

The dot between two molecules indicates that they are bound together, as in an enzyme-substrate complex. The globular head of myosin is attached to the fibrous tail at a hinged pivot point. The energy released by ATP causes the head to undergo a conformational change and pivot into the energized state, shown schematically in Figure 7.6. As we will see shortly, the energy stored in this energized form of myosin fuels the sliding of the filaments past each other during contraction.

Interaction Between Myosin and Actin

When actin combines with energized myosin, the stored energy in the myosin molecule is released. The myosin molecule then returns to its resting state, and the globular head pivots about its hinged attachment point to the thick filament. The pivoting motion requires that the thick and thin filaments move longitudinally with respect to one another, as illustrated in Figure 7.7.

How is the bond between actin and myosin broken so that a new cycle of sliding can be initiated? In the scheme presented so far, each myosin molecule on the thick filament could interact only once with an actin molecule on the thin filament, and the total excursion of sliding would be restricted to that produced by a single piv-

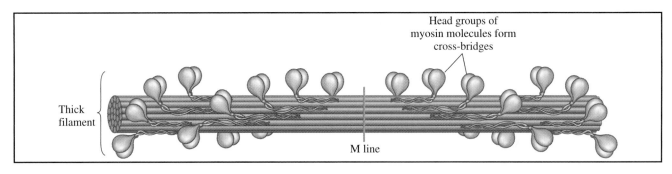

Figure 7.4.

The structure of a thick filament. The fibrous tails of individual myosin molecules polymerize to form the backbone of the filament. The globular heads extend to the side, perpendicular to the long axis of the filament, and form cross-bridges that attach to the thin filament. The myosin molecules reverse orientation at the M line, at the midpoint of the filament.

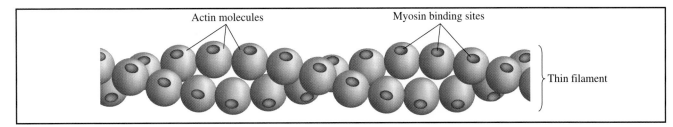

Figure 7.5.

The structure of a thin filament. The backbone of the filament is formed by two entwined chains of actin molecules. Each myosin molecule includes a binding site for the globular head of myosin molecules.

oting of the globular head. To produce the large filament movements that actually occur, the attachment of the cross-bridges must be broken so that the cycle of my-osin energization, binding to actin, and movement can be repeated.

The full cycle during contraction is summarized in Figure 7.8. When energized myosin binds to actin and releases its stored energy, ADP bound to the globular

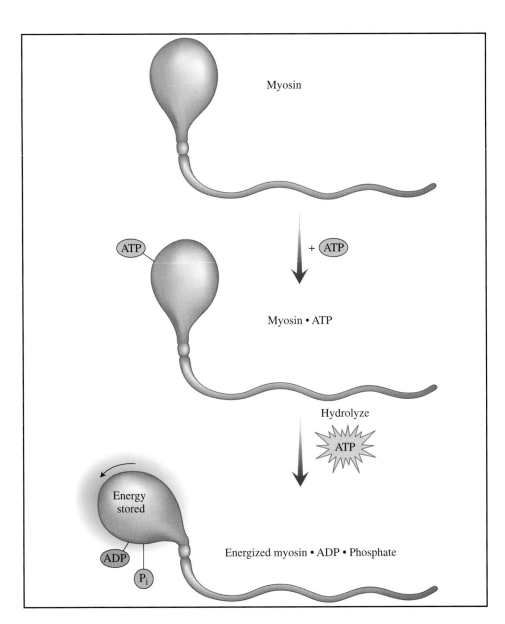

Figure 7.6.

Myosin is an ATPase. Adenosine triphosphate (ATP) binds to the globular head of myosin, which catalyzes hydrolysis of ATP to adenosine diphosphate (ADP) plus inorganic phosphate (P_i). Energy released by ATP hydrolysis is stored in myosin, which is transformed into an energized form. The transition from the resting to the energized state of myosin involves rotation of the globular head around its flexible attachment to the fibrous tail.

143

Figure 7.7.

A schematic representation of the mechanism of filament sliding during contraction of a myofibril. The globular head of energized myosin binds to a specific binding site on actin, and the energy stored in myosin is released. The resulting relaxation of the myosin molecule entails rotation of the globular head, which induces longitudinal sliding of the filaments.

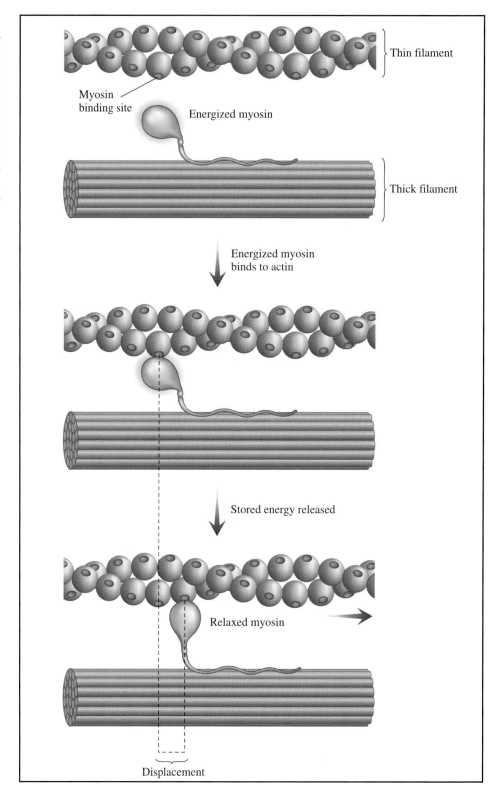

head is liberated. This frees the ATP binding site of the globular head, and a new molecule of ATP can then bind to myosin. Binding of ATP induces the bond between actin and myosin to break, presumably because the interaction between ATP and myosin alters the structure of the globular head. The new ATP molecule is then split by myosin to restore the energized state, which is then free to interact with another actin molecule on the thin filament. Note that ATP has two roles in this scheme: it provides the energy to "cock" myosin for movement, and it breaks the

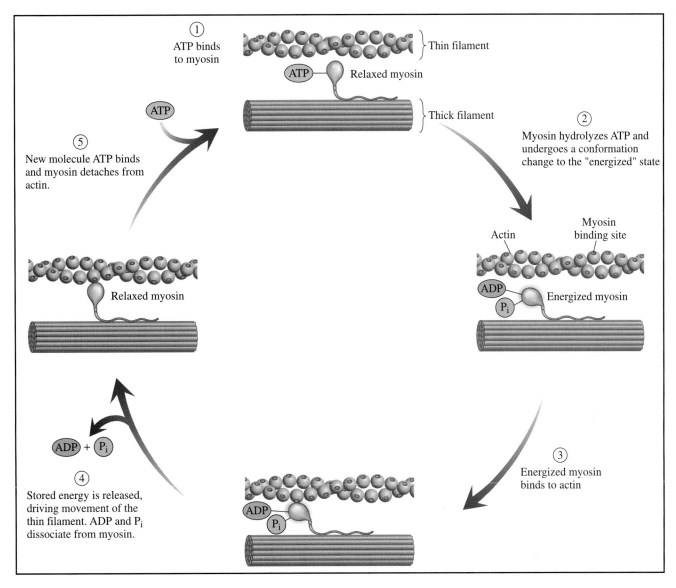

① ATP binds to myosin

Thin filament

ATP — Relaxed myosin

Thick filament

⑤ New molecule ATP binds and myosin detaches from actin.

ATP

② Myosin hydrolyzes ATP and undergoes a conformation change to the "energized" state

Actin

Myosin binding site

ADP Pᵢ — Energized myosin

Relaxed myosin

③ Energized myosin binds to actin

ADP + Pᵢ

④ Stored energy is released, driving movement of the thin filament. ADP and Pᵢ dissociate from myosin.

ADP Pᵢ

Figure 7.8.

The cycle of cross-bridge formation and dissociation between myosin and actin during fila-ment sliding. 1. A molecule of adenosine triphosphate (ATP) binds to myosin. 2. Myosin hydrolyzes the ATP molecule and undergoes a conformational change into a high-energy state. 3. The head group of myosin binds to actin on an adjacent thin filament, forming a cross-bridge between the two filaments. 4. Energy stored by myosin is released, and adenosine diphosphate (ADP) and inorganic phosphate dissociate from myosin. Relaxation of myosin drives sliding of the thin filament. 5. Binding of a new molecule of ATP induces relaxed myosin to detach from actin, returning the cycle to the beginning.

interaction between actin and myosin after movement has occurred. If ATP is ab-sent, actin and myosin become stuck together and a rigid muscle results (as in rigor mortis).

Each of the many myosin heads on an individual thick filament independently goes through repetitive cycles of energization by ATP, binding to actin, release of stored energy to produce sliding, and detachment from actin. Each cycle splits one molecule of ATP into ADP and inorganic phosphate. The orientation of the myo-sin heads reverses at the midpoint of the thick filament, the M line (see Fig. 7.4), providing the proper orientation to pull both Z lines at the boundary of a sarcomere toward the center, as illustrated in Figure 7.9. The thin filaments

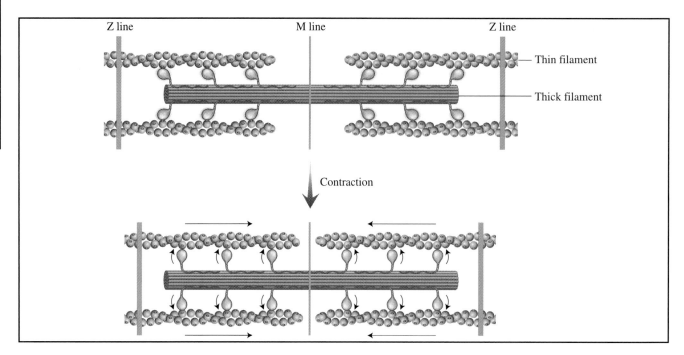

Figure 7.9.

The mechanism of sarcomere shortening during contraction. For clarity, the myosin heads are shown acting in concert, although in reality they behave independently.

attached to the left Z line will be pulled to the right by the cyclical pivoting of the myosin cross-bridges. Similarly, the thin filaments attached to the right Z line will be pulled to the left. Thus, each sarcomere in each myofibril shortens, as does the muscle as a whole.

Regulation of Contraction

How is the contraction of a muscle cell triggered and terminated?

The contraction scheme summarized in Figure 7.8 includes no mechanism to control the interaction between actin and myosin. As long as ATP is present, every muscle in the body would be maximally contracted. We will now examine the molecular mechanisms that prevent myosin from interacting with actin except when contraction is triggered by an action potential in the muscle cell.

Thin filaments also contain the proteins troponin and tropomyosin, which regulate the interaction between myosin and actin molecules. The regulatory scheme is summarized in Figure 7.10. In the resting muscle, tropomyosin covers the myosin binding site on actin, blocking myosin's access to the site. The position of tropomyosin on the actin polymer is in turn regulated by troponin. In the resting state, troponin locks tropomyosin in the blocking position. Thus, tropomyosin acts like a trapdoor covering the myosin binding site, and troponin acts like a lock to keep the door from opening.

The signal that initiates contraction is the binding of calcium ions to troponin, which unlocks the door and causes tropomyosin to reveal the myosin binding site on actin. Each troponin molecule contains a specific binding site for Ca^{2+}. Normally, the concentration of calcium inside the cell is very low, and the binding site is not occupied. In the calcium-free state, troponin locks tropomyosin in the blocking position, and myosin cannot reach its binding site on actin. An action potential in the muscle cell triggers a large increase in the concentration of calcium ions inside the cell, and calcium binds to troponin. Binding of calcium causes a structural change in the troponin molecule, which alters the interaction between

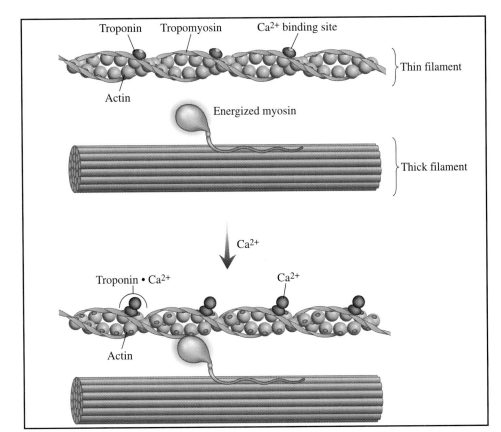

Troponin   Tropomyosin   Ca²⁺ binding site

Thin filament

Actin

Energized myosin

Thick filament

Ca²⁺

Troponin · Ca²⁺   Ca²⁺

Actin

Figure 7.10.

The regulation of the interaction between actin and myosin by calcium ions, troponin, and tropomyosin. In the absence of calcium ions, tropomyosin blocks access to the myosin binding site of actin (*upper diagram*). In the absence of calcium ions, troponin locks tropomyosin in the blocking position. When calcium binds to troponin, the positions of troponin and tropomyosin are altered on the thin filament, and myosin then has access to its binding site on actin. The cycle of filament sliding is then free to begin.

troponin and tropomyosin as shown in Figure 7.10. Tropomyosin then uncovers the myosin binding site on actin, and the cycle depicted in Figure 7.8 is allowed to proceed.

The Sarcoplasmic Reticulum

In the case of neurotransmitter release, which is also triggered by an increase in intracellular calcium concentration, extracellular calcium ions enter the synaptic terminal through voltage-sensitive calcium channels in the plasma membrane (see Chapter 5). In the case of skeletal muscle, however, calcium ions that trigger contraction do not come from outside the cell. Instead, calcium is released from a separate intracellular compartment called the **sarcoplasmic reticulum**, which is illustrated in Figure 7.11. The sarcoplasmic reticulum is an intracellular sack that surrounds the myofibrils of a muscle cell. The membrane of the sarcoplasmic reticulum is not continuous with the plasma membrane of the muscle cell.

The concentration of calcium ions inside the sarcoplasmic reticulum is much higher than that in the rest of the intracellular space. Calcium is accumulated inside the sarcoplasmic reticulum by a calcium pump in the membrane of the sarcoplasmic reticulum. Like the sodium pump of the plasma membrane, the calcium pump of the sarcoplasmic reticulum hydrolyzes ATP and uses the released energy to transport calcium ions into the sarcoplasmic reticulum against a large concentration gradient. To initiate a contraction, a puff of calcium ions is released from the sarcoplasmic reticulum, which is strategically located surrounding the contractile apparatus of the myofibrils. Calcium then binds to troponin to allow cross-bridge interaction to occur. Contraction is terminated when calcium ions are pumped back into the sarcoplasmic reticulum by the calcium pump. Thus, another important role for ATP in muscle contraction is to terminate contraction by providing fuel for the calcium pump that removes calcium from the space surrounding the myofibrils.

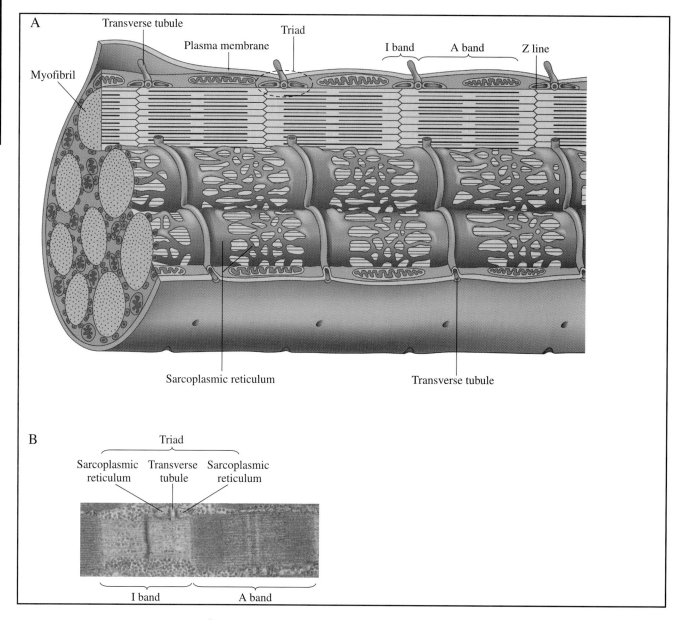

A. Transverse tubule, Triad, Plasma membrane, I band, A band, Z line, Myofibril, Sarcoplasmic reticulum, Transverse tubule

B. Triad, Sarcoplasmic reticulum, Transverse tubule, Sarcoplasmic reticulum, I band, A band

Figure 7.11.

The sarcoplasmic reticulum and transverse tubules. **A.** The transverse tubules are invaginations of the plasma membrane of the muscle cell. Depolarization during an action potential can spread along the transverse tubules to the interior of the fiber. The sarcoplasmic reticulum is an intracellular compartment surrounding each myofibril in the muscle cell. Calcium ions that trigger contraction are released from the sarcoplasmic reticulum. The membranes of the transverse tubules and the sarcoplasmic reticulum come close together at the triad. Depolarization of the membrane of the tubules triggers calcium release from the sarcoplasmic reticulum. **B.** The triad near a single myofibril, viewed through the electron microscope. Electron micrograph provided by B. Walcott of the State University of New York at Stony Brook.

Calcium is released from the sarcoplasmic reticulum via calcium-selective ion channels in the membrane of the sarcoplasmic reticulum. These calcium channels differ from the voltage-dependent calcium channels we encountered previously in our discussion of synaptic transmission. Rather than being activated by depolarization, the calcium channels in the sarcoplasmic reticulum are activated by an increase in cytoplasmic calcium concentration. For this reason, they are known as **calcium-induced calcium-release channels**. If calcium is released from the sarcoplasmic reticulum via channels that are themselves activated by an increase in calcium, then the calcium-release process exhibits positive feedback reminiscent of the rising phase of the action potential (where depolarization opens sodium channels, which in turn produce further depolarization). This positive feedback ensures that calcium release is large and rapid, producing fast and complete activation of the contractile apparatus.

The Transverse Tubule System

How does an action potential in the plasma membrane of a muscle cell trigger the release of calcium from the sarcoplasmic reticulum, whose membrane is separate from the plasma membrane? The crucial aspect of the action potential in triggering contraction is depolarization of the plasma membrane. However, to affect the sarcoplasmic reticulum surrounding the myofibrils deep within the muscle cell, the depolarization produced by the action potential at the outer surface of the cell must somehow be transmitted to the interior of the muscle cell. To accomplish this task, the plasma membrane of the muscle cell forms periodic infoldings, called **transverse tubules**, that extend into the depths of the muscle fiber (see Fig. 7.11). The transverse tubules provide a path for depolarization during an action potential in the surface membrane to influence events in the interior of the cell.

In most species, the transverse tubules are located at the boundary between the A band and the I band of the myofibrils making up the muscle fiber. This location represents the edge of overlap between the thick and thin filaments in a resting muscle fiber, and it makes sense that calcium release should be triggered first at this position at the leading edge of filament sliding. Where transverse tubules encounter the sarcoplasmic reticulum surrounding a myofibril, the tubule membrane and the sarcoplasmic reticulum membrane come close together but do not touch. Because the two membranes are separated by a small gap, the depolarization produced by an action potential cannot spread directly to the sarcoplasmic reticulum. Therefore, some indirect signal is required to link depolarization of the transverse tubule to calcium release by the sarcoplasmic reticulum.

Because calcium is released from the sarcoplasmic reticulum through calcium-induced calcium-release channels, it is natural to suppose that an influx of external calcium ions provides the link between the transverse tubules and the sarcoplasmic reticulum. Indeed, the membrane of the transverse tubules contains voltage-dependent calcium channels that are opened by depolarization, and these calcium channels are known to be necessary for initiation of contraction. In cardiac-muscle cells, influx of extracellular calcium through voltage-activated calcium channels in the transverse tubules is in fact the initial trigger for calcium release from the sarcoplasmic reticulum.

However, in skeletal-muscle cells calcium influx via calcium channels of the transverse tubules is not required to trigger contraction, and some other linkage mechanism is needed. Figure 7.12 illustrates the current view of the role of the voltage-activated calcium channels in the initiation of contraction in skeletal muscle. The calcium channels of the transverse tubule act as voltage sensors that detect the depolarization produced by the action potential. A direct physical link extends through the intracellular gap separating the transverse tubule from the sarcoplasmic reticulum and connects individual calcium channels in the transverse tubule to calcium-release channels in the sarcoplasmic reticulum. Through this physical link, a conformational change in the transverse-tubule calcium channel upon depolarization is thought to induce a conformational change in the calcium-induced calcium-release channel. The sarcoplasmic reticulum channel then opens, locally releasing calcium and initiating the explosive calcium-induced release of calcium from the sarcoplasmic reticulum as a whole.

How is the depolarization produced by the muscle action potential communicated to the sarcoplasmic reticulum?

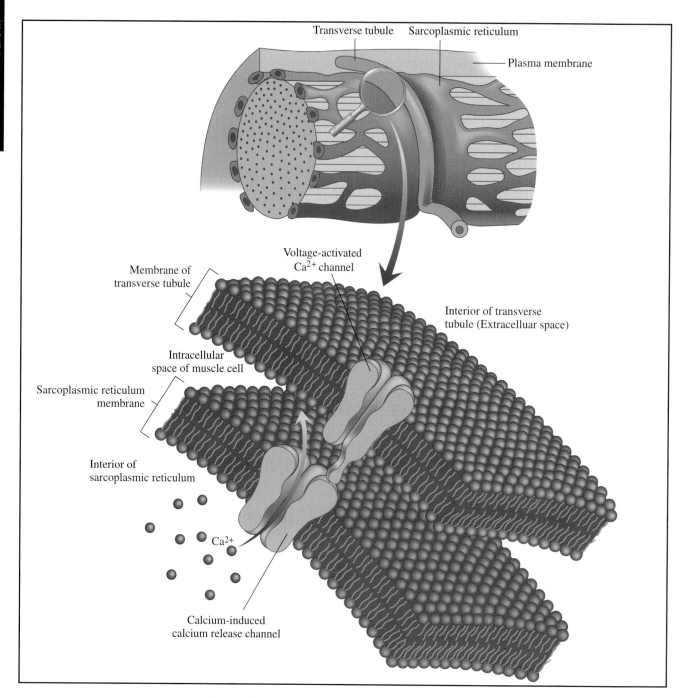

Figure 7.12.

The interaction between the membranes of the transverse tubules and sarcoplasmic reticulum. The two membranes come close together but do not fuse. At the contact point, calcium channels in the transverse tubule are coupled to calcium-release channels in the sarcoplasmic reticulum. Depolarization of the transverse tubule causes a conformational change in the calcium channel, which communicates with the calcium-release channel. The calcium-release channel then opens, allowing calcium ions to flow out of the sarcoplasmic reticulum.

Summary of Excitation-Contraction Coupling

Figure 7.13 summarizes the sequence of events leading to contraction of a skeletal-muscle fiber after stimulation of its motor neuron. The sequence is as follows:

- Acetylcholine released from the presynaptic terminal depolarizes the end-plate region of the muscle fiber.
- The depolarization initiates an action potential in the muscle fiber, which propagates along the entire length of the fiber.
- Depolarization produced by the action potential spreads to the interior of the fiber along the transverse tubules.
- Depolarization of the transverse tubules causes the release of calcium ions by the sarcoplasmic reticulum.
- Released calcium ions bind to troponin molecules on the thin filaments.
- When calcium combines with troponin, tropomyosin uncovers the myosin binding site of actin.
- Globular heads of myosin molecules, which have been energized by hydrolyzing ATP, attach to actin at the uncovered binding site.
- The stored energy of the activated myosin is released and propels the thick and thin filaments past each other. The spent ADP is then released from myosin.
- A new ATP molecule binds to myosin, breaking its attachment to the actin molecule.
- The new ATP molecule is split to reenergize myosin, which again binds to actin and repeats the contraction cycle.
- Contraction is maintained as long as the internal calcium concentration remains elevated. The calcium concentration declines as calcium ions return to the sarcoplasmic reticulum via an ATP-dependent calcium pump.

CONTRACTION OF WHOLE MUSCLE

At this point, we have examined in detail the mechanism responsible for the twitch contraction of a muscle cell. We will now consider how the nervous system is able to produce smooth, graded movements of muscles from the all-or-none twitches of single muscle fibers making up the muscle.

The Motor Unit

A single motor neuron makes synaptic contact with a number of muscle fibers. The actual number varies considerably from one muscle to another and from one motor neuron to another within the same muscle. A single motor neuron may contact as few as 10 to 20 muscle fibers or more than 1000. In mammals, a single muscle fiber normally receives synaptic contact from only one motor neuron. Therefore, a single motor neuron and the muscle fibers to which it is connected form a basic unit of motor organization called the **motor unit**, shown schematically in Figure 7.14.

Recall from Chapter 5 that the synapse between a motor neuron and a muscle fiber is a one-for-one synapse—that is, a single presynaptic action potential produces a single postsynaptic action potential and hence a single twitch of the muscle cell. As a result, all muscle cells in a motor unit contract together as group. Thus, the fundamental unit of contraction of the whole muscle is not the contraction of a

What is a motor unit?

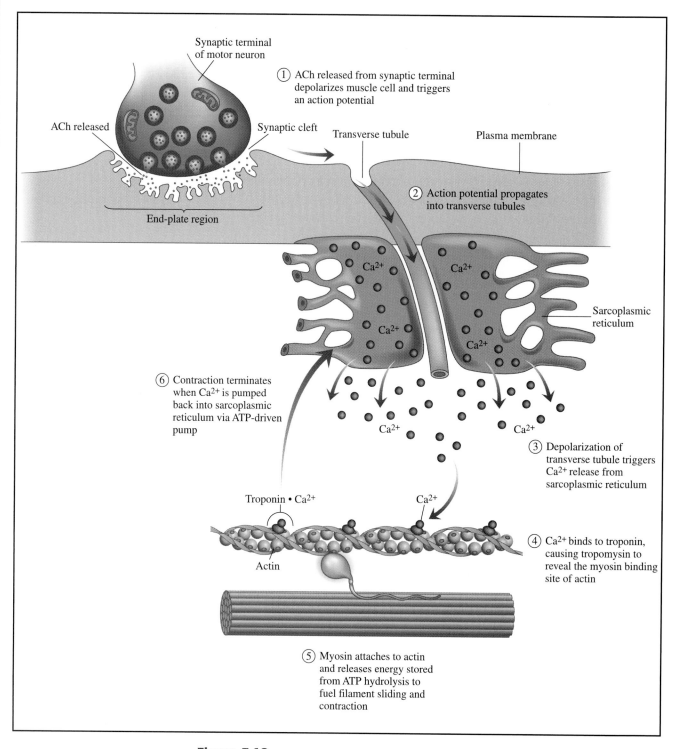

Figure 7.13.

A summary of the sequence of events during excitation-contraction coupling in a skeletal-muscle cell. Events labeled 1 through 6 represent in order the major steps in the process.

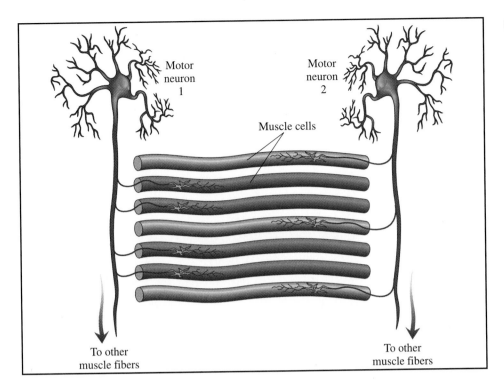

Figure 7.14.

Portions of two motor units. The motor unit consists of a single motor neuron and all of the muscle fibers that receive synaptic contact from that motor neuron.

single muscle fiber, but rather the contraction produced by all the muscle cells in a single motor unit.

Gradation in the overall strength of a muscle contraction is controlled by the nervous system. The nervous system produces graded contraction by two basic methods:

- Variation in the total number of motor neurons activated, and hence in the total number of motor units contracting
- Variation in the frequency of action potentials in the motor neuron of a single motor unit

The greater the number of motor units activated, the greater the strength of contraction. Also, within broad limits, the greater the rate of action potentials within a motor unit, the greater the strength of the resulting summed contraction.

The Mechanics of Contraction

When the nerve controlling a muscle is stimulated, the resulting action potentials in the muscle fibers initiate filament sliding in the individual myofibrils within the muscle cells. This sliding generates a force that tends to shorten the muscle fibers, and hence the muscle as a whole. Whether the muscle actually shortens, however, depends on the load attached to the muscle. While we might attempt to order the muscles in our arms to lift an automobile, it is unlikely that they would be able to shorten against such a load. The force developed in an activated muscle is called the muscle **tension**, and the muscle will shorten and lift the load only if the tension equals the weight of the load.

We can distinguish between two kinds of responses to activation of a muscle. If the muscle tension is less than the load, the contraction is said to be **isometric** ("same length") because the length of the muscle does not change even though the tension increases. That is, the force exerted on the load by the muscle is insufficient to move the load, so the muscle cannot shorten. In the isometric contraction diagrammed in Figure 7.15A, an isolated muscle is attached to a load it cannot lift. The tension developed by the muscle is registered by a strain gauge that measures the minuscule flexing of the strut to which the muscle is attached. A single activation of the muscle triggers a transient increase in tension, typically lasting about 0.1 sec. You can easily feel the tension developed in an isometric contraction by placing your palms together with your arms flexed in front of your chest and pushing with both hands, one against the other.

If the tension is great enough to overcome the weight of the load, the contraction is said to be **isotonic** ("same tension") because the tension remains constant

IN THE CLINIC

BOX 1

A wide variety of human diseases affect the motor unit. Because the motor neuron and its innervated muscle fibers constitute the final output path for control of the skeletal muscles, anything that disrupts the functioning of the motor unit produces muscle weakness in mild cases or paralysis in severe cases. Proper functioning of the motor unit requires the structures at four transmission stages to be intact: the cell body of the motor neuron in the spinal cord, the axon of the motor neuron as it courses through the peripheral nerve to the muscle, the neuromuscular junction, and the muscle cells themselves. Diseases of the motor unit are distinguished based on which of the transmission stages is affected. Diseases that affect the muscle are collectively called myopathies, whereas diseases that affect the motor neuron or the peripheral nerve are referred to as neuropathies. Diseases of the neuromuscular junction are usually considered a separate category. Because neurogenic diseases often lead to atrophy of the muscle, the distinction between neuropathy and myopathy is often blurred, however.

Perhaps the best-known example of a disease that affects the motor neurons is amyotrophic lateral sclerosis (Lou Gehrig's disease), which is an inherited disorder that leads to death of the motor neurons in the spinal cord. The genetic defect has been localized to a gene that encodes an enzyme involved in the removal of highly toxic free radicals, which are by-products of certain oxidation reactions. Exactly why the presumed abnormal buildup of free radicals preferentially affects the motor neurons is not yet clear.

Neuropathies of the peripheral nerve often interfere with motor unit function by blocking the conduction of action potentials from the spinal cord to the muscle. An example is Guillain-Barré syndrome, which is thought to be an autoimmune disease in which the patient produces antibodies that attack and destroy the myelin sheath of axons in peripheral nerves.

Duchenne muscular dystrophy is an example of an inherited disorder that leads to progressive degeneration of skeletal muscle cells. The underlying defect is a mutation in the gene for a muscle protein called dystrophin, which is involved in linking plasma membrane proteins (including cell adhesion molecules and acetylcholine receptors) to the cytoskeleton.

Diseases that block neuromuscular synaptic transmission also disrupt the function of motor units. Two examples of autoimmune diseases that target the neuromuscular junction are myasthenia gravis, in which antibodies attack the acetylcholine receptors, and Lambert-Eaton myasthenic syndrome, in which patients produce antibodies against the voltage-dependent calcium channels of the motor nerve synaptic terminal.

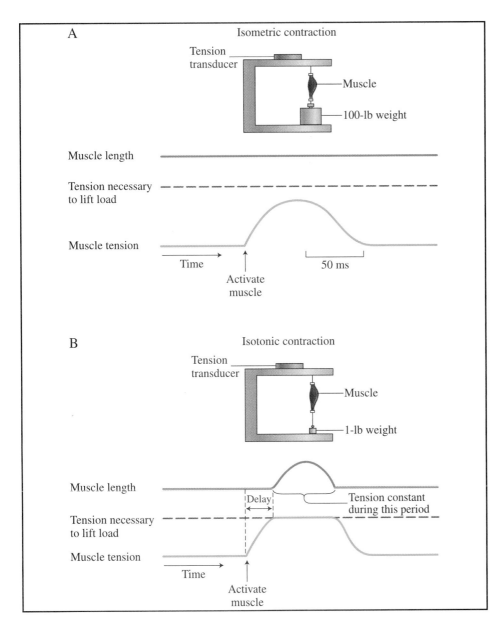

Figure 7.15.

Measurements of muscle length and muscle tension during isometric (**A**) and isotonic contractions (**B**). At the *upward arrow*, the nerve innervating the muscle is stimulated, which activates contraction of the muscle.

once it reaches the level necessary to move the load. In Figure 7.15B, the strain gauge again records the increase in tension, as with the isometric contraction. When the tension reaches the threshold necessary to lift the load, it levels off and the muscle begins to shorten as the load is lifted. During the change in muscle length, the tension remains constant and equal to the weight of the load. The weight hanging from the muscle and support strut determines the flexing measured by the strain gauge. In an isotonic contraction, the force developed by the sliding filaments in the myofibrils making up the muscle produces work in the form of moving the load through space.

In Figure 7.15B, note the delay between activation of the muscle and the change in muscle length during the isotonic contraction. The tension begins to rise within a few milliseconds, which is the time required for the excitation-contraction process to take hold. Muscle length changes only after tension rises to the point where the load is lifted, and the delay between activation and shortening depends on the size of the load. With light loads, shortening begins quickly, but with heavier loads, the onset of shortening is progressively delayed. With sufficiently heavy loads, no shortening occurs, and the contraction becomes isometric. In addition, with heavier loads the duration of shortening decreases, and the maximum speed of shortening is slower. In a sense, the measurement of tension during an isometric contraction gives a more direct view of the contractile state of the muscle, and for this reason we will focus on isometric contractions.

The Relationship Between Isometric Tension and Muscle Length

To relate the tension developed by a muscle to the microscopic contractile apparatus within each muscle fiber, we will consider the relationship between the magnitude of isometric tension and the muscle length at which the tension is measured. Suppose the experiment diagrammed in Figure 7.15A is repeated at a variety of muscle lengths, as set by varying the distance between the upper support bar and the weight. As the muscle is stretched beyond its normal resting length, the tension developed upon stimulating the muscle falls off rapidly, reaching zero at about 175% of resting length. Figure 7.16A shows the peak isometric tension as a function of muscle length, expressed as a percentage of the resting length of the unstimulated muscle. The decline in maximum tension with increasing muscle length can be understood in terms of the underlying state of the thick and thin filaments. As the distance between Z lines increases in the stretched muscle, the degree of overlap between thick and thin filaments declines, and thus the number of myosin head groups available to form cross-bridges diminishes. Finally, with sufficient stretch, no overlap occurs (see Fig. 7.16B, number 3) and no tension develops.

If the muscle is artificially shortened, maximum isometric tension also declines, falling to zero at about 50% of resting length. If the distance between successive Z lines becomes sufficiently short, thin filaments attached to neighboring Z lines begin to overlap (see Fig. 7.16B, number 1). This overlap distorts the necessary spatial relation between thin and thick filaments that is required for cross-bridge attachments to form, once again leaving fewer cross-bridges available to develop tension. In addition to this geometrical effect, reduced coupling between depolarization of the membrane and release of calcium from the sarcoplasmic reticulum might contribute to the reduced peak tension at short muscle lengths.

The drop in tension with both increasing and decreasing length means that an optimal range of length exists for the development of tension. Within this range, there is a maximal overlap of thin filaments with the cross-bridges of the thick filament (see Fig. 7.16B, number 2). For maximum efficiency, the range of length over which a muscle operates should be close to this optimal range. This is in fact the case—the length of a functioning skeletal muscle in the body remains within about 30% of the optimal length (the shaded region in Fig. 7.16A). To ensure that this range is not exceeded, precise arrangements of muscle-fiber length, tendon length and attachment sites, and joint geometry have evolved to be appropriate for the functional task of each muscle.

CONTROL OF MUSCLE TENSION BY THE NERVOUS SYSTEM

Recruitment of Motor Neurons

How are all-or-none twitches of single muscle cells integrated to produce smooth, graded movements?

A single muscle typically receives inputs from hundreds of motor neurons. As a result, tension in the muscle can be increased by increasing the number of motor neurons that are firing action potentials. The tension produced by activating individual motor units sums to produce the total tension in the muscle. A simplified ex-

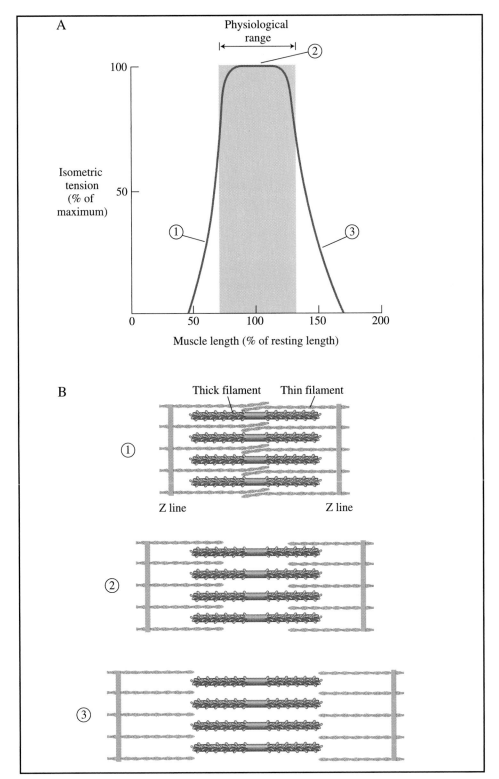

Figure 7.16.
The relationship between muscle length and strength of isometric tension in a skeletal muscle. **A**. Graph showing the isometric tension developed when a muscle is stimulated, as a function of the length of the muscle. Tension is expressed as a percentage of the maximum tension, and muscle length is expressed as a percentage of resting length. The *shaded area* shows the range of muscle length over which the muscle actually operates in the body. **B**. Diagrams showing the states of the thick and thin filaments within a sarcomere at each of the three numbered positions marked in **A**.

ample is shown in Figure 7.17. The increase in the number of active motor neurons—called **recruitment** of motor neurons—is an important physiological means of controlling muscle tension.

When motor neurons are recruited during naturally occurring motor behavior, such as locomotion or lifting loads, the order of recruitment is determined by the size of the motor unit. As the tension in a muscle is increased from the relaxed state, motor units containing a small number of muscle fibers are the first to be re-

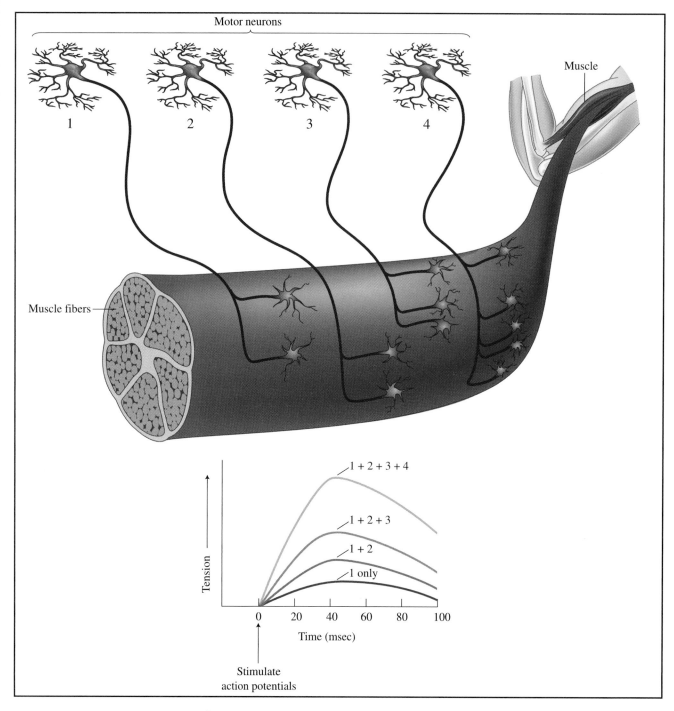

Muscle

Muscle fibers

1 + 2 + 3 + 4

1 + 2 + 3

1 + 2

1 only

Tension

0   20   40   60   80   100

Time (msec)

Stimulate
action potentials

Figure 7.17.

Motor units are recruited in order of their size. Four motor neurons innervate different numbers of muscle cells, resulting in four motor units of varying size. Motor neurons 1 and 2 innervate few muscle fibers, motor neuron 3 innervates an intermediate number, and motor neuron 4 innervates the largest number of muscle fibers. The graph shows isometric tension in response to simultaneous action potentials (at the *arrow*) in different combinations of the motor neurons, as marked.

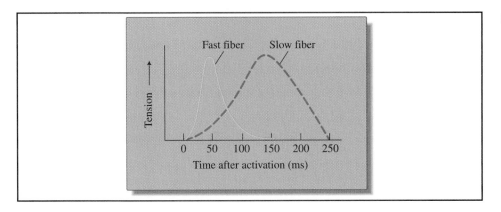

Figure 7.18.

A comparison of the speed of development of isometric tension in fast and slow muscle fibers.

cruited, followed by later recruitment of larger motor units. When there is little activity in the pool of motor neurons controlling a muscle and muscle tension is low, small motor units are recruited to produce an increase in tension. This ensures that tension is added in small increments first, thus preventing large jerky increases in tension when the tension is low. As tension increases, however, further increases in tension must be larger to make a significant difference. Consequently, larger motor units are added, resulting in larger increments of tension when the background tension is already high. In Figure 7.17, for example, the tension would increase by adding the smaller motor units (numbers 1 and 2) first and the largest unit (number 4) last.

Fast and Slow Muscle Fibers

The time delay between the action potential in a muscle fiber and the peak of the resulting tension is not constant across all muscle fibers. The delay to peak tension can be as short as 10 msec or as long as 200 msec. In general, muscle fibers can be grouped into two classes—fast and slow—on the basis of this speed. Figure 7.18 shows samples of isometric contractions in fast and slow fibers. Both slow and fast fibers are found in most muscles, but slow fibers predominate in muscles that must maintain steady contraction, such as those involved in keeping the human body standing upright. Fast muscle fibers are more common in muscles that require rapid contraction, such as those involved in jumping and running. The fastest muscle fibers are those in muscles that move the eyes in rapid jumps, like the movements made by your eyes as you scan the words on this page.

Temporal Summation of Contractions Within a Single Motor Unit

When motor neurons are activated during naturally occurring movement, they typically do not fire just a single action potential. Instead, action potentials tend to occur either in rapid bursts or as steady discharges at a relatively constant rate. In many cases, action potentials within a burst are separated by 10 msec or less. Under normal conditions, each action potential in a motor neuron produces a corresponding action potential in each of the motor unit's muscle fibers. Because the tension resulting from a single muscle action potential commonly lasts for many tens or hundreds of milliseconds, the tension from successive action potentials summates, as illustrated in Figure 7.19. This temporal summation of individual twitches represents another major strategy by which the nervous system controls tension in skeletal muscles.

Figure 7.19.

Isometric tension in response to a series of action potentials in a muscle. The *dashed lines* show the expected response if only the first action potential of a series occurred.

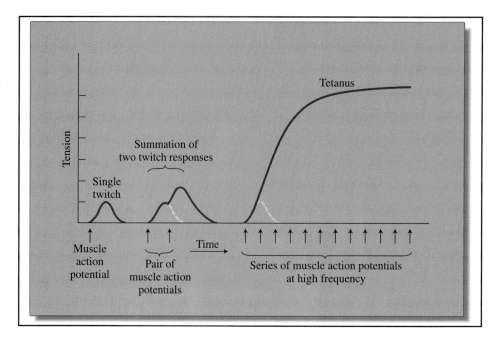

The amount of summation within a burst of muscle action potentials depends on the frequency of action potentials: the higher the frequency, the greater the resulting summed tension. When the frequency is sufficiently high, however, the individual tension responses of the muscle fuse together into a plateau of tension, shown in Figure 7.19. A further increase in frequency beyond this point does not increase tension, because the muscle has reached its maximum response. This plateau state is called **tetanus**. As expected from the examples shown in Figure 7.18, the frequency of stimulation required to produce tetanus varies considerably depending on whether slow or fast muscle fibers are involved. A frequency of more than 100 action potentials per second may be required for fast fibers, while a frequency of 20 action potentials per second may suffice for slow fibers.

Asynchronous Activation of Motor Units During Maintained Contraction

How does the nervous system avoid muscle fatigue during a maintained contraction?

As anyone who has exercised vigorously can attest, muscle contractions cannot be maintained indefinitely—muscles fatigue and must be rested. Thus, the state of tetanus shown in Figure 7.19 could not be maintained in a single motor unit for very long without allowing the muscle fibers in the motor unit to relax. Some muscles—such as those involved in maintaining body posture—must contract for prolonged periods, however. As you might expect, there is a mechanism that helps prevent muscle fatigue during these prolonged contractions.

When tension is maintained in a muscle, not all motor neurons of the muscle are active simultaneously. The activity of the motor units occurs in bursts separated by quiet periods, with the activity of different motor units staggered in time. An example of this kind of asynchronous activity during steady contraction is shown in Figure 7.20. In the example, the summation of the tensions produced by activity of only three motor units—each active only half the time—results in a reasonably smooth, steady tension. With hundreds of motor units available in many muscles, a much smoother and larger steady tension can be maintained with less effort on the part of any one motor unit. In this manner, asynchronous activation of motor neurons to a muscle allows a prolonged contraction with reduced fatigue of individual muscle motor units.

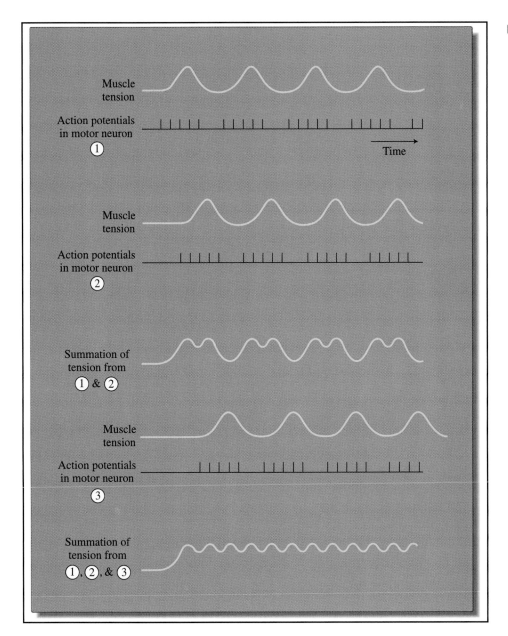

Figure 7.20.
Summation of muscle tension during asynchronous activation of three motor units in a muscle.

SUMMARY

Skeletal muscles are made up of striated-muscle cells (muscle fibers). Individual muscle cells are bundles of smaller fibers called myofibrils. Myofibrils exhibit a regularly repeating pattern of crosswise light and dark stripes (striations), called the A band, I band, and Z line. The I band is a predominantly light region with a dark Z line at its center, while the A band is a darker region separating two I bands of the repeating pattern. At the center of the A band is the M line. The basic unit of the repeating striation pattern is called the sarcomere, which is defined as extending from one Z line to the next Z line. The striation pattern of a myofibril arises from the arrangement of two kinds of longitudinally oriented filaments, the thick filaments and the thin filaments, which make up each myofibril. Thick filaments are aggregates of a protein called myosin, which consists of a fibrous tail region and a globular head region. The aggregated tails of the myosin molecules form the backbone of the thick filament, and the globular heads extend to the side to form cross-bridges that connect with the adjacent thin filaments. Thin filaments consist largely of the protein actin, together with the associated proteins troponin and tropomyosin.

During contraction, the thin and thick filaments slide past each other, propelled by movements of the myosin cross-bridge. Myosin is an ATPase that hydrolyzes ATP and uses the released energy to drive filament sliding. In the resting muscle, the interaction between myosin and actin is prevented by tropomyosin and troponin. Tropomyosin blocks the binding site for myosin on actin molecules, and troponin locks tropomyosin in the blocking position. To trigger contraction, calcium ions are released from the sarcoplasmic reticulum and bind to troponin, altering the position of tropomyosin on the thin filament and uncovering the myosin binding site on actin. Depolarization of the plasma membrane during an action potential spreads to the interior of the muscle cell along deep invaginations of the plasma membrane, called the transverse tubules, which come into close contact with the membrane of the sarcoplasmic reticulum. Depolarization of the transverse tubules activates calcium-release channels in the membrane of the sarcoplasmic reticulum.

The basic unit of contraction of a skeletal muscle is the group of muscle fibers making up a single motor unit, which consists of a single motor neuron and all the muscle fibers receiving synaptic connections from that neuron. When the motor neuron fires an action potential, all muscle fibers in that motor unit twitch together. The magnitude of the contraction generated by activation of a motor unit depends on the number of muscle fibers in that motor unit. The number of fibers in a unit—and hence the magnitude of the tension produced by activation of the unit—varies considerably among the motor neurons innervating a particular muscle.

The type of contraction produced by activation of a whole muscle depends on the load against which the muscle is contracting. If the load is too great for the muscle to move, the length of the muscle does not change during the contraction, which is then called an isometric contraction. If the tension is sufficient to overcome the weight of the load, the contraction will be accompanied by a shortening of the muscle. The tension in the muscle then remains constant and equal to the weight of the load during shortening. Such a contraction is called an isotonic contraction.

The overall tension developed by a muscle depends on the number of motor units activated and the frequency of action potentials within a motor unit. Increasing muscle tension by increasing the number of active motor neurons is called motor neuron recruitment. When the frequency of action potentials within a motor unit is increased, the resulting muscle tension rises to a steady plateau state, called tetanus. Normally, all motor neurons of a muscle are not active simultaneously during a maintained contraction. Instead, the activity of individual motor neurons is restricted to periodic bursts that occur asynchronously among the pool of motor neurons controlling a muscle. This asynchrony reduces fatigue in the muscle by allowing individual motor units to rest periodically during a maintained contraction.

1. Draw the structure of a single sarcomere and label the bands and lines that make up the striation pattern.
2. Describe why the A band remains constant but the I band becomes thinner during contraction of a muscle cell.
3. List the four proteins that constitute the thin and thick filaments of a myofibril and describe the function of each protein.
4. What is the sarcoplasmic reticulum and what role does it play in muscle contraction?
5. Describe three distinct roles for ATP in muscle contraction.
6. What steps link an action potential in a muscle fiber to activation of the contractile apparatus?
7. What is the difference between an isometric contraction and an isotonic contraction?
8. Gradation in the overall strength of contraction of a muscle is achieved by what mechanisms?
9. Define asynchronous activation of motor units and explain why it is important in avoiding fatigue during sustained contraction of a muscle.

INTERNET ASSIGNMENT   CHAPTER 7

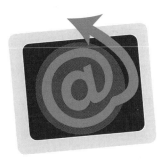

1 Search the Internet for images, cartoons, and animation related to muscle contraction. Try using the following search terms: myofibril, thick filament, myosin, and sarcoplasmic reticulum.

2 Hugh Huxley is a name associated with the sliding filament hypothesis of muscle contraction. Describe his contributions. (Note: A. F. Huxley, who together with Alan Hodgkin established the mechanism of the action potential, also worked on muscle contraction and made important contributions to the sliding filament hypothesis. Do not confuse the two Huxleys.)

SPINAL CORD MOTOR MECHANISMS

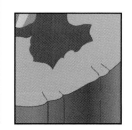

As we learned in Chapter 2, the hierarchical organization of the nervous system is one of the emergent trends during the evolution of increasingly complex forms of neural organization. Motor control systems provide a particularly clear example of hierarchical organization. In complex nervous systems, such as those of mammals, the lowest level of the motor hierarchy is the spinal cord, which contains the motor neurons that directly control the muscles. In this chapter, we will examine some of the spinal cord circuits that serve as building blocks for the motor hierarchy.

HIERARCHICAL ORGANIZATION OF MOTOR CONTROL SYSTEMS

Each segment of the spinal cord includes thousands of motor neurons, controlling a wide variety of different skeletal muscles. Even a simple movement, such as turning a page in this book, involves the careful temporal programming of excitation in large numbers of these motor neurons. If the brain had to precisely time the activation of each motor neuron for each movement, the brain motor centers would have to carry out massive computations. Instead, motor neurons are organized into larger functional units, so that complex movements can be programmed by selecting from among a more manageable number of alternatives. These fundamental circuits dramatically reduce the number of possible choices for descending commands, restricting the alternatives to those that make functional sense for the particular set of muscles and joints controlled by a particular spinal segment.

Consider the simplified scheme diagrammed in Figure 8.1. In this example, each of four pools of motor neurons within a spinal cord segment controls a separate skeletal muscle. If circuit A is activated by the brain, motor neurons controlling the extensor muscle for joint 1 and the flexor muscle for joint 2 will be excited, while motor neurons for the antagonistic muscles of each joint will be inhibited. Thus, circuit A produces extension of joint 1 combined with flexion of joint 2. Circuit B, on the other hand, has the opposite effect, producing flexion of joint 1 and extension of joint 2.

In addition, each of the inputs from a circuit to a given pool of motor neurons may be active at different times, so that the activation and inhibition of different sets of motor neurons may be asynchronous. For instance, imagine what would happen if circuits A and B in Figure 8.1 were activated in alternation. If joints 1 and 2 are located in limbs on opposite sides of the body, alternating activation of circuits A and B would produce repetitive stepping motions in the two limbs. First one limb would flex and the other extend, then the opposite pattern would occur. Circuits A and B thus might be part of larger circuits that produce alternating limb movements involved in locomotion. The main point here is that *complex sets of motor neuron activity can be selected by higher motor centers without having to specify the detailed pattern of activation. The details are inherent in the intraspinal connections of the spinal cord circuits.*

Spinal circuits are also organized so as to compensate automatically for the mechanical properties of the particular muscle groups and joints controlled by the circuits. Thus, the temporal order of activation of motor neuron pools is fine-tuned in different circuits depending on the muscle mass, size of the bones, rotation angle of the joint, and so on. In a hierarchical system, these details of organization need not be specified by higher motor centers when desired motor actions are selected.

In addition to reducing the required complexity of descending commands from higher motor centers, the spinal motor circuits also allow automation of commonly required motor activities, without the intervention of higher motor centers. For example, the maintenance of body posture is a fundamental function of the skeletal-muscle control system for any animal, and such fundamental aspects need not occupy the command resources of higher motor centers. Although the spinal motor systems can carry out the "automated" functions without intervention from higher centers, the correct functioning of the spinal circuits requires more than just the selection of prepatterned groups of motor neurons. For example, the mechanisms that maintain body posture must take into account information about the deviation of joint position and muscle length from the desired values—that is, sensory information is also required. Independent of postural concerns, maintaining muscle length under changing muscle load is commonly required for many muscle actions, and this task also requires sensory information. Thus, automation

What are the advantages of a hierarchical organization in motor systems of the central nervous system?

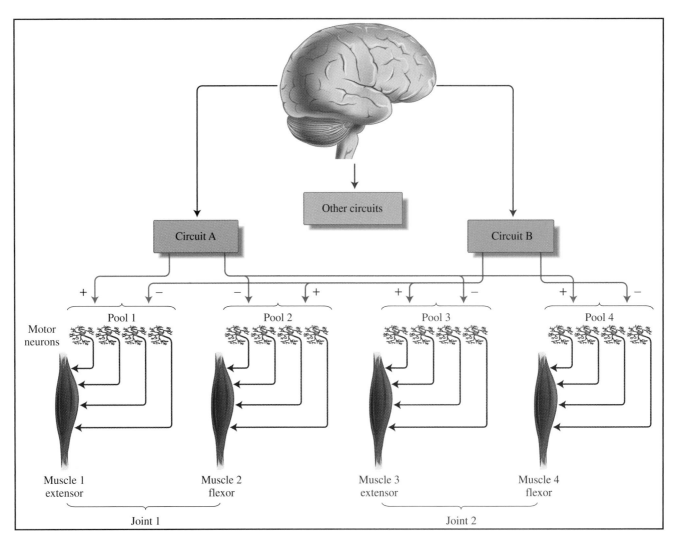

Figure 8.1.

A schematic diagram of the hierarchical organization of the motor control system. The brain directs movements by selecting among spinal cord circuits, which consist of interneurons that control various combinations of motor neurons. In this example, four pools of motor neurons control the flexor and extensor muscles of two limb joints. Circuit A produces extension of joint 1 combined with flexion of joint 2, while circuit B produces the opposite movement. The *arrows* in circuits A and B indicate synaptic connections, the *plus signs* indicate excitatory synapses, and the *minus signs* indicate inhibitory synapses. The motor neurons always produce excitation of the muscles they control.

of commonly used motor functions requires that the underlying neural circuits include sensory information, which forms the basis for many spinal cord reflexes.

ANATOMICAL ORGANIZATION OF THE SPINAL CORD

The spinal cord is a long chain of repeated segments, one segment for each spinal vertebra. As shown in Figure 8.2, nerve fibers and neuronal cell bodies are spatially segregated within the spinal cord. The cell bodies are concentrated in the more central regions, while the outer layers predominantly consist of connecting axons of sensory neurons and interneurons. Because of the large amount of insulating myelin in the areas where axons dominate, these areas are more opaque than

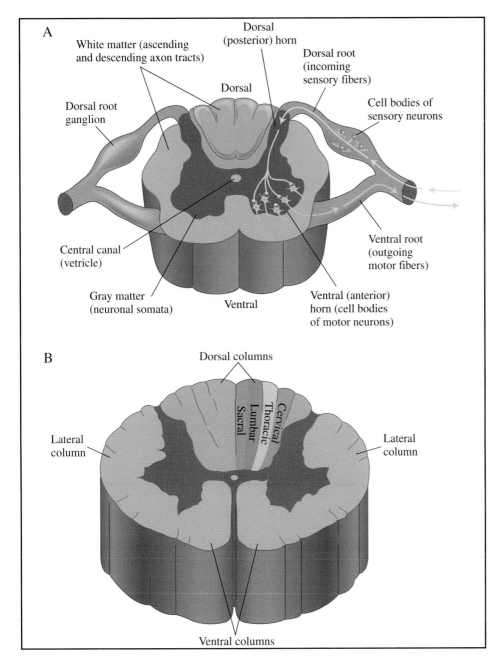

A

White matter (ascending and descending axon tracts)

Dorsal root ganglion

Dorsal

Dorsal (posterior) horn

Dorsal root (incoming sensory fibers)

Cell bodies of sensory neurons

Central canal (vetricle)

Gray matter (neuronal somata)

Ventral

Ventral (anterior) horn (cell bodies of motor neurons)

Ventral root (outgoing motor fibers)

B

Dorsal columns

Cervical
Thoracic
Lumbar
Sacral

Lateral column

Lateral column

Ventral columns

Figure 8.2.

The anatomical organization of the spinal cord. The diagrams show transverse views of the mammalian spinal cord at a lower spinal level (**A**; lumbar spinal cord) and at a higher spinal level (**B**; cervical spinal cord).

the regions where cell bodies dominate, giving the axon-containing regions a whiter appearance. Thus, the fiber tracts are called **white matter**, while the central neuron-containing region is called **gray matter**.

The incoming sensory fibers enter the spinal cord via the dorsal roots, and the outgoing motor neuron axons exit via the ventral roots. The dorsal and ventral roots merge within the vertebral column just outside the spinal cord to form the mixed motor and sensory spinal nerve exiting each vertebral segment. The spinal cord is divided into four regions, each named for the corresponding groups of vertebrae in the spinal column. From upper to lower, these regions are the cervical, thoracic, lumbar, and sacral segments of the spinal cord.

After they enter the spinal cord, the sensory fibers ramify, with some branches extending to interneurons and motor neurons in the same spinal segment, and other branches extending through the white matter to make connections with neurons in adjoining spinal segments. Axon branches from the sensory neurons also extend into the brain where they deliver sensory information to the higher sensory processing centers involved in the conscious perception of body sensations, including touch, pressure, temperature, limb position, and pain.

Because the white matter consists of longitudinal fiber tracts ascending and descending along the spinal cord, the white matter is also referred to as spinal **columns**. The butterfly-shaped gray matter divides the white matter in each half of the spinal cord into three regions, the **dorsal column**, the **lateral column**, and the **ventral column** (see Fig. 8.2). These columns can be subdivided further into various ascending and descending tracts, based on their points of origin in the brain (in the case of descending motor fibers) or their projection targets in the brain (in the case of sensory fibers).

The spinal columns pick up progressively larger numbers of sensory fibers from the sensory neurons at each successive spinal segment beginning from the lower part of the spinal cord up toward the brain. Moving from the top of the spinal cord to the bottom, the spinal columns contain progressively fewer descending motor fibers, as the axons targeted for each successive spinal segment leave the white matter and terminate on the neurons in the gray matter. As a result, the white matter accounts for a progressively smaller proportion of the cross-sectional area of the spinal cord descending from cervical to sacral levels. For instance, the overall pattern of white and gray matter shown in Figure 8.2A is typical of a section through the human spinal cord in the lower lumbar region. In the cervical region, however, the amount of white matter is greater (see Fig. 8.2B).

The sensory axons added to the ascending columns at each segmental level of the spinal cord do not intermingle randomly among the preexisting sensory fibers. Instead, the branches of the sensory neurons that ascend to the brain at each segment join the dorsal columns at the lateral edge of the column. Thus, at the higher levels of the cord, the ascending sensory fibers from the sacral region of the spinal cord occupy the most medial part of the dorsal columns, followed by the lumbar and thoracic sensory axons at intermediate positions and the cervical sensory axons at the most lateral position, as shown in Figure 8.2B.

The amount of gray matter also varies along the length of the spinal cord. In the parts of the spinal cord that innervate the forelimbs and the hindlimbs, extra motor and sensory neurons are needed to supply the muscle and skin of the limbs, as well as the more medial portions of the body. By contrast, the middle part of the spinal cord (thoracic levels) contains only the neurons that innervate the trunk. Thus, the gray matter in the cervical and lumbosacral parts of the spinal cord is larger than the gray matter in the thoracic region of the cord.

REFLEXES CONTROLLING MUSCLE LENGTH AND TENSION

Myotatic Reflex

What synaptic connections underlie the myotatic (stretch) reflex?

Within the spinal cord, sensory inputs activate local spinal reflexes. The stretch reflex is a particularly simple example of the coupling between sensory and motor systems in the spinal cord. The circuitry of a stretch reflex is summarized in Figure 8.3. Passive stretch of the muscle is signaled by the sensory neurons, which make excitatory connections onto motor neurons that activate the same muscle and onto interneurons that make inhibitory connections with the motor neurons of the antagonist muscles of the same joint. In addition, the stretch-activated sensory neurons also make direct excitatory connections onto motor neurons that control the synergistic (agonist) muscles of the same joint. This combination of connections tends to maintain a constant muscle length—and thus a fixed joint position—by stimulating the muscles that restore the joint position, while relaxing the muscles

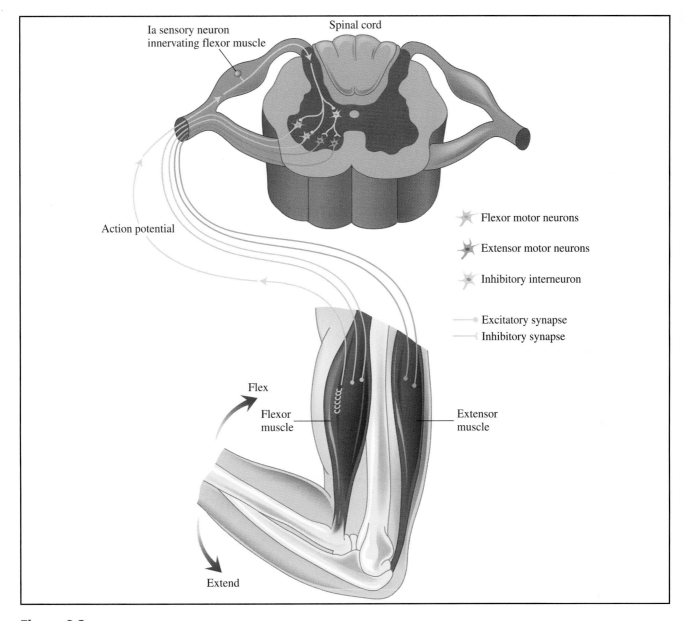

Figure 8.3.

The neuronal circuitry of the myotatic reflex. This diagram illustrates the circuit for a *flexor* reflex (the patellar reflex is an *extensor* reflex), a reminder that stretch reflexes are a general mechanism and are not restricted to extensor muscles.

that oppose the desired movement. This type of reflex, which is found in almost all skeletal muscles, is called the **myotatic reflex**. The patellar reflex is a specific example of a myotatic reflex.

The axons of the stretch-activated sensory neurons are the largest axons in the spinal nerve and thus conduct action potentials most rapidly. The sensory axons within peripheral nerves are classified according to conduction speed, and the fastest group is called **group I**. Because the stretch-activated sensory axons are among the fastest axons in group I, these sensory neurons are referred to as **Ia neurons**. The motor neurons that receive direct excitatory connections from the Ia sensory neurons are among the largest motor neurons, called **α motor neurons**. Because the axons of the α motor neurons are also large and conduct action potentials rapidly, both the sensory and motor signals in the stretch reflex take a minimum amount of time to travel up to the spinal cord and return to the muscle. This rapid conduction speed and the direct excitatory connection between sensory and motor neurons allow muscle length to be controlled rapidly and automatically.

Most joints have a wide range of possible positions, each corresponding to different lengths of the muscles that control the joint. Therefore, the nervous system requires a mechanism to reset the stretch sensors to detect a change in muscle length over a wide range of length. To understand this mechanism, we must examine the structure of the sensory receptors in the muscle.

Muscle Spindles: The Sensory Receptors for Muscle Stretch

How do muscle spindles provide information about muscle stretch?

In schematic diagrams of the circuitry underlying the stretch reflex (for example, see Fig. 8.3), we have portrayed the sensory ending in the muscle as a spiral wrapped around muscle fibers like a spring. The endings of Ia sensory fibers in the muscle really do form such spirals around individual muscle fibers, as illustrated in more detail in Figure 8.4.

The muscle fibers contacted by the sensory endings differ from those that make up the bulk of the skeletal muscle and provide the power for moving loads. A specialized subset of muscle fibers (the **intrafusal muscle fibers**) receive the sensory endings. The intrafusal fibers are functionally and anatomically distinct from the other muscle fibers (the **extrafusal muscle fibers**) that make up the muscle. Scattered throughout skeletal muscles, in parallel with the extrafusal muscle fibers, are specialized structures called **muscle spindles** (so-named because of their shape, fat in the middle, thin at the two ends). Inside the fibrous capsule surrounding each muscle spindle are several intrafusal muscle fibers (see Fig. 8.4), which are similar to extrafusal muscle fibers except that the contractile machinery is absent from the central portion of each fiber. The Ia sensory fibers form their spiral endings (called **annulospiral endings**) around the muscle fibers in this central region.

The intrafusal muscle fibers also receive inputs from axons of motor neurons, as do extrafusal muscle fibers. However, because the intrafusal muscle fibers are few in number and short in length, activation of their motor neurons produces no detectable contraction of the muscle. We will discuss the functional importance of the motor inputs to the intrafusal muscle fibers shortly.

The mechanical behavior of intrafusal muscle fibers and the resulting response of the sensory neuron are illustrated schematically in Figure 8.5. The extrafusal muscle fibers parallel the intrafusal fibers. When the length of the intrafusal fibers matches the resting length of the muscle as a whole (see Fig. 8.5A), the sensory neurons discharge action potentials at a slow steady rate. If a weight is then attached to the muscle, causing a passive stretch of both the extrafusal and the intrafusal fibers, the stretch of the intrafusal fibers is detected by the annulospiral ending of the sensory neurons, which increase their firing rate. The activation of the sensory neuron arises because the annulospiral endings contain stretch-sensitive ion channels that open upon mechanical deformation, depolarizing the sensory ending and stimulating action potentials. (Mechanosensitive ion channels are discussed in more detail in the description of sensory systems in Part IV.)

Figure 8.5B shows what happens to the sensory response of the muscle spindle when the motor neurons supplying the extrafusal muscle fibers are stimulated to fire action potentials. The muscle actively contracts, but the intrafusal muscle fibers remain the same length, relieving the resting stretch of the intrafusal fibers. The resting discharge of the sensory neurons therefore halts when the muscle contracts. If the contracted muscle is then passively stretched by adding a weight, the mismatch in length of the intrafusal and extrafusal muscle fibers prevents the stretch from deforming the annulospiral endings. Therefore, during active contraction, the stretch sensors are unable to detect increased muscle length and the nervous system is unable to regulate muscle length.

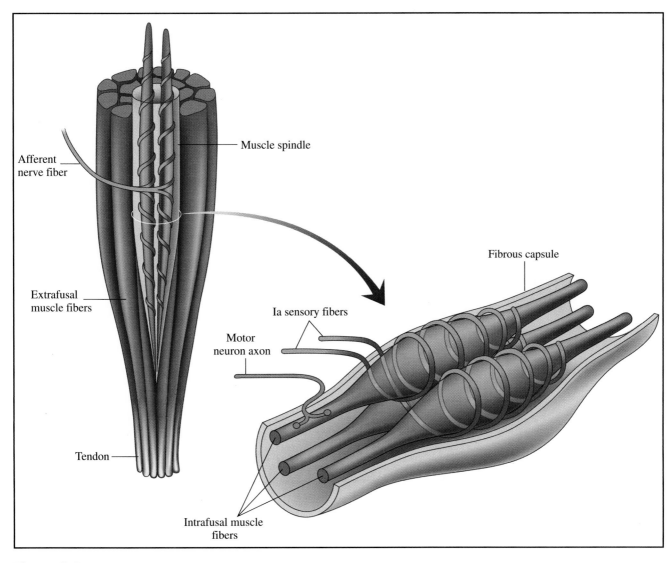

Figure 8.4.

The anatomical organization of the muscle-spindle stretch receptor. Muscle spindles are encapsulated structures that parallel the muscle fibers making up the bulk of the muscle (extrafusal muscle fibers). As shown in the magnified view on the right, the capsule of the spindle contains specialized muscle fibers (intrafusal muscle fibers) that receive sensory fibers from group Ia sensory neurons. The sensory fibers spiral around the muscle fibers. The intrafusal muscle fibers also receive inputs from motor neurons.

Motor Innervation of Intrafusal Muscle Fibers

The motor neurons of the intrafusal muscle fibers, however, allow the nervous system to restore sensitivity to passive stretch during active contraction. The effect of stimulating the intrafusal motor neurons, together with the extrafusal motor neurons, is illustrated in Figure 8.5C. If the intrafusal muscle fibers also contract, the resting level of stretch of the central mechanosensory region is maintained, and the slow resting discharge of the sensory neurons is retained during the active contraction. When the intrafusal motor neurons are stimulated, passive stretch of the muscle can be detected, because the length of the intrafusal fibers is matched to the new, reduced length of the extrafusal fibers during active contraction. The active response of the intrafusal muscle fibers—stimulated by the intrafusal motor neurons—is the key to maintaining the ability of the stretch sensor system to respond to changes in muscle length across the entire operating range of muscle length.

Why is the motor innervation of the intrafusal muscle fibers important for proper maintenance of muscle length by the nervous system?

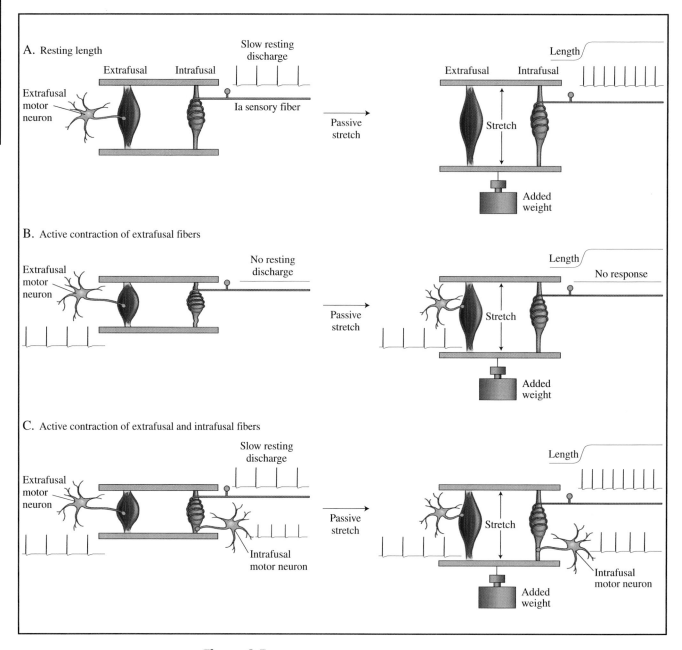

Figure 8.5.

The response of the muscle-spindle sensory neuron to stretch of the muscle under various conditions. Extrafusal and intrafusal muscle fibers are arranged in parallel. **A.** When passive stretch is applied to a resting muscle in which the length of the intrafusal muscle fibers matches the resting length of the extrafusal fibers, the rate of action potential in the sensory neuron increases. **B.** During active contraction of the extrafusal muscle fibers, the muscle shortens and the load on the intrafusal muscle fibers is removed. The firing of action potentials in the sensory neuron ceases, and the sensory neuron fails to respond to a passive stretch of the muscle superimposed on the contracted muscle. **C.** The resting discharge and the sensitivity to stretch of the sensory neuron are restored if the intrafusal muscle fibers are stimulated to contract along with the extrafusal muscle fibers during contraction of the muscle.

The motor neurons that supply the intrafusal muscle fibers form a separate pool within the population of motor neurons controlling a particular muscle. This segregation allows motor centers of the nervous system to regulate separately the activity of extrafusal and intrafusal motor neurons supplying a muscle. In mammals, the intrafusal pool can be distinguished from the extrafusal pool on the basis of axon diameter and hence conduction velocity of action potentials. Whereas the extrafusal fibers are supplied by large-diameter fibers of α motor neurons, the intrafusal fibers are supplied by slower-conducting, smaller fibers of the **γ motor neurons**.

The intrafusal pool of motor neurons can be subdivided further according to the properties of the intrafusal muscle fibers they activate. Muscle fibers within the muscle spindle fall into two classes: static fibers and dynamic fibers. **Static fibers** and the sensory neurons that innervate them provide the sustained action potentials that give a steady indication of muscle length. **Dynamic fibers** and their sensory neurons are most sensitive to the rapid changes in length that accompany the onset of a muscle stretch.

Tendon Reflex

In addition to muscle spindles, skeletal muscles are supplied with another type of specialized sensory receptor, called **tendon organs** or **Golgi tendon organs**. Tendon organs are located at the junction between extrafusal muscle fibers and the tendon that connects the muscle to other body structures. Each tendon organ is an encapsulated structure containing a mesh of collagen fibers connected to the ends of the muscle fibers. Branches of sensory axons innervating the tendon organ entwine among the mesh of collagen fibers. The axons of sensory neurons of the tendon organ are members of the fast-conducting group I, like the sensory neurons of muscle spindles. Because the sensory neurons of tendon organs conduct action potentials a bit more slowly than the muscle-spindle receptors, however, they are called group Ib sensory neurons, to distinguish them from the faster-conducting group Ia fibers.

The tendon-organ sensory neurons respond to passive and active muscle stretch differently from muscle-spindle sensory neurons. Figure 8.6A shows the response of a tendon-organ receptor neuron during passive stretch. At the resting muscle length, the sensory neuron fires action potentials at a rate that depends on the resting tension in the muscle. When the muscle is passively stretched, the firing rate of the tendon-organ sensory neuron changes little. In contrast, the muscle-spindle sensory neuron (Fig. 8.5A) fires briskly when the muscle is passively stretched from the resting length.

During active contraction, the two types of sensory neurons also respond quite differently. Figure 8.6B shows the response of the tendon-organ receptor neuron during active contraction. In this case, the rate of action potentials in the sensory neuron of the tendon organ increases when the muscle contracts and exerts tension on the tendon. In contrast, muscle-spindle sensory neurons either cease firing during active contraction (in the absence of co-activation of the intrafusal motor neuron; see Fig. 8.5B) or maintain their resting firing rate (during co-activation of the intrafusal motor neuron; see Fig. 8.5C).

You might wonder what accounts for these important differences in the sensitivity of tendon-organ sensory neurons and muscle-spindle sensory neurons to passive and active stretch of the muscle. The answer lies in the different mechanical properties of the muscle fibers and tendon and in the different arrangement of the sensory structure relative to the extrafusal muscle fibers in the two cases. The tendon and muscle fibers of the muscle are arranged *in series*. When a weight is applied to passively stretch the muscle-tendon combination, most of the stretch is confined to the muscle fibers, and the length of the tendon changes little. The tendon

What synaptic connections underlie the inverse myotatic (tendon-organ) reflex?

What mechanical factors account for the different ways muscle spindles and tendon organs respond to active muscle contraction and passive muscle stretch?

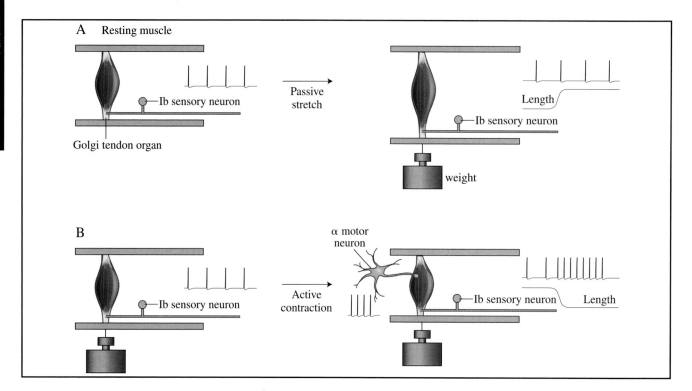

Figure 8.6.

The response of the Golgi tendon-organ sensory neuron during passive stretch and active contraction of the muscle. The Golgi tendon organ is arranged in series with the extrafusal muscle fibers. (Contrast this arrangement with that of the muscle spindle, shown in Fig. 8.5.) **A.** During passive stretch of the muscle, the increase in length is absorbed by the muscle fibers but not by the tendon. Thus, the rate of action potentials in the group Ib sensory neuron is unaffected by passive stretch. **B.** During active contraction, the force generated by the muscle is transmitted to the joint via the tendon, which deforms the Golgi tendon organ and increases the rate of action potentials in the sensory neuron.

is much stiffer than unstimulated muscle fibers. The longitudinally oriented contractile filaments of the muscle cells can slide past each other readily, allowing the muscle fibers to stretch easily. Because the intrafusal muscle fibers of the muscle spindles are aligned *in parallel* with the other muscle fibers, they also increase in length during passive stretch, and the Ia afferent fibers signal the stretch to the nervous system. On the other hand, the collagen mesh within the Golgi tendon organ is not significantly distorted during passive stretch, and the intertwined branches of the sensory fiber will not be activated.

During active contraction, the mechanical situation is quite different. In this case, the muscle fibers themselves *generate* the force applied to the muscle. Because the muscle fibers transfer their force to the attached body structures via the tendons, the contracting muscle fibers pull the collagen mesh within the Golgi tendon organ, distort the mesh, and squeeze the entwined branches of the innervating Ib sensory fibers. The amount of tendon-organ distortion during active contraction depends on the amount of force applied to the tendon by the contracting muscle. If the muscle tension is high, as in lifting a heavy weight, the tendon organ will be highly distorted, and the sensory neuron of the tendon organ will fire action potentials at a high rate. If the muscle tension is low, however, the collagen mesh within the tendon organ will not be distorted very much, and the sensory neuron will fire action potentials at a lower rate.

Because of their different mechanical arrangements relative to the muscle fibers of a muscle, the group Ia sensory neurons of the muscle spindles and the group Ib

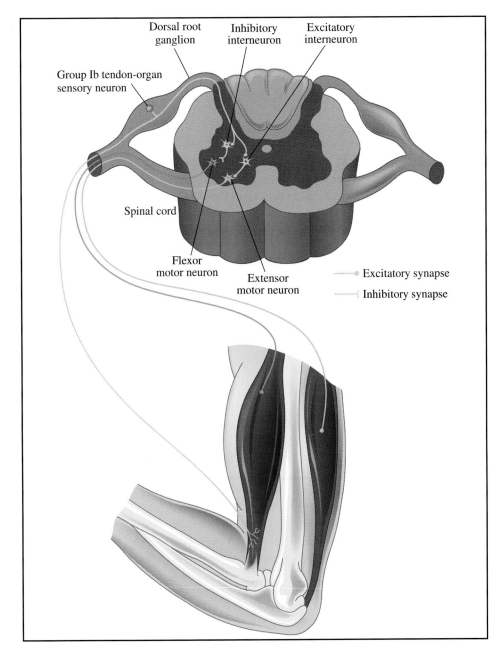

Dorsal root
ganglion

Inhibitory
interneuron

Excitatory
interneuron

Group Ib tendon-organ
sensory neuron

Spinal cord

Flexor
motor neuron

Extensor
motor neuron

Excitatory synapse

Inhibitory synapse

Figure 8.7.

The neuronal circuitry underlying the tendon reflex, or inverse myotatic reflex. The
sensory neuron makes excitatory synapses on interneurons. The interneurons then
make inhibitory synaptic connections on the motor neurons controlling the same
muscle and excitatory synaptic connections onto motor
neurons controlling the antagonist muscles of the joint.

sensory neurons of the Golgi tendon organs provide the nervous system with different kinds of information about the state of the muscle. The muscle-spindle sensory neurons give information about *muscle length*, while the tendon-organ sensory
neurons give information about *muscle tension*.

Figure 8.7 shows a schematic diagram of the tendon reflex circuit, demonstrating how the sensory information provided by the tendon organ is used in reflex circuits in the spinal cord. Like other sensory neurons of spinal nerves, the cell bodies
of the tendon-organ sensory neurons are located in the dorsal root ganglion, just
outside the spinal cord. Group Ib afferent fibers branch after entering the spinal
cord and make excitatory synaptic connections with inhibitory and excitatory
interneurons. The inhibitory interneurons make inhibitory synaptic connections
onto the pool of motor neurons controlling the same muscle from which the tendon-organ sensory fiber originated. When tension in the muscle rises, the sensory
neuron of the tendon organ fires action potentials at a higher rate, stimulating the
inhibitory interneurons and inhibiting motor neurons of the same muscle. Reduced

activity in the motor neurons decreases tension in the muscle. Therefore, the tendon-organ reflex represents a **negative feedback loop** that reduces tension in a muscle.

The tendon reflex allows the nervous system to set and maintain a desired muscle tension, just as the muscle-spindle system allows the nervous system to set and maintain a desired muscle length. The inhibitory interneurons in the tendon reflex receive inhibitory and excitatory connections from other spinal interneurons and from higher motor control centers in the brain, which allow the nervous system to set the desired tension. If a large amount of tension in a muscle is required for a particular movement, the inhibitory interneurons for that muscle can be strongly inhibited by higher motor systems. In this case, a large amount of excitation from the group Ib sensory fibers from the muscle, corresponding to high muscle tension, will be required to activate inhibitory feedback of the tendon reflex. Conversely, if low muscle tension is required, then the inhibitory interneurons can be excited by other neural circuits, so that a relatively small amount of excitation from the group Ib fibers will be sufficient to activate the reflex.

Tendon-organ sensory neurons also make excitatory synaptic connections onto excitatory interneurons, which in turn excite motor neurons controlling antagonist motor neurons of the same joint. Thus, the tendon reflex produces inhibition of the same muscle and excitation of the antagonist muscle, whereas the stretch reflex results in excitation of the same muscle and inhibition of the antagonist. Because the two reflexes have opposite actions, the tendon reflex is also referred to as the **inverse myotatic reflex**.

The stretch reflex involves a direct synaptic connection from the sensory neuron onto motor neurons. For this reason, the stretch reflex is an example of a **monosynaptic reflex**. By contrast, the sensory neurons in the tendon reflex connect only with interneurons, which then form the appropriate connections with motor neurons. The tendon reflex is therefore an example of a **polysynaptic reflex**, because the signal from the sensory neurons must pass through more than one synaptic relay before reaching the motor neurons. Monosynaptic reflexes have greater speed because they involve the minimum number of relay steps before the signal returns to the muscle. Polysynaptic reflexes, however, provide greater opportunity for modifying and altering the behavior of the reflex by allowing integration of multiple signals within the interneurons interposed between sensory and motor neurons.

Self-inhibition of Motor Neurons: Renshaw Cells

In Chapter 7, we learned that the nervous system can avoid fatigue within a motor unit if the motor neuron fires action potentials in bursts separated by quiet periods. By staggering the bursts in different pools of motor neurons, smooth and steady increases in muscle tension can be attained without fatiguing the muscle as a whole and without significant jitter in tension. A simple feedback circuit in the spinal cord, involving a type of inhibitory interneuron called the **Renshaw cell**, helps produce the desired oscillations in the firing rate of motor neurons. Before the axon of a motor neuron exits the spinal cord through the ventral root, it gives off a collateral branch that remains within the spinal cord and makes excitatory synaptic connections with local inhibitory interneurons, the Renshaw cells. As shown in Figure 8.8, the Renshaw cells then make an inhibitory synaptic connection back onto the motor neuron. This kind of self-inhibitory synaptic connection is called **recurrent inhibition**.

The effect of recurrent inhibition via Renshaw cells is summarized in Figure 8.8B. If a motor neuron is stimulated by strong excitatory input from some neural source, it will fire action potentials at a high rate. This firing triggers summated

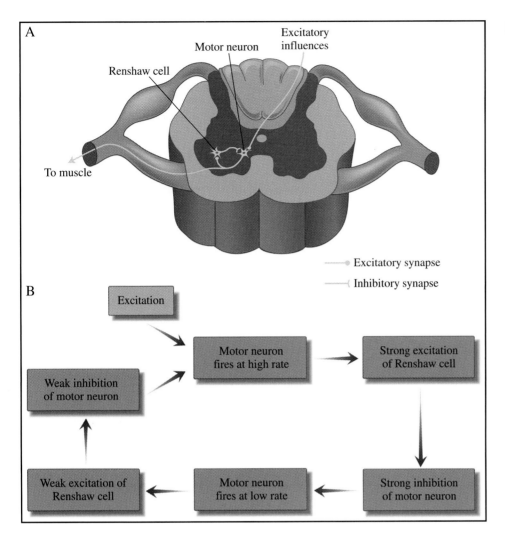

Figure 8.8.

Renshaw cells produce self-inhibition of motor neurons. **A.** The axons of motor neurons send branches that make excitatory synaptic connections onto Renshaw cells. The Renshaw cells in turn make inhibitory synaptic connections back onto the same motor neurons. **B.** A summary of the cyclical effect of this circuit on firing of the motor neuron.

contraction of the muscle fibers making up the motor unit controlled by the motor neuron. In addition, the motor neuron strongly excites Renshaw cells, which in turn produce strong inhibition of the motor neuron. The recurrent inhibition reduces the firing rate of the motor neuron, which translates into weaker excitation of the Renshaw cell and thus into weaker recurrent inhibition. If the excitatory input from other sources persists, the motor neuron will fire again at a faster pace, returning to the beginning of the cycle shown in Figure 8.8B. Thus, the motor neuron oscillates between periods of high firing rate and periods of low firing rate.

THE WITHDRAWAL REFLEX

At one time or another, everyone has had the unpleasant experience of eliciting another type of spinal reflex, the limb withdrawal reflex. If you accidentally touch a hot object, your hand will rapidly jerk away from the object without a conscious command and indeed before the perception of pain reaches a conscious level. Similarly, if you step on a piece of glass hidden in the sand while walking barefoot on the beach, your leg will rapidly flex to withdraw the foot—again without conscious control. In concert with the flexion of the injured leg, the other leg will extend, to take the weight of the body and keep you from falling over. A variety of other reflexive rearrangements of upper-limb and trunk musculature will also occur to shift the body weight off the injured leg and onto the other leg. Thus, two different aspects of limb withdrawal reflexes are triggered by noxious stimuli: with-

How does the spinal cord coordinate withdrawal of an injured limb with extension of the contralateral limb when a noxious stimulus is applied to a limb?

drawal of the stimulated limb and extension of the contralateral limb together with postural rearrangements to maintain support of the body.

Withdrawal of the Stimulated Limb

Let us consider first the withdrawal component of the reflex circuit, diagrammed in Figure 8.9. If the hand encounters a hot object, pain-sensitive sensory neurons will be stimulated. Like other sensory neurons, the cell bodies of these sensory neurons are located in the dorsal root ganglia, just outside the spinal cord. The axons of the pain-sensitive sensory cells branch within the spinal cord and make excitatory synaptic connections with various types of spinal interneurons, including two types illustrated in Figure 8.9. Both interneuron types then make excit-

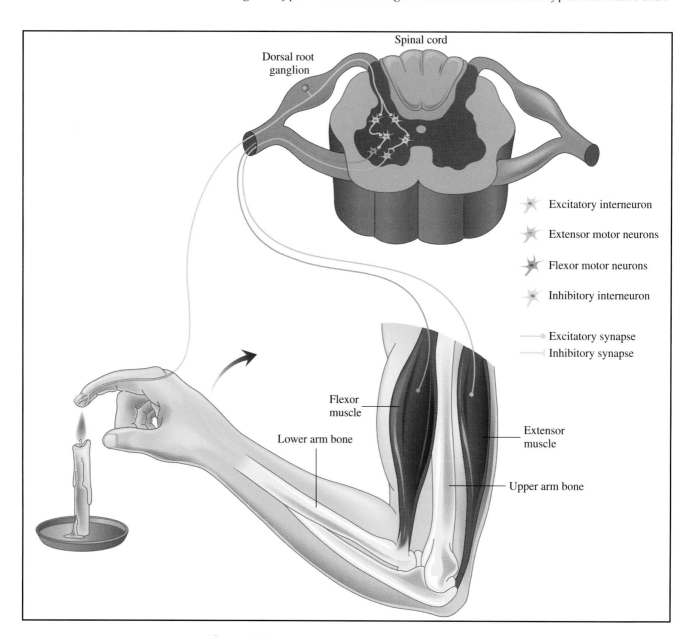

Figure 8.9.

The neuronal circuitry underlying limb withdrawal in response to a painful stimulus. The sensory neuron makes excitatory synaptic connections onto pools of excitatory interneurons in the spinal cord. These interneurons then excite other interneurons, which in turn excite the flexor motor neurons of the injured limb and inhibit the extensor motor neurons.

atory connections with the next interneurons in the circuit. In one case, the target interneurons excite the flexor motor neurons of the limb receiving the painful stimulus. In the other case, the target interneurons inhibit the motor neurons controlling the extensor muscles of the limb receiving the stimulus. Stimulation of the sensory neuron thus activates two parallel circuits, culminating in contraction of the flexor muscles and relaxation of the extensor muscles. This reflex produces the rapid, involuntary withdrawal of the limb from the pain-inducing object.

For simplicity, Figure 8.9 shows only the muscles of a single joint. In reality, the pain-sensitive sensory neurons make similar connections with all of the flexor and extensor motor neurons controlling all of the joints in the limb (e.g., fingers, wrist, elbow, and shoulder joints in the case of a human arm). The connections with the motor neurons are indirect, involving a polysynaptic pathway through at least two layers of intervening interneurons.

Extension of the Contralateral Limb

During the withdrawal reflex, extension of the contralateral limb requires additional neuronal circuitry in the spinal cord to activate and inhibit the appropriate motor neurons controlling the contralateral limb (Fig. 8.10). Because the motor neurons controlling the contralateral limb are located on the other side of the spinal cord, the sensory neuron must stimulate interneurons that cross the midline of the spinal cord and terminate on the other side. As shown in Figure 8.10, the pain-sensitive sensory neurons make excitatory synaptic connections with a group of interneurons, which then activate another pool of interneurons that send axons to the contralateral side of the spinal cord. There, the interneurons make excitatory synaptic connections with the pools of inhibitory and excitatory interneurons that control the flexor and extensor motor neurons for the contralateral limb. In this case, however, the activated pools of interneurons are the opposite of those described for the ipsilateral side of the spinal cord. That is, the inhibitory interneurons of the flexor motor neurons and the excitatory interneurons of the extensor motor neurons are activated. This leads to contraction of the muscles that extend the limb, while the opposing flexor muscles relax. In this way, the flexion of the stimulated limb is accompanied by extension of the contralateral limb.

The circuitry of the withdrawal reflex is actually more complicated than illustrated in Figure 8.10, which shows only a single segment of the spinal cord. The intermediate interneurons send connections to both higher and lower spinal cord segments, contacting appropriate pools of interneurons on both sides of the spinal cord to maintain stable body posture during the withdrawal of the injured limb. These connections in complex reflex circuits are much more elaborate than the simple myotatic reflex controlling the length of a single skeletal muscle. Indeed, because the withdrawal reflex involves the coordinated activity of many pools of motor neurons, it serves as a transition between purely reflexive circuits and more general spinal circuits that underlie voluntary, coordinated activity of the organism. Examples of this second type of spinal circuit are the spinal circuits involved in locomotion.

SPINAL CIRCUITS CONTROLLING LOCOMOTION

In reflex circuits, pools of spinal neurons that carry out a particular function form components of a variety of neuronal circuits. For instance, consider the pools of inhibitory and excitatory spinal interneurons that make synaptic connections with motor neurons controlling an extensor muscle of a limb. In the stretch reflex,

What is a central pattern generator?

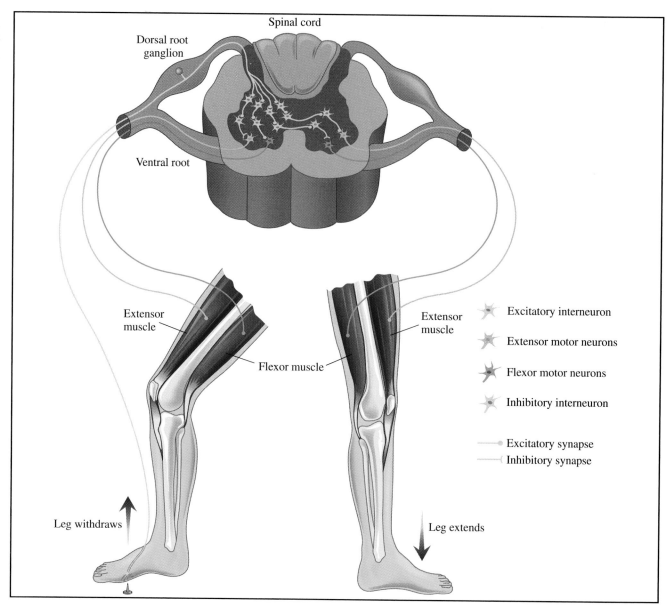

Spinal cord

Dorsal root
ganglion

Ventral root

Extensor
muscle

Flexor muscle

Extensor
muscle

Excitatory interneuron

Extensor motor neurons

Flexor motor neurons

Inhibitory interneuron

Excitatory synapse
Inhibitory synapse

Leg withdraws

Leg extends

Figure 8.10.

The expanded circuitry for the withdrawal reflex, combining flexion of the injured limb with extension of the contralateral limb. The ipsilateral portion of the circuit is the same as in Figure 8.9, and this portion of the circuit produces excitation of the flexor motor neurons combined with inhibition of the extensor motor neurons of the ipsilateral limb. The sensory neurons also stimulate two additional pools of interneurons, which make excitatory synaptic connections onto excitatory interneurons that cross to the other side of the spinal cord and connect with pools of interneurons controlling the motor neurons of the contralateral limb. These interneurons produce the opposite effect on the contralateral limb, exciting the extensor motor neurons and inhibiting the flexor motor neurons.

interneurons that inhibit extensor-muscle motor neurons are excited by the Ia sensory neurons from the flexor muscle (see Fig. 8.3). In addition, the same extensor-muscle inhibitory interneurons are excited during the withdrawal reflex for the limb (see Fig. 8.9). The excitatory interneurons for the same extensor muscle participate in still other reflex circuits. For example, the excitatory interneurons for an extensor muscle are excited by stimulating the Golgi tendon organ of the antagonist flexor muscle (see Fig. 8.7) and by stimulating the withdrawal reflex for the contralateral limb (see Fig. 8.10). This flexibility in tapping pools of interneurons is one advantage of hierarchical motor control, as discussed earlier in this chapter (see Fig. 8.1).

Groups of interneurons like those used in spinal reflex circuits can also be utilized in other kinds of spinal motor circuits to control movement of the organism through space—the process of **locomotion**. The circuitry of the withdrawal reflex produces flexion of a limb combined with extension of the contralateral limb. For the contralateral limb, a mirror-image withdrawal circuit produces the reverse effect. The nervous system can produce alternating limb movements of the type used in quadruped locomotion by alternately exciting the populations of interneurons on the two sides of the spinal cord that are used in the withdrawal circuits for the two limbs. Of course, locomotion involves more than just alternating stepping motions of the limbs, but the basic pattern can be produced by circuitry of the type shown in Figure 8.10.

In mammals and in other vertebrates, the spinal cord contains not only circuits required for the basic alternating stepping pattern but also circuits that produce interlimb coordination under changing conditions of locomotion. If the spinal cord is transected at a high level to eliminate all descending commands from the brain, patterns of limb movements similar to those during voluntary locomotion can still be evoked. Even in the absence of sensory inputs from the limbs, alternating stepping movements still occur in animals with spinal cord transections. Thus, the basic pattern of motor output during locomotion is produced by **central pattern generators** (CPGs) that do not require sensory information from the limbs to generate the correct motor pattern.

Although sensory information is not required for stepping motions, sensory input from the limbs is normally used to adapt the motor pattern to the changing conditions that are encountered as the animal moves through the world. Without sensory information, the CPGs can generate alternating cycles of flexion and extension, but the movements are stereotyped and easily disrupted. Thus, both automatic generators of motor patterns and sensory information are required to produce normal locomotion.

BOX 1

IN THE CLINIC

Spinal reflexes are a mainstay of the basic neurological examination. Diseases of the spinal cord can often be detected by their effects on reflexes such as the stretch reflex or the tendon reflex, often before more severe symptoms appear. Because reflexes involve both excitatory and inhibitory pathways in the spinal cord, hyperactive reflexes can be a sign of spinal cord disease, as well as loss of reflexes. The location of the affected muscles provides information about the level of the spinal cord where a lesion is located. For instance, a loss of the knee-jerk reflex would be consistent with a lesion in the lumbar region of the spinal cord. In addition to local reflex circuits, the spinal cord includes sensory pathways ascending to the brain and descending motor pathways from brain motor centers. Thus, spinal cord lesions often result in a complex mix of sensory and motor disturbances, which in combination can provide precise clues about the location of the lesion. The pattern of sensory and motor disturbances can also establish whether a lesion affects primarily white matter or gray matter in the spinal cord. Modern imaging techniques, such as magnetic resonance imaging (MRI), can then be used to confirm the location and extent of the damage in the central nervous system.

The Spinal Circuits Underlying Central Pattern Generators

The CPGs and interlimb coordination circuits that produce locomotion probably include the same spinal interneurons that govern simpler spinal reflexes. These spinal circuits are not yet understood in detail in quadruped vertebrates. In less complex vertebrates such as fish, however, the body movements required for locomotion (that is, swimming) are somewhat simpler, and the underlying spinal circuits are correspondingly easier to understand. Thus, we will describe the neural circuits controlling swimming in fish, as an example of spinal locomotion mechanisms.

In keeping with the principle of hierarchical organization, the brain does not directly program the alternating activation of motor neurons on the two sides of the body during swimming. Instead, the brain issues a general command to the spinal cord, and spinal cord circuits cooperate to produce the correct sequence of muscle contractions. The brain says "swim," and the spinal cord obliges.

The details regarding the motion required to produce effective swimming depend on the exact situation, including body position, water currents, and so on. Nevertheless, the basic pattern for a prototypical fish is shown in Figure 8.11A. A wave of contraction propagates from the head to the tail along each side of the body, with the waves on each side out of phase with each other. These alternating waves produce an undulating motion that propels the animal through the water. Many fish also have various fins that contribute to propulsion through the water, as well as to steering

Figure 8.11.

The neuronal circuitry that produces alternating contractions on the two sides of the body when the lamprey swims. Although the circuitry for a single spinal cord segment is shown, the same pattern of connections is repeated along the entire spinal cord. **A.** A schematic diagram of the undulating motion during swimming in the lamprey. At time 1, the right-side muscles are contracting, producing bending to the right at positions 1 and 3. In the middle of the animal, the left side is contracting, at position 2. At a later time (time 2), the contraction of the right side has moved to a more posterior position (position 1), as has the contraction on the left side (position 2). A new wave of contraction has just begun on the left side (position 4). Still later (time 3), the waves of contraction on the two sides of the body have moved to more posterior positions. **B.** A circuit diagram for the central pattern generator of swimming at a single spinal cord segment. The circuits on the two sides of the spinal cord (enclosed in *dashed boxes*) are mirror images of one another. The network is activated by descending excitatory inputs that arise from swimming command centers in the brain. MN = motor neuron; CI = crossed interneuron; EI = excitatory interneuron; II = inhibitory interneuron.

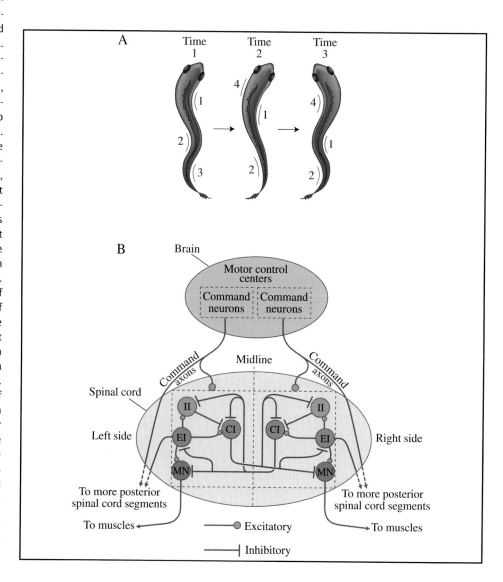

and body orientation during locomotion; however, we will simplify the situation by considering only the generation of the propagating wave of contraction.

Comparing the positions of the body undergoing contraction at times 1 and 3 in Figure 8.11A, we see that the swimming movement is produced by alternating contractions of the muscles on the two sides of the body. Figure 8.11B shows the basic circuit that generates these undulating contractions in the lamprey, a primitive jawless fish. Swimming is initiated by action potentials in motor command axons descending along both sides of the spinal cord from brain command centers located bilaterally in the brainstem. These motor command axons make excitatory synaptic connections with the pattern generator neurons (see Fig. 8.11B) on the two sides of the spinal cord at each spinal segment. Although the diagram shows only a single spinal segment for simplicity, the circuit is actually repeated at each segment along the spinal cord. The command neurons provide a steady level of excitation that adds to the inputs arising from the connections among the pattern generator neurons themselves and from other spinal sources (for example, sensory inputs). The pattern of action potentials in the command axons does not provide information about the alternating rhythm of output from the motor neurons on the two sides of the spinal cord. However, the rate of action potentials in the command axons does affect the overall level of excitability in the pattern generators and thus the period of oscillation.

How does the circuit in Figure 8.11B produce alternating excitation to the muscles on the two sides of the body? The swimming command axons make excitatory connections onto four types of neurons on each side of the spinal cord: the motor neurons themselves, and three kinds of interneurons. A crossed interneuron sends an axon to the opposite side of the spinal cord, where it makes inhibitory synapses onto all four types of neurons in the contralateral circuit. An excitatory interneuron makes excitatory synapses onto the other three types of neurons on the same side of the spinal cord, and an inhibitory interneuron makes inhibitory synapses onto the crossed interneuron on the same side of the spinal cord.

During swimming, action potentials are triggered in the command axons on both sides. As a result, the bilateral pattern generator circuits receive steady excitation on both sides of the spinal cord. At the onset of swimming, however, the generator circuit on one side will reach the threshold to initiate a burst of action potentials before the circuit on the other side is triggered. The side that fires first will be determined by other excitatory influences (such as sensory inputs) and by modulatory inputs onto the brainstem command centers. If the right-side neurons fire first, for example, the combination of the direct excitatory input from the command axons and the excitatory input from the excitatory interneuron will cause the motor neurons on the right to fire, contracting the muscles on that side and causing the body to bend to the right. This would correspond to time 1, position 1 in Figure 8.11A, for instance. In addition, the summed excitation from the command axons and from the excitatory interneuron activates the crossed interneuron. Action potentials in the crossed interneuron suppress activity in the contralateral generator circuit, ensuring that the contralateral muscles will relax. Therefore, bending to the right is a consequence of a burst of action potentials in the right-side motor neurons combined with a corresponding silent period in the left-side motor neurons.

To produce alternating bursts of action potentials in the motor neurons on the two sides, the burst on the right side must be terminated. Nothing in the synaptic circuitry of the network shown in Figure 8.11B would appear capable of halting the activation of the motor neurons once the process has begun. Burst termination occurs principally because of the membrane electrical properties of the motor neurons and the excitatory interneurons themselves. The action potentials of these neurons exhibit pronounced after hyperpolarizations caused by calcium-activated potassium channels (see Chapter 4). As calcium accumulates inside the neurons during a burst of action potentials, the after hyperpolarizations summate, causing the frequency of action potentials to decline and finally to cease altogether. Thus, the motor neurons and excitatory interneurons fire action potentials in discrete bursts, separated by quiet periods, even in the presence of sustained excitatory input from the command axons.

This example clearly indicates the importance of cellular mechanisms in determining the behavior of neural networks. *In general, a diagram of the connections between neurons is not sufficient to predict the behavior of the circuit.* Additional information about the ion channels and electrical characteristics of the individual neurons making up the circuit is essential to understand the function of the nervous system.

As the burst of activity on the right side proceeds, the activation of the crossed interneuron falls off because of the declining excitation provided by the excitatory interneurons and the delayed inhibition arising from the inhibitory interneuron, which is excited by the command axons and the excitatory interneuron. Thus, coincident with the declining burst activity on the right side, inhibition of the contralateral network decreases. This reduced inhibition allows the continuing excitation supplied to the contralateral network by the descending command axons to reach the threshold for activation of the network on the left side of the spinal cord. As soon as the burst of action potentials in the left network begins, activation of the crossed interneuron from that side produces inhibition of the right network and ensures termination of the right-side burst. At this stage, the state of the network is a mirror image of the starting condition, with excitation of the left-side motor neurons and inhibition of the right-side motor neurons. The resulting body position is also the mirror image (see, for example, time 3, position 4 in Fig. 8.11A).

Intersegmental Control of Central Pattern Generators

Effective locomotion requires not only alternating contraction on both sides of the body at each segment, but also anterior-to-posterior propagation of the contraction along each side (see Fig. 8.11A). To produce this pattern, the CPG networks at more posterior positions must be activated progressively later than the networks at more anterior positions. The axons from the brainstem motor command centers descend the entire length of the spinal cord and deliver excitation to all of the segmental pattern generators. However, not all of the segmental pattern generators are equally excitable, and the segmental network with the highest excitability will be the first to be activated. The level of excitability of a segmental network is influenced by the activity of additional excitatory or inhibitory spinal interneurons, which generate excitatory postsynaptic potentials (e.p.s.p.'s) and inhibitory postsynaptic potentials (i.p.s.p.'s) that sum with the e.p.s.p.'s produced by the command axons. Under ordinary conditions, the most excitable pattern generators are those at the rostral (anterior) end of the spinal cord. Thus, alternating contraction of the body musculature typically starts at the anterior end.

In addition, the excitatory interneuron of each segmental oscillator sends an axon branch that makes excitatory synapses onto the neurons of the ipsilateral oscillators in adjacent spinal cord segments (see Fig. 8.11B). The excitation descending from the anterior pattern generator sums with the excitation from the command axons to initiate activity in the next most posterior segmental pattern generator. The activity of the excitatory interneuron in this segment is then transmitted to the next posterior segment, initiating activity in the pattern generator network at that location. In this manner, activity of the pattern generators sweeps down the spinal cord, producing a propagating wave of contraction.

When the activity in the first-activated network (that is, at the anterior end) switches over to the contralateral side, the excitatory interneuron on that side will excite the more posterior ipsilateral network, and a wave of contraction will sweep down that side of the body. In this way, the segmental pattern generators of the spinal cord program the oscillating contractions of each body segment, while the intersegmental excitatory connections couple the oscillators in the proper sequence to produce effective swimming.

Sensory Inputs Modulate the Central Pattern Generators

The CPG circuitry can produce swimming motions in the absence of any sensory input about muscle length or body posture. Thus, rhythmic behaviors can be generated by the central nervous system, without requiring sensory information to produce the pattern. This fact does not mean that sensory inputs have no effect on the rhythmic behavior, however. In the lamprey swimming circuit, for example, sensory neurons sensitive to the stretching of the body reinforce and adjust the timing of the alternating bursts of action potentials within the swimming circuits on the two sides of the spinal cord. In Figure 8.11A, note that when the right side of the body is contracting at a particular position, the left side is being stretched (see, for example, time 1, position 1). Stretch-sensitive sensory neurons are activated whenever the body is stretched in this manner.

In the lamprey, the stretch-sensitive neurons are located within the spinal cord itself and are stimulated by the bending of the spinal cord during the undulations, rather than by the stretching of the muscles of the body wall. The stretch-sensitive neurons and their synaptic connections are diagrammed in Figure 8.12. To make the wiring diagram less confusing, the oscillator circuitry shown in detail in Figure 8.11B is lumped together on each side of the spinal cord and labeled *CPG* (for "central pattern generator"). The stretch-sensitive neurons are located along the lateral edges of the spinal cord (and are called **edge cells** for that reason) and have dendrites that spread laterally along the margin of the cord. When the muscles on the right side contract and bend the body toward the right, the left side of the spinal cord stretches and the edge cells on the left side fire action potentials.

Two types of edge cells are found on each side of the spinal cord: excitatory and inhibitory. The excitatory cells make excitatory synaptic connections onto the neurons of the CPG circuit on the same side of the spinal cord. The inhibitory cells make inhibitory connections onto the neurons of the CPG on the contralateral side of the spinal cord, including the inhibitory edge cells on the other side. When the right-side CPG is active and the body bends to the right, the left-side stretch-sensitive cells become active. The left-side excitatory edge cells add excitation to the left-side CPG, just at the time when the burst of activity in the right-side CPG begins to wane. This additional excitation, combined with decreasing inhibition crossing from the contralateral CPG, ensures that a burst of activity

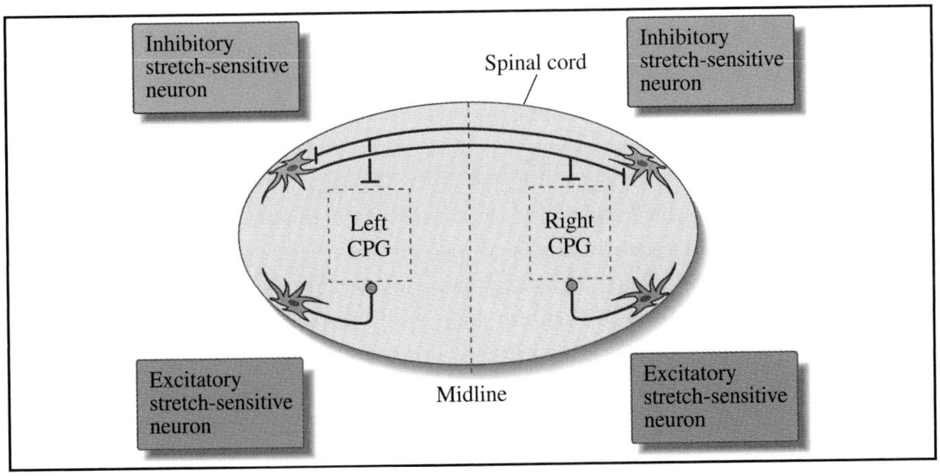

What role is played by sensory information in the generation of rhythmic motor output?

Figure 8.12.

The effects of stretch-sensitive sensory neurons on the swimming pattern generator in the spinal cord of the lamprey. The stretch-sensitive neurons are located within the spinal cord, at the lateral edges. The *dashed boxes* represent the bilateral central pattern generator (CPG) networks detailed in Figure 8.11.

begins in the left-side CPG, producing the next phase of the alternating cycle of activity on the two sides of the spinal cord. When the body bends to the right, the inhibitory edge cells on the left are also activated, inhibiting the right-side CPG and helping to end the burst of activity on the right side. Thus, the stretch-sensitive sensory neurons help coordinate the network, ensuring that bursts of activity in the segmental swimming circuits alternate in the proper way.

In the generation of rhythmic behavior, the basic motor pattern results from the synaptic wiring diagram of the neurons in the CNS and the cellular properties of the neurons in the network. Sensory information serves to reinforce the pattern and ensure that activity in the circuit is tailored to the environment in which the movement occurs.

SUMMARY

Hierarchical organization of motor control systems allows higher centers to control complex movements without having to specify the details of the activity of individual motor neurons. The spinal cord contains circuits that automate commonly needed motor functions. The stretch reflex, or myotatic reflex, is a simple example of such an automated function, allowing the nervous system to automatically maintain a fixed muscle length.

In the stretch reflex, sensory information about muscle length originates from specialized muscle fibers called intrafusal muscle fibers, which are contained within an encapsulated sensory structure known as the muscle spindle. The annulospiral endings of group Ia sensory neurons fire action potentials when the length of the muscle spindle increases as a result of passive stretch of the muscle. The intrafusal muscle fibers are innervated by γ motor neurons, which stimulate active contraction of the intrafusal muscle fibers and allow the muscle spindle to signal passive stretch over a wide range of resting muscle length.

The Golgi tendon organ is a muscle sensory structure that gives the nervous system information about the tension of a muscle. This information is transmitted to the spinal cord by group Ib sensory neurons and is used in the tendon reflex (also called the inverse myotatic reflex).

Pools of excitatory and inhibitory interneurons that make synaptic connections onto motor neurons are activated by sensory neurons as part of the reflex circuits controlling muscle length and tension. In addition, motor neurons make self-inhibitory synaptic connections via a class of inhibitory interneurons called Renshaw cells. The withdrawal reflex is an example of a more complex reflex circuit involving interneurons on both sides of the spinal cord. In this reflex, flexion of the stimulated limb is combined with extension of the contralateral limb and with postural adjustments.

Interneuron circuits similar to those found in the withdrawal reflex are also likely involved in nonreflex spinal cord networks such as those controlling movements during locomotion. The basic patterns of rhythmic movements are produced by CPGs located in the spinal cord. For example, alternating contractions on the two sides during swimming are produced by interneuron networks in the spinal cord that depend on both synaptic connections and intrinsic electrical properties of the neurons to generate alternating activation of the motor neurons on the two sides of the spinal cord. Excitatory coupling among segmental pattern generators along the spinal cord produces propagation of contractions along the body as required for effective swimming. Although the basic pattern is produced by intrinsic properties of the central network, sensory input from stretch receptors helps to reinforce and coordinate this pattern.

1. True or false: In the myotatic reflex, the sensory neurons from muscle spindles make direct inhibitory synaptic connections with the motor neurons of antagonist muscles. Explain your answer.

2. How does the nervous system ensure that muscle spindles provide information about stretch of a muscle throughout the range of length over which the muscle operates?

3. Contrast the responses of muscle spindles and Golgi tendon organs to active contraction and passive stretch of a muscle. How do you account for the different responses?

4. Draw the neural circuit of the inverse myotatic reflex. Explain why this circuit is an example of negative feedback.

5. In the withdrawal reflex, pain-sensitive sensory neurons make excitatory synapses with four distinct pools of interneurons in the spinal cord. Describe these four pools and their functional roles in the reflex.

6. Define the following: α motor neuron, γ motor neuron, group Ia sensory fiber, group Ib sensory fiber, extrafusal muscle fiber, intrafusal muscle fiber.

7. In the lamprey spinal cord, what are edge cells and how do they affect the central pattern generators for swimming?

8. Draw the bilateral circuits that generate alternating contractions on the two sides of the body during swimming in the lamprey. Label all of the neuron types, and indicate excitatory and inhibitory connections.

9. Describe the mechanisms that contribute to termination of a burst of activity within the central pattern generator for swimming on one side of the lamprey spinal cord.

10. Speculate about how the spinal circuits for swimming in the lamprey spinal cord might be generalized to locomotion in the mammalian spinal cord, based on what you know about the pools of interneurons utilized in spinal reflex circuits.

INTERNET ASSIGNMENT CHAPTER 8

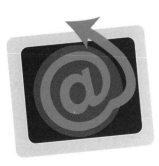

Search the Internet for pictures of segmental cross sections of the spinal cord at the sacral, lumbar, thoracic, and cervical levels. Identify the gray matter and the white matter at each level, and describe why the gray and white matter change in relative proportion at different positions along the spinal cord.

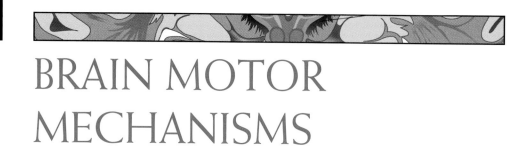

BRAIN MOTOR MECHANISMS

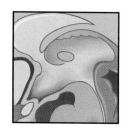

In Chapter 8, we discussed some of the spinal cord circuits that regulate and coordinate movement. These circuits can generate both simple behavior, such as stretch and tendon reflexes, and complex coordinated activities, such as locomotion. As an animal moves and interacts with its environment, however, these low-level control circuits are normally combined in ever-changing ways to produce appropriate actions. These less stereotypical, goal-directed actions are the responsibility of motor control systems found in higher parts of the brain. In this chapter, we present an overview of the higher motor systems and their functional interconnections.

MOTOR CONTROL CENTERS ARE FOUND IN THE BRAINSTEM, MIDBRAIN, AND FOREBRAIN

One of the evolutionary trends described in Chapter 2 is the trend toward increasing cephalization. The brainstem is the most phylogenetically primitive part of the brain, and it contains many of the brain circuits that regulate motor mechanisms in the spinal cord and modulate motor activity based on sensory information. In simple vertebrates like the lamprey, the brainstem circuits perform virtually all of the integrative motor functions responsible for guiding the animal's motor behavior. During the course of brain evolution, the forebrain increased in size and complexity, but the brainstem motor mechanisms were retained, providing an intermediate level of control in the motor hierarchy. Thus, the brainstem contains regions that act independently to control spinal motor systems, but in addition the brainstem is used by forebrain motor centers as a go-between in guiding motor behavior.

In mammalian brains, the trend toward increasing importance of the forebrain is manifested principally in the evolution of proportionally larger amounts of the brain devoted to the cerebral cortex. In addition to the forebrain-to-brainstem route of descending motor control (called the **corticobulbar system**), the evolution of larger cortical areas is accompanied by development of a second, direct route of descending motor control (called the **corticospinal system**) that bypasses the brainstem areas and projects directly to the spinal cord. In general, the larger the cortex, the greater the influence of the corticospinal system on motor behavior. Although exceptions exist, the brainstem motor systems tend to govern more global motions, such as swimming and walking. In contrast, the corticospinal system provides finer motor control, such as the motions of fingers typing on a keyboard.

Figure 9.1 shows a block diagram of some connections among motor system components in the mammalian nervous system. The core of the system consists of

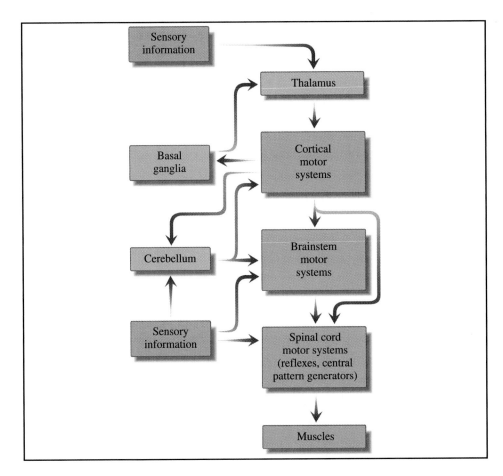

Figure 9.1.

A block diagram of the flow of information in the hierarchy of motor systems. The *arrows* indicate the direction of connections but do not imply monosynaptic connections. In all cases, information transfer at the cellular level involves a combination of excitatory and inhibitory synaptic influences. The term "sensory information" is used generically—that is, sensory information about the body and the environment enters the network at several levels, and the different types of sensory information are not distributed equally among all parts of the network.

the central axis of cortical, brainstem, and spinal cord motor systems. At the spinal cord level, the motor system provides the basic circuitry for controlling the muscles, including the reflexes and central pattern generators discussed in Chapter 8. The spinal cord in turn receives commands from both the brainstem and the motor cortex. In addition to the connections to the spinal cord, the cortex sends descending axons that terminate in the brainstem motor centers. This central axis receives inputs from other brain regions involved in motor coordination—most notably the **cerebellum**, which is part of the hindbrain, and the **basal ganglia**, which span the border between the forebrain and midbrain. Each of these modulatory motor systems will be discussed later in this chapter.

Motor output must be altered based on sensory information. For example, during locomotion, the orientation of the body in space constantly changes, and the movements of body parts must be updated to take this into account. Thus, sensory information provides input to the motor control systems at every level of the hierarchy. In the spinal cord, information about muscle length and muscle tension is employed in spinal reflexes, and information about body bending or limb position influences the activity of central pattern generators (see Chapter 8). Sensory information also helps to determine the outputs from brain motor centers. The cerebellum, for instance, monitors ongoing activity in the core motor control systems and reinforces or suppresses that activity, based on sensory information. Maintenance of balance and proper body posture during locomotion is one example of motor modulation involving the cerebellum.

BRAINSTEM MOTOR AREAS

What descending tracts from the brainstem are involved in the control of spinal motor circuits?

In the lamprey, swimming is initiated in response to excitatory inputs descending in the spinal cord from command centers in the brainstem (see Chapter 8). Similar motor command centers for locomotion are also found in higher vertebrates. Electrodes can be placed into brainstem nuclei to deliver brief electrical stimuli that stimulate action potentials in nearby neurons and axons, thereby mimicking the effect of natural activation of this part of the brain. If trains of electrical stimuli are applied in this way to certain regions in the midbrain of a mammal, coordinated locomotion can be induced and the animal can be made to walk on a treadmill. It is worth emphasizing again that the pattern of the electrical stimuli carries no inherent information about the pattern of the stepping motion. Instead, the stimulation in the brainstem serves only as a trigger for spinal cord networks that produce the appropriate motions. If the brainstem stimulation is strengthened by increasing either the electrical current or the frequency of stimulus pulses, the speed of locomotion increases accordingly. In other words, an animal can be induced to walk, trot, or gallop, depending on the strength of electrical stimulation applied to the brainstem initiator regions.

Reticulospinal System

The brainstem locomotor region is located at the upper end of the midbrain, near the anterior end of a diffuse network of neurons called the **reticular formation** (Fig. 9.2). The reticular formation (*reticulum* means "net" or "mesh") runs along the lower part of the brainstem from the midbrain into the medulla. It contains neurons that carry out a variety of sensory and motor functions, including the regulation of arousal. Neurons in the reticular formation also send axons down into the spinal cord, forming the **reticulospinal tract**. These axons make synaptic connections onto interneurons and motor neurons involved in spinal reflexes. In the lamprey, reticulospinal neurons carry the motor commands for initiating swimming. In

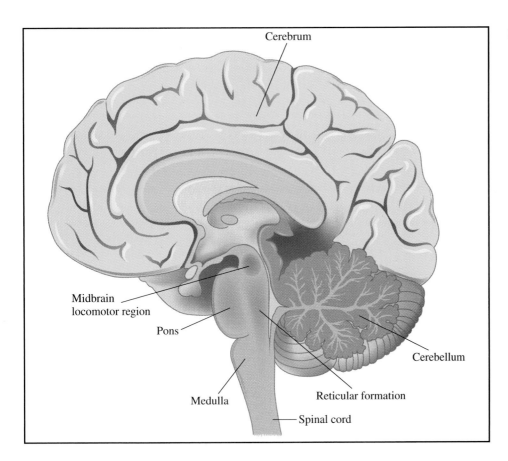

Figure 9.2.

The location of the midbrain locomotor region and the reticular formation in the human brain. The reticular formation extends from the midbrain into the medulla.

Labels in figure: Cerebrum; Midbrain locomotor region; Pons; Medulla; Cerebellum; Reticular formation; Spinal cord

mammals, similar neural systems originating in the reticular formation are also important in relaying locomotor commands.

The neurons of the reticular formation receive sensory information from several sources, including the sensory projections ascending into the brain from the spinal cord. These ascending sensory axons carry information about limb position, muscle length, muscle tension, and so on. This sensory information modifies the motor commands descending in the reticulospinal axons, providing the sensory feedback necessary to alter the strength of motor excitation as required by the locomotor state of the animal.

In a swimming lamprey, for example, bending of the body sends sensory signals from the spinal cord to the swimming command centers in the reticular formation. If the muscles on the right side are contracted and those on the left relaxed, then the level of excitation in right-side reticulospinal command neurons will decline and excitation in left-side reticulospinal neurons will increase. This change in activity of the descending command neurons reduces activation of the right-side central pattern generators in the spinal cord and promotes activation of left-side central pattern generators. The contraction on the right will be terminated and the alternating contraction on the left initiated. Thus, sensory information about the bending of the body reinforces the swimming pattern not only by influencing the pattern generators at each spinal segment (see Fig. 8.12), but also by modulating the activity of the brainstem neurons that provide excitation to the spinal cord.

Vestibulospinal System

Another type of sensory information that is important in modulating motor output is vestibular information. The vestibular system includes sensory receptors that give information about the orientation of the body with respect to gravity and also about acceleration (see Chapter 10). Such information helps an animal steer and maintain balance as it moves through the environment. Indeed, specialized sensory receptors that respond to tilt of the organism with respect to the Earth's gravity are found in even the most primitive mobile multicellular organisms, such as jellyfish. Thus, vestibular sensory input to motor command systems is an ancient evolutionary adaptation.

In primitive vertebrates, like the lamprey, the vestibular apparatus strongly influences the activity of reticulospinal neurons, which in turn make widespread connections on interneurons and motor neurons throughout the spinal cord. In other vertebrates, additional pathways carry vestibular information to the spinal cord via the **vestibulospinal tract**. Sensory neurons of the vestibular sense organs send axons into the brainstem, where they terminate in the **vestibular nuclei** (Fig. 9.3).

Figure 9.3.

The location of the vestibular nuclei in the brainstem. The block diagram summarizes some of the connections made by neurons of the vestibular nuclei. The vestibular nuclei send axons to the cerebellum and to the reticular motor systems, in addition to the spinal cord.

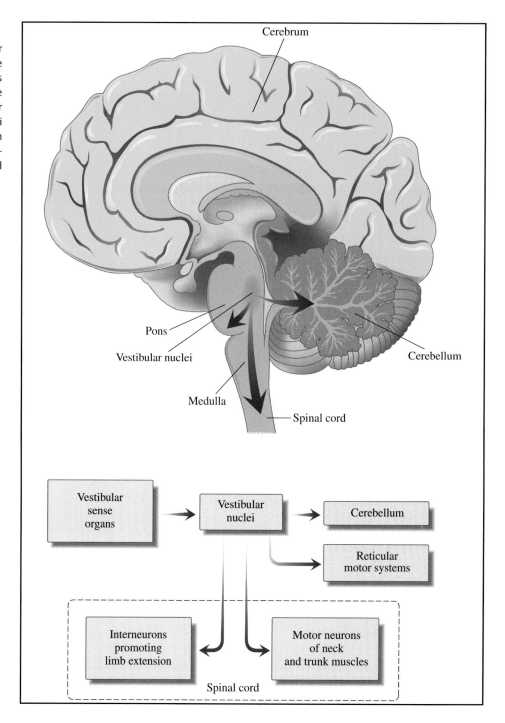

The neurons of the vestibular nuclei send axons down into the spinal cord, where they make two different types of synaptic connections, summarized in Figure 9.3. First, excitatory synaptic connections are made onto pools of interneurons that control the motor neurons of limb muscles. These pools consist of excitatory interneurons for extensor motor neurons and inhibitory interneurons for flexor motor neurons. Thus, action potentials descending from the vestibular nuclei polysynaptically excite extensor motor neurons and inhibit flexor motor neurons, promoting extension of all four limbs. Second, axons of neurons in the vestibular nuclei make direct excitatory and inhibitory synaptic connections onto motor neurons that control the muscles of the neck and trunk. These connections provide reflexive adjustments of head and body position in response to tilt and rotation, both of which commonly occur during locomotion.

The vestibular nuclei also send axons to the cerebellum (see Fig. 9.3), which aids in the maintenance of balance and body posture. The vestibular nuclei also make other connections not shown in Figure 9.3, including an important connection to the motor neurons controlling the eye muscles. (The role of this vestibular input in oculomotor reflexes is discussed in Chapter 10.) The vestibular input to the cerebellum plays a role in these oculomotor reflexes, especially in the modification of oculomotor reflexes based on experience (see Chapter 20).

Rubrospinal System

The **red nucleus** is another brainstem region that contributes to descending control of spinal cord motor functions. This nucleus is located near the anterior end of the midbrain, as shown in Figure 9.4. A major source of input to the red nucleus is the cerebellum. The neurons of the red nucleus send axons that descend into the spinal cord, forming the **rubrospinal tract**. In the spinal cord, the rubrospinal axons make excitatory synapses with interneurons that excite flexor

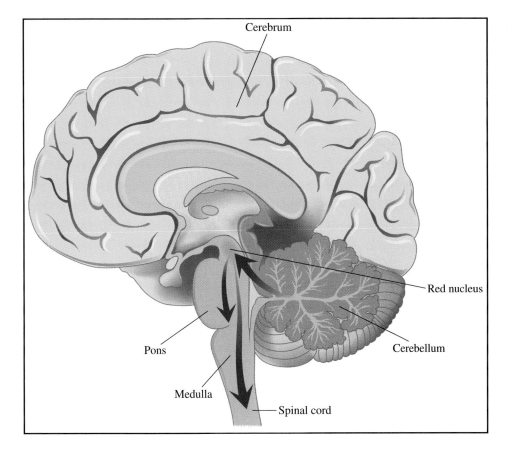

Figure 9.4.

Location of the red nucleus in the human brain. The red nucleus receives inputs from the cerebellum and sends outputs to the spinal cord via the rubrospinal tract and to brainstem motor regions.

motor neurons of the limbs. Thus, activation of the neurons in the red nucleus promotes limb flexion. Activation of the vestibulospinal tract has the opposite effect, promoting limb extension. The balance between activity in the red nucleus and in the vestibular nuclei is important, therefore, in determining the overall equilibrium between flexor and extensor muscle systems of the limbs.

CORTICAL MOTOR AREAS

What parts of the cerebral cortex give rise to the corticospinal and corticobulbar tracts?

In many animals (particularly in more primitive vertebrates), the brainstem motor areas provide all the circuitry necessary to initiate and coordinate movement. As the forebrain blossomed during the course of evolution, however, other control mechanisms associated with the forebrain came on the scene. As discussed earlier in this chapter, motor regions of the cerebral cortex arose to augment and, in some cases, partly supplant the motor control function of the more primitive brainstem. As shown in Figure 9.1, the descending motor commands from the cortex project directly to the spinal cord via the corticospinal tract, bypassing the brainstem and giving the cortex direct control of spinal circuits. The cortex also sends inputs to the brainstem via the corticobulbar tract, providing further indirect control of spinal circuits.

An important source of the descending cortical tracts is the primary motor cortex, which is illustrated in Figure 9.5. The primary motor cortex is located on the **gyrus** (outfolding of the cortex) just in front of the deep groove (**sulcus**) that runs laterally across the surface of the brain about halfway between its front and back. This groove is called the **central sulcus**. The primary motor area is also called the **precentral cortex** to indicate its location in the precentral gyrus, just in front of the central sulcus. Based on microscopic differences in the cellular architecture of different parts of the cortex, neuroanatomists divide the human cortex into broad areas designated by numbers, and primary motor cortex corresponds to **area 4** in the commonly used numbering scheme of Brodmann.

Representation of the Body in the Primary Motor Cortex

What is the somatotopic organization of the primary motor cortex?

In the nineteenth century, a combination of anecdotal observations on human patients with head wounds and experimental observations on the brains of experimental animals provided evidence that motor function is localized in the precentral gyrus. Stimulation of the primary motor cortex on the left side of the brain gave rise to movements on the right side of the body, while stimulation of the right precentral gyrus caused movements on the left side. This contralateral control of the body arises because the descending axons of the corticospinal tract cross (or **decussate**) from one side of the brain to the other as they pass through the medulla, just before entering the spinal cord. Thus, the axons from the right motor cortex enter the left side of spinal cord, where they make synaptic connections onto motor neurons controlling the muscles of the left half of the body. The reverse holds true for the axons from the left motor cortex. In the medulla, the axons from motor cortex form large bundles, called the **pyramids**, and the point of crossing is called the **pyramidal decussation**.

In addition to the gross functional organization into regions controlling the left and right sides of the body, the primary motor cortex on each side of the brain is subdivided into regions that control specific parts of the body. There is an orderly progression from the most medial to the most lateral portions of the motor cortex. Figure 9.5 shows the organizational scheme, which is known as the **somatotopic organization** of the primary motor cortex. The most medial parts of precentral cortex control the foot and leg (or the hindlimb in four-legged animals), and the most

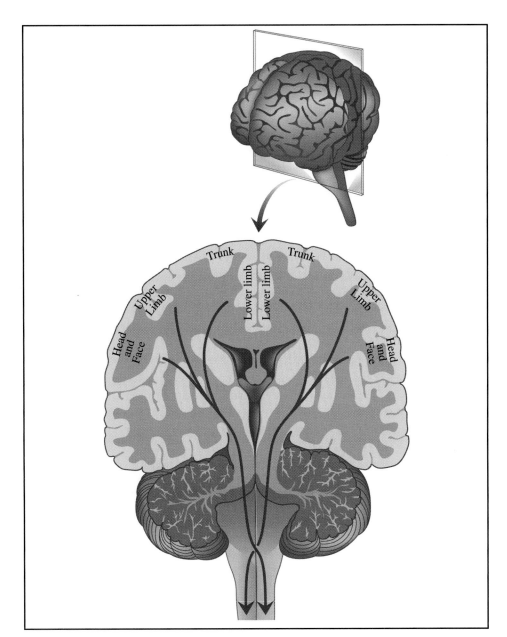

Figure 9.5.

The primary motor cortex is a strip of cortex located just in front of the central sulcus on both sides of the brain. The *upper diagram* shows a three-dimensional view of the motor cortex, and the *lower part* shows the organization of the cortex, viewed in cross section. The plane of the cross section is indicated above. The motor cortex exhibits a somatotopic organization. Neurons located in the most medial portion, near the midline, control the muscles of the lower limbs, and successively more lateral portions of the cortex control the trunk, upper limb, head, and face. The descending axons from the motor cortex cross the midline in the medulla and descend in the contralateral spinal cord.

lateral parts control the head and mouth. The trunk of the body, the arm, and the hand are controlled by the intermediate parts of motor cortex. Within the region devoted to the lower limb, an orderly progression is observed from the toes in the most medial portion, to the hip in the most lateral portion. Similarly, in the region controlling the upper limb, there is a progression from the medial portion to the lateral portion, but in the opposite direction. That is, the shoulder is controlled by the most medial part of the region, and the fingers (or forepaw) by the most lateral portion.

Although this basic somatotopic scheme is universal in the motor cortex, the amount of cortex in a specific species that is devoted to a particular muscular group reflects the relative importance of that muscle group for that species. For instance, in primates—and especially in humans—the amount of motor cortex devoted to the control of the hand and fingers is particularly large, in keeping with the great importance of the hand in primate motor behavior. Similarly, in the region devoted to the face in primate motor cortex, the majority of the neurons are involved in movements of the jaw, lips, and tongue.

Microscopic Anatomy of the Motor Cortex

The primary motor cortex (Brodmann's area 4) is only one small part of the overall cerebral cortex. The cortex is a thin sheet of cells, a few millimeters thick, that forms the outer surface of the cerebral hemispheres, like the rind of an orange. Like other parts of the cortex, the motor cortex has a layered structure. The layers are defined based on microscopic examination of the types of cells and their densities, as summarized in Figure 9.6. At the outermost edge of the cortex, layer I consists primarily of incoming axons that synapse onto dendrites of neurons found in deeper layers. Layers II and III, the next deepest layers, contain large numbers of neuronal cell bodies, whose axons project predominantly to other cortical regions, either nearby or some distance away. The neurons in layers II and III have cell bodies that are shaped like pyramids, with a broad base that tapers into a long dendrite extending toward the cortical surface (see Fig. 9.6B). Consequently, this type of neuron is called a **pyramidal cell**. The apical dendrites receive numerous synaptic connections from the incoming axons running through layer I. Although the distinction between layer II and layer III is not readily apparent in most parts of cortex, the cell bodies of the pyramidal neurons in layer II tend to be smaller than those in layer III.

Layer IV contains neurons with multiple dendrites that radiate out from a roughly spherical cell body. These star-shaped neurons are called **stellate cells** (see Fig. 9.6B). Unlike the pyramidal cells, whose axons can project long distances to make connections with other regions of the central nervous system, the axons of stellate cells remain in the same vicinity, making synapses predominantly with nearby neurons. The stellate cells receive inputs from axons carrying sensory information into the cortex. For this reason, cortical regions that focus on sensory processing have greater numbers of stellate cells and a thicker, more pronounced layer IV. The primary motor cortex (Brodmann's area 4) is principally an output region that sends motor commands to noncortical motor areas. Consequently, layer IV is not well developed in area 4—an anatomical aspect that prompted Brodmann to distinguish the precentral gyrus as a separate cortical region.

By contrast, layer V is particularly prominent in the primary motor cortex. This layer contains pyramidal neurons whose cell bodies are the largest among the pyramidal cells. These neurons give rise to axons that descend long distances to carry motor commands to the brainstem and spinal cord. In the motor cortex, the largest of the pyramidal neurons in layer V (called **Betz cells**) give rise to the largest and fastest-conducting axons that descend through the medullary pyramids into the spinal cord. In the nonmotor portions of the cortex, the pyramidal cells of layer V also are a major source of outputs from the cortex to other brain regions, including the thalamus and basal ganglia (see below). The axons of pyramidal cells in layer V commonly give rise to one or more collateral branches that remain within the cortex (see Fig. 9.6B), providing information about the outgoing activity to local cortical circuits.

Layer VI—the final cellular layer—contains neurons that send axons to other noncortical areas of the central nervous system. An important target of descending connections from layer VI is the **thalamus**. As we will learn in more detail in chapters focusing on sensory systems, the thalamus is a complex group of nuclei that process and relay various kinds of sensory information. In addition, some areas of the thalamus receive extensive inputs from brain motor control systems, including the motor cortex, and are important in the regulation of motor output. Layer VI of the motor cortex is a major source of axons that project to the motor parts of the thalamus.

Beneath layer VI, the outgoing axons form the myelinated fiber tracts of the cerebral white matter. As with the white matter in the spinal cord, the whitish color

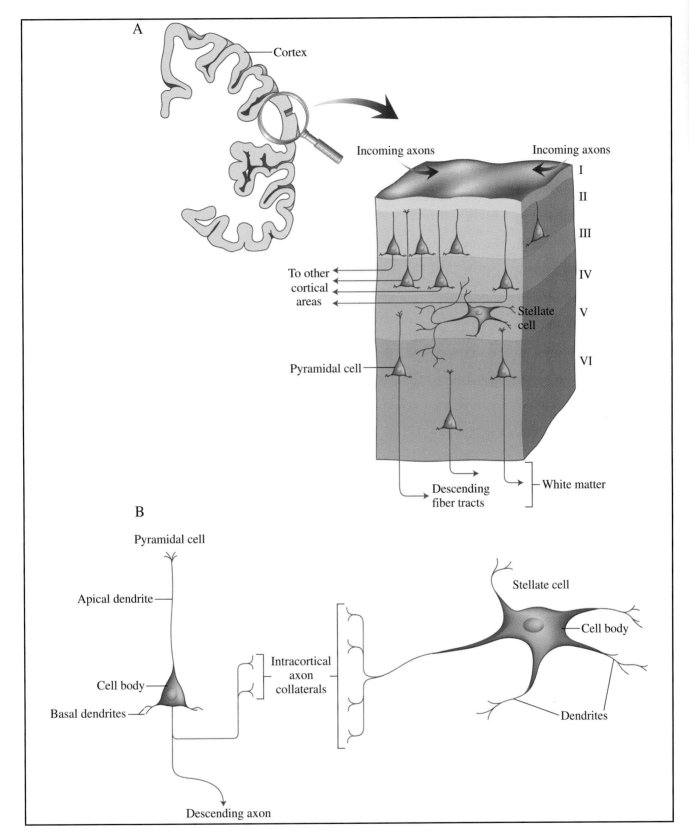

Figure 9.6.

The microscopic anatomy of the cerebral cortex. **A.** The cortex is organized in cellular layers, numbered with Roman numerals I through VI (*right*). Pyramid-shaped pyramidal cells are found in layers II, III, V, and VI. Star-shaped stellate cells are found in layer IV. **B.** Schematic drawings of the structures of pyramidal cells (*left*) and stellate cells (*right*) of cerebral cortex.

arises because the densely packed myelin sheaths of the axon bundles make the tissue more opaque than the overlying layers containing neuronal cell bodies.

Encoding of Movement by Neurons of the Primary Motor Cortex

In what way is the desired direction of movement encoded by neurons in the cortical motor areas?

Electrical stimulation can be applied to the motor cortex using microelectrodes, which activate a small number of pyramidal neurons in a specific subregion of the motor cortex and at different depths within the cortex. Experiments using this microstimulation technique showed that individual cortical neurons cause contractions in either a single muscle or a group of related muscles. In addition, when stimulation is applied at various vertical distances below the surface of the cortex, all of the stimulated cells at different depths cause contractions in the same muscle or group of muscles. Thus, the motor cortex consists of a series of vertically oriented columns, and all cells within a column have similar connections to motor neurons in the spinal cord. As we will see in more detail in Chapter 16, this columnar organization of functionally related cells is commonly found throughout the cerebral cortex. Neighboring columns cause contraction in closely related muscles or muscle groups, and in a medial to lateral progression through the primary motor cortex, the locations of the controlled muscles vary consistently according to the overall somatotopic map (see Fig. 9.5).

Electrical stimulation experiments provide information about the parts of the motor cortex that control movements of particular body parts. They do not, however, establish how normally occurring action potential activity in neurons of the primary motor cortex is related to the direction and strength of movement. To establish this relationship, we must record the action potential activity of neurons in the primary motor cortex during production of a defined movement. Such studies typically employ awake experimental animals (usually monkeys) that have been trained to make simple movements. Because the primate wrist joint offers a wide range of motion and is well represented in the motor cortex, deflection of a joystick handle is often used as the motor task.

As expected given that neurons in the motor cortex *initiate* movement, the rate of action potential firing in the cortical neurons increases about a tenth of a second *before* the onset of contraction in the relevant muscles. Figure 9.7A shows an example of the increased firing of a cortical spinal neuron, relative to the onset of the movement it triggers. The cortical neuron fires more frequently when the amount of force required to move the handle is greater (see Fig. 9.7A). In other words, the neurons in the motor cortex send signals that determine not only which muscles are activated, but also how much force the muscles exert.

One interesting characteristic of the neurons in the primary motor cortex is that they fire most strongly for movements in a particular direction (for example, flexion of the wrist joint) and cease firing for movements in the opposite direction (for example, extension of the wrist joint). In Figure 9.7B, for instance, the corticospinal neuron fires most strongly for movements of the joystick to the left (180°, using the angular coordinate system shown in the figure) and becomes silent for movements to the right (0°). Notice, however, that the neuron also fires quite strongly for upward movement (90°). In this example, then, the neuron becomes active for any wrist movement in the range of approximately 90° to 180°. In general, activation of a particular neuron in the primary motor cortex is associated with a relatively broad range of movement directions, and thus a single neuron cannot be said to specify a unique direction of movement.

The direction of movement of a limb is thought to be specified by the overall pattern of activity in the entire population of corticospinal neurons controlling the

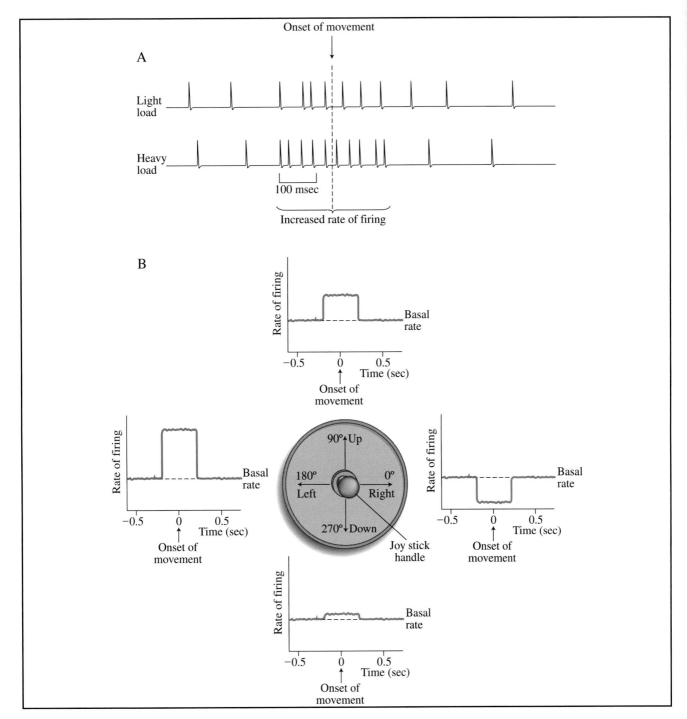

Figure 9.7.

The firing characteristics of corticospinal neurons in the primary motor cortex. **A.** An example of action potential firing in a cortical neuron. The *arrow* and *dashed line* indicate the time of onset of the movement triggered by the neuron. The *upper trace* shows the activity when the muscle must move a light load, and the *lower trace* shows the activity when the muscle must move a heavy load. **B.** The firing rate of a corticospinal neuron depends on the direction of movement. The diagram in the *center* shows the directions of motion of a joystick handle, which is deflected by movements of the wrist joint. The four graphs show the changes in firing rate of a neuron in the part of the motor cortex that controls the wrist joint. The neuron fires most strongly for movements to the left but also fires prior to upward movements. The firing rate decreases during movements to the right. Downward movements are associated with little change in firing rate.

relevant muscles. Recording from the entire population of cortical neurons that control the wrist, for instance, would reveal some neurons that fire strongest for upward movements, some for downward movements, some for motion to the right, and some for movement to the left. In the population of cells, all preferred directions from 0° to 360° would be represented. The pattern of firing in the population will vary, depending on the intended direction of movement, as shown in Figure 9.8. For a movement direction of 180°, the cells whose preferred direction is 180° will be most active, while those whose preferred direction is 0° will be most strongly inhibited. Cells with intermediate preferred directions will be less strongly affected. This pattern of activity in the corticospinal inputs to the spinal cord will then most strongly activate the spinal motor neurons controlling muscles that move the wrist joint to the left (that is, 180°). For an intended movement direction of 90°, the pattern of activity in the cell population will shift to that shown by the blue curve in Figure 9.8. Thus, the pattern of excitation reaching the spinal motor neurons will shift, and a different set of muscles controlling the wrist joint will be most strongly activated.

This scheme provides a simplified representation of the complex actions of the corticospinal system in the spinal cord. Nevertheless, it should serve to demonstrate that the encoding of movement direction is a population characteristic of the cortical neurons, rather than being uniquely determined by a small group of cells.

Other Cortical Areas Involved in Motor Control

Electrical stimulation of the precentral gyrus produces well-defined movements of particular muscles or muscle groups, with the topographical organization described earlier (see Fig. 9.5). However, stimulation of other parts of the brain also produces movement.

Just anterior to the primary motor cortex is Brodmann's cortical area 6, and electrical stimulation applied in this area elicits movements. In addition, pyramidal neurons in area 6 send axons both to the primary motor cortex and to brainstem and spinal cord motor circuits, indicating that they exert both direct influence on

Figure 9.8.

The pattern of action potential activity in the entire population of corticospinal neurons controlling the wrist joint. The x-axis shows the preferred direction for the cells making up the population (that is, the direction of movement at which the firing rate is highest for a given cell). The *yellow curve* shows the pattern of firing in the population for movement of the joystick handle to the left (180° in the diagram of Fig. 9.7B). The *blue curve* shows the pattern of activity for upward movement (90°).

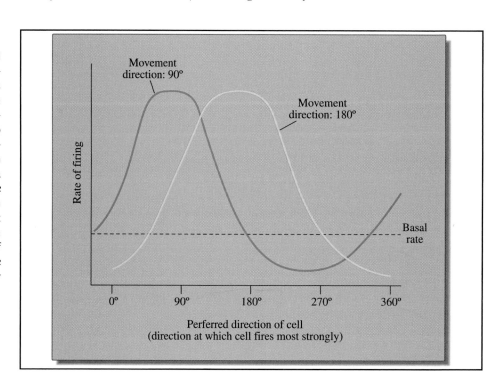

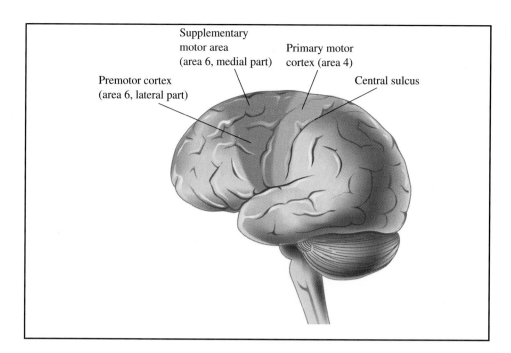

Figure 9.9.

The location of the supplementary motor area and the premotor cortex in cortical area 6. The primary motor cortex is also indicated.

lower motor centers and indirect influence via the primary motor cortex. Figure 9.9 shows the location of these additional cortical motor regions in the human brain.

Area 6 is divided into two functionally distinct regions: the **supplemental motor area**, which is located more medially, and the **premotor cortex**, which is located laterally. The movements produced by stimulation of area 6 tend to be more complex than the discrete muscle movements evoked by stimulation of area 4. For instance, stimulation of area 4 might cause movement of a single finger, while stimulation in area 6 might produce coordinated movement of all the fingers of the hand. Consequently, the supplemental motor area and the premotor cortex are thought to be used in programming sequences of movements and in integrating sensory information with motor commands so that movements of limbs and the body produce actions that "make sense" within the environment. Exactly how the neurons of these cortical regions interact with each other and with the neurons of area 4 to program and initiate an appropriate plan of action remains poorly understood. Nevertheless, it is clear that lesions in area 6 interfere with the ability to make complex coordinated movements in primates.

THE BASAL GANGLIA

Although the cerebral cortex is the most prominent and visible forebrain structure, other parts of the forebrain are also important in motor control. In the central part of the telencephalon are three interconnected groups of neurons, collectively called the **basal ganglia**. Their locations are shown schematically in Figure 9.10A. The three components of the basal ganglia are the **caudate nucleus**, the **putamen**, and the **globus pallidus**. Together, the caudate nucleus and the putamen are known as the **striatum**.

Unlike other motor systems we have discussed so far, the basal ganglia have no direct connections with either the spinal cord or brainstem motor systems. Instead, the basal ganglia exert their motor effects principally by altering the output of cortical motor areas. As shown in Figure 9.10B, the basal ganglia do not themselves project directly to the motor cortex; instead, they interact with the parts of the thalamus that in turn provide inputs to the motor cortex. Thus, the basal ganglia monitor the output from the motor cortex, via the corticostriatal connections, and

What are the interconnections between the basal ganglia and the motor cortex?

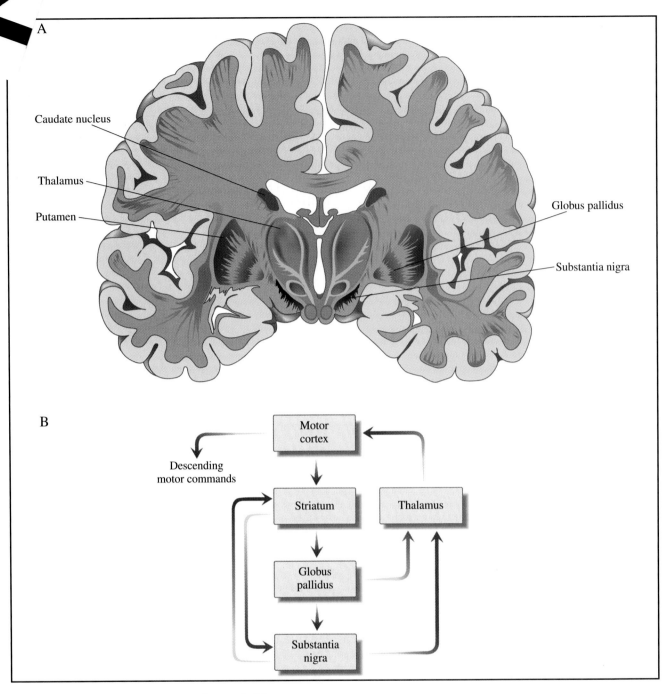

Figure 9.10.

The organization of the basal ganglia. **A.** Locations of the basal ganglia within the core of the forebrain. The three nuclei of the basal ganglia (caudate, putamen and globus pallidus) are arrayed around the thalamus. The substantia nigra is located in the midbrain. **B.** Connections of the basal ganglia and substantia nigra. The striatum consists of the caudate and putamen.

control the inputs that generate activity in the voluntary motor output path. In keeping with this central position in the motor command pathway, damage to the basal ganglia produces severe deficits in motor behavior.

Another brain region intimately associated with the basal ganglia is the **substantia nigra**, which is located in the midbrain (see Fig. 9.10). Many neurons of the substantia nigra contain high concentrations of the neurotransmitter dopamine, which oxidizes to form a dark pigment in freshly cut brain sections. This pigment makes the area appear black, giving rise to the name of the nucleus. As diagrammed in Figure 9.10B, the substantia nigra both receives inputs from and sends outputs to the striatum. In addition, some parts of the substantia nigra project to the same thalamic nuclei that relay outputs from the basal ganglia to the motor cortex. Although the synaptic inputs from the substantia nigra to the striatum release the neurotransmitter dopamine, the substantia nigra neurons that project to the thalamus use the neurotransmitter γ-aminobutyric acid, or GABA. Exactly how these synaptic inputs alter motor commands is not yet understood in detail.

Degeneration of the dopamine-releasing neurons of the substantia nigra destroys the synaptic inputs to the striatum, severely impairing motor activity. In humans, degeneration of the substantia nigra neurons leads to **Parkinson's disease**, a condition associated with muscle tremor and difficulty in initiating and sustaining locomotion. Thus, the dopamine-releasing neurons of the substantia nigra are important in the translation of motor plans into actual motor commands.

THE CEREBELLUM

The cerebellum forms an evagination of the midbrain on the dorsal surface of the brain at the level of the pons (Fig. 9.11). Although its size varies across animal species, the cerebellum is a major brain structure in mammals and plays important roles in sensorimotor integration. From its strategic position astride the ascending sensory pathways and descending motor pathways in the brainstem, the cerebellum monitors both sensory and motor information and provides feedback control of motor outflow.

How does the cerebellum influence motor outputs from the brain to the spinal cord?

BOX 1

IN THE CLINIC

The importance of the substantia nigra and the basal ganglia in motor behavior is clearly demonstrated by Parkinson's disease. Patients with this condition exhibit muscle tremors and have difficulty with locomotion. For instance, afflicted people sometimes "freeze up" while walking. The cause of Parkinson's disease is unknown, but the motor symptoms are caused by a degeneration of neurons in the substantia nigra that project to the striatum (the nigrostriatal projection). Loss of this synaptic input severely impairs motor activity, by disrupting the normal synaptic circuitry of feedback loops involving the basal ganglia.

The neurons of the substantia nigra that project to the striatum release the neurotransmitter dopamine, and drugs that mimic the missing dopamine or that potentiate the action of remaining dopamine inputs can reduce the symptoms of Parkinson's disease. The most commonly used treatment is L-dopa, which is the immediate precursor of dopamine in the synthesis pathway for the neurotransmitter (L-dopa is converted to dopamine by the enzyme L-aromatic acid decarboxylase).

Patients with Parkinson's disease report that they intend to carry out simple motor acts, such as standing up or walking, but the intended action does not occur or is executed slowly and haltingly. Because of these deficits, it appears that the dopamine-releasing neurons of the substantia nigra are somehow important in the translation of motor plans into actual motor commands.

Figure 9.11.

The location of the cerebellum in the brainstem. The three-dimensional view (*above*) represents the cerebellum and cerebrum of a rodent brain. The cross section (*below*) shows the division of the cerebellum into the deep nuclei and the cerebellar cortex

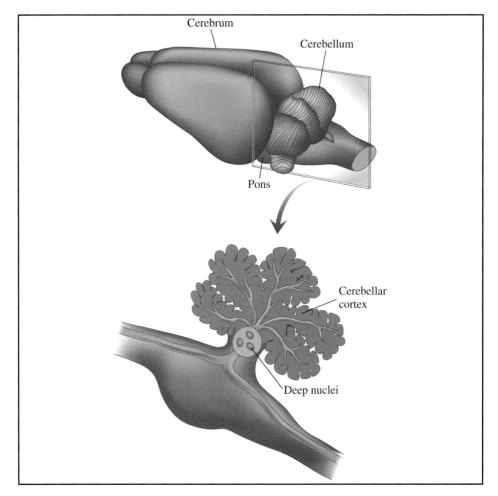

A major sensory input to the cerebellum is from sensory systems that provide information about the orientation and acceleration of the body during locomotion, such as the vestibular apparatus and, in fish, the lateral line system (which gives information about water movement over the body surface). The cerebellum appears to have evolved as an adjunct to the locomotor command centers in the brainstem that are involved in swimming, for the purpose of adjusting motor commands based on sensory feedback about the organism's position in space. In terrestrial animals, additional information about joint position, muscle length, and muscle tension must also be monitored by the cerebellum to fine-tune motor output based on performance. Also, the evolution of motor control systems in the forebrain provided additional sources of inputs and targets for outputs for the cerebellum. Therefore, these evolutionary developments are associated with the expansion of the brain tissue devoted to the cerebellar circuitry.

In keeping with the idea that the cerebellum modulates motor output to make fine adjustments based on performance, lesions of the cerebellum do not prevent movement but do interfere with balance and coordination. As a result, movements become awkward and less effective.

In vertebrates with a well-developed cerebellum, the cerebellum consists of two highly convoluted hemispheres overlying the brainstem, and three pairs of **deep nuclei** hidden within. The deep nuclei are called the **dentate nucleus**, the **emboliform nucleus**, and the **fastigial nucleus**. The cerebellar hemispheres have an organization analogous to that of the cerebral hemispheres, with a densely packed cellular layer, the cerebellar cortex, on the outside and white matter containing incoming and outgoing axons underneath.

The deep nuclei receive synaptic inputs from axons carrying sensory information and from axons carrying information about commands issued by cortical and brainstem motor centers. This same sensory and motor information is also sent on to the cerebellar cortex for further processing. As a result, the cerebellar cortex is able to compare motor commands with sensory information of various kinds. The processed output from the cerebellar cortex is then relayed back to the deep nuclei. This information flow is diagrammed in Figure 9.12. The exact nature of the calculation being performed in the deep nuclei has not been unraveled yet, and it remains unknown exactly how the sensory and motor signals are combined and compared in the cerebellar cortex. In general, however, the information flow shown in Figure 9.12 seems well suited to a comparison, carried out in the deep nuclei, between an outgoing motor command and an altered form of the motor command that has been passed through the neuronal network of the cerebellar cortex.

The outputs from the cerebellar deep nuclei project to all of the brain motor systems (see Fig. 9.12), as might be expected for a structure that is involved in the modulation of motor performance. The vestibular nuclei provide a major sensory input to the cerebellum, giving information necessary to maintain balance and body posture during locomotion. The cerebellum sends outputs back to the vestibular nuclei to regulate the outputs of the vestibulospinal motor system. The red nucleus also receives a major input from the cerebellum, which helps control the activity of the rubrospinal motor system. The cortical motor system is also targeted by outputs of the cerebellum. As with the basal ganglia, the cerebellum exerts an indirect influence on the motor cortex. The cerebellar deep nuclei project to the same thalamic nuclei that receive inputs from the basal ganglia, and the thalamus in turn sends inputs to the cortical motor areas. In this way, the cerebellum influences both the corticospinal and the corticobulbar motor systems indirectly, via the thalamic neurons that provide inputs to the motor cortex.

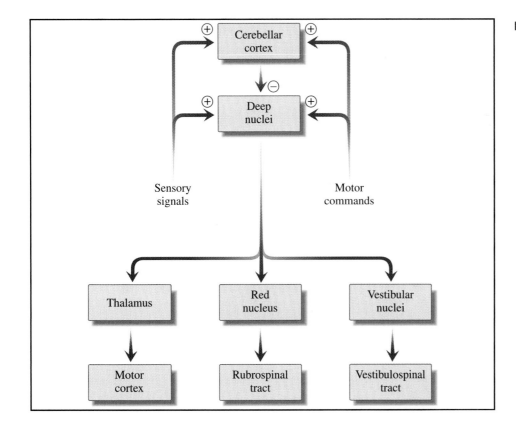

Figure 9.12.

Connections of the cerebellum. Excitatory connections are indicated with a *plus sign* (+) and inhibitory connections are indicated with a *minus sign* (−).

The cerebellum is thought to play an important role in motor learning—the process by which the timing and amplitude of motor commands are altered based on experience with prior motor outcomes. The pattern of sensory and motor connections to and from the cerebellum appears to be well suited to such a role. The wide range of sensory inputs received by the cerebellum provides a source of information about the sensory consequences of motor acts, and the cerebellum also receives inputs from motor centers related to their outgoing motor commands. The role of the cerebellum in motor learning will be discussed in more detail in Chapter 20, when we consider how reflexes can be modified.

ORGANIZATION OF DESCENDING MOTOR TRACTS IN THE SPINAL CORD

Where in the spinal cord are the axons of brain motor systems located?

The principal target of the outputs from brain motor areas is ultimately the spinal cord. The motor neurons that control most of the somatic musculature are located in the gray matter of the spinal cord, and the brain motor systems must connect with these motor neurons in order to affect the activity of those muscles. The descending axons from the brain form a large portion of the white matter of the spinal cord (see Chapter 8), with ascending sensory axons accounting for the remainder (see Chapter 14). The axons coming from each brain motor region travel together in discrete bundles, or tracts, that occupy characteristic positions in the white matter of the spinal cord. Figure 9.13 shows the organization of these tracts. The axons from the motor cortex form two tracts: the **lateral corticospinal tract** in the lateral portion of the white matter, and the **ventral corticospinal tract**, which occupies the medial portions of the ventral white matter. The axons of neurons in the red nucleus (the **rubrospinal tract**) also descend in the lateral portion of the white matter (see Fig. 9.13), near the lateral corticospinal tract. The vestibular nuclei and the reticular formation in the brainstem give rise to descending fibers that occupy ventral portions of the white matter, as shown in Figure 9.13.

As the tracts from all of the higher motor centers descend in the spinal cord, axons leave the tracts and enter the gray matter. There, the axons make synaptic connections either directly onto motor neurons or onto spinal interneurons that then affect the activity of the motor neurons.

Figure 9.13.

The location in the spinal cord white matter of the descending axon tracts from the brain motor control areas.

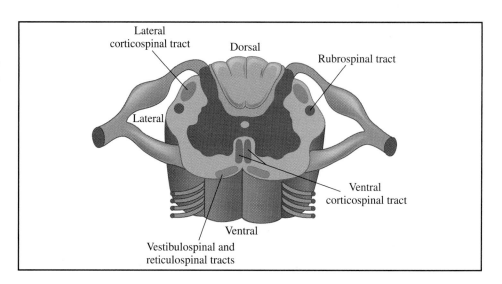

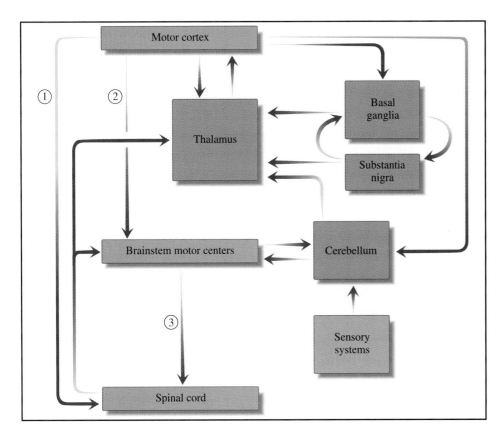

Figure 9.14.

A summary of the interconnections of the brain motor control systems. The central hierarchy is shaded blue. *Arrow 1* is the corticospinal tract, *arrow 2* is the corticobulbar tract, and *arrow 3* represents the reticulospinal, vestibulospinal, and rubrospinal tracts. Brainstem motor centers and cortical motor areas are grouped together into single boxes to simplify the wiring diagram. The connection from the cortex to the cerebellum is indirect via brainstem relay nuclei.

Now that we have discussed the major components of the motor control system of the brain, we can return to our summary diagram in Figure 9.1 and add some of the functional interconnections we have described in this chapter. In the more detailed block diagram in Figure 9.14, the hierarchical core of the motor outflow path (consisting of the motor cortex, the brainstem motor centers, and the spinal cord) is shaded blue. Ascending sensory information about muscles and joints is distributed to the brainstem and the thalamus. At the top of the hierarchy is the motor cortex. For simplicity, we have lumped together the primary motor cortex, the supplementary motor cortex, and the premotor cortex (see Fig. 9.9) into a single box in Figure 9.14. In general, the primary motor cortex (cortical area 4) produces discrete movements of single muscles or related groups of muscles, while the supplementary motor area and premotor cortex (cortical area 6) produce more global movements of larger body regions.

Two main tracts of axons descend from the motor cortex: the corticospinal tract (labeled 1 in Fig. 9.14), and the corticobulbar tract (labeled 2 in Fig. 9.14). The axons running in these tracts originate from pyramidal neurons in layer V of the cortex. The descending axons from the brainstem motor centers to the spinal cord (labeled 3 in Fig. 9.14) fall into three major groups. First, the reticulospinal tract originates in the reticular formation of the brainstem and makes synaptic connections onto motor neurons and interneurons throughout the spinal cord. Excitatory inputs from reticulospinal neurons drive the central pattern generators of the spinal cord to initiate locomotion. Second, the vestibulospinal tract originates in the vestibular nuclei of the brainstem. Activation of this tract promotes extension of the limbs and inhibits flexion. Third, the rubrospinal tract originates in the red nucleus. Activation of this tract promotes flexion of the limbs and inhibits extension. The balance of activity

SUMMARY

in the vestibulospinal system and the rubrospinal system is therefore important in governing the flexion-extension equilibrium of the limbs.

In addition to the hierarchically arranged central core of the motor pathways, other components monitor and regulate the motor commands to coordinate movements based on sensory information. These regulatory regions are also important in initiating motor commands during voluntary movements. The basal ganglia in the forebrain receive inputs from the motor cortex and project back to the motor cortex indirectly via the parts of the thalamus that send axons to the cortical motor areas. The basal ganglia are divided into the globus pallidus and the striatum, with the latter consisting of the caudate nucleus and the putamen. The basal ganglia are also closely associated with a midbrain region called the substantia nigra.

Together with the thalamus, the basal ganglia and substantia nigra form three interconnected feedback loops that affect the cortical motor areas. First, a local feedback loop extends from the basal ganglia to the substantia nigra and then back to the basal ganglia. A second loop circles from the motor cortex, to the basal ganglia, to the thalamus, and then back to the motor cortex. Third, a slightly longer path goes from the motor cortex, to the basal ganglia, to the substantia nigra, to the thalamus, and then back to the motor cortex. These interrelated feedback loops allow the basal ganglia and the substantia nigra, acting via the thalamus, to influence the motor outputs from the cortex. The importance of these connections is evident in Parkinson's disease, in which patients experience problems in the initiation of movement caused by a destruction of dopamine-containing neurons in the substantia nigra.

The other important brain component involved in motor coordination is the cerebellum, which is part of the brainstem. The cerebellum consists of two principal divisions: the deep cerebellar nuclei and the cerebellar cortex. Both divisions receive sensory information from a variety of sensory systems, as well as copies of the motor commands sent by the cortical and brainstem motor centers. The deep nuclei then send information back to these same motor centers. The feedback is direct in the case of the brainstem centers and indirect (via the thalamus) in the case of cortical centers. Fine coordination of limb movements and maintenance of balance during locomotion are among the functions of the cerebellum in mammals. The cerebellum also plays a role in motor learning.

1. Describe the dual descending pathways from the primary motor cortex to the spinal cord.
2. Contrast the actions of the rubrospinal and vestibulospinal tracts on spinal motor systems.
3. Locate the primary motor cortex, the supplemental motor area, and the premotor cortex on a map of the cortical surface.
4. Describe the somatotopic organization of the primary motor cortex?
5. Starting with the outermost layer, describe the characteristics of the layers found in the motor cortex.
6. What nuclei make up the basal ganglia?
7. Define the following: substantia nigra, precentral gyrus, striatum, dentate nucleus.
8. Draw the locations of the corticospinal, rubrospinal, and vestibulospinal tracts in the white matter of the spinal cord.

INTERNET ASSIGNMENT CHAPTER 9

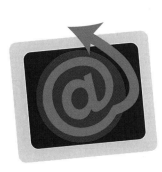

Locate an atlas of neuroanatomy on the Internet (see Internet Assignment for Chapter 2) and use it to find the locations of the following brain structures related to the control of movement: red nucleus, basal ganglia, primary motor cortex, and pyramidal tract.

SENSORIMOTOR INTEGRATION

The importance of sensory information in motor control has surfaced repeatedly in our consideration of motor systems in the spinal cord and brain. This ubiquitous process of converting sensory information into appropriate motor action is known as **sensorimotor integration**. We have already encountered several examples of sensorimotor integration. In the spinal cord, the reflexes we have considered are triggered in response to specific events that

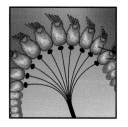

are detected by specialized sensory receptor neurons. The reflex response is determined by the pattern of synaptic connections made by those sensory neurons within the spinal cord, which governs the populations of motor neurons that are excited and inhibited during the reflex. In the stretch reflex (myotatic reflex), for example, the group Ia sensory neurons innervating the muscle spindles make monosynaptic excitatory connections with the motor neurons of the same muscle. By means of this simple yet elegant synaptic arrangement, sensory information (in this case, that the muscle has been passively stretched) is integrated within the spinal cord to produce the desired motor consequence (contraction of the muscle to oppose the passive stretch). Even in the case of more complex reflexes, such as the withdrawal reflex (see Chapter 8), the pattern of synaptic connectivity within the spinal cord can account in a rather straightforward way for the translation of sensory information into motor commands.

When we consider brain motor mechanisms, however, the rules that govern sensorimotor integration become less clear. Sensory information usually reaches the brain motor systems only after passing through numerous synaptic relay stages. At each of these stages, the synaptic processing is more complex and the calculations and transformations performed are less well understood than in the spinal reflex circuits. An exception is the system controlling the movements of the eyes: the **oculomotor system**. Because the oculomotor system offers a clear view of several aspects of sensorimotor integration, this chapter will explore this brain motor system as a model of how sensory information influences motor output in the brain.

As a model system, eye movements offer several advantages. First, humans are highly visual animals, and so students of neurobiology (and research neurobiologists) have an intuitive comprehension of many of the neuronal phenomena under consideration. Second, the relevant sensory pathways (visual system and vestibular system), although complex, have been thoroughly studied, and good information is available about the sensory side of the control pathways. Third, the complement of muscles that produce the coordinated movements of the eyes is relatively small, and thus the number of motor neuron pools is rather limited, simplifying the neurophysiological analysis. In addition, the object being moved—the eyeball—is not a limb or skeletal joint, and so the motor control mechanisms need not compensate for widely varying amounts of load on the muscles, unlike motor systems regulating joint movements. Finally, because both reflexive and voluntary movements are involved, the oculomotor system provides examples of both cortical and subcortical control systems. We will begin by considering reflexive eye movements, and then we will describe some properties of the voluntary control mechanisms.

Reflexive Eye Movements: Vestibulo-Ocular Reflex

As we walk, the position of our heads—and thus the position of our eyes—is constantly shifting in three-dimensional space. Despite this movement, the world we see does not shift and blur as we move, and we have no trouble maintaining a constant view of the world. The **vestibulo-ocular reflex** (**VOR**) is one of the control systems that keep the eyes pointed in the same direction in external space during head motion. It is easy to demonstrate the operation of this system on yourself as you are reading these words. Focus on this *word*, and then slowly rotate your head first to the right and then to the left. You should be able to keep the word in sharp focus during the rotation. Do the same while rotating your head vertically, instead of horizontally. If you repeat this exercise while watching the reflection of your own eyes in a mirror, you will readily see the large changes in eye position within the orbit that occur to keep the fixated object in the center of the field of view (Fig. 10.1A). Note that the direction of eye motion is the opposite of the direction of head motion, as required to keep the eyes pointed at the same location in space.

The visual system could provide, in principle, the sensory information used to control the eye movements in these examples. A shift in image position on the retina could generate an error signal that is passed to the motor neurons controlling the eye muscles, producing a compensating movement to cancel the image shift.

Figure 10.1.

The vestibulo-ocular reflex keeps the eyes pointing at the same point in space as the head rotates. **A.** A frontal view, similar to what you would see if you look at your own reflection in a mirror while turning your head to the side. **B.** A top view, showing that the eyes change position in the appropriate way to keep light from the external world on the same portion of the retina at the back of the eyes.

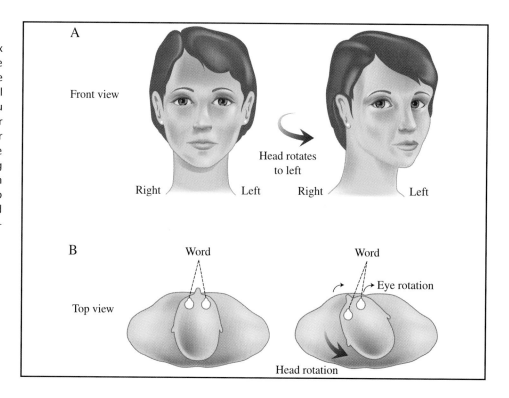

Indeed, visual information is used in this way to help position the eyes, as we will discuss later in this chapter. However, in the case of horizontal and vertical rotations of the head, the sensory signals instead come from the parts of the vestibular apparatus that are sensitive to rotation: the semicircular canals. To understand this reflex, we must first become familiar with the eye muscles and their neuronal control, as well as the vestibular sensory system.

The Eye Muscles and Their Motor Neurons

What muscles control the movements of the human eye?

The eyes of most vertebrates are capable of four different types of motion, summarized in Figure 10.2. The eye can be moved to the left and right in the horizontal plane and up and down in the vertical plane. In addition, it can be rotated in the eye socket, and it can be retracted into the socket (for example, when the eyes are tightly closed in anticipation of a blow). The exact arrangement of the muscles necessary to achieve these movements varies across species, depending on the anatomy of the eye socket and on the relative importance of each type of motion for the animal. In humans, the first two motions (horizontal and vertical) are the most important in stabilizing the visual world during head rotation, and we will concentrate primarily on these two directions of movement.

The muscles that move the human eye (the **extraocular muscles**) are shown in Figure 10.2. The **superior rectus muscle** attaches to the top of the eyeball and moves the eyeball upward. The antagonist of this muscle is the **inferior rectus**, which attaches to the bottom of the eyeball and moves the eyeball down. Horizontal movements are produced by a pair of muscles that attach to sides of the eyeball. The **medial rectus muscle** attaches on the nasal side and rotates the eye toward the nose. The **lateral rectus muscle** attaches on the temporal side of the eyeball and produces horizontal rotation toward the temple. Rotation of the eye in the socket is controlled by another pair of opposed muscles, the **superior oblique** and **inferior oblique muscles**. The extraocular muscles fan out and form broad attachment points on the surface of the eyeball (see Fig. 10.2). Because these attachments are not precisely located at the horizontal and vertical meridians of the

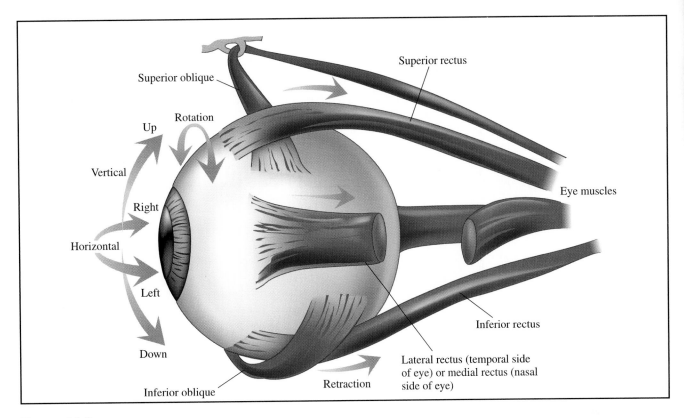

Figure 10.2.

The organization of the extraocular muscles. The six muscles are arranged to pull the eye in various directions. The four rectus muscles (inferior, superior, lateral, and medial) move the eyes in the vertical and horizontal planes. The two oblique muscles (superior and inferior) rotate the eye. Acting in concert, all of the muscles retract the eye into the socket for protection.

eyeball, each muscle produces components of motion in both horizontal and vertical axes. For our purposes, however, we can neglect the minor vertical movements produced by the medial and lateral rectus muscles and the minor horizontal movements produced by the superior and inferior rectus muscles.

All of the extraocular muscles are attached to a common tendon at the back of the orbit, except for the inferior oblique muscle, which attaches on the nasal side of the orbit. The muscle fibers of the extraocular muscles produce the fastest contractions of all the muscles in the body. By activating various combinations of this small set of muscles, the nervous system can rapidly and precisely position the eyes to center the gaze on any portion of the visual field.

Like other striated muscles, the extraocular muscles are controlled by motor neurons. The motor neurons of the extraocular muscles are located within the brain itself, in the **oculomotor nuclei** of the brainstem (Fig. 10.3). In the spinal cord, the axons of motor neurons exit the spinal cord via the segmental spinal nerves. In the brain, however, the outgoing axons of motor neurons exit the brain case (cranium) via a set of nerves called the **cranial nerves**. In humans, there are 12 pairs of cranial nerves, numbered with Roman numerals. Axons of oculomotor neurons are carried in three different cranial nerves. The appropriately named **oculomotor nerve** (nerve III) carries axons that innervate most of the extraocular muscles, including the superior and inferior rectus muscles, the medial rectus muscle, and the inferior oblique muscle. The superior oblique muscle is supplied via cranial nerve IV (the **trochlear nerve**), while the lateral rectus muscle receives its motor innervation through cranial nerve VI (the **abducens nerve**).

What parts of the brainstem contain ocular motor neurons?

Figure 10.3.

A lateral view of the human brain, showing the approximate anterior-posterior locations of the three cranial nerve nuclei containing motor neurons that control the extraocular muscles. The Roman numerals refer to the numbers of the corresponding cranial nerves.

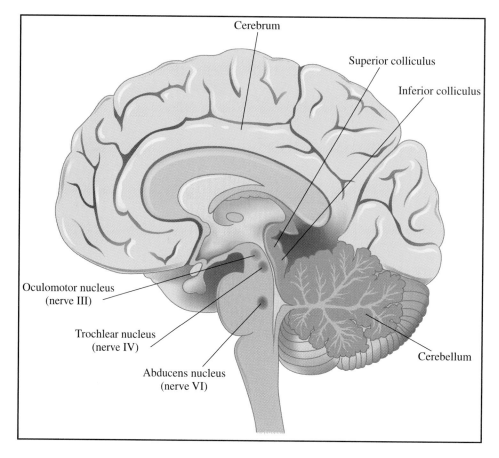

Each of these cranial nerves innervating the eye muscles has its own motor nucleus. The most anterior of the oculomotor nuclei is the motor nucleus of the oculomotor nerve, which lies near the midline of the midbrain at the level of the superior colliculus (see Fig. 10.3). As we will discuss later, the superior colliculus is also involved in the control of eye movements. The motor neurons of the trochlear nerve also lie along the midline of the brainstem, slightly posterior to the motor neurons of nerve III, at the level of the inferior colliculus. The motor neurons of the abducens nerve are found even further posterior, just beneath the floor of the fourth ventricle.

The Semicircular Canals

How does the sensory apparatus of the vestibular system respond to head rotation?

We now turn to the sensory end of the VOR and examine the structures that give rise to the information about head movement: the vestibular apparatus. Sensory structures that give information about the position of the organism with respect to gravity and about acceleration of the organism during locomotion are among the phylogenetically most ancient sensory systems. These sensory structures are based on a specialized type of sensory cell called the **hair cell**, which will be described in detail in Chapter 17. Hair cells change their membrane potential in response to deflections of fine cilia that project from one end of the cell, as shown in Figure 10.4. The cilia increase in length from one end of the cell to the other. Deflection of the cilia toward the longest cilium depolarizes the hair cell, while deflection in the opposite direction (away from the longest cilium) hyperpolarizes the hair cell. The amount of depolarization or hyperpolarization depends on the amount of deflection. The hair cell makes a synaptic connection onto a sensory neuron that then projects into the brain. As in other synapses, the hair cell releases more neurotransmitter upon depolarization and stops releasing neurotransmitter

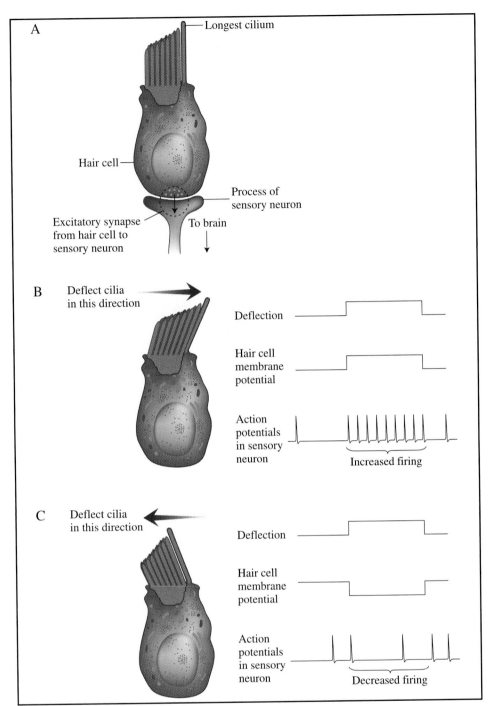

Figure 10.4.
The response of a hair cell to deflection of the cilia. **A.** Changes in the membrane potential of the hair cell cause changes in the release of excitatory neurotransmitter at a synapse between the hair cell and the peripheral end of the sensory neuron that connects the hair cell to the brain. **B.** The response when cilia are deflected toward the longest cilium. The *traces on the right* show the timing of the deflection, the change in membrane potential of the hair cell, and the action potentials in the sensory neuron. **C.** The response when the cilia are deflected away from the longest cilium. In this case, the hair cell hyperpolarizes and the rate of action potentials in the sensory neuron decreases.

during hyperpolarization. Because the neurotransmitter excites the sensory neuron, the rate of action potentials in the sensory neuron increases when the cilia are deflected in the direction that depolarizes the hair cell and decreases when the cilia are deflected in the opposite direction (see Fig. 10.4).

Hair cell organs that detect the position of the organism with respect to gravity are found universally among multicellular, mobile animals. The basic vertebrate position-sensing organ is the **otolith organ**, which is essentially a closed sack of fluid, with hair cells located on the interior surface. The cilia of the hair cells project into the interior of the sack, where they are embedded in a gel-like material containing tiny crystals of calcium carbonate—the **otoliths** ("ear stones"). The crystals add mass to the gel, and the force of gravity shifts the whole structure when the animal tilts to the side, as shown in Figure 10.5.

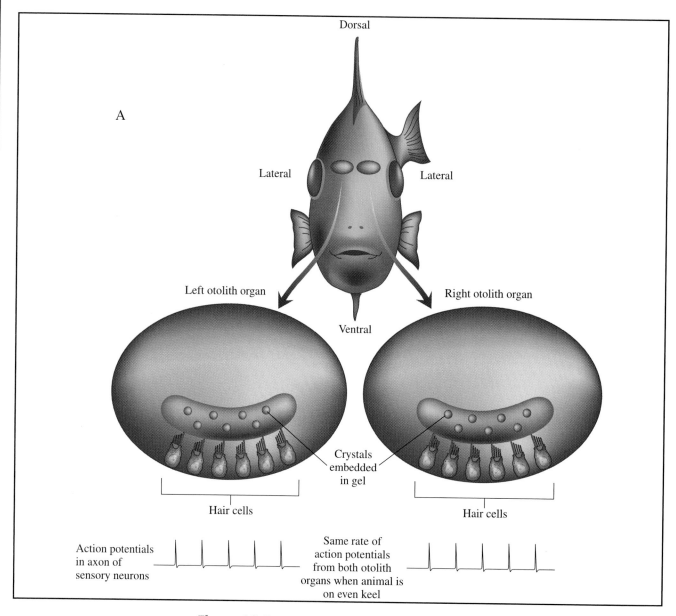

Figure 10.5.

The response of sensory neurons of the otolith organs when an animal tilts vertically. **A.** When the animal is level, the otoliths rest evenly on top of the hair cells. The sensory neurons from the otolith organs on both sides fire action potentials at the same, steady rate. **B.** When the animal tilts to the right, the otoliths shift as indicated. The cilia of the hair cells deflect in opposite directions, relative to the longest cilium. In this case, the hair cells on the left depolarize, and the hair cells on the right hyperpolarize. The sensory neurons on the left fire action potentials more frequently, while those on the right fire less frequently.

When the animal is upright, the gel rests directly over the hair cells, and the cilia are not deflected significantly in either direction. Under these conditions, transmitter is released from the hair cell at a moderate rate, and the sensory neurons that receive synapses from the hair cells fire action potentials at a correspondingly moderate rate. The rate of firing is the same on the two sides of the animal (see Fig. 10.5A). When the animal tilts to the right, however, both otolith-containing gels shift to the right (see Fig. 10.5B). Because the two otolith organs are mirror images of each other, the cilia in the left otolith organ deflect toward the longest cilium, but the cilia in the right organ deflect in the opposite direction, toward the

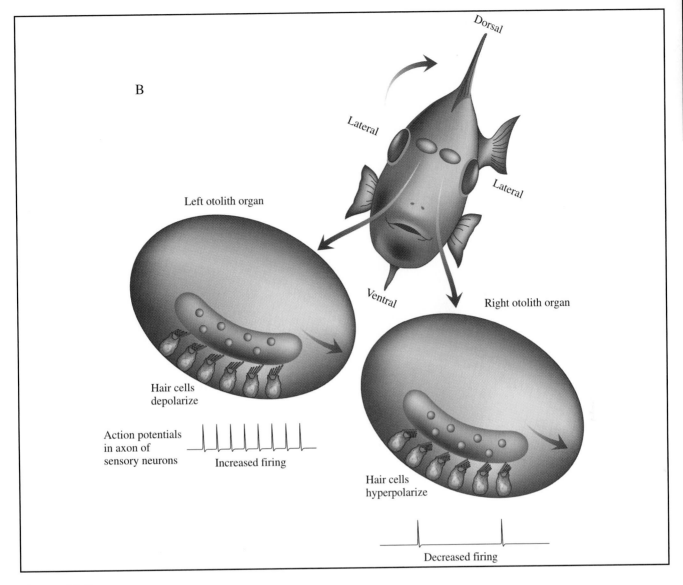

Figure 10.5.

(continued)

shortest cilium. Thus, the hair cells on the left depolarize, and the hair cells on the right hyperpolarize. The increased release of excitatory neurotransmitter on the left side increases the rate of action potentials in the sensory neurons on that side. Conversely, the rate of action potentials declines in sensory neurons on the right side. By comparing the rate of action potentials on the two sides, the nervous system can determine the relative tilt of the body in space.

The hair cells of the otolith organs provide a steady signal during sustained tilting. As long as the tilt persists, the hair cell cilia remain deflected as shown in Figure 10.5B. The same shift in the cilia would also occur if the animal remained upright but accelerated at a constant rate to the left. Thus, the otolith organs provide information about both static tilt and acceleration. In humans, as in most other vertebrates, the otolith organs are divided into two parts: the horizontally oriented **saccule** and the vertically oriented **utricle**.

During the course of vertebrate evolution, the simple otolith organ became more elaborate and gave rise to two additional fluid compartments: the **cochlea** and the **semicircular canals**. The otolith organs, the cochlea, and the semicircular canals are collectively called the **labyrinth**, shown in Figure 10.6. The cochlea first

Figure 10.6.

The response of the semicir-cular canals to rotation of the head. When the head turns to the left, the labyrinth rotates, setting up a counterflow in the endolymph fluid within the horizontal semicircular ca-nal. This flow bends the cupula inside the ampulla of the canal, which deflects the cilia of the hair cells embed-ded in the cupula. Deflection of the cilia alters the rate of action potentials in the sen-sory neurons contacted by the hair cells.

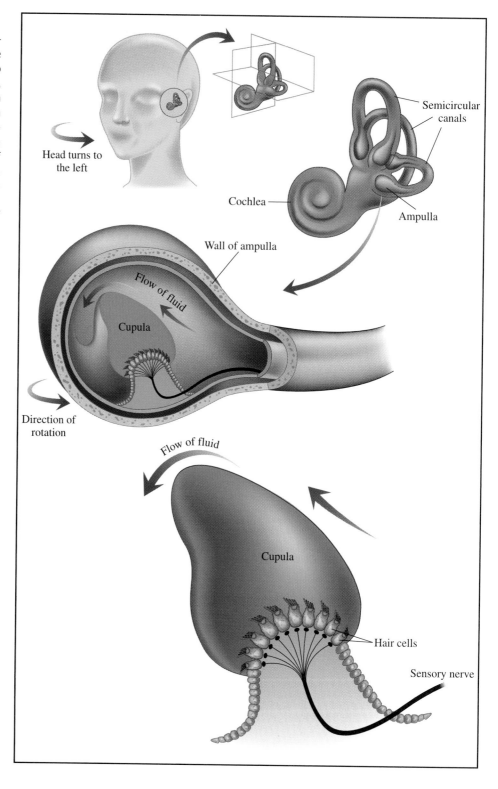

appeared in amphibians and is responsible for the sense of hearing in terrestrial vertebrates (see Chapter 17). The semicircular canals form three loops, oriented at right angles with respect to one another. One loop parallels the horizontal plane of the head, one is oriented vertically, and the third lies in the anterior-posterior plane. The semicircular canals provide information about acceleration of the head, as detailed in Figure 10.6.

Each semicircular canal is a tube filled with a fluid called the **endolymph**. When the head rotates, the solid outer wall of the canal rotates as well. The fluid inside the tube, however, does not immediately follow suit. Because of inertia, the endolymph fluid initially stays in place while the tube rotates. This discrepancy creates motion of the fluid with respect to the wall of the tube, in the direction opposite to the direction of head rotation (see Fig. 10.6). Motion of the fluid is sensed by hair cells within a specialized swelling, called the **ampulla**, located at the end of each semicircular canal, where the canal joins the utricle. The cilia of the hair cells in the ampullae are embedded in a gelatinous structure called the **cupula**, which sticks out into the endolymph from the wall of the canal, like a sail in the wind. As the head rotates, the cupula is dragged through the endolymph, producing a flow of endolymph up and over the cupula. This flow deflects the cupula and the embedded cilia of the underlying hair cells (see Fig. 10.6). Depending on the direction of rotation—and hence the direction of ciliary deflection—the hair cells will either depolarize or hyperpolarize. In the example shown in Figure 10.6, the deflection is toward the longest cilium, and the hair cells would depolarize during the head movement. As with the otolith organ, changes in the membrane potential of the ampullar hair cells affect the rate of action potentials in the sensory neurons that receive synapses from the hair cells. Because the semicircular canals on the two sides of the head are mirror images of each other, the endolymph flows in opposite directions with respect to the cupula on the left and right sides. Therefore, as with the otolith organs (see Fig. 10.5), the rate of action potentials in the vestibular sensory neurons increases on one side and decreases on the other side during rotation in a given direction.

If rotation continues in the same direction at the same speed, inertia in the endolymph fluid is overcome, and the fluid inside the canal eventually moves at the same speed as the wall of the canal. When the fluid and the wall move at the same speed, there is no flow of the endolymph relative to the wall, and thus the cupula is not deflected. For this reason, the signal from the semicircular canals is strongest at the onset of rotation, when the head is accelerating from rest. As a result of the physical properties of the detection apparatus, the signal progressively declines during sustained rotation.

Translating Vestibular Information into Oculomotor Output

How does the sensory signal from the semicircular canal connect appropriately with the motor neurons controlling the extraocular muscles? The hair cells of the canals make excitatory synapses with vestibular sensory neurons, whose cell bodies are located just outside the labyrinth, in the **vestibular ganglion**. In animals that have a cochlea, the axons leaving the vestibular ganglion join with those of the cochlear neurons and enter the brain as the **eighth cranial nerve** (nerve VIII; often called the auditory nerve, but more correctly called the vestibulocochlear nerve). The incoming axons from the vestibular ganglion terminate in the **vestibular nuclei** of the brainstem. As described in Chapter 9, the vestibular nuclei give rise to the vestibulospinal tract and are also an important source of sensory input to the cerebellum. The vestibular nuclei are located beneath the cerebellum in the brainstem, as illustrated in Figure 10.7.

The vestibular nuclei contain several different types of neurons concerned with eye movements. The neuron types are distinguished based on the semicircular canal from which they receive inputs and the ocular motor neuron pool to which they project. Stimulation of the horizontal semicircular canal produces horizontal eye movements, and stimulation of the vertical canal results in vertical eye movements. Thus, the neurons in the vestibular nuclei that receive inputs from the horizontal canal must project to the motor neurons of the medial and lateral rectus

How are synaptic connections in the vestibulo-ocular system arranged to produce appropriate reflexive movements of the eye to compensate for head motion?

Figure 10.7.

The location of the vestibular nuclei within the brainstem. **A**. Lateral view. **B**. Top view.

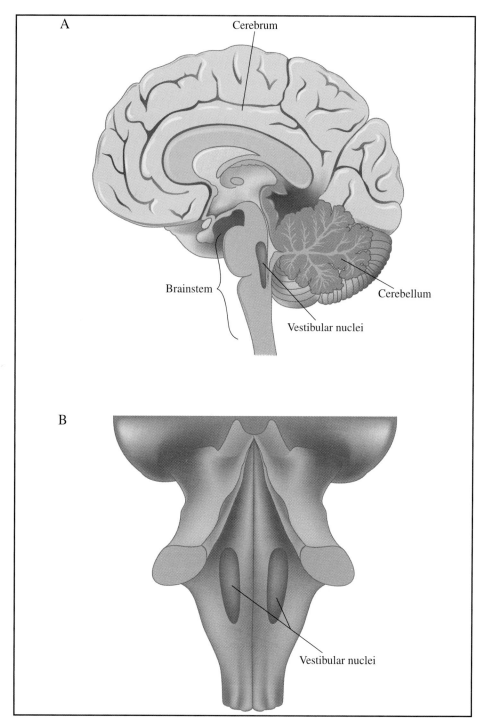

muscles. Figure 10.8 summarizes this set of connections for the horizontal canal. The motor neurons of the medial rectus muscle for each eye are located in the ipsilateral oculomotor nucleus, while the motor neurons for each lateral rectus muscle are found in the ipsilateral abducens nucleus. The vestibular ganglion neurons make excitatory synaptic connections on the interneurons of the vestibular nuclei. Some of these interneurons then project to the ipsilateral oculomotor nucleus, where they make excitatory synaptic contact with motor neurons of the ipsilateral medial rectus muscle. Other vestibular nucleus interneurons send axons that cross the midline and make excitatory synapses with lateral rectus motor neurons in the contralateral abducens nucleus.

In addition to the excitatory interneurons, the vestibular nuclei also contain in-

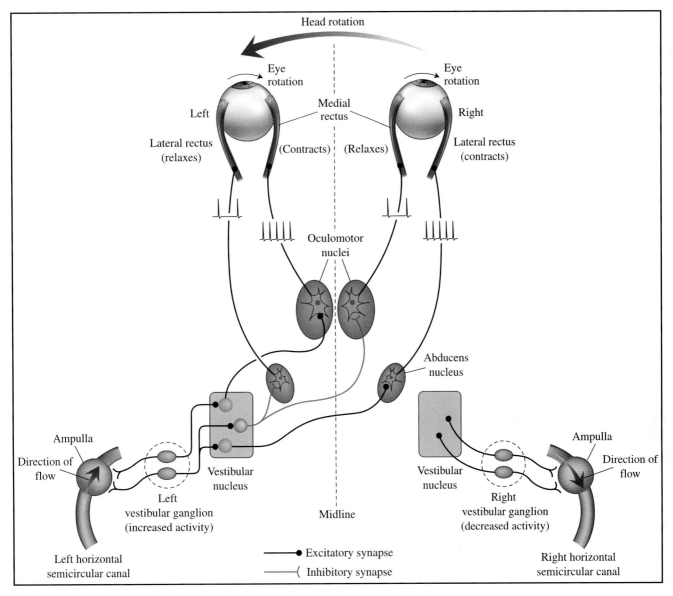

Figure 10.8.

The circuitry of the vestibulo-ocular reflex. Head rotation to the left elicits eye movement to the right. Sensory information from the horizontal semicircular canal is distributed to the appropriate motor neurons by the interneurons of the vestibular nuclei. The cranial nerve nuclei are shaded in *blue*. Inhibitory neurons are in *red*. The right vestibular nuclei contain the same sets of interneurons as on the left. For clarity, the mirror-image connections of the interneurons on the right are not shown.

hibitory interneurons. For the horizontal semicircular canal, these inhibitory interneurons project to the ipsilateral abducens nucleus and to the contralateral oculomotor nucleus. (The connection from the inhibitory interneurons to the medial rectus motor neurons is probably indirect, but it is shown as direct in Fig. 10.8 for simplicity.) Thus, excitation of this subset of vestibular ganglion neurons rapidly inhibits the ipsilateral lateral rectus motor neurons and the contralateral medial rectus motor neurons.

Figure 10.8 illustrates the action of the circuit for the horizontal canal when the head rotates to the left. In the horizontal canal on the left, endolymph flows toward the ampulla, depolarizing the hair cells and increasing the rate of action potentials in the vestibular ganglion neurons on the left. The vestibular ganglion neurons then make excitatory connections with pools of interneurons in the vestibular nuclei on the left side of the brainstem. One group of interneurons excites the motor neurons of the lateral rectus muscle of the right eye, and another group excites motor neurons of the medial rectus muscle of the left eye. The contractions of these muscles rotate the eyes to the right, in the direction opposite to the direction of head rotation. A third group of interneurons in the vestibular nucleus inhibits the motor neurons of the left-eye lateral rectus muscle and the right-eye medial rectus muscle. This inhibition reduces the tension in the muscles that oppose rotation of the eyes to the right. The diagram in Figure 10.8 shows only the connections for the left horizontal semicircular canal. The horizontal canal on the right gives rise to a similar set of synaptic connections via the vestibular nuclei on the right side of the brainstem, producing a circuit that is the mirror image of the one shown.

In the horizontal canal on the right, endolymph flows away from the ampulla when the head rotates to the left. This direction of flow hyperpolarizes the hair cells and reduces the rate of action potentials in the vestibular ganglion neurons on the right side. The *reduced* firing rate on the right reinforces the effect of the *increased* activity in the left-side vestibular ganglion neurons. Less excitation is supplied by interneurons of the right vestibular nuclei to the motor neurons of the left lateral rectus muscle and the right medial rectus muscle. The decreased excitation acts together with the inhibition of these same motor neurons by inhibitory interneurons from the vestibular nuclei on the left side, further relaxing the muscles that oppose the desired eye motion. Decreased activity on the right also removes inhibition supplied to motor neurons of the right-eye lateral rectus and left-eye medial rectus muscles. A motor neuron innervating the lateral rectus muscle of the right eye, for example, is doubly excited because of increased excitation from excitatory interneurons in the vestibular nuclei on the left side of the brain and because of decreased inhibition coming from inhibitory interneurons in the vestibular nuclei on the right side of the brain.

Connections for the other semicircular canals follow the same basic scheme shown for the horizontal canals in Figure 10.8, but the pattern of synaptic connections to motor neurons differs as appropriate for the required direction of the reflexive eye movements. The vestibular ganglion neurons for each canal project to a specific subset of interneurons within the vestibular nuclei, and these interneurons then provide the appropriate connections with the motor neurons in the three cranial nerve nuclei (nerves III, IV, and VI) that control the extraocular muscles.

The Vestibulo-Ocular Reflex Lacks Feedback Control

The reflex pathway from the semicircular canals to the motor neurons of the eye muscles is very short, requiring only two synapses to reach from the neurons of the vestibular ganglion to the motor neurons. This short path ensures a rapid response for the VOR: the conduction delay to the motor neurons is only about 15 thousandths of a second after the vestibular hair cells detect head movement. This high speed is one reason why the nervous system uses vestibular information—rather than visual information—to stabilize eye position. Monitoring head movement allows the nervous system to anticipate blurring of the image before it actually occurs. If visual information were used instead, then the blur would have to occur before it could be detected.

Another striking feature of the VOR is the absence of feedback control in the pathway. In this regard, the VOR differs dramatically from stretch reflexes, which inherently involve a feedback mechanism: the sensory signal (passive stretch of the intrafusal muscle fibers) results in a motor output that reduces the input signal, until the length set point is restored. The circuit shown in Figure 10.8, however, lacks sensory feedback about the success of the eye movements. This type of reflex is called an **open loop reflex** to indicate the lack of feedback that would close the loop between output and input. By contrast, reflexes with feedback, like the stretch reflex, are called **closed loop reflexes**. The ability of the VOR to hold the eyes steady depends on the precision of the excitatory and inhibitory synaptic connections with the motor neurons and interneurons, which must be exactly balanced to produce the correct eye motions over a wide range of amplitude, speed, and direction of head movement.

To ensure that eye movements produced by the VOR are in fact matched correctly to head rotation, the nervous system monitors the performance of the VOR and modifies the strength of the excitatory and inhibitory connections to maximize stability of the visual world. The motor signals in the VOR are continually compared with both vestibular and visual information, and additional synaptic signals are added both in the vestibular nuclei and in the ocular motor nuclei to adjust the accuracy of performance. If the eye movements are smaller or larger than required to balance head movement, an error signal is added to or subtracted from the vestibular signal, compensating for the mismatch. The cerebellum plays an important role in modification of the VOR based on experience, which represents a simple form of learning, as described in more detail in Chapter 20.

REFLEXIVE EYE MOVEMENTS: OPTOKINETIC REFLEX

The **optokinetic reflex** (OKR) is another ocular reflex that maintains a constant retinal position for images during movement. In the VOR, reflexive movement of the eyes is triggered by head movement—not by movement of the visual image on the retina. Unlike the VOR, the OKR is triggered by motion of the external world, with the head position fixed. We commonly experience this type of eye movement while riding in a car or train. If we look out the side window while passing a series of telephone poles or fence posts, our eyes tend to track a single pole until the eyes reach their limit within the orbit. The eyes then flick back rapidly in the opposite direction, followed by resumption of the slower tracking movement. This type of eye motion, with slow steady movement in one direction followed by a rapid return movement in the opposite direction, is called **nystagmus**. The OKR or similar visual following responses are found in virtually all animals that have eyes.

The same groups of interneurons in the vestibular nuclei that are excited by inputs from the semicircular canals receive inputs from the visual system and can be excited by moving visual stimuli. Figure 10.9 illustrates the effects of vestibular and visual stimulation on the firing of action potentials in the vestibular nucleus. An animal is placed at the center of a rotating drum with vertical stripes. If the animal is rotated while the drum is stationary, the VOR is activated, and if the drum is rotated while the animal is stationary, the OKR is elicited. A neuron in the vestibular nucleus that is excited when the animal is rotated to the left (see Fig. 10.9B) will also be excited when the animal remains stationary and the drum rotates to the right (see Fig. 10.9C). In both cases, the stimulus elicits eye movements toward the right in the orbit, compensating for the head movement in the one case and following the moving stimulus in the other. If the directions of rotation were reversed (that is, if the animal were rotated to the right or the drum were rotated to the left), the same neuron would be inhibited by both stimuli, and the rate of firing action potentials would decline during the stimulus.

Because they respond to visual stimuli, the interneurons of the vestibular nuclei can be viewed as part of a visual pathway, as well as the vestibular pathway. This duality exemplifies one of the central features of sensorimotor integration: information from more than one sensory system is combined to produce appropriate motor output. In the oculomotor system, the integration of multiple sensory inputs occurs at a particularly low level in the motor pathway—only one synapse away from the motor neurons of the extraocular muscles. Such rapid and low-level combination of vestibular and visual information is important for ocular motor control, because under normal conditions we move both our head and our eyes as we follow

What is the difference between the optokinetic reflex and the vestibulo-ocular reflex?

Figure 10.9.

The optokinetic reflex (OKR) and the vestibulo-ocular reflex (VOR) act on the same set of interneurons in the vestibular nuclei. In this experiment, an animal is placed on a rotating stool in the center of a rotating drum. **A.** A schematic diagram of the recording arrangement and the synaptic connections. **B.** Rotating the head to the left elicits the VOR and increases the firing of action potentials in the interneuron. **C.** Rotating the drum to the right elicits the OKR and also increases the firing of action potentials in the interneuron.

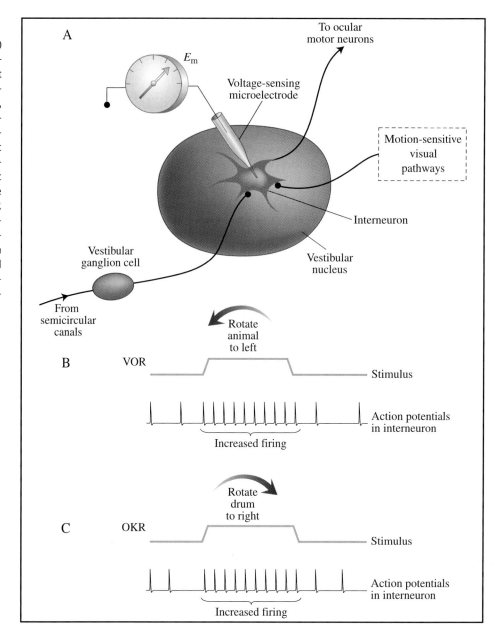

objects. Thus, accurate eye movements to follow moving visual stimuli require information about head motion.

The vestibular nuclei can be thought of as a general machine that computes the amount of excitation and inhibition of the various oculomotor neurons required to produce particular eye movements. The nervous system can reuse this computational machine for other systems that influence eye movements, such as the OKR, without having to recreate and recalibrate the synaptic machinery controlling the motor neurons. In addition, by tapping into this machinery, other parts of the nervous system can access the supervisory circuitry in the cerebellum that generates error signals, which are used to ensure that eye movements produce the desired result.

The Accessory Optic System

What is the source of the visual information about movement in the OKR?

Visual information leaves the eye in the optic nerve and is passed via the thalamus to regions of the cerebral cortex that decipher the signals (see Chapter 16). In addition to this thalamic-cortical path, other projections of the optic nerve

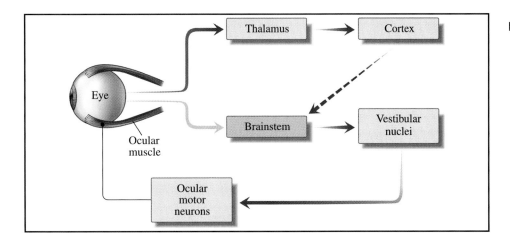

Figure 10.10.

A diagram of visual system inputs to the oculomotor systems in the brainstem. The accessory optic system is shown in *pink*. The retina projects to the thalamus and to the brainstem. The brainstem also receives indirect projections from the visual portions of the cerebral cortex (*dashed line*).

bypass the thalamus and connect directly with brainstem neurons, forming a noncortical path called the **accessory optic system** (Fig. 10.10). The brainstem neurons of the accessory optic system are excited by moving visual stimuli. The visual projection to the brainstem likely represents a phylogenetically more primitive system for detecting movement, used in the reflexive control of eye position. The neurons of the accessory optic system send axons to the vestibular nuclei on both sides of the brain, where they make synaptic connections with the interneurons of the vestibular nuclei.

In many species, the accessory optic system is the principal source of visual motion information for the control of eye movements. In animals with a more developed cerebral cortex, such as primates, cortical areas also pass along information about moving visual stimuli to the oculomotor system in the brainstem (see Fig. 10.10). In addition to providing signals used in the optokinetic reflex, the cortical

IN THE CLINIC

BOX 1

The eye movement system includes components in several parts of the brain, and the movements of the eyes are readily observed and tested in routine clinical examinations. Therefore, disorders of eye movement can be used to indicate the nature of the defect in several neurological conditions. Because of the vestibulo-ocular reflex, defects of the vestibular system can cause abnormal eye movements, such as nystagmus. Nystagmus is a normal component of the optokinetic reflex, and it refers to a slow steady movement in one direction (as when following a moving stimulus during the optokinetic response) followed by a rapid saccade in the opposite direction to recenter the eyes. Normally, when the head is still, there is a small amount of resting activity in the vestibular ganglion neurons on both sides of the head, but the amount of activity is the same on the two sides and so the eyes remain still. If the semicircular canals or the nerve fibers from the vestibular ganglion are damaged on one side, however, the reduced activity on that side produces an imbalance between the two sides that mimics rotation of the head away from the damaged side and causes the eyes to drift in the opposite direction just as they would if the head were moving. When the eyes reach the extreme position in the orbit, a rapid saccade is executed to recenter the gaze, and the process begins again. Thus, nystagmus when the head is still is one sign of peripheral or central disease of the vestibular pathway.

visual centers are important in generating other types of eye movements, which we will discuss next.

VOLUNTARY EYE MOVEMENTS: SACCADES

As you read the words of this sentence, your eyes scan the page in a series of rapid jumps, fixating first on one group of words and then making a rapid lateral movement to fixate on the next group of words. These rapid jumps, called **saccades**, are the eye movements most commonly used by primates to scan the visual world. Eye movement during a saccade is extremely rapid. A small saccade (for example, a shift of 10° in the angle of the eyes with respect to the head) is complete in 50 msec or less, and even a large saccade (approximately 30°) requires only about 100 msec.

Saccades bring different portions of the visual environment into the center of the visual field, so that light coming from objects of interest falls on the fovea of the retina, where visual acuity is highest (see Chapter 15). Saccades are also found in animals that do not have a fovea. The neural machinery that produces the rapid movement probably evolved first as a component of reflex systems, acting as a reset mechanism to return the eyes to the central position in the orbit. For example, saccades are a normal component of the optokinetic nystagmus, producing the rapid phase of movement in the opposite direction after the eyes reach their extreme horizontal positions in the orbits during the OKR. Later in evolution, the basic machinery of the saccade came under the control of higher centers involved in voluntary control of eye movements, allowing different visual targets to be brought rapidly to the fovea.

The Saccade Generator

What neuronal circuitry in the brainstem programs the contractions of the ocular muscles during a saccade?

In keeping with the idea that the saccade circuit is an old evolutionary development, the neurons of the circuit are found within the brainstem reticular formation, in various nuclei stretching from the pons to the midbrain. As with all oculomotor circuits, the output of the saccade generator is carried by the ocular motor neurons—the final common path for control of the extraocular muscles.

If we record the action potentials of an ocular motor neuron during a saccade, we would observe a firing pattern like that shown in Figure 10.11. At the onset of the saccade, the motor neuron fires a burst of action potentials at a very high rate, approaching 400 action potentials per second. This initial burst of activity, called the **pulse phase**, produces a strong and rapid contraction of the muscle. The strong contraction rapidly overcomes the inertia of the eyeball and pulls the eye quickly into a new position within the orbit. The pulse phase lasts only 100 msec or less and rapidly dies out as the eyeball approaches its new position. The rate of action potentials in the motor neuron does not decline to zero, however. Instead, the pulse phase is followed by a sustained plateau of firing at a moderate rate, called the **step phase**. This phase holds the eye steady at its new position and prevents relaxation caused by the elastic properties of the supporting tissues of the eyeball.

The basic organization of the neuronal connections that account for the initial pulse of activity in the ocular motor neurons is summarized in Figure 10.12. As in our previous examples, we will consider the circuit only for a horizontal movement, which involves the medial and lateral rectus muscles. An equivalent set of neurons accounts for vertical saccades. The diagram in Figure 10.12 shows only the circuitry for a saccade toward the right, which is controlled by interneurons located in the right side of the brain. On the left side, a mirror-image circuit drives saccades toward the left in the horizontal plane.

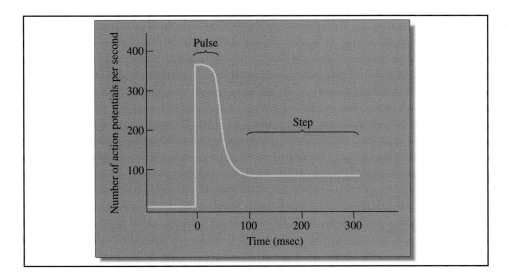

Figure 10.11.

The pattern of action potentials in a motor neuron of an extraocular muscle during a saccade. The saccade is triggered at time 0 on the time axis. Initially, the motor neuron fires a burst of action potentials at a high rate (pulse phase). This high rate is maintained for a short time, followed by a decline to a lower rate (step phase).

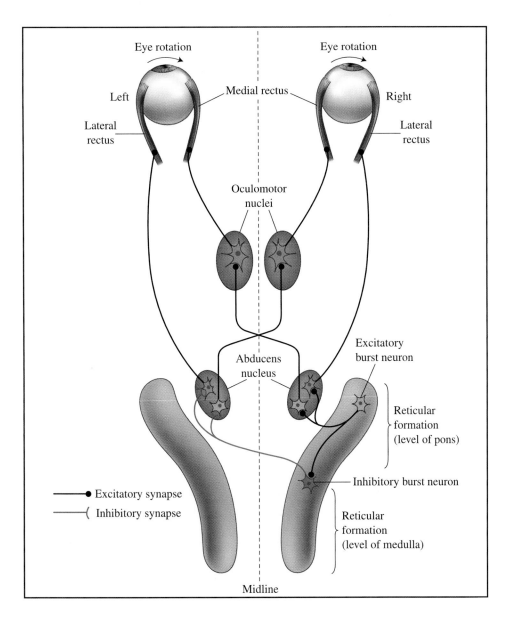

Figure 10.12.

A schematic diagram of the basic circuitry for generating a saccade to the right. The cranial nerve nuclei are shaded *blue*. The inhibitory burst neuron is *red*.

The trigger neuron for the burst phase is a type of interneuron called the **excitatory burst neuron**, which is located in the pontine reticular formation. Excitatory burst neurons fire a rapid burst of action potentials just before the onset of a saccade, producing strong excitation of lateral rectus motor neurons in the abducens nucleus on the same side of the brain. This strong excitatory connection triggers the burst phase of action potentials in the lateral rectus motor neurons for the right eye. In addition, the excitatory burst neurons make excitatory synapses with interneurons within the abducens nucleus that project to the contralateral nucleus of the oculomotor nerve. There, the interneurons make excitatory connections onto the motor neurons of the medial rectus muscle of the left eye, triggering the pulse phase for that group of motor neurons. Through this set of connections, shown in Figure 10.12, the excitatory burst neurons trigger a strong contraction of the left-eye medial rectus muscle and the right-eye lateral rectus muscle.

The excitatory burst neurons also send collateral branches of their axons to more posterior parts of the reticular formation, where they make excitatory synaptic contact with another class of interneurons involved in the control of saccades, the **inhibitory burst neurons**. The input from the excitatory burst neurons triggers a burst of action potentials in the inhibitory burst neurons, whose axons cross the midline and make inhibitory synaptic connections with the lateral rectus motor neurons in the contralateral abducens nucleus. This strong inhibitory input silences the motor neurons of the antagonistic horizontal muscle of the left eye, preventing it from opposing the strong pull produced by the contraction of the medial rectus muscle on that side. The inhibitory burst neurons also inhibit interneurons in the left abducens nucleus that provide excitatory inputs to medial rectus motor neurons of the right eye. Silencing this source of excitatory input to the medial rectus motor neurons reduces tension in the medial rectus muscle of the right eye, preventing it from opposing the desired movement. An equivalent set of excitatory and inhibitory burst neurons is found on the left side of the brain. These neurons are responsible for producing the pulse phase of saccades toward the left. Thus, stimulation of the excitatory burst neurons on a particular side of the brain will produce a saccade toward that side of the brain.

The burst of action potentials produced by the excitatory burst neurons triggers the rapid phase of the eye movement. For a large-amplitude saccade, the required strength and duration of muscle contraction are greater than those for a smaller saccade. To produce the stronger contraction, the pulse phase of activity in the motor neurons must also be larger and longer. A larger saccade also requires a higher rate of firing during the step phase, to overcome the larger passive resistance of supportive tissues and antagonistic muscles during a larger movement. In other words, whenever the pulse phase is greater, the step phase is also greater. Figure 10.13A shows examples of the time course of activity in ocular motor neurons during large and small saccades.

To monitor the size of the pulse phase, the nervous system sums (or integrates) the action potential activity during the pulse phase. In Figure 10.13A, the shaded areas show the integral of activity during the pulse phase for the small and large saccades. The pulse phase is produced by the burst of action potentials in excitatory burst neurons, whose axons provide excitatory input to a neuronal integrator circuit (see Fig. 10.13B) as well as to ocular motor neurons. The integrator circuit converts the burst of input action potentials into a sustained train of output action potentials. The rate of action potentials in the output of the integrator is proportional to the number of action potentials in the driving burst from the excitatory burst neurons. The neurons of the neuronal integrator then make excitatory synapses with the same ocular motor neurons that receive inputs from the excitatory burst neurons. Thus, the output from the motor neuron to the muscle consists of both the rapid burst and the sustained train of activity.

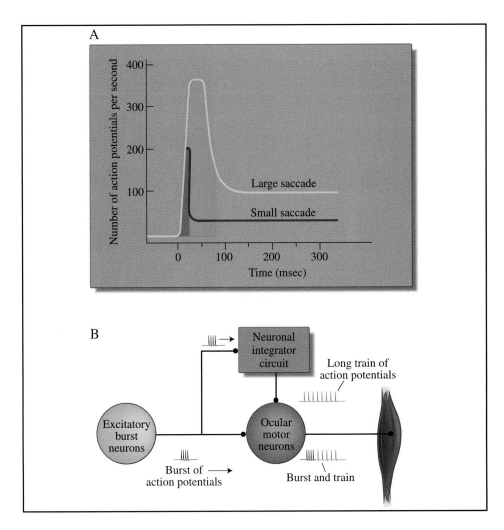

Figure 10.13.
The circuitry for generating pulse and step phases of ocular motor neuron activity during a saccade. **A.** The time courses of pulse and step phases during large and small saccades. The large saccade is shown in *yellow*, and the small saccade in *red*. The area of the pulse phase is indicated in *dark green* for the small saccade and in *light green* for the large saccade. **B.** The neuronal connections for generating the step phase by integrating the activity during the burst of firing by the excitatory burst interneurons. The action potentials from the integrator circuit are shown in *red*. The action potentials in the ocular motor neuron arise from excitatory inputs from the excitatory burst neurons (*black* action potentials) and from the integrator circuit (*red* action potentials).

Control of the Saccade Generator: Pause Neurons

We now move up the control hierarchy and examine the neural systems that regulate the lower-level saccade generator. Saccade production is prevented by a general-purpose saccade inhibition system, which consists of **omnidirectional pause neurons** in the **raphe nucleus** along the midline of the brainstem at the level of the abducens nerves. Omnidirectional pause neurons fire continuously at a steady rate, except just prior to and during a saccade (hence, the name *pause neuron*). They cease firing during a saccade in any direction, without directional specificity (hence, the name *omnidirectional* pause neuron). Omnidirectional pause neurons make inhibitory synaptic contact with excitatory burst neurons, providing a sustained inhibition that keeps the burst neurons from firing, except during a saccade.

Thus, the release from inhibition by the omnidirectional pause neurons is one trigger for activation of the saccade generator. If the raphe nucleus is stimulated electrically to activate the omnidirectional pause neurons, animals are unable to produce saccades, although slower eye movements are unaffected. If the omnidirectional pause neurons are stimulated artificially during the performance of a saccade, the saccade terminates prematurely. Thus, cessation of activity in the omnidirectional pause neurons is obligatory for the triggering of a saccade.

In addition to the inhibitory input from the omnidirectional pause neurons, the excitatory burst neurons receive inputs from higher motor control centers that are involved in planning and programming saccades. These descending commands excite the burst neurons and inhibit the pause neurons, and this combination activates the burst neurons and initiates the saccade. The omnidirectional pause neurons act as an overall gate that permits the saccade to be activated by the descending excitatory command. The selection among the various possible saccade directions is then determined by the subset of saccade circuits that receive excitation from the eye movement command centers, as shown in Figure 10.14.

Control of the Saccade Generator: The Superior Colliculus

What brain regions control the saccade generator circuits in the brainstem?

The superior colliculus (see Fig. 10.3) is a major source for the descending motor commands that are shown in Figure 10.14. Neurons of the superior colliculus receive extensive inputs from the visual system and send axons to the areas of the brainstem where excitatory burst neurons are found. The superior colliculus is organized into several layers. The dorsal layers (near the surface of the brainstem) receive visual inputs, including direct input from the retina. The ventral layers (deeper within the brainstem) give rise to the descending axons that connect with the oculomotor systems in the reticular formation. This arrangement is shown in Figure 10.15.

Both the dorsal layers and the ventral layers are organized into two-dimensional maps: a sensory map of the visual fields in the dorsal region, and a motor map of relative eye position in the ventral region. For example, a visual stimulus appearing in the upper part of the visual field would excite neurons in the medial portion of the dorsal layers of the superior colliculus. Similarly, electrical stimulation of the medial portion of the ventral layers would elicit a saccade upward. Thus, electrical stimulation in the ventral layers produces eye movement toward the point in the visual field represented by the corresponding, overlying portion of the dorsal layers. The direction and magnitude of the eye movement are independent (within the limits of the possible range of motion) of the absolute eye position within the orbit. Thus, there is a topographical correspondence between the maps in the ventral and dorsal layers.

Figure 10.14.

A schematic diagram for the connections of the saccade command centers with the excitatory burst neurons responsible for the four saccade directions. The omnidirectional pause neurons make inhibitory connections on all of the excitatory burst neurons. The higher centers also inhibit the pause neurons.

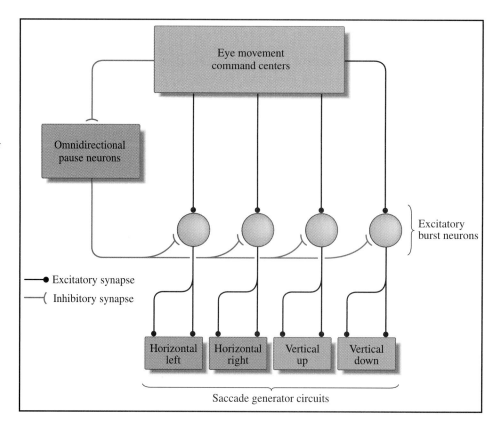

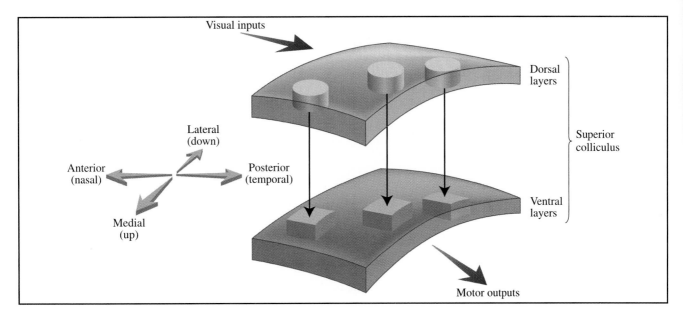

Figure 10.15.

Schematic diagram of the layers of the superior colliculus. Visual inputs arrive in the dorsal layers (*tan*) and are relayed to the output layers (*red-brown*). The process of translating a sensory map of the external world into a set of motor commands is indicated by the *arrows* connecting the two layers. The three-dimensional spatial orientation within the superior colliculus is indicated by the *compass arrows*. The parts of the visual field that correspond to the spatial regions are given in *parentheses* next to the compass arrows.

The superior colliculus is thought to translate a sensory map of the external world (projected onto the neurons of the dorsal layers) into a set of motor commands that move the eyes so that the fovea is centered at the corresponding position in the visual field (see Fig. 10.15). How this translation process is carried out by the synaptic interactions among the layers is not yet understood. Some neurons in the superior colliculus respond to both auditory and visual stimulation, which suggests that the superior colliculus might be important for generating eye movements toward external auditory targets, as well as visual targets.

Control of the Saccade Generator: Cortical Eye Movement Centers

Cortical regions are also important in programming saccades, especially in primates. A major cortical area involved in saccades is the **frontal eye field**, which is located bilaterally in the frontal cortex (in part of Brodmann's area 8), just in front of the primary motor cortex (Fig. 10.16). Neurons of the frontal eye fields fire action potentials prior to saccades. These neurons send connections to the superior colliculus and directly to the oculomotor system in the reticular formation. The frontal eye fields also send outputs to the basal ganglia. The interconnections of the cortical and subcortical eye movement systems are summarized in Figure 10.17.

Electrical stimulation applied to the frontal eye field on one side of the brain elicits a saccade of both eyes toward the opposite side. For example, stimulation of the left frontal eye field causes the eyes to move to the right. The latency of this response to electrical stimulation is less than 0.1 sec, which suggests that the neurons of the frontal eye fields are closely connected to the saccade generator circuitry. Direct projections from the frontal eye fields to the superior colliculus and the brainstem reticular formation are consistent with this rapid motor response. The

Figure 10.16.

The approximate locations of the cortical areas that affect eye movements.

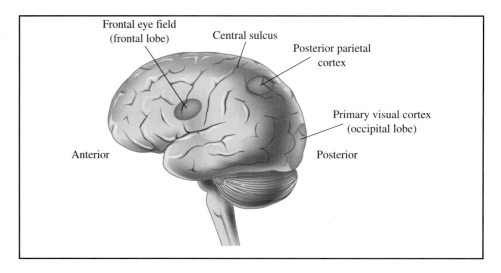

frontal eye fields are thought to issue the command that initiates a saccade. Individual neurons within the frontal eye fields fire action potentials just before the onset of a saccade in a particular direction. Thus, the cells of the frontal eye fields appear to select the desired direction of a saccade by exciting the appropriate saccade generators in the brainstem.

The frontal eye fields receive inputs from another cortical region involved in the eye movements—the **posterior parietal cortex** (see Fig. 10.16). Although electrical stimulation in this part of the cortex can elicit saccades, the latency is longer and more variable than when the stimulation is applied directly to the frontal eye fields. The parietal cortex is thought to carry out higher-level integration of

Figure 10.17.

The connections among the cortical eye movement areas (*tan*) and subcortical systems. The *minus signs* indicate inhibitory connections.

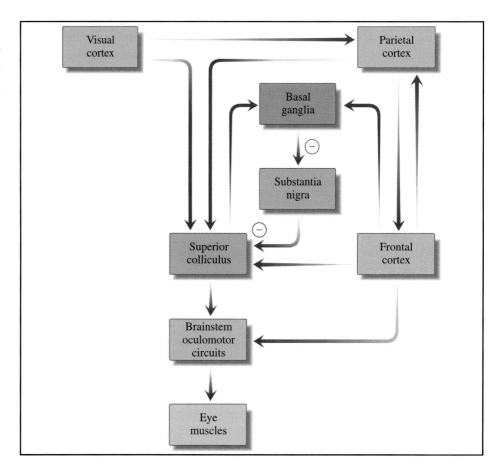

sensorimotor information related to the planning of eye movements, including the selection of visually detected objects to which saccades will be directed (visual attention). Of particular interest is a portion of the parietal cortex buried within the folds of one of the deep sulci. This region, called the **lateral intraparietal area**, contains neurons that fire action potentials in response to visual stimuli and in association with saccades. The axons of neurons in the lateral intraparietal area project to both the superior colliculus and the frontal eye fields. Like the superior colliculus, the lateral intraparietal area appears to connect sensory information with motor outputs related to voluntary saccades. Individual neurons within the lateral intraparietal area fire for saccades of a particular direction and amplitude.

Unlike the superior colliculus, the lateral intraparietal area is not closely tied to the immediate production of saccades. In fact, some neurons in the lateral intraparietal area, called **intended-movement neurons**, apparently encode the *intention* to make a saccade of a particular size and direction, rather than actually triggering the saccade itself. This characteristic of the intended-movement neurons was revealed in experiments that required trained monkeys to make a delayed saccade to the remembered location of a target. In this task, the animal must look at a central fixation point while a visual target is briefly flashed elsewhere in the visual field. After a delay, the animal must make a saccade to the remembered position of the target, which is no longer present. Intended-movement neurons that code for saccades in the appropriate direction begin firing shortly after the target appears, and they continue to fire action potentials throughout the delay period (even though the target is absent) until the saccade actually occurs. These interesting neurons thus seem to be signaling the intention to make the saccade, supporting a motor-planning role for the lateral intraparietal area.

Control of the Saccade Generator: The Role of the Basal Ganglia

In Chapter 9, we discussed the role of the basal ganglia and the substantia nigra in the coordination and initiation of locomotion. These motor control centers also influence the eye movement systems. The superior colliculus, for example, receives an important input from a portion of the substantia nigra. This connection seems to be required for the inhibition of saccades (see Fig. 10.17). The inhibitory input from the substantia acts as a brake to prevent saccades until they are ordered by the cortical centers. To release the brake and initiate a saccade, an inhibitory input from the basal ganglia to the substantia nigra is activated. The saccade command descends from the frontal eye fields to the superior colliculus and to the caudate nucleus of the basal ganglia, which contains neurons that make inhibitory synaptic connections with the substantia nigra. In this way, the superior colliculus is activated directly (by the excitatory command from the frontal eye fields) and indirectly (by removal of the inhibitory influence from the substantia nigra).

The somatic nervous system controls the skeletal musculature. The autonomic nervous system controls other organ systems involved in homeostasis, including the cardiovascular system, the respiratory system, and the digestive system. The motor neurons of the autonomic nervous system are located outside the central nervous system, in autonomic ganglia. The somatic motor neurons, by contrast, are located in the gray matter of the spinal cord, within the central nervous system. The autonomic nervous system is divided into the parasympathetic and the sympathetic divisions. The parasympathetic ganglia are located close to or in the target organs

SUMMARY

SUMMARY

themselves. The sympathetic ganglia are typically located close to the central nervous system, primarily in two chains of ganglia (the paravertebral ganglia) that parallel the spinal column on each side of the spinal cord.

The nerve terminals of the parasympathetic postganglionic neurons release the neurotransmitter ACh, whereas sympathetic postganglionic neurons release norepinephrine. In organs that receive both sympathetic and parasympathetic innervation, ACh and norepinephrine usually have opposite actions on the target cells. In the heart, for example, ACh decreases the heart rate and reduces the cardiac output, while norepinephrine increases the heart rate and the cardiac output.

In addition, the heart contains specific structures that coordinate the heart beat, including the SA node, AV node, and Purkinje fibers. The SA node is the master pacemaker of the heart, controlling the heart rate. The AV node provides the electrical connection between the atria and the ventricles and is responsible for the delay between atrial and ventricular contractions. The Purkinje fibers provide a rapidly conducting pathway for distributing excitation throughout the ventricles during the power stroke of the heartbeat.

The heart is controlled by the sympathetic and parasympathetic divisions of the autonomic nervous system. ACh released by the parasympathetic nerve terminals in the heart slows the heart rate by opening potassium channels. Norepinephrine released by the sympathetic nerve terminals increases the response of voltage-dependent calcium channels to depolarization, which then increases the rate of beating and the strength of contraction. Both neurotransmitters activate G-protein–coupled receptor molecules: muscarinic receptors in the case of ACh and β-adrenergic receptors in the case of norepinephrine. β-Adrenergic receptors increase cyclic AMP inside the cardiac cells, which promotes phosphorylation of calcium channels by protein kinase A.

REVIEW QUESTIONS

1. Describe the components of the labyrinth and their sensory roles.

2. What is the effect of deflection of hair cell cilia toward and away from the longest cilium, and how do these deflections affect action potential activity in neurons that receive synapses from the hair cells?

3. What is the difference between the vestibular ganglion and the vestibular nuclei?

4. List the muscles that control movements of the eyeball and describe their effects.

5. What cranial nerves include axons of the motor neurons for the extraocular muscles? Where are the cell bodies of the corresponding motor neurons located?

6. Draw the synaptic connections for the VOR activated by horizontal rotation of the head. Include excitatory and inhibitory connections on one side of the brain, and name the nuclei involved in the reflex.

7. Identify the following and describe their roles in saccade generation: excitatory burst neurons, inhibitory burst neurons, omnidirectional pause neurons.

8. What are the roles of the basal ganglia and substantia nigra in saccade generation?

9. Describe the organization of the superior colliculus with respect to the topographical maps in the dorsal and ventral layers.

10. Describe the roles of the frontal eye fields and lateral intraparietal area in saccades.

INTERNET ASSIGNMENT   **CHAPTER 10**

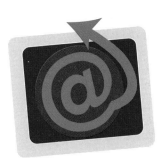

The oculomotor neurons that control the extraocular muscles are found in three cranial nerve nuclei in the brainstem: the oculomotor, trochlear, and abducens nuclei. Use your knowledge of neuroanatomy resources on the Internet to find the locations of these nuclei in cross sections of the human brainstem.

THE AUTONOMIC NERVOUS SYSTEM

The motor functions we have described so far in this part of the book have been concerned with the control of skeletal muscles. These muscles produce overt movements of the body and give rise to the observable external actions that we normally think of as the "behavior" of an animal. However, even in an animal that appears to an external observer to be quiescent, the nervous system is quite busy coordinating many ongoing motor actions that are as impor- 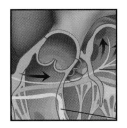 tant for survival as skeletal-muscle movements. These motor activities include such things as regulating digestion, maintaining the proper glucose balance in the blood, regulating heart rate, and so on. The part of the nervous system that controls these functions is called the **autonomic nervous system**. The motor targets of the autonomic nervous system include gland cells, cardiac-muscle cells, and smooth-muscle cells such as those found in the gut. To distinguish it from the autonomic nervous system, the parts of the nervous system we have been discussing up to this point—whose motor targets are the skeletal muscles—are collectively called the **somatic nervous system**.

In addition to the differences in their target cells, there are other differences between the autonomic and somatic nervous systems. As we have seen, in the somatic nervous system, the cell bodies of the motor neurons are located within the central nervous system, either in the spinal cord or in the nuclei of cranial nerves in the brainstem. By contrast, the cell bodies of the motor neurons in the autonomic nervous system are located outside the central nervous system altogether, in a system of **autonomic ganglia** distributed throughout the body. The central nervous system controls these autonomic ganglia by way of output neurons called **preganglionic neurons**, which are located in the spinal cord and brainstem. This arrangement is illustrated in Figure 11.1. The motor neurons in the autonomic ganglia are also called **postganglionic neurons**. The axons of the preganglionic neurons entering the ganglia are referred to as the **preganglionic fibers**, while the axons of the autonomic motor neurons carrying the output to the target cells are called the **postganglionic fibers**. Thus, in the somatic nervous system, the motor commands exiting from the central nervous system go directly to the target cells, while in the autonomic nervous system, the motor commands from the central nervous system are relayed via an additional synaptic connection in the peripheral nervous system.

The autonomic and somatic nervous systems also differ in the effects that the motor neurons have on the target cells. In Chapter 7, we discussed in detail the synaptic interaction between motor neurons and skeletal-muscle cells at the neuromuscular junction. All of the somatic motor neurons release acetylcholine (ACh) as their neurotransmitter, and the effect on the skeletal-muscle cells is al-

Where are the motor neurons of the autonomic nervous system located?

What neurotransmitters are used by the motor neurons of the sympathetic and parasympathetic divisions of the autonomic nervous system?

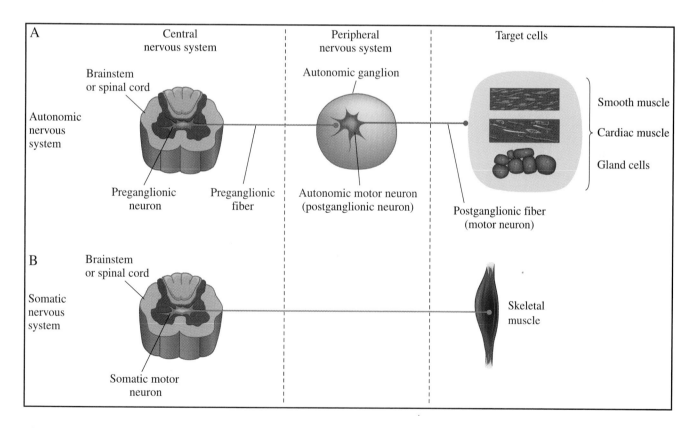

Figure 11.1.

Differences between the autonomic and somatic nervous systems. **A.** In the autonomic nervous system, the motor neurons are located outside the central nervous system, in autonomic ganglia. The motor neurons contact smooth-muscle cells, cardiac-muscle cells, and gland cells. The central nervous system controls the ganglia via preganglionic neurons. **B.** In the somatic nervous system, the motor neurons are located within the central nervous system and contact skeletal-muscle cells.

ways excitatory: contraction is stimulated. In the autonomic nervous system, however, some motor neurons release ACh and other motor neurons release the neurotransmitter norepinephrine (see Chapter 8), instead of ACh. Further, an autonomic motor neuron may either excite or inhibit its target cell. In general, if norepinephrine excites the target cells, then ACh inhibits them, and vice versa. For example, norepinephrine increases the heart rate, whereas ACh decreases the heart rate, as we will examine in detail shortly.

The norepinephrine-releasing and ACh-releasing motor neurons are organized into anatomically distinct divisions of the autonomic nervous system, called the **sympathetic division** (norepinephrine-releasing) and the **parasympathetic division** (ACh-releasing). The ganglia containing the sympathetic motor neurons are called **sympathetic ganglia**, and those containing parasympathetic motor neurons are called **parasympathetic ganglia**. Most of the sympathetic ganglia are arrayed parallel to the spinal cord, one ganglion on each side just outside the vertebral column. There is one pair of **paravertebral ganglia** for each vertebral segment. The ganglia are interconnected by thick, longitudinal bundles of axons containing the preganglionic fibers exiting from the spinal cord. Because of these connectives, the paravertebral ganglia form two long chains parallel to the spinal column, sometimes referred to as the **sympathetic chains**. In addition to the paravertebral ganglia that make up the chains, there are also sympathetic ganglia called the **prevertebral ganglia**, located within the abdomen.

The parasympathetic ganglia are distributed more diffusely throughout the body and tend to be located closer to their target organs. In some cases, the parasympathetic ganglia are actually located within the target organ itself. This is the case, for example, in the heart. Because the sympathetic ganglia are located predominantly near the central nervous system while the parasympathetic ganglia are located mostly near to their target organs, the preganglionic fibers of the sympathetic nervous system are usually much shorter than the preganglionic fibers of the parasympathetic nervous system, which must extend all the way from the central nervous system to the vicinity of the target organ in order to reach the postganglionic neurons. Conversely, the postganglionic fibers are typically much longer in the sympathetic nervous system than in the parasympathetic nervous system.

Most target organs receive inputs from both the sympathetic and the parasympathetic division of the autonomic nervous system. As noted earlier, the sympathetic and parasympathetic inputs produce opposing effects on the target. In general, excitation of the sympathetic nervous system has the overall effect of placing the organism in "emergency mode," ready for vigorous activity. The parasympathetic nervous system has the opposite effect of placing the organism in a "vegetative mode." For example, sympathetic activity increases the heart rate and blood pressure, diverts blood flow from the skin and viscera to the skeletal muscles, and reduces intestinal motility, all of which are appropriate for rapid reaction to an external threat. Parasympathetic activity, on the other hand, decreases heart rate and blood pressure and promotes blood circulation to the gut and intestinal motility. These actions are appropriate for resting and digesting, in the absence of any threatening situation in the environment.

AUTONOMIC CONTROL OF THE HEART

As an example of the actions of the autonomic nervous system, we will examine the neural control of the heart. The heart consists of muscle cells that differ in some important ways from skeletal-muscle cells (see Chapter 7). First, we will discuss the electrical and mechanical properties of the heart muscle, before returning to the modulation of these properties by sympathetic and parasympathetic inputs.

The Pattern of Cardiac Contraction

The contractile apparatus of cardiac-muscle cells is similar to that of other striated-muscle cells, consisting of bundles of myofilaments as described in Chapter 7. Unlike other striated muscles, however, the heart muscle is specialized to produce a rhythmic and coordinated contraction that drives the blood efficiently through the blood vessels, providing oxygen to the cells of the body. To accomplish this task, the heart must receive oxygen-poor blood returning from the body tissues via the venous circulation and send that blood to the lungs for oxygenation. It also must receive the oxygenated blood from the lungs and send it out through the arterial circulation to the rest of the body. These steps require precise timing of the contractions of the chambers of the heart. Otherwise, the flow of oxygenated blood will not occur efficiently or will cease altogether.

Figure 11.2 illustrates the flow of blood through a human heart during a single contraction cycle. The human heart consists of four chambers: the left and right **atria** (singular: atrium) and the left and right **ventricles**. The two atria can be thought of as the receiving chambers, or "priming" pumps, of the heart. The two ventricles are the "power" pumps of the circulatory system. The right atrium receives the blood returning from the body through the veins, and the left atrium receives the freshly oxygenated blood from the lungs.

During the phase of the heartbeat when the atria are filling with blood, the valves connecting the atria with the ventricles remain closed, preventing the flow of blood into the ventricles. When the atria become filled with blood, they contract. The valves leading to the ventricles open, allowing the blood to be driven from the atria into the ventricles. At this point, the muscle of the ventricles is relaxed, and the valves connecting the ventricles to the vessels leaving the heart are closed. When the ventricles have filled with blood, they contract, opening these valves and delivering the power stroke to drive the blood out to the lungs and to the rest of the body (see Fig. 11.2B). Thus, during a normal heartbeat, the two atria contract together, followed by the simultaneous contraction of the two ventricles.

Coordination of Contraction Across Cardiac-Muscle Fibers

To expel fluid, all of the individual muscle fibers making up the walls of a heart chamber must contract in synchrony. This unified contraction constricts the cavity of the chamber and propels the blood into the circulatory system. In skeletal muscles, an action potential in one muscle fiber remains confined to that fiber and does not influence neighboring fibers; therefore, contraction is restricted to the particular fiber undergoing an action potential. In cardiac muscle, however, the situation is quite different. An action potential in a cardiac-muscle fiber triggers action potentials in neighboring fibers, which in turn set up action potentials in their neighbors. Thus, excitation spreads rapidly through the muscle fibers of the chamber, ensuring that all of the fibers contract together.

Figure 11.3 illustrates the mechanism by which the action potential spreads from one fiber to another. At the ends of each cardiac cell, the plasma membranes of neighboring cells come into close contact at specialized structures called **intercalated disks**. The contact at this point allows electrical current flowing in one fiber to cross directly into the neighboring cell; in electrical terms, the neighboring muscle cells can be considered to form one larger cell.

Electrical current does not normally flow from one cell into its neighbors because the plasma membranes of the cells form an insulating barrier. At the intercalated disk, however, the resistance to current flow across the two cell membranes is low. Thus, depolarization during an action potential in one cell can spread directly into the neighboring cell, setting up an action potential in the neighbor. The low-resis-

What role does electrical coupling play in coordinated contraction of the heart?

Figure 11.2.

Schematic drawings of the state of the heart valves and the direction of blood flow during two stages in a single heartbeat. **A**. The atria contract, expelling blood into the relaxed ventricles. **B**. The valves between the atria and ventricles close and the ventricles contract, forcing blood out to the lungs (right ventricle) and to the arteries supplying the rest of the body (left ventricle).

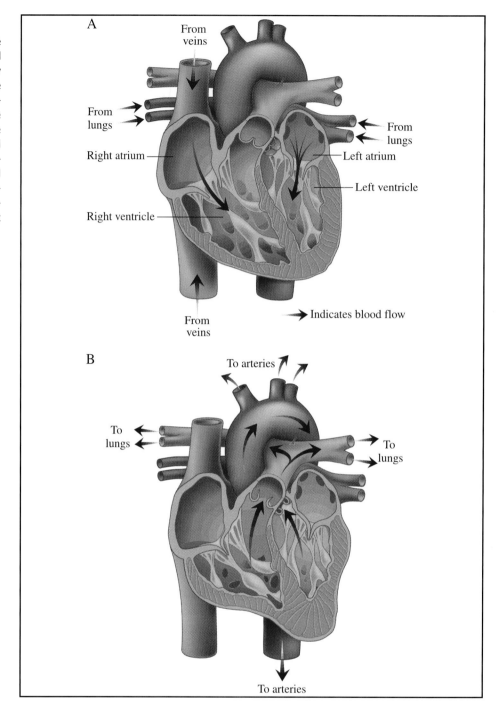

tance path from one cell to another is provided by **gap junctions**, which consist of arrays of small pores directly connecting the interiors of the joined cells. The pores are formed by pairs of protein molecules, one in each cell, that attach to each other and bridge the small extracellular gap between the two cell membranes (see Fig. 11.3). The pores at the center of each of these **gap junction channels** are aligned, permitting small molecules like ions to pass directly from one cell to the other.

When electrical current can pass from one cell to another (as in cardiac-muscle cells), the cells are said to be **electrically coupled**. Figure 11.4 illustrates the behavior of electrically coupled cells connected by gap junctions. When current is injected into a cell, no response occurs in a neighboring cell if the cells are not electrically coupled (see Fig. 11.4B). If the two cells are coupled via gap junctions, however, the membrane potential of both cells changes when current is injected

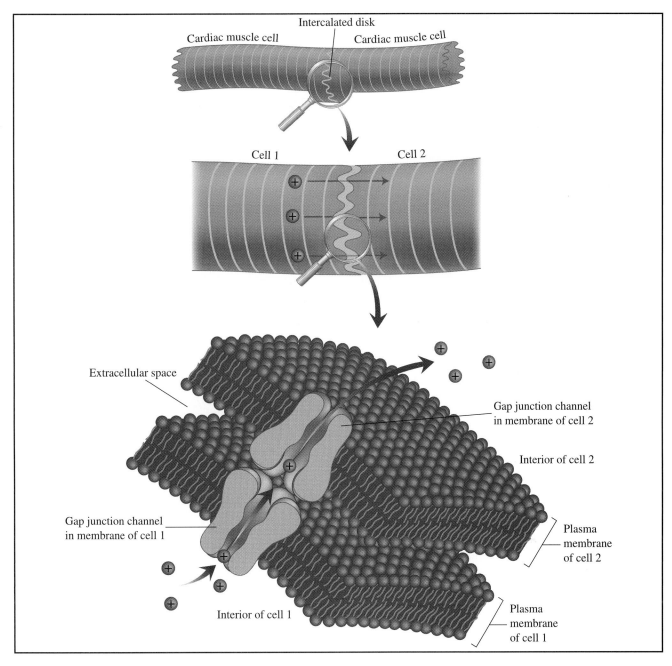

The following labels appear in the figure:

Intercalated disk

Cardiac muscle cell   Cardiac muscle cell

Cell 1   Cell 2

Extracellular space

Gap junction channel
in membrane of cell 2

Interior of cell 2

Gap junction channel
in membrane of cell 1

Plasma
membrane
of cell 2

Interior of cell 1

Plasma
membrane
of cell 1

Figure 11.3.

Electrical current can flow from one cardiac-muscle cell to another through specialized membrane junctions located in a region of contact called the intercalated disk. The current flows through pores formed by pairs of gap junction channels that bridge the extracellular space at the intercalated disk.

into one member of the pair (see Fig. 11.4C). Ions carrying electrical current can pass freely through the gap junction channels from one cell to the other. If the depolarization is large enough to trigger an action potential in one cell, an action potential will also occur in the coupled partner.

Generation of Rhythmic Contractions

Electrical coupling among cardiac-muscle cells explains how contractions can occur synchronously in all cells of a heart chamber. We will now consider the mechanisms responsible for the repetitive contractions that produce the beating of the heart.

If the heart is removed from the body and placed in an appropriate artificial environment, it will continue to contract repetitively even though it is isolated from the nervous system. In contrast, a skeletal muscle isolated under similar conditions will

Figure 11.4.

Electrical coupling allows depolarization to spread directly from one cell to another. **A.** The membrane potentials (E_m) of two neighboring cells are measured simultaneously with intracellular microelectrodes. Depolarizing current is injected into cell 1. **B.** If the cells are not electrically coupled, the depolarization occurs only in the cell in which the current was injected (cell 1). The membrane potential of cell 2 does not change. **C.** If the cells are electrically coupled via gap junctions, depolarization occurs in both cells when current is injected into only one of the cells. An action potential occurring in either cell would spread to both.

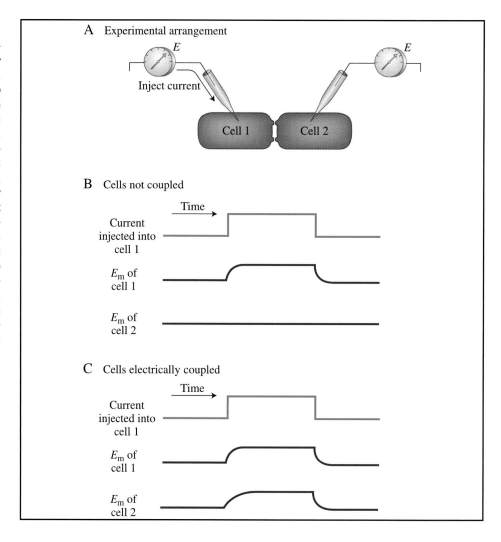

A   Experimental arrangement

Inject current

Cell 1   Cell 2

B   Cells not coupled

Time

Current injected into cell 1

E_m of cell 1

E_m of cell 2

C   Cells electrically coupled

Time

Current injected into cell 1

E_m of cell 1

E_m of cell 2

not contract unless its nerve is activated. The rhythmic activity of the heart muscle is an inherent property of the individual muscle fibers making up the heart—another important difference between cardiac- and skeletal-muscle fibers. If muscle tissue is dissociated into individual cells, muscle cells from skeletal muscles remain quiescent and do not contract spontaneously. Cells from cardiac muscle, however, continue to contract rhythmically even in isolation. Thus, rhythmic contractions of the heart muscle are generated by built-in properties of the cardiac-muscle cells.

The Cardiac Action Potential

How does the cardiac action potential differ from the action potential of neurons and skeletal-muscle cells?

The action potential of skeletal-muscle cells is similar to neuron action potentials (see Chapter 4). The cardiac action potential, however, differs in several important ways. Figure 11.5 compares the characteristics of action potentials of skeletal- and cardiac-muscle cells.

One striking difference is that cardiac action potentials can last several hundred milliseconds, while skeletal-muscle action potentials are typically only 1 to 2 msec in duration. A long-lasting action potential like the cardiac action potential can arise when voltage-dependent calcium channels contribute to the action potential (see Chapter 4). In cardiac-muscle cells, calcium channels open upon depolarization and allow an influx of positively charged calcium ions, which produces a long-lasting plateau of depolarization. In addition, reduced potassium permeability contributes to the plateau of the cardiac action potential. Cardiac-muscle cells possess a type of potassium channel that remains open when the membrane potential

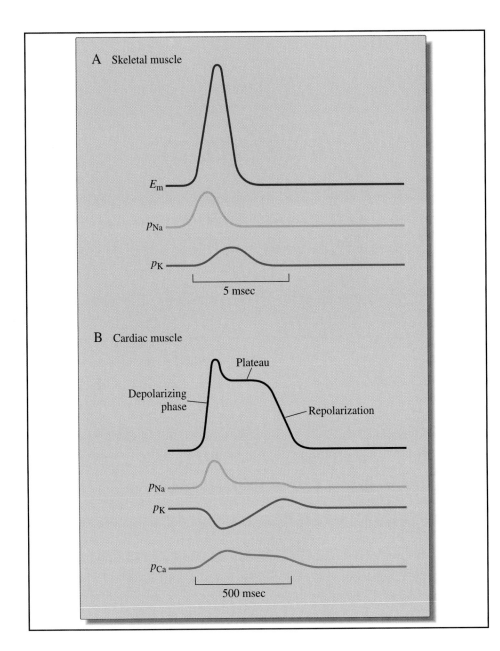

A Skeletal muscle

E_m

p_{Na}

p_K

5 msec

B Cardiac muscle

Plateau

Depolarizing phase

Repolarization

p_{Na}

p_K

p_{Ca}

500 msec

Figure 11.5.

The sequence of permeability changes underlying the action potentials of skeletal-muscle fibers (**A**) and cardiac-muscle fibers (**B**). Note the different time scales of the two action potentials. E_m = membrane potential; p_{Na} = sodium permeability; p_K = potassium permeability; p_{Ca} = calcium permeability.

is near its normal resting level and closes upon depolarization. The reduction in potassium permeability caused by the closing of this channel tends to depolarize the cardiac-muscle fiber. Both the opening of the calcium channels and the closing of the potassium channels contribute to the prolonged action potential in cardiac-muscle cells (see Fig. 11.5B).

The initial rising phase of the cardiac action potential is produced by voltage-dependent sodium channels very much like those found in neurons. These sodium channels rapidly depolarize the cardiac-muscle cell and are responsible for the brief initial spike before the plateau phase of the cardiac action potential. Like the sodium channel of neurons, cardiac sodium channels inactivate during maintained depolarization, but inactivation is not total. A small, maintained increase in sodium permeability persists during the plateau of the cardiac action potential (see Fig. 11.5B).

Two factors contribute to the termination of the prolonged plateau phase of the cardiac action potential. First, the calcium permeability of the plasma membrane slowly declines during the maintained depolarization. This decline is a consequence of accumulation of internal calcium as calcium ions enter the muscle fiber through the open calcium channels. Internal calcium ions interact directly or indi-

Figure 11.6.

The duration of the action potential controls the duration of contraction in a cardiac-muscle cell, but not in a skeletal-muscle cell. **A.** In a skeletal-muscle fiber, the action potential is much briefer than the resulting contraction. Thus, the action potential acts only as a trigger for the contraction, which proceeds independently of the duration of the action potential. **B.** In a cardiac-muscle fiber, the duration of the contraction is closely related to the duration of the action potential, because calcium influx during the plateau of the action potential sustains the contraction. Thus, characteristics of the action potential can influence the duration and strength of the cardiac contraction. E_m = membrane potential.

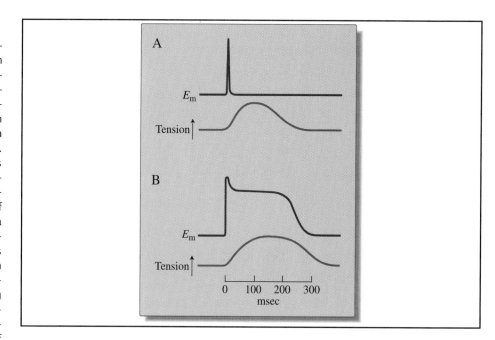

What ionic mechanisms underlie the generation of spontaneous contractions by the heart?

rectly with the calcium channels, causing them to close. Second, the potassium permeability of the plasma membrane increases, which drives the membrane potential toward the potassium equilibrium potential and results in repolarization of the muscle cell. The increase in potassium permeability is partly due to voltage-sensitive potassium channels that open during the plateau phase of the action potential. Calcium-activated potassium channels (see Chapter 4) also contribute to the delayed rise in potassium permeability.

One functional implication of the prolonged cardiac action potential is that the duration of the action potential controls the duration of the contraction in cardiac-muscle cells. Figure 11.6 compares the action potential and contraction of cardiac-muscle fibers with those of skeletal-muscle fibers. In skeletal muscle, the action potential only triggers the contractile events; the duration of the contraction is controlled by the timing of the calcium release and calcium reuptake by the sarcoplasmic reticulum, not by the duration of the action potential. In cardiac-muscle fibers, however, only the initial part of the contraction is controlled by calcium from the sarcoplasmic reticulum; the contraction is maintained by the influx of calcium ions across the plasma membrane during the plateau phase of the cardiac action potential. For this reason, the duration of the contraction in the heart can be altered by changing the duration of the action potential in the cardiac-muscle fibers. Thus, changing the action potential duration is an important mechanism for modulating the pumping action of the heart.

The Pacemaker Potential

Although the cardiac action potential differs in important ways from other action potentials, these differences do not account for the endogenous beating of isolated heart cells discussed earlier. Spontaneous contractions of heart cells are produced by spontaneous action potentials, as illustrated in Figure 11.7. After each action potential, the membrane potential reaches its normal negative resting value, then begins to depolarize slowly. This slow depolarization, called a **pacemaker potential**, is caused by spontaneous changes in the membrane ionic permeability.

Voltage-clamp experiments on single isolated cardiac-muscle fibers show that the pacemaker potential arises from the combination of a slow decline in potassium permeability and a slow increase in sodium and calcium permeability. When the depolarization reaches threshold, it triggers an action potential in the fiber. Both

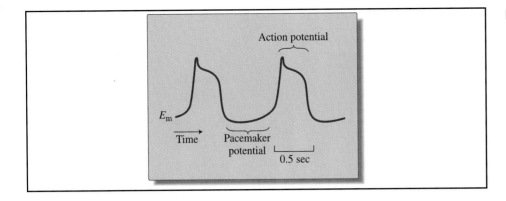

Figure 11.7.

Changes of membrane potential (E_m) during repetitive, spontaneous beating in a single cardiac-muscle fiber. The repolarization at the end of one action potential is followed by a slow, spontaneous depolarization called the pacemaker potential. When this depolarization reaches threshold, it triggers a new action potential.

voltage-dependent sodium channels and voltage-dependent calcium channels contribute to the action potential.

Part of the early phase of the pacemaker potential represents the normal undershoot period of an action potential, when potassium channels that were opened by depolarization during the action potential slowly close again. As these potassium channels close, the membrane potential will move in a positive direction, away from the potassium equilibrium potential. Later phases of the pacemaker potential represent increases in sodium and calcium permeability, both of which move the membrane potential in a positive direction, toward the sodium and calcium equilibrium potentials. The increase in sodium permeability during the pacemaker potential arises from nonspecific cation channels that open at more hyperpolarized membrane potentials. As with the ACh-activated channels at the neuromuscular junction (see Chapter 5), channels that are equally permeable to sodium and potassium ions depolarize the muscle cell. These hyperpolarization-activated cation channels open in response to the membrane hyperpolarization during the undershoot of the action potential. The resulting influx of sodium ions moves the membrane potential of the cardiac-muscle cell in a positive direction, toward the threshold for firing an action potential. As the membrane potential becomes more positive during the pacemaker potential, voltage-dependent calcium channels open in response to the depolarization. The resulting influx of positively charged calcium ions produces even greater depolarization, ultimately triggering the next action potential in the series.

The rate of spontaneous action potentials in isolated heart cells varies from one cell to another; some cells beat rapidly, while others beat slowly. In the intact heart, however, the electrical coupling among the muscle cells guarantees that they all contract together, with the overall rate being governed by the fibers with the fastest pacemaker activity. Normally, a special set of pacemaker cells, called the **sinoatrial (SA) node**, determine the overall heart rate. Figure 11.8 illustrates the location of the SA node in the upper part of the right atrium.

In the resting human heart, the cells of the SA node generate spontaneous action potentials at a rate of approximately 70 per minute. These action potentials spread through the electrical connections among fibers throughout the two atria, generating simultaneous contraction of the atria. The spread of excitation from the right atrium to the left atrium is facilitated by a bundle of muscle fibers, called **Bachmann's bundle**, that are specialized for more rapid conduction of action potentials. This helps ensure that the two atria contract together.

The atrial action potentials do not spread directly to the muscle fibers of the ventricles, however. The contraction of the ventricles is delayed, allowing the relaxed ventricles to fill with blood pumped into them by the atrial contraction. In terms of electrical conduction, the heart behaves as two isolated units, as shown in Figure 11.8. The two atria contract together as one unit, and the two ventricles form a second unit. Another specialized group of muscle fibers, called the

Figure 11.8.

The spread of action potentials across the heart during a single heartbeat. The excitation originates in the sinoatrial (SA) node of the right atrium and spreads throughout the atria via electrical coupling among the atrial-muscle fibers. The spread is facilitated by special conducting fibers in Bachmann's bundle. The fibers of the atria are not electrically connected to those of the ventricles. The action potential spreads to the ventricles via the atrioventricular (AV) node, which introduces a delay between the atrial and ventricular action potentials. When the wave of action potentials leaves the AV node, its spread throughout the ventricles is aided by the rapidly conducting Purkinje fibers of the bundle of His.

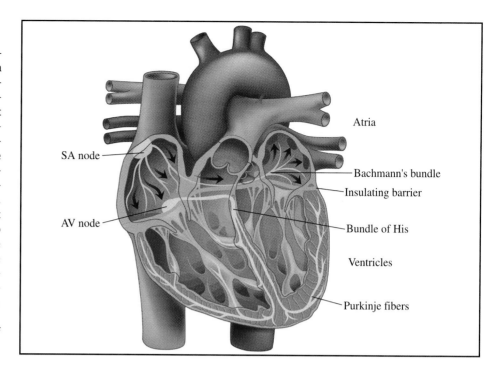

How do the neurotransmitters of the autonomic nervous system affect the target organs?

atrioventricular (**AV**) **node**, provides the electrical connection between the atria and ventricles. Excitation in the atria must travel through the AV node to reach the ventricles. The fibers of the AV node are small in diameter compared with other cardiac-muscle fibers, and action potential conduction is slower in small-diameter fibers. Therefore, conduction through the AV node introduces a time delay sufficient to retard the contraction of the ventricles relative to the contraction of the atria. Excitation leaving the AV node does not travel directly through the muscle fibers of the ventricles but moves along specialized muscle fibers that are designed for rapid conduction of action potentials. These **Purkinje fibers** form a fast-conducting pathway through the ventricles called the **bundle of His**. The Purkinje fibers carry the excitation rapidly to the base of the heart, where it spreads out through the ventricular muscle fibers to produce the contraction of the ventricles.

Actions of Acetylcholine and Norepinephrine on Cardiac-Muscle Cells

Each skeletal-muscle fiber receives direct synaptic input from a particular motor neuron; without this synaptic input, a skeletal fiber does not contract unless stimulated directly by artificial means. On the other hand, cardiac-muscle fibers generate spontaneous contractions that are coordinated into a functional heartbeat by the electrical conduction mechanisms inherent in the heart itself. Although the basic heartbeat is generated by the heart itself without neural influence, the rate and strength of the spontaneous contractions are regulated by the nervous system. The heart receives two opposing neural inputs from neurons of the parasympathetic and sympathetic divisions of the autonomic nervous system.

Parasympathetic motor neurons in the heart release the neurotransmitter ACh, which slows the rate of depolarization during the pacemaker potential of the SA node. Thus, activation of the parasympathetic input increases the interval between successive action potentials and slows the rate at which the master pacemaker in the SA node drives the heartbeat. ACh increases potassium permeability in cardiac-muscle cells, which allows increased potassium efflux and retards the growth of the pacemaker potential toward the threshold for triggering an action potential.

Sympathetic motor neurons release the neurotransmitter norepinephrine in the heart. Norepinephrine speeds the heart rate and increases the strength of contraction, by increasing the number of calcium channels that open during depolarization. Thus, the parasympathetic and sympathetic divisions of the autonomic nervous system have opposite effects on the heart.

Both ACh and norepinephrine indirectly affect ion channels in cardiac-muscle cells. Neurotransmitters can affect ion channels either directly, by binding to ligand-gated ion channels, or indirectly via intracellular second messengers (see Chapter 6). In the heart, ACh activates a type of ACh receptor molecule called the **muscarinic acetylcholine receptor** (because it is activated by the drug muscarine and related compounds, as well as by ACh). By contrast, the ligand-gated ACh receptor molecule at the neuromuscular junction is called the **nicotinic acetylcholine receptor** (because it is activated by the drug nicotine and related compounds).

Muscarinic receptors are not ion channels. Instead, the activated receptor stimulates guanosine triphosphate (GTP)–binding proteins (G-proteins; see Chapter 6) that are attached to the inner surface of the membrane near the receptors. The sequence of events linking muscarinic receptor molecules to potassium channels is summarized in Figure 11.9. When ACh binds to the muscarinic receptor, the receptor activates G-proteins by stimulating the replacement of guanosine diphosphate (GDP) by GTP at the GTP-binding site on the alpha-subunit of the G-protein. With GTP bound, the alpha-subunit then dissociates from the beta- and gamma-subunits. Because the G-protein consists of three distinct protein subunits, this type of G-protein is referred to as a **heterotrimeric G-protein**.

The free beta- and gamma-subunits of the activated G-proteins are thought to interact directly with potassium channels, causing the channels to open. The increase in potassium permeability then slows the rate of cardiac action potentials. The activated alpha-subunit, with GTP bound, may also increase potassium permeability by stimulating intracellular production of arachidonic acid, a second messenger produced by enzymatic cleavage of membrane lipids. The action of the G-protein is terminated by intrinsic GTPase activity of the alpha-subunit, which hydrolyzes the terminal phosphate of GTP, converting it to GDP. With GDP bound, the alpha-, beta-, and gamma-subunits recombine into an inactive form of the G-protein

The linkage between norepinephrine receptor molecules and calcium channels is also mediated via G-proteins in cardiac-muscle cells, as summarized in Figure 11.10. The norepinephrine receptor is a type called the **β-adrenergic receptor** (a different class of norepinephrine receptor, called the α-adrenergic receptor, is also present, but is not involved in the effects of norepinephrine on calcium channels described here). β-Adrenergic receptor molecules are members of the same general family of receptors as the muscarinic cholinergic receptors. Like the muscarinic receptor, the β-adrenergic receptor is not itself an ion channel. Instead, the binding of norepinephrine to the receptor activates G-proteins inside the cell. In this case, the activated alpha-subunit, with GTP bound, stimulates the synthetic enzyme for cyclic adenosine monophosphate (AMP), **adenylyl cyclase**, causing cyclic AMP levels to rise inside the cardiac cell. Cyclic AMP activates **protein kinase A** (also called **cyclic AMP–dependent protein kinase**), which in turn **phosphorylates** (that is, attaches a phosphate group to) specific amino acid groups of the calcium channel protein. Phosphorylation of the calcium channel is thought to be required for opening of the channel during depolarization. Thus, by promoting phosphorylation, a rise in cyclic AMP increases the number of calcium channels that open when the cardiac-muscle cell depolarizes. In addition, each channel remains open for a longer time, on average, during depolarization. Thus, phosphorylation of the calcium channels greatly potentiates the influx of calcium into cardiac-muscle cells during depolarization.

In the SA node, the triggering of the action potential depends on calcium channels. Norepinephrine lowers the threshold potential for triggering the action po-

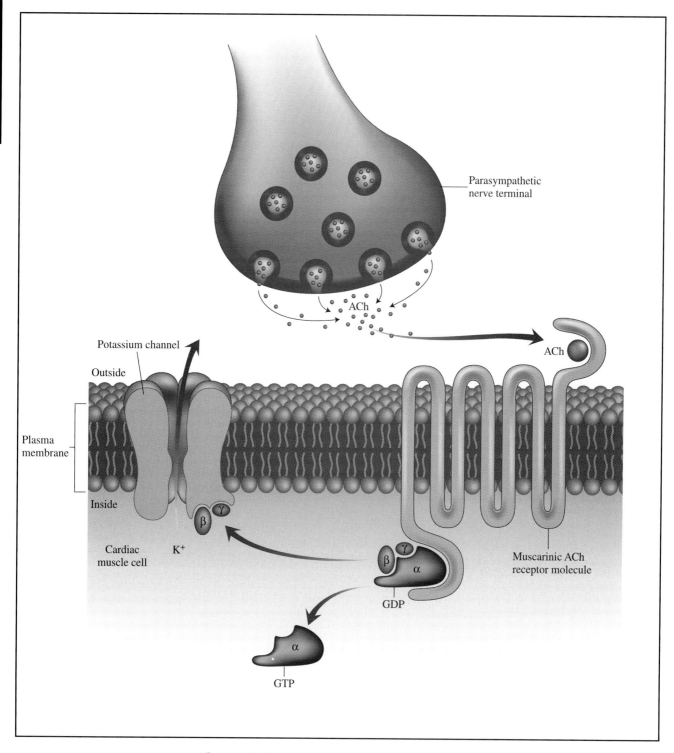

Figure 11.9.

Acetylcholine (ACh) indirectly opens potassium channels in cardiac-muscle cells. The synaptic terminals of parasympathetic neurons release ACh, which binds to muscarinic ACh receptor molecules in the membrane of the postsynaptic muscle cell. The receptor then activates G-proteins, by catalyzing the replacement of guanosine diphosphate (GDP) by guanosine triphosphate (GTP) on the GTP-binding site on the alpha-subunit of the G-protein. The beta- and gamma-subunits dissociate from the alpha-subunit when GTP binds. The potassium channel is thought to open when the beta- and gamma-subunits directly interact with the channel.

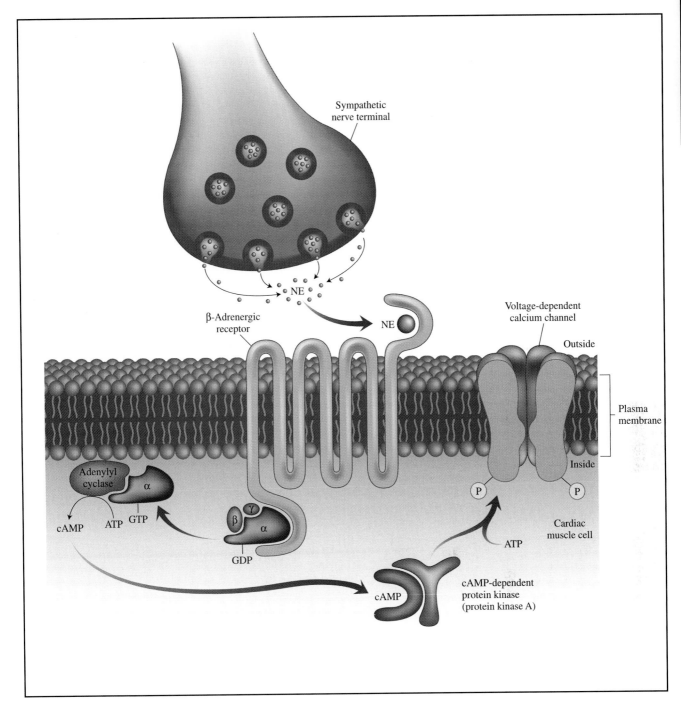

Figure 11.10.

Norepinephrine (NE) promotes the activation of voltage-dependent calcium channels in cardiac-muscle cells. When norepinephrine is released from the synaptic terminals of sympathetic neurons, it combines with β-adrenergic receptors in the postsynaptic membrane of the cardiac-muscle cells. The activated receptor stimulates G-proteins, by catalyzing binding of guanosine triphosphate (GTP) to the alpha-subunit, which then dissociates from the beta- and gamma-subunits. The alpha-subunit of the G-protein activates adenylyl cyclase, an enzyme that converts adenosine triphosphate (ATP) into cyclic adenosine monophosphate (cAMP). Cyclic AMP then stimulates protein kinase A, which phosphorylates calcium channel molecules. Phosphorylated calcium channels open more readily during depolarization and also remain open for a longer time. As a result, calcium influx increases during depolarization of the heart cell. P = phosphate.

tential by increasing the number of calcium channels that open in response to depolarization. Thus, in the presence of norepinephrine the action potential occurs earlier during the pacemaker potential, and the heart rate increases correspondingly. Outside of the SA node, in the muscle cells of the atria and ventricles, calcium channels contribute to the plateau phase of the action potential and allow calcium influx that sustains the muscle contraction. In the atria and ventricles, therefore, norepinephrine increases calcium influx during the action potential, which in turn strengthens the contraction of the overall heart muscle.

The combination of increased heart rate and strength of contraction makes β-adrenergic receptors powerful regulators of the amount of blood volume circulated per minute through the heart. As a result, the β-adrenergic receptors are targeted by many drugs that are used clinically to increase the heart output in human patients whose heart muscle has been damaged by disease.

Because the autonomic neurotransmitters exert their actions through G-protein–linked receptors, rather than by direct binding to ion channels, the parasympathetic and sympathetic motor neurons produce long-lasting effects on the heart without a continuing neural signal. Once the G-proteins are activated, their action continues for up to several seconds, until GTP is hydrolyzed and the G-protein returns to the resting state. By contrast, somatic motor neurons are tightly temporally coupled to the activation of their targets, the skeletal-muscle fibers. The ligand-gated ion channels at the neuromuscular junction allow subsecond control of skeletal-muscle activity by somatic motor neurons. In general, the targets controlled by the autonomic nervous system are involved in slower activities that are typically sustained for longer periods. Therefore, the slower and more sustained activation produced by G-protein–coupled neurotransmitter receptors is well suited for the autonomic nervous system.

Table 11.1 summarizes a number of differences between skeletal-muscle cells and cardiac-muscle cells. These differences help account for the ability of the heart to pump blood through the circulatory system.

ORGANIZATION OF PREGANGLIONIC AUTONOMIC NEURONS

What parts of the central nervous system control the autonomic ganglia?

We now consider the neural systems in the brain and spinal cord that control the peripheral autonomic ganglia. The motor neurons (postganglionic neurons) of the autonomic nervous system are located outside the central nervous system, in the autonomic ganglia. In the case of the heart, the sympathetic postganglionic neurons are located in sympathetic chain ganglia that parallel the spinal column in the cervical and upper thoracic regions. In keeping with the general rule that the parasympathetic postganglionic neurons are located in or near their target organs, the parasympathetic neurons of the heart are found in a diffuse network within the heart muscles. The preganglionic neurons of the sympathetic and parasympathetic divisions are located in the central nervous system, but the two divisions have different anatomical organizations, shown in Figure 11.11. The parasympathetic preganglionic neurons are found in the brain—in cranial nerve nuclei of the midbrain, pons, and medulla—and in the sacral segments of the spinal cord. The sympathetic preganglionic neurons are distributed along the spinal cord throughout the thoracic and upper lumbar regions.

Parasympathetic Preganglionic Neurons

The parasympathetic preganglionic neurons in the brain are found in the nuclei of cranial nerves III (oculomotor nerve), VII (facial nerve), IX (glossopharyngeal

Property	Skeletal muscle	Cardiac muscle
Striated	Yes	Yes
Electrically coupled	No	Yes
Spontaneously contracts in absence of nerve input	No	Yes
Duration of contraction is controlled by duration of action potential	No	Yes
Action potential is similar to that of neurons	Yes	No
Calcium ions make an important contribution to the action potential	No	Yes
Effect of neural input	Excite	Excite or inhibit
Division of nervous system that provides neural control	Somatic	Autonomic (parasympathetic and sympathetic)
Neurotransmitter released onto muscle fibers by neurons	ACh	ACh (parasympathetic) or norepinephrine (sympathetic)
Effect of neurotransmitter on postsynaptic ion channels	Direct	Indirect (via G-proteins)

Table 11.1

Comparison of selected properties of skeletal- and cardiac-muscle fibers

ACh = acetylcholine.

nerve), and X (vagus nerve) (see Fig. 11.11). The nucleus of the vagus nerve in the medulla is the dominant source of parasympathetic preganglionic fibers in the body. The vagus nerve distributes parasympathetic fibers to most of the viscera, including the heart, lungs, and abdominal organs. The nuclei of the glossopharyngeal nerve in the medulla and the facial nerve in the pons contain the parasympathetic preganglionic neurons controlling the parasympathetic ganglia of exocrine secretory glands in the mouth, nose, and eye orbits (for example, the salivary and lacrimal glands). The parasympathetic ganglia that control the ciliary and iris muscles in the eye receive their preganglionic input from the oculomotor nuclei of the midbrain. The sacral region of the spinal cord contains the parasympathetic preganglionic neurons controlling the lower part of the bowel, the bladder, and the genital organs. Like the parasympathetic postganglionic neurons, the parasympathetic preganglionic neurons release the neurotransmitter ACh.

Sympathetic Preganglionic Neurons

The sympathetic preganglionic neurons are located within the gray matter of the spinal cord (see Fig. 11.11). The axons of sympathetic preganglionic neurons exit the spinal cord via the ventral roots, together with the axons of somatic motor neurons. The preganglionic axons then enter the connectives of the sympathetic chain and extend for some distance within the connectives before making synaptic contact with postganglionic neurons within the paravertebral sympathetic ganglia (see Fig. 11.11). Sympathetic preganglionic neurons are located in the **intermediolateral gray matter**, between the ventral and dorsal horns of the spinal gray

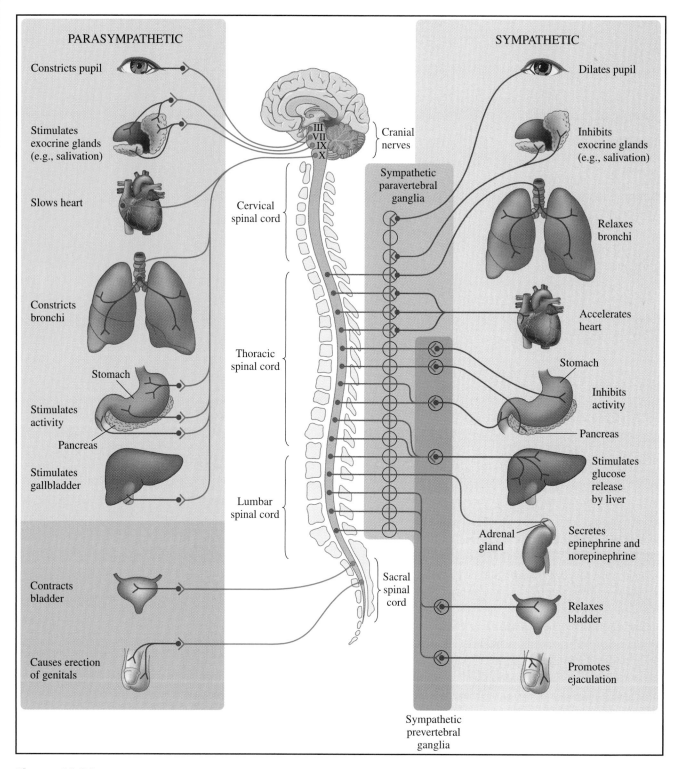

Figure 11.11.

The locations of preganglionic neurons of the parasympathetic division and the sympathetic division of the autonomic nervous system. The cranial nerve nuclei of nerves III (oculomotor), VII (facial), IX (glossopharyngeal), and X (vagus) contain the parasympathetic preganglionic neurons (*red*) in the midbrain, pons, and medulla. These preganglionic neurons send fibers through the corresponding cranial nerves to peripheral parasympathetic ganglia (*blue*) in or near the target tissues. Parasympathetic preganglionic neurons are also found in the sacral part of the spinal cord. The preganglionic neurons of the sympathetic division (*purple*) are located in the gray matter of spinal cord, distributed diffusely along the length of the cord from the thoracic to the lumbar region. The sympathetic preganglionic fibers travel along the chain of paravertebral sympathetic ganglia and extend for several spinal segments above and below the position of the preganglionic neuron. The prevertebral ganglia also receive direct synaptic connections from the preganglionic fibers exiting the spinal cord. The postganglionic neurons (*green*) in the sympathetic ganglia then send axons to the target organs. The exception is the adrenal gland, which receives direct synaptic input from sympathetic preganglionic neurons.

matter, as shown in Figure 11.12. The cell bodies of the sympathetic preganglionic neurons form a diffusely organized column of cells, called the **intermediolateral cell column**, throughout the thoracic and upper lumbar regions of the spinal cord.

Most sympathetic preganglionic axons immediately enter the paravertebral chain after exiting the spinal cord and make synaptic connections in paravertebral ganglia. However, some preganglionic neurons send axons to the prevertebral sympathetic ganglia, which innervate the abdominal organs and the sex organs. Sympathetic preganglionic neurons also make excitatory synaptic connections in the adrenal gland with **chromaffin cells**, which secrete epinephrine and norepinephrine into the bloodstream. The chromaffin cells therefore may be thought of as altered sympathetic postganglionic neurons that have taken on an endocrine function (releasing transmitter into the circulation, thus reaching diffuse and diverse target organs) rather than a typical neuronal function (releasing transmitter directly onto specific target organs). Alternative names for epinephrine and norepinephrine are **adrenaline** and **noradrenaline**, reflecting the fact that these hormones/neurotransmitters are released by the adrenal gland.

Neighboring sympathetic preganglionic neurons within a single segment of the spinal cord control the sympathetic innervation of diverse postsynaptic targets and produce physiological changes in widely distributed target organs. Particular regions of the body are not mapped onto specific parts of the intermediolateral cell

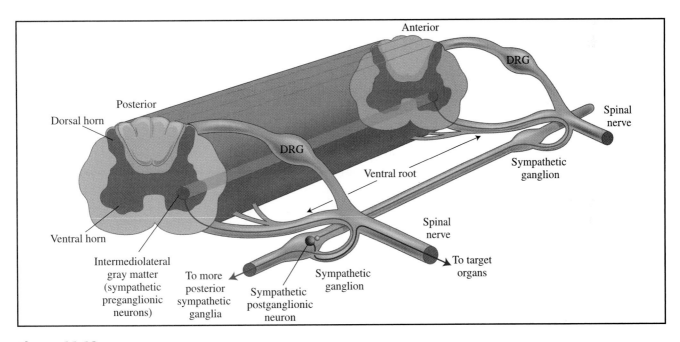

Figure 11.12.

The location of sympathetic preganglionic neurons within the gray matter of the spinal cord. The diagram shows two successive spinal segments. The cell bodies of the sympathetic preganglionic neurons are located at an intermediate level in the gray matter, called the intermediolateral gray matter (shown in *red*). The preganglionic neurons are scattered all along the spinal cord in the intermediolateral gray matter, although the figure shows only two neurons, one at each spinal nerve. The axons of the sympathetic preganglionic neurons (*red*) leave the spinal cord via the ventral roots and enter the paravertebral sympathetic chain. Within the sympathetic chain ganglia, the preganglionic axons make excitatory synaptic contact with the sympathetic postganglionic neurons. The postganglionic axons exit the ganglia and enter the spinal nerves to travel to their target organs in the periphery. Although the preganglionic neurons and sympathetic chain are shown on only one side of the spinal cord, the same circuitry is duplicated on the other side. The axons of some sympathetic preganglionic neurons continue through the spinal nerve to the prevertebral sympathetic ganglia (see Fig. 11.11), which are not shown in this diagram. DRG = dorsal root ganglion.

column. This scheme differs from the organization of somatic motor neurons. The motor neurons that innervate a particular skeletal muscle are located near one another within a single spinal cord segment, whereas the sympathetic preganglionic neurons whose corresponding postganglionic neurons innervate a particular organ are scattered along several spinal segments. The diffuse organization of the sympathetic preganglionic neurons is consistent with the diffuse actions of the sympathetic nervous system on many different organ systems during "flight-or-fight" responses.

Like the parasympathetic preganglionic neurons, the sympathetic preganglionic neurons release the neurotransmitter ACh. Both nicotinic and muscarinic ACh receptor molecules are found in the postganglionic neurons. The nicotinic receptors produce a fast excitatory postsynaptic potential via an increase in sodium and potassium permeability. The muscarinic receptors produce a slower excitatory postsynaptic potential via internal second messengers, by closing a particular type of potassium channel. The resulting reduction in potassium permeability increases the repetitive firing of action potentials during synaptic excitation, producing a stronger sympathetic response in the target organs. In addition to ACh, the synaptic terminals of sympathetic preganglionic neurons contain a variety of neuropeptides that are thought to act as neurotransmitters, producing slow synaptic responses in the postsynaptic neurons via intracellular second messengers.

BRAINSTEM CONTROL OF THE AUTONOMIC NERVOUS SYSTEM

What synaptic circuitry underlies the cardiac baroreceptor reflex?

In the somatic nervous system, fast intraspinal reflex loops connect sensory information from the muscles to the skeletal motor neurons. In the stretch reflex, for instance, this connection is as direct as possible, with the sensory neuron making a monosynaptic connection onto the motor neuron from the same muscle. In the autonomic nervous system, however, reflex loops are commonly much longer, with many synapses intervening between sensory neurons and autonomic preganglionic neurons. For example, the sympathetic preganglionic neurons in the spinal cord receive sensory information predominantly from descending axons of neurons located in the brainstem, which themselves are only indirectly connected to sensory neurons.

An example of the organization of the autonomic reflexes is the **cardiac baroreceptor reflex**, which is summarized in Figure 11.13. Increased blood pressure is sensed by stretch receptor neurons (baroreceptors) that innervate the walls of the carotid artery in a specialized region called the **carotid sinus**. Additional baroreceptors innervate the walls of the aorta, the main artery leaving the heart. When blood pressure rises, the walls of the blood vessels expand, increasing action potential firing in the stretch receptor neurons. Increased activity in the baroreceptors reflexively decreases the sympathetic input to the heart and increases the cardiac parasympathetic input. These changes in autonomic activity decrease the heart rate and cardiac output, lowering blood pressure. Conversely, if blood pressure drops below normal, the arterial walls will be less stretched, and activity in the baroreceptors declines. Inhibition of cardiac sympathetic preganglionic neurons in the spinal cord is reduced, as is the excitation supplied to the parasympathetic preganglionic neurons in the nucleus of the vagus nerve. Thus, activity increases in the sympathetic input to the heart and decreases in the parasympathetic input, raising both the heart rate and cardiac output. In this manner, the reflex maintains the arterial blood pressure at a particular set point, adjusting the heart rate and cardiac output as required to prevent changes in the blood pressure.

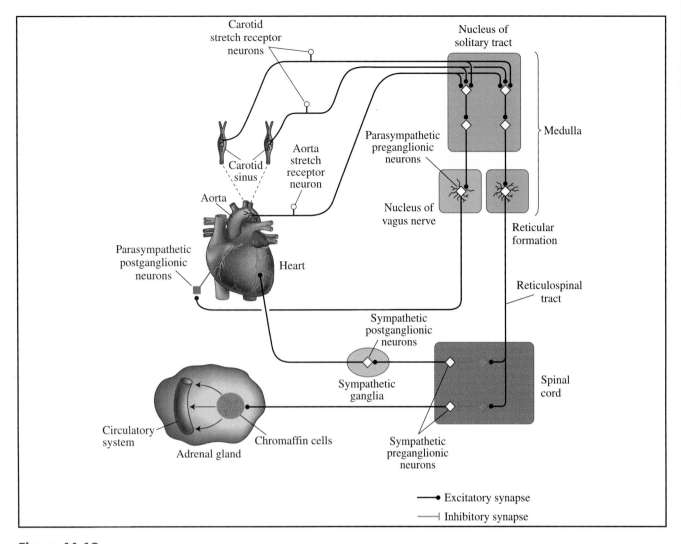

Figure 11.13.

The cardiac baroreceptor reflex. Stretch receptor neurons innervate the arterial walls of the aorta and specialized regions of the carotid arteries, the carotid sinuses. The blood pressure stretches the artery wall and activates the stretch receptor neurons, which make excitatory connections onto neurons within the nucleus of the solitary tract in the medulla. The solitary tract neurons in turn project via additional interneurons to the parasympathetic preganglionic neurons of the heart, located in the nucleus of the vagus nerve, and to reticulospinal neurons that send axons to the spinal cord. Increased activity of the stretch receptors excites the parasympathetic preganglionic neurons, which in turn excite the parasympathetic neurons of the heart and increase the release of acetylcholine. The reticulospinal neurons excite interneurons in the spinal cord, which then inhibit sympathetic preganglionic neurons involved in control of the heart.

The axons of the arterial stretch receptor neurons enter the brain in the medulla, where they make excitatory synapses with interneurons in the **nucleus of the solitary tract**. This nucleus is a multipurpose area that receives inputs from a variety of sensory systems and regulates automatic homeostatic functions of the body, including cardiac function. After passing through one or more excitatory interneurons within the nucleus of the solitary tract, activity in the stretch receptor neurons is relayed to the parasympathetic preganglionic neurons of the heart, in the nucleus of the vagus nerve (cranial nerve X). These parasympathetic preganglionic neurons then make excitatory synaptic contact with the parasympathetic postganglionic neurons in the heart, which release ACh and inhibit cardiac activity by activating muscarinic cholinergic receptors.

Other interneurons in the nucleus of the solitary tract make excitatory synapses with reticulospinal tract neurons in the medullary reticular formation. The reticulospinal neurons excite groups of inhibitory interneurons in the spinal cord that inhibit the sympathetic preganglionic neurons. This inhibition reduces activity in the sympathetic input to the heart, and norepinephrine release decreases. The release of epinephrine and norepinephrine from the adrenal chromaffin cells is also reduced via the same inhibitory pathway (see Fig. 11.13). The confluence of these parasympathetic, sympathetic, and adrenal influences reduces the cardiac output and blood pressure.

At the normal blood pressure, the walls of the arteries are somewhat stretched, producing ongoing action potential activity in the baroreceptors. This resting activity contributes a steady level of excitation to the cardiac parasympathetic pathway and a steady level of inhibition to the cardiac sympathetic pathway, by means of the synaptic connections shown in Figure 11.13. Within the central nervous system, other sources of excitation to both parasympathetic and sympathetic preganglionic neurons ensure a resting level of action potential activity in both pathways. Thus, the heart rate and cardiac output at any moment represent the sum of competing influences. A fall in arterial pressure below the normal level leads to decreased activity of the baroreceptors and hence reduced excitation in the parasympathetic pathway and reduced inhibition in the sympathetic pathway. The balance between the parasympathetic and sympathetic inputs to the heart then shifts to increase the cardiac output and restore the blood pressure. In this manner, the baroreceptor reflex opposes both increases and decreases in blood pressure from the normal set point.

IN THE CLINIC

BOX 1

Because the autonomic nervous system controls so many physiological functions that are fundamental to survival, many clinically useful drugs target the cholinergic and adrenergic receptors that are used by parasympathetic and sympathetic postganglionic neurons to regulate organ systems. A premier example is the cardiovascular system. In patients with high blood pressure (hypertension), treatment commonly includes drugs (for example, propranolol) that block the β-adrenergic receptors of the heart, reducing cardiac output. One common cause of hypertension is stress, which causes an overall increase in the activity of the sympathetic division of the autonomic nervous system. It is also thought that an abnormally high "set point" of the baroreceptor reflex might underlie some cases of high blood pressure, causing the reflex circuitry to regulate the blood pressure at too high a level (like a thermostat set to make a room too warm). This abnormal set point might arise from synaptic influences in the central nervous system or from altered sensitivity of the arterial stretch receptor neurons to extension of the vessel walls.

Another example of drugs that target postsynaptic receptors of the autonomic nervous system is the group of drugs that block muscarinic ACh receptors to produce dilation of the pupils (mydriasis), which facilitates ophthalmological examination of the retina. The diameter of the pupil is controlled by two antagonistic sets of muscles: circularly arranged sphincter muscles that constrict the pupil, and radial dilator muscles that increase the pupillary opening. The constrictor muscles are activated by the parasympathetic input to the iris, and the dilator muscles are activated by the sympathetic input. Blocking the muscarinic receptors of the constrictor muscles therefore causes the pupil to dilate.

The somatic nervous system controls the skeletal musculature. The autonomic nervous system controls other organ systems involved in homeostasis, including the cardiovascular system, the respiratory system, and the digestive system. The motor neurons of the autonomic nervous system are located outside the central nervous system, in autonomic ganglia. The somatic motor neurons, by contrast, are located in the gray matter of the spinal cord, within the central nervous system. The autonomic nervous system is divided into the parasympathetic and the sympathetic divisions. The parasympathetic ganglia are located close to or in the target organs themselves. The sympathetic ganglia are typically located close to the central nervous system, primarily in two chains of ganglia (the paravertebral ganglia) that parallel the spinal column on each side of the spinal cord.

The nerve terminals of the parasympathetic postganglionic neurons release the neurotransmitter ACh, whereas sympathetic postganglionic neurons release norepinephrine. In organs that receive both sympathetic and parasympathetic innervation, ACh and norepinephrine usually have opposite actions on the target cells. In the heart, for example, ACh decreases the heart rate and reduces the cardiac output, while norepinephrine increases the heart rate and the cardiac output.

In addition, the heart contains specific structures that coordinate the heart beat, including the SA node, AV node, and Purkinje fibers. The SA node is the master pacemaker of the heart, controlling the heart rate. The AV node provides the electrical connection between the atria and the ventricles and is responsible for the delay between atrial and ventricular contractions. The Purkinje fibers provide a rapidly conducting pathway for distributing excitation throughout the ventricles during the power stroke of the heartbeat.

The heart is controlled by the sympathetic and parasympathetic divisions of the autonomic nervous system. ACh released by the parasympathetic nerve terminals in the heart slows the heart rate by opening potassium channels. Norepinephrine released by the sympathetic nerve terminals increases the response of voltage-dependent calcium channels to depolarization, which then increases the rate of beating and the strength of contraction. Both neurotransmitters activate G-protein–coupled receptor molecules: muscarinic receptors in the case of ACh and β-adrenergic receptors in the case of norepinephrine. β-Adrenergic receptors increase cyclic AMP inside the cardiac cells, which promotes phosphorylation of calcium channels by protein kinase A.

The central nervous system controls the neurons of the autonomic ganglia via output neurons called preganglionic neurons. The parasympathetic preganglionic neurons are located in the brainstem and the sacral region of the spinal cord. The parasympathetic preganglionic fibers exit the brain via cranial nerves III, VII, IX, and X. The sympathetic preganglionic neurons are located in the intermediolateral gray matter of the spinal cord, from the thoracic to the lumbar level. Most sympathetic preganglionic fibers exit the spinal cord and enter the chain of paravertebral sympathetic ganglia on either side of the spinal column. Unlike many reflexes in the somatic nervous system, sensory input in autonomic reflexes reaches the preganglionic neurons only indirectly, after passing through a number of interneurons.

1. List the three different synaptic targets of neurons in the intermediolateral cell column of the spinal cord.

2. Describe the linkage between muscarinic cholinergic receptors and potassium channels in the heart.

3. Describe the linkage between β-adrenergic receptors and calcium channels in the heart.

4. What ionic mechanisms in cardiac-muscle cells account for spontaneous contractions?

5. List at least three functional differences between skeletal-muscle cells and cardiac-muscle cells.

6. Identify the following and provide a brief functional description: SA node, AV node, Purkinje fibers.

7. Draw the circuit of the baroreceptor reflex and describe the response of the reflex to an increase in blood pressure above the normal level.

8. What neurotransmitters are released by the preganglionic and postganglionic neurons of the parasympathetic and sympathetic divisions of the autonomic nervous system?

9. List the cranial nerve nuclei that contain parasympathetic preganglionic neurons.

INTERNET ASSIGNMENT   CHAPTER 11

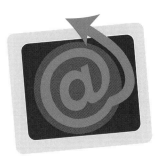

GTP binding proteins (G-proteins) are important in linking certain types of neurotransmitter receptors to their cellular actions in the nervous system. Two examples in the autonomic nervous system are the actions of norepinephrine and acetylcholine on the heart. G-proteins were first discovered outside the nervous system, however, in studies of hormone actions. Martin Rodbell and Alfred G. Gilman are two scientists who first worked the central role of G-proteins in linking receptor molecules to cellular actions. Research the Internet for the biographies and scientific contributions of these two scientists.

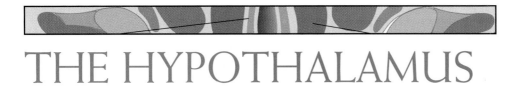
THE HYPOTHALAMUS

**ESSENTIAL
BACKGROUND**

Anatomy of the brain
and spinal cord
(Chapter 2, Chapter 8)

Endocrine glands
in mammals

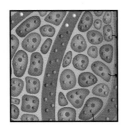

Many of the functions carried out by the autonomic nervous system (see Chapter 11) are important in regulating the internal environment of the organism. Under a wide variety of external environmental conditions, the internal environment of the body remains remarkably constant, including such factors as body temperature, water content of the tissues and blood, availability of energy derived from food, and so on. The maintenance of this constant internal environment is called **homeostasis**, and it requires both internal actions, involving the endocrine system and the autonomic nervous system, and external actions such as avoiding unfavorable temperature environments and seeking and ingesting food and water. The brain mechanisms that maintain homeostasis often involve the hypothalamus, which can be regarded as a master control center for the autonomic nervous system. In addition to its actions on the autonomic nervous system, the hypothalamus also maintains homeostasis by regulating the master gland of the body, the pituitary. In this chapter we will examine both of these roles of the hypothalamus.

The hypothalamus is also important in generating **circadian** ("approximately a day") **rhythms**. Many physiological factors vary with an approximately 24-hour cycle, even in the absence of external time clues provided by the normal day-night cycle. As we will discuss in this chapter, the internal clock required for these circadian cycles is present in the molecular machinery of single cells throughout the body, but in mammals a portion of the hypothalamus is pivotal for the overall coordination of circadian rhythms for the animal as a whole.

THE HYPOTHALAMUS IS PART OF THE LIMBIC SYSTEM

Where is the hypothalamus located and what are its subdivisions?

Figure 12.1 shows the location of the hypothalamus, which extends along the floor of the diencephalon from the mammillary bodies at the posterior end to the most anterior edge of the diencephalon, just overlying the optic chiasm, at the anterior end. Although the subdivisions are not very distinct, the hypothalamus can be divided broadly into anterior, middle, and posterior hypothalamic nuclei in the anterior-posterior direction, as shown in Figure 12.1B. In the medial-lateral direction, the hypothalamus is divided into periventricular, medial, and lateral groups of nuclei (see Fig. 12.1C). The periventricular nuclei surround the third ventricle of the brain, which runs along the center of diencephalon. Another brain region closely associated with the hypothalamus is the preoptic area, which is located just anterior and slightly dorsal to the most anterior part of the hypothalamus (see Fig. 12.1B). Although technically part of the telencephalon rather than the diencephalon, the preoptic area is extensively interconnected with the hypothalamus and is usually considered on functional grounds to be part of the hypothalamus.

The hypothalamus is part of a diverse set of brain regions called the **limbic system,** which is involved in a variety of actions related to homeostasis, emotion, and sexual behavior. Limbic system structures are responsible for motivations or drives, which cause animals to engage in complex goal-directed behaviors required to satisfy basic needs. Examples include the subjective states of hunger or thirst, which impel ingestive behaviors (feeding and drinking), and the sex drive, which motivates animals to seek out and mate with appropriate partners. In addition, activation of particular parts of the limbic system elicits emotional states, such as anger, fear, and anxiety.

What parts of the brain form the limbic system?

The basic core of the limbic system is formed by a neural loop (also called the Papez circuit) that extends from the cingulate gyrus of the neocortex through the entorhinal paleocortex to the hippocampus, continuing on through the hypothalamus and the thalamus and then back to the cingulate gyrus to complete the loop (Fig. 12.2). The **cingulate gyrus** runs front to back in each cerebral hemisphere within the interhemispheric fissure separating the two hemispheres at the midline. The axons projecting from the cingulate gyrus to the entorhinal cortex run in a fiber bundle called the **cingulum**. The **entorhinal cortex** is part of the olfactory cortex (see Chapter 18), and its axons connect to the hippocampus by means of the **perforant path**. The **hippocampus** is a C-shaped structure tucked deep within the lower and posterior lip of the neocortex, near the border between the cerebrum and the midbrain (see Fig. 12.2B). As described in Chapter 20, the hippocampus is thought to play a role in certain types of learning and memory, as well as in emotional behavior. The output axons of the hippocampus form a large fiber bundle called the **fornix**, which has numerous synaptic targets in the brain, including the mammillary bodies of the hypothalamus. Within the hypothalamus, the fornix forms the dividing line between the medial and lateral subdivisions of hypotha-

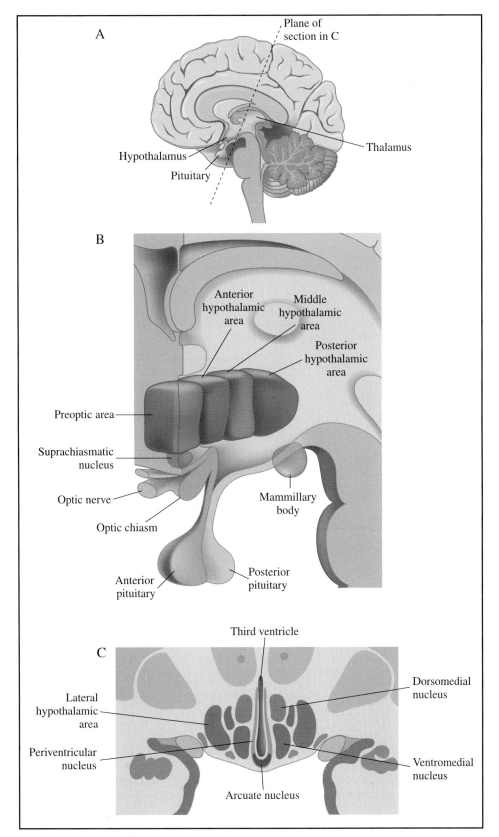

Figure 12.1.

The location of the hypothalamus. **A**. A diagram of the human brain cut along the midline to reveal internal structures. The location of the hypothalamus is marked at the base of the brain, just above the pituitary gland and below the thalamus. **B**. A closer view of the hypothalamus, with some important subdivisions indicated. **C**. A diagram of the subdivisions of the hypothalamus from medial to lateral, at the level of the middle of the hypothalamus (plane of section shown in **A**).

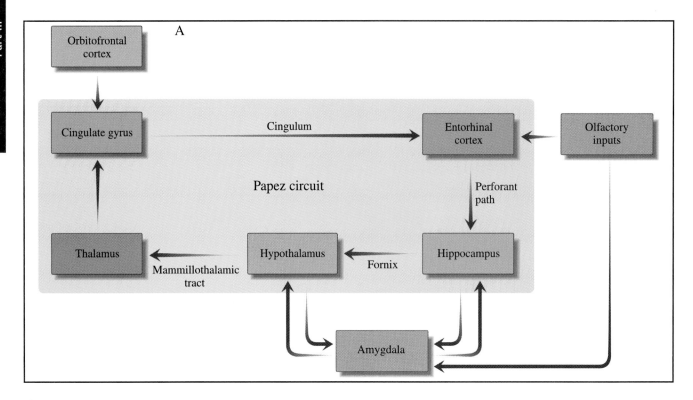

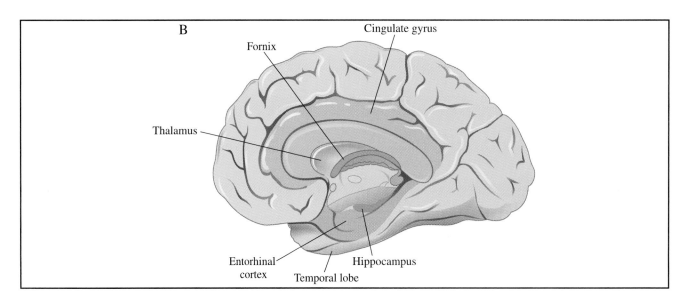

Figure 12.2.

The organization of the limbic system. **A**. A block diagram of some brain structures that make up the limbic system. The core of the limbic system is a set of structures called the Papez circuit (*shaded area*). **B**. The location of some limbic system structures in the human brain. The diagram shows a brain divided along the midline, with part of the inferior temporal lobe and midbrain structures removed to reveal the location of the hippocampus.

lamic nuclei. In the Papez circuit, the output axons of the mammillary bodies run in the **mammillothalamic tract** to the anterior nuclei of the thalamus, which then send axons to the cingulate gyrus to complete the loop.

In addition to the core Papez circuit, other structures associated with the limbic system include the orbitofrontal neocortex, the parahippocampal gyrus of the neocortex, the amygdala, the septal area, and parts of the midbrain reticular formation. The amygdala is a group of nuclei at the medial tip of the temporal lobe of the cortex. The neurons of the amygdala receive inputs from and send outputs to the hypothalamus and the hippocampus. Also, the amygdala is part of the olfactory cortex and thus provides an important route for olfactory information to enter the limbic system. Olfactory information is important for a number of the behavioral functions of the limbic system, such as sexual behavior and feeding.

HYPOTHALAMIC CONTROL OF THE PITUITARY GLAND

In the autonomic nervous system, motor neurons contact a variety of different target tissues, including endocrine glands. In keeping with the close association between the hypothalamus and the autonomic nervous system, neurons of the hypothalamus also are involved directly in the control of the endocrine system. A particularly important target for the hypothalamus is the pituitary gland, which hangs from the bottom of the hypothalamus on a connecting stalk called the **infundibulum** (Fig. 12.3). The pituitary is a master control gland for the endocrine system, and it is in turn controlled by a special subset of neurons in the hypothalamus, called **neurosecretory neurons**. Neurosecretory neurons have modified synaptic terminals that directly release hormones into the bloodstream. Thus, neurosecretory neurons act much like endocrine cells.

As shown in Figure 12.3, the pituitary gland consists of two lobes: the anterior lobe (also called the **adenohypophysis**) and the posterior lobe (the **neuro-**

BOX 1

IN THE CLINIC

Because of the wide variety of functions served by the limbic system, symptoms arising from pathology of the limbic system range from simple, such as fever, to complex, such as emotional disorders. Fever results from an increase in the temperature set point, so that body temperature is regulated at an elevated level. Pyrogens released into the bloodstream during the immune response to infection act directly on the preoptic area to affect the set point. Perhaps the most notorious example of a clinical use of the knowledge of the roles the limbic system plays in emotion is frontal lobotomy. Surgical lesions of orbitofrontal cortex or the cutting of fiber tracts connecting the orbitofrontal and cingulate cortex to the rest of the limbic system was found to reduce aggression and anger and make experimental animals more placid. Therefore, the same procedures were performed on psychiatric patients to control emotional disorders. The advent of psychoactive drugs, coupled with concerns about effectiveness and side effects of the surgery, put an end to the practice.

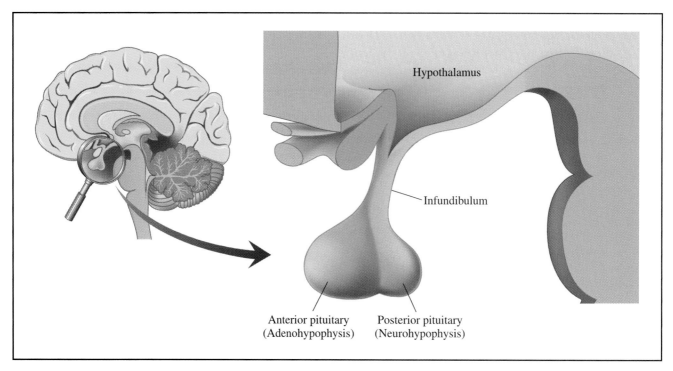

Figure 12.3.

The subdivisions of the pituitary gland. The pituitary hangs from the base of the brain, as shown in the overview on the *left*. The connecting stalk is the infundibulum. The anterior lobe of the pituitary is also called the adenohypophysis, and the posterior lobe is also called the neurophypophysis.

hypophysis). Hormones are released in the two lobes by different mechanisms. Axons of **magnocellular** (large-cell) **neurosecretory cells** of the hypothalamus project directly to the posterior pituitary, where they release the peptide hormones **vasopressin** (also called antidiuretic hormone, or ADH) and **oxytocin** into the general systemic circulatory system for distribution throughout the body, as illustrated in Figure 12.4. Vasopressin promotes the constriction of blood vessels and the retention of water by the kidneys. Oxytocin stimulates milk ejection from the mammary glands in mammals and also causes uterine contraction.

The hormones released by the neurohypophysis are synthesized and secreted by the magnocellular neurosecretory cells of the hypothalamus, and not by a separate group of endocrine cells. By contrast, the anterior lobe of the pituitary contains endocrine cells that release seven different hormones into the bloodstream (Table 12.1). The release of these anterior pituitary hormones in turn is controlled by regulatory substances (stimulatory or inhibitory **release factors**) secreted by **parvocellular** (small-cell) **neurosecretory neurons** of the hypothalamus into special portal capillaries, located at the base of the hypothalamus in a structure called the **median eminence**. These **portal vessels** then transport the release factors to the target endocrine cells in the anterior pituitary, as illustrated in Figure 12.5. The pituitary hormones, their actions in the body, and their regulation by the hypothalamus are summarized in Table 12.1.

The cell bodies of magnocellular neurosecretory cells are located in both the supraoptic nucleus and the paraventricular nucleus of the hypothalamus. The parvocellular neurosecretory cells are scattered among several hypothalamic nuclei, including the arcuate nucleus, the preoptic area, the periventricular area, and the paraventricular nucleus, among others. Note that the paraventricular nucleus

Which hormones are released in the anterior and posterior lobes of the pituitary gland?

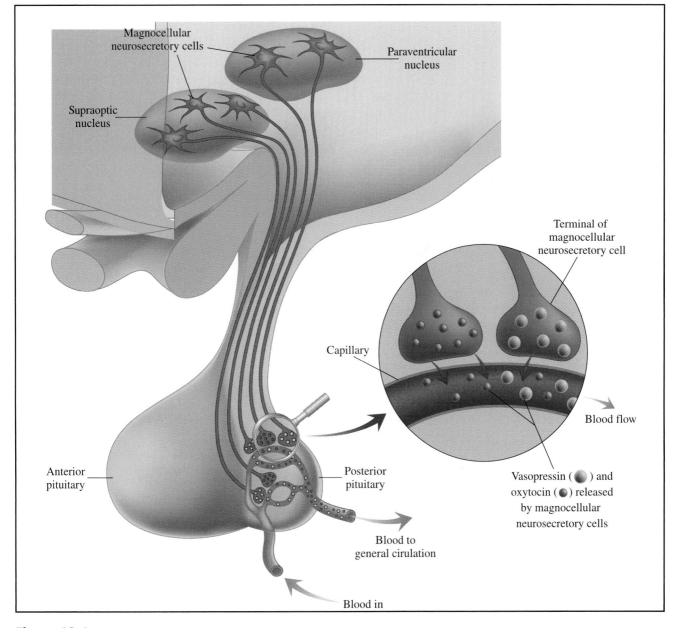

Figure 12.4.

The hormones of the posterior lobe of the pituitary gland are released from the terminals of hypothalamic magnocellular neurosecretory cells. The cell bodies of the magnocellular neurosecretory cells are located in the paraventricular nucleus and the supraoptic nucleus of the hypothalamus. Their axons project through the infundibulum and form terminals near capillaries within the posterior lobe of the pituitary gland. The hormones vasopressin and oxytocin are released from the terminals into the bloodstream for distribution throughout the body.

contains both magnocellular neurosecretory cells, which project to the posterior lobe of the pituitary, and parvocellular neurosecretory cells, which project to the portal vessels and control the anterior lobe of the pituitary. This functional diversity within a nucleus is a common pattern in the hypothalamus, and nuclei of the hypothalamus typically contain neurons that are involved in a variety of homeostatic processes. Because each hypothalamic nucleus serves several functions, the neural circuitry of the hypothalamus is complex and difficult to unravel experimentally.

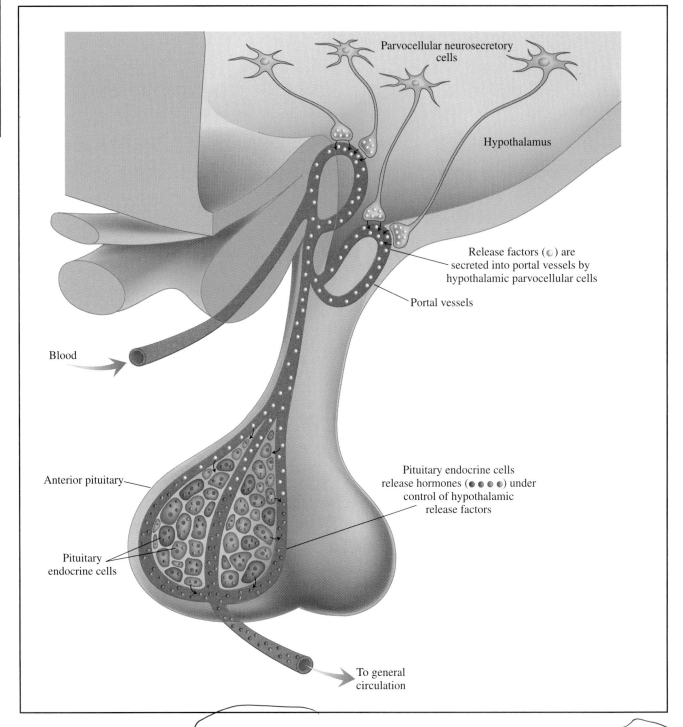

Parvocellular neurosecretory cells

Hypothalamus

Release factors (○) are secreted into portal vessels by hypothalamic parvocellular cells

Portal vessels

Blood

Pituitary endocrine cells release hormones (● ● ● ●) under control of hypothalamic release factors

Anterior pituitary

Pituitary endocrine cells

To general circulation

Figure 12.5.

The hormones of the anterior lobe of the pituitary gland are released by endocrine cells. The endocrine cells are controlled by release factors that are secreted by parvocellular neurosecretory cells of the hypothalamus. The axons of the parvocellular neurosecretory cells project to a special set of capillaries, the portal vessels, at the upper portion of the infundibulum. The portal vessels then carry the release factors to the anterior lobe of the pituitary gland. The seven different hormones released by the various kinds of anterior pituitary cells are then carried throughout the body by the circulatory system.

Table 12.1.

Pituitary hormones, their actions, and hypothalamic control of their release.

	Released hormone	Effect of released hormone	Hypothalamic regulation of released hormone
Posterior pituitary hormones	vasopressin (antidiuretic hormone)	water retention; vasoconstriction	direct: released by magnocellular neurosecretory neurons
	oxytocin	milk ejection from mammary glands; uterine contraction	direct: released by magnocellular neurosecretory neurons
Anterior pituitary hormones	thyrotropin (TSH)	increased thyroxin release from thyroid gland	thyrotropin releasing hormone (+)
	adrenocorticotropic hormone (ACTH)	increased cortisol release from adrenal gland	corticotropin releasing hormone (+)
	growth hormone (somatotropin)	whole body growth	growth hormone releasing hormone (+) somatostatin (−)
	gonadotropins (LH, FSH)	development of reproductive cells and release of sex hormones from gonads	gonadotropin releasing hormone (+)
	prolactin	milk production by mammary glands	prolactin releasing hormone (+) dopamine (−)
	melanocyte stimulating hormone (MSH)	melanocytes and body coloration changes	MSH releasing factor (+) MSH release inhibiting factor (−)

LH = luteinizing hormone; FSH = follicle stimulating hormone.

HYPOTHALAMIC NEURONS REGULATE BODY TEMPERATURE

Regulation of body temperature is another important homeostatic function of the hypothalamus. The anterior hypothalamus, preoptic area, and posterior hypothalamus are involved in temperature regulation. The actions of the anterior and posterior temperature-regulating regions are summarized in Figure 12.6. Electrical stimulation applied to the anterior hypothalamus produces both behavioral (for example, panting) and autonomic responses (for example, dilation of skin blood vessels) that dissipate heat. Stimulation of the posterior hypothalamus produces opposing responses (vasoconstriction and shivering) that favor heat production and conservation. Thus, activation of neural systems in the anterior hypothalamic region reduces body temperature, whereas activation of the posterior hypothalamic system increases body temperature. Consistent with these actions, damage to the anterior part of the hypothalamus produces elevated body temperature (hyperthermia) because heat-dissipating responses are impaired. Conversely, dam-

What parts of the hypothalamus are involved in regulating body temperature?

267

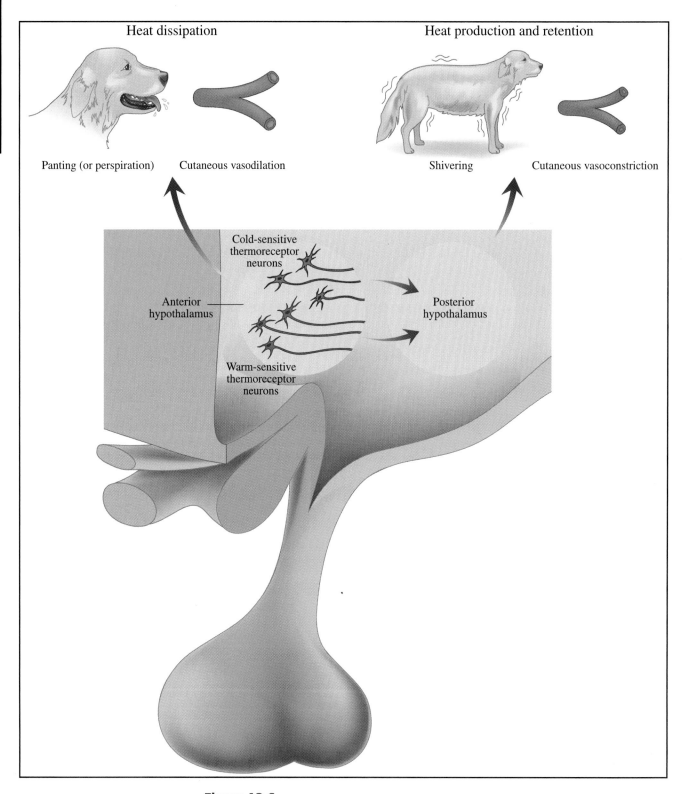

Figure 12.6.

The location of hypothalamic regions involved in temperature regulation. Stimulation applied to the anterior hypothalamus produces responses that promote heat dissipation. Stimulation applied to the posterior hypothalamus produces responses that lead to heat retention and heat production. The anterior hypothalamus contains neurons that respond directly to cooling or heating of the brain.

age to the posterior part produces an inability to maintain normal body temperature (hypothermia) in a cold environment because heat-generating responses are impaired. Fever results from an increase in the temperature set point, so that body temperature is regulated at an elevated level. Pyrogens released into the bloodstream during the immune response to infection act directly on the preoptic area to affect the set point.

Interestingly, the hypothalamus contains its own set of temperature-sensitive neurons (thermoreceptors) that respond to changes in local brain temperature (see Fig. 12.6). Cold-sensitive neurons in the anterior hypothalamic and preoptic areas are activated when brain temperature falls below normal body temperature. A separate set of warm-sensitive neurons in the same hypothalamic regions is activated when brain temperature exceeds the normal body temperature. The temperature-sensitive hypothalamic neurons are also activated by corresponding changes in skin temperature, indicating that the brain thermoreceptors receive inputs from the thermoreceptors of the somatosensory system (see Chapter 14), as well as have intrinsic temperature sensitivity. Thermoreceptors have not been found in the posterior hypothalamus, and so the heat-generating circuitry of the posterior region must obtain its temperature information from other brain systems.

HYPOTHALAMIC CONTROL OF FOOD AND WATER INTAKE

The hypothalamus is also involved in the initiation of drinking,. Terrestrial animals continually lose water to the environment through such normal physiological events as humidifying inspired air in the lungs, cooling the body through evaporation, and producing urine. When water intake is insufficient to replace the water lost, the osmolarity of the extracellular fluid rises and the fluid volume of the blood decreases. Both of these stimuli activate hypothalamic neurons that generate the thirst drive and promote water retention. As summarized in Figure 12.7, specialized osmoreceptor cells in the hypothalamus become active when the osmolarity of the extracellular fluid in the brain rises. We learned in Chapter 3 that increased external osmolarity causes cells to lose water and shrink. Shrinkage increases the firing rate of the hypothalamic osmoreceptor cells. The osmoreceptor cells in turn promote water retention, by stimulating the vasopressin-secreting magnocellular neurosecretory cells described earlier. The osmoreceptors also activate thirst circuitry of the limbic system, motivating the animal to drink water to restore the correct osmolarity.

Loss of vascular volume is signaled to the hypothalamus by both neural and chemical messages, summarized in Figure 12.8. Baroreceptors (pressure sensors) in the walls of blood vessels provide the neural signal, which stimulates vasopressin release and also activates the circuits of the hypothalamus that generate the thirst drive. When the volume of the fluid in the circulatory system is below normal, the walls of blood vessels are not properly distended, and the change in vessel shape is detected by stretch-sensitive vascular baroreceptors. The chemical signal for reduced vascular volume originates from the kidney, which releases the protein renin into the bloodstream in response to a fall in blood volume. Renin is a protease that cleaves the plasma protein angiotensinogen, releasing a fragment called **angiotensin I**, which is then further converted into **angiotensin II** as the blood passes through the lungs. Angiotensin II is detected by specialized receptor neurons in the subfornical organ, which is located within the third ventricle. The capillaries of the subfornical organ allow the angiotensin II peptide to diffuse out of the blood and be detected by the neurons of the subfornical organ, which then pass the signal to neurons of the preoptic area.

What parts of the hypothalamus are involved in regulating feeding and drinking?

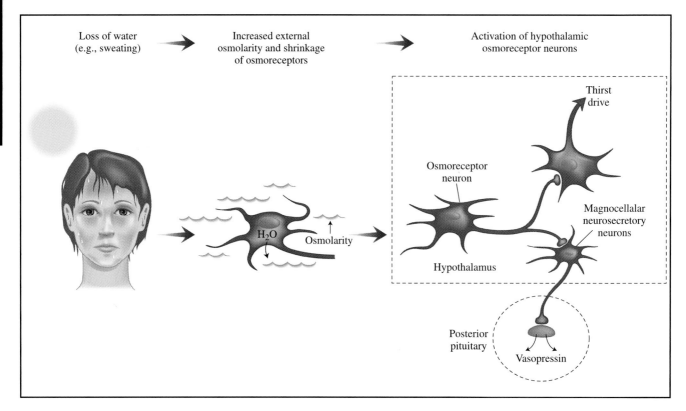

Loss of water
(e.g., sweating) → Increased external
osmolarity and shrinkage
of osmoreceptors → Activation of hypothalamic
osmoreceptor neurons

Thirst
drive

Osmoreceptor
neuron

Magnocellalar
neurosecretory
neurons

H₂O   Osmolarity

Hypothalamus

Posterior
pituitary
Vasopressin

Figure 12.7.

Loss of body water promotes drinking and water retention by increasing the osmolarity of the extracellular fluid. Osmoreceptor neurons in the hypothalamus are activated by increased external osmolarity. The osmoreceptor neurons in turn activate thirst circuits in the hypothalamus and magnocellular neurosecretory cells that release vasopressin in the posterior pituitary.

Hypothalamic neural circuits also regulate feeding behavior. . Normally, animals regulate body weight at a relatively steady level and adjust food intake appropriately to maintain that weight. The set point of desired body weight is encoded in the hypothalamus, by means of the interaction of hypothalamic nuclei that stimulate and inhibit feeding (Fig. 12.9). Damage to the ventromedial nucleus of the hypothalamus produces overeating and obesity, whereas damage to the neighboring lateral hypothalamic area causes undereating and weight loss. In severe cases, damage to the lateral hypothalamic area produces **aphagia** (absence of feeding). Neurons in the lateral hypothalamic area are thought to be involved in activating the hunger drive, which motivates animals to seek out and ingest food. A neuropeptide called **orexin** is produced by certain neurons in the lateral hypothalamic area and may be released to stimulate feeding. Damage to these orexin-containing neurons may explain the aphagia produced by lesions in the lateral hypothalamic area.

To regulate body weight, the hypothalamus must receive some signal that gives information about how much the animal weighs. Less is known about this body weight signal than about the signals underlying other regulatory processes, such as water balance and temperature regulation. One signal related to the maintenance of body weight may be hormonal. Fat cells in the body produce a peptide hormone called leptin. Interfering with leptin production results in overeating and obesity. Also, receptor molecules that respond to leptin are found in the hypothalamic areas involved in the regulation of feeding, including the ventromedial nucleus. Leptin therefore may be a **satiety signal** that inhibits food intake by activating the ventromedial nucleus of the hypothalamus.

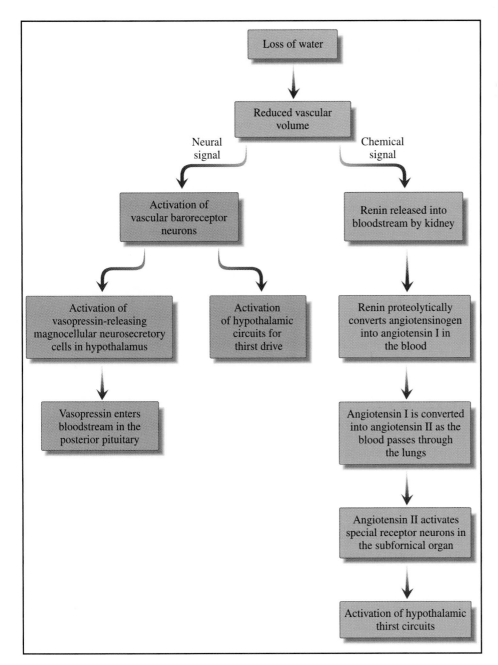

Figure 12.8.
Loss of body water promotes drinking and water retention by reducing the volume of blood in the circulatory system. Both direct neural signals (*left limb of the diagram*) and chemical signals (*right limb of the diagram*) link a loss of blood volume to the release of vasopressin and the activation of the thirst drive.

CIRCADIAN RHYTHMS AND THE HYPOTHALAMUS

Many behavioral, physiological, and biochemical processes vary during the course of the day. During daylight, diurnal animals—such as humans—are more active, have higher body temperature, and secrete hormones that mobilize the body's energy stores. Conversely, at night these animals are inactive, their body temperature is lower, and hormones that promote restoration of energy stores are secreted. The reverse holds true for nocturnal animals. Such rhythmic cycles that have a period of 24 hours are called **circadian rhythms**. Circadian rhythms are a ubiquitous characteristic of living systems and are found in organisms as diverse as bacteria, plants, and people. Ordinarily, the timekeeping for daily cycles is governed by the day-night cycle imposed by the rotation of our planet. However, circadian rhythms are actually produced by an internal, biological clock within the cellular machinery of the organism. If the external day-night cycle is eliminated by

What is the important behavioral role of the suprachiasmatic nucleus of the hypothalamus?

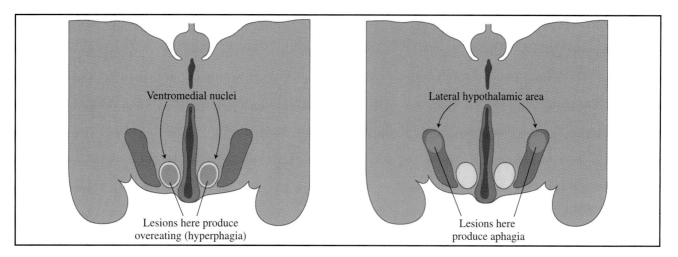

Ventromedial nuclei

Lesions here produce
overeating (hyperphagia)

Lateral hypothalamic area

Lesions here
produce aphagia

Figure 12.9.

Locations of hypothalamic nuclei involved in the regulation of feeding. Lesions in the ventromedial nucleus (*left*) produce hyperphagia and weight gain, whereas lesions in the lateral hypothalamus (*right*) produce aphagia and weight loss.

keeping an animal in constant dim light, for example, circadian rhythms of behavior, physiology, and biochemistry continue unabated. Such rhythms in the absence of external time cues are called **free-running rhythms**.

The biological clock that maintains the rhythms is not precisely accurate, however, and it produces a cycle period slightly longer or shorter than 24 hours in the absence of external time cues. As Figure 12.10 illustrates, the active period of a nocturnal animal (for example, a rat) kept in constant darkness gradually shifts with respect to the true time of day. However, if a brief light stimulus (or some other stimulus) is presented at a set time each day, the activity of a free-running animal rapidly shifts to lock in with the external time cue. This synchronization of the endogenous rhythm to a regular external stimulus is called **entrainment**, and the external cue is called a **zeitgeber** (German for "time giver"). Entrainment occurs naturally during the year, as the time of sunrise and sunset shifts with the progression of Earth in its orbit around the sun.

If circadian rhythms are found in unicellular organisms and in multicellular organisms without a nervous system, such as bacteria and plants, then you might wonder why we are discussing this topic in a chapter devoted to the hypothalamus. The answer is that in mammals, a part of the hypothalamus contains the master clock that governs circadian rhythms of many behavior and physiological processes. The hypothalamic master clock is located in the base of the anterior region of the hypothalamus, just above the optic chiasm, as shown in Figure 12.11. The nucleus is called the suprachiasmatic nucleus (SCN) because of its location superior to the chiasm. The neurons of the SCN receive direct synaptic input from a special subset of retinal ganglion cells, whose axons form the **retinohypothalamic tract**. These retinal ganglion cells provide photic information for synchronizing circadian rhythms with the natural light-dark cycle.

A variety of evidence shows that the SCN controls circadian rhythms in mammals. If the neurons of the SCN are destroyed on both sides of the brain, normal cycles of activity, body temperature, and so on are abolished (Fig. 12.12). Normal rhythms are restored if SCN tissue from a donor animal or immortalized SCN cells grown in culture are transplanted into the hypothalamus of an animal whose own SCN has been destroyed. It is interesting that the cycle length of the restored circadian rhythm in the transplant recipient is characteristic of the cycle length of the

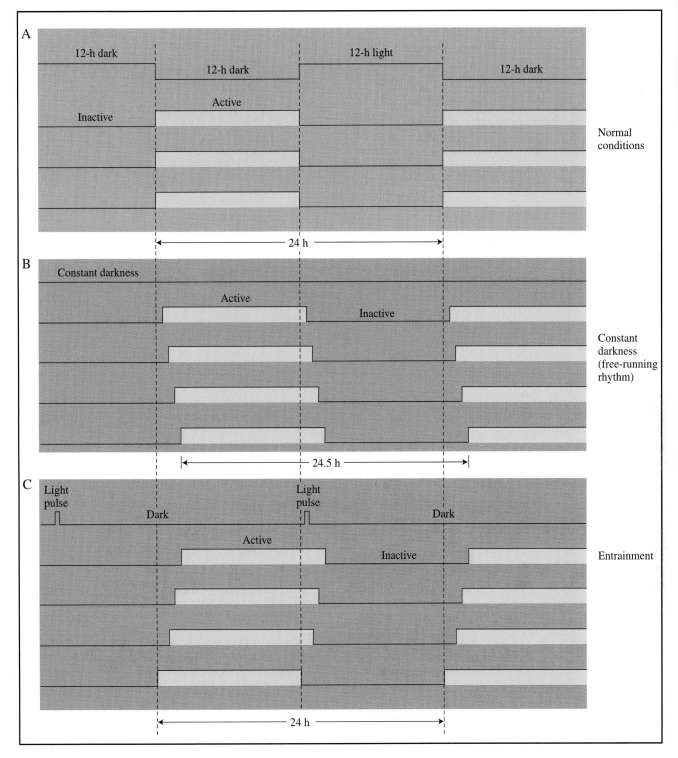

Figure 12.10.

The characteristics of circadian rhythms of activity. **A.** Under normal illumination conditions, a nocturnal animal is active during the dark phase of the light-dark cycle and inactive during the light phase. **B.** Without an external lighting cycle, the cycle of activity continues as a free-running rhythm. The time between the onset of successive active periods is typically not exactly 24 hours, however. In this example, the length of the cycle is 24.5 hours. **C.** A brief light pulse given every 24 hours causes the rhythm of activity to become synchronized, or entrained, with an interval of exactly 24 hours between successive active periods.

Figure 12.11.

The location of the supra-chiasmatic nucleus. The diagram shows a cross section through the human brain at the level of the optic chiasm.

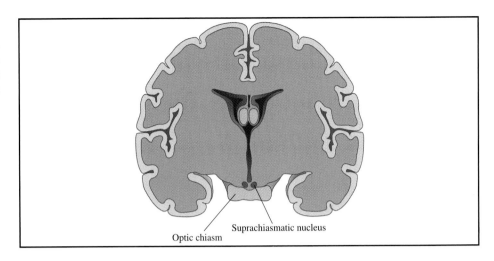

Suprachiasmatic nucleus

Optic chiasm

donor animal. For example, if the transplant is derived from an animal with an abnormally short circadian rhythm (for example, 20 hours instead of 24 hours), then the recipient also adopts the abnormally short cycle under free-running conditions (see Fig. 12.12). This experiment demonstrates that the SCN is indeed the master clock that sets the pace for circadian rhythms.

When SCN neurons are removed from the brain and placed in cell culture, they retain circadian rhythms of action potential activity, neuropeptide secretion, and metabolic activity. Also, immortal cell lines derived from embryonic precursors of SCN neurons have similar circadian patterns in cell culture. These findings demonstrate that individual neurons of the hypothalamic master clock have an endogenous cellular timekeeper that persists when the neurons are isolated from the rest of the brain and from each other. The molecular basis of this cellular oscillator underlying the circadian pacemaker is our next subject.

Molecular Basis of Circadian Rhythms

What is the molecular mechanism underlying the generation of circadian rhythms in single cells?

Key information about the molecular mechanisms of circadian timekeeping has come from genetic studies of mutations that affect circadian rhythms in the fruit fly, genus *Drosophila*, and in bread mold, genus *Neurospora*. More recently, molecular biological studies have also given information about molecular clocks in mammals. The molecular mechanisms of the circadian oscillator are remarkably similar in these diverse species, although this should not be surprising for a fundamental feature of life such as circadian rhythms.

A timekeeping device must contain an oscillator with a defined cycle period that can be used to keep track of time (for example, the pendulum of a mechanical clock). In biological systems, oscillations within cells are typically produced by negative feedback, in which a signal feeds back to inhibit its own production. For instance, see Chapter 17 for a description of how such a feedback mechanism accounts for the generation of oscillatory responses in hair cells of the ear. The circadian oscillator also involves feedback, but the 24-hour time scale for the oscillation dictates the types of cellular mechanisms appropriate to form the feedback oscillator. The time scale of hours is best matched to slow cellular events like gene transcription and protein translation. Indeed, it turns out that transcriptional control of gene expression is a central part of the circadian clock in cells.

Figure 12.13 shows the general scheme thought to generate the pacemaker oscillation for circadian rhythms in the fruit fly, which is probably the best-studied circadian mechanism. Mutation experiments showed that two genes, called *period*

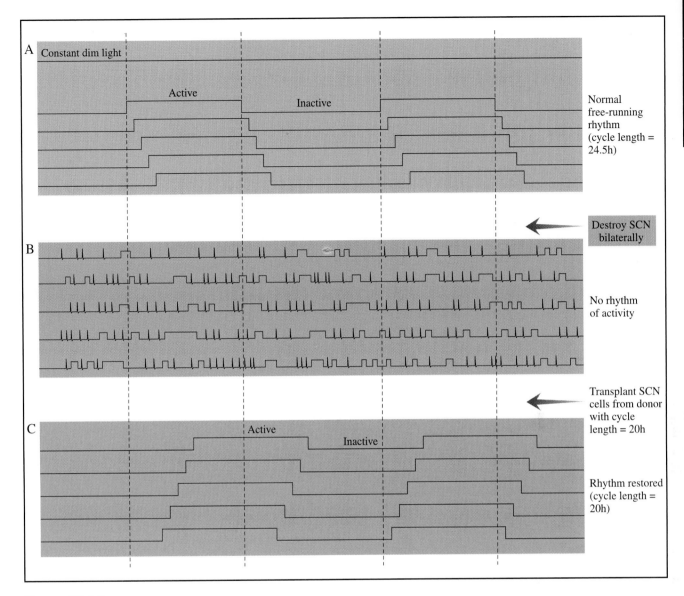

A Constant dim light

Active   Inactive

Normal
free-running
rhythm
(cycle length =
24.5h)

Destroy SCN
bilaterally

B

No rhythm
of activity

Transplant SCN
cells from donor
with cycle
length = 20h

C   Active
                         Inactive

Rhythm restored
(cycle length =
20h)

Figure 12.12.

Neurons of the suprachiasmatic nucleus are required for circadian rhythms. **A.** In constant illumination, a free-running rhythm of activity is observed, with a cycle length of 24.5 hours in this example. **B.** Destruction of the suprachiasmatic nucleus on both sides of the brain abolishes the free-running rhythm of activity. **C.** Transplantation of cells from the suprachiasmatic nucleus of a donor animal restores the free-running rhythm of activity. The new cycle length (20 hours in this example) is characteristic of the donor animal rather than the recipient.

(*per*) and *timeless* (*tim*), are necessary for circadian rhythms in the fruit fly.* The levels of messenger RNA (mRNA) and proteins (**PER** and **TIM**) produced from these genes rise and fall with a 24-hour cycle. The PER and TIM proteins bind to each other, forming a dimer that then enters the nucleus of the cell. There, PER and TIM inhibit the transcription of their own genes, producing negative feedback. Be-

*Note on gene terminology. In genetics, as each gene is characterized, it is given a more or less clever name by its discoverers, usually reflecting in some way the effect of mutating the gene. Gene names are written in italics using lowercase letters (even at the beginning of a sentence) and are abbreviated with a three-letter abbreviation derived from the name, also in italics. The protein made from the gene is given the same name and abbreviation as the gene but is written in capital letters, without italics. Thus, *period* or *per* refers to the gene itself, and PERIOD or PER refers to the protein encoded by the gene.

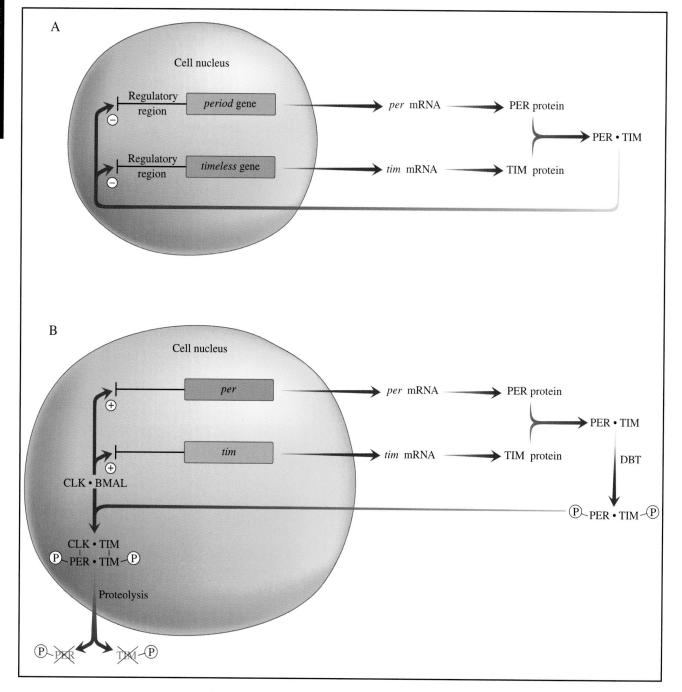

Figure 12.13.

The molecular mechanism of the cellular clock underlying circadian rhythms. **A**. PERIOD (PER) and TIMELESS (TIM) are proteins that inhibit the transcription of messenger RNA (mRNA) from their own genes (*per* and *tim*). Thus, the levels of PER and TIM protein in the cell rise and fall. **B**. The mechanism of inhibition of *per* and *tim* genes by PER and TIM proteins. PER and TIM form a dimer, which is phosphorylated by DOUBLETIME (DBT) and is then able to enter the cell nucleus. In the nucleus, the PER·TIM dimer binds to the transcription factors CLK and BMAL and prevents the transcription factors from activating the *per* and *tim* genes. The proteins PER and TIM are then destroyed by proteolysis, restoring the starting conditions for a new round of PER and TIM synthesis.

cause the existing PER and TIM proteins are degraded by proteolysis, the absence of mRNA transcription to form new proteins means that the levels of PER and TIM then begin to fall. As the levels fall, inhibition of transcription is removed, mRNA is produced, and PER and TIM levels rise again. These cycles take about 24 hours for completion.

The proteins PER and TIM do not directly bind to DNA and so do not directly affect their own genes. As Figure 12.13B illustrates, the PER·TIM dimer in the nucleus instead binds to another protein dimer, formed by the transcription factors **CLOCK (CLK)** and **BMAL1**. BMAL1 was discovered in mammalian cells, and the homologous protein in the fruit fly is called **CYCLE (CYC)**; however, here we will refer to the protein by its mammalian name. CLOCK and BMAL1 bind to the regulatory regions of *per* and *tim* and activate transcription of the genes. When PER and TIM bind to the CLK·BMAL1 dimer, the transcription factors no longer activate *per* and *tim* transcription, thus forming the negative feedback part of the daily PER·TIM cycle.

Phosphorylation of TIM and PER is required for the formation of PER·TIM dimers and subsequent movement to the nucleus. The protein kinase that performs the necessary phosphorylation is the product of a gene called *doubletime (dbt)*, as illustrated in Figure 12.13B. Mutations of any of the genes whose protein products are shown in Figure 12.13B interfere with the core cycle of circadian timekeeping and thus abolish circadian rhythms in the fruit fly.

Setting and Reading the Clock

Although the basic circadian oscillator is endogenous to cells, the circadian rhythm is normally entrained to external stimuli such as the day-night cycle. Also, cycling of PER and TIM is of little use unless the cycle is coupled to signals that can be passed on to other cells to coordinate physiological and behavioral responses (a clock needs hands to indicate time). The molecular mechanisms of entrainment and clock output are less well understood than those of the cellular clock itself.

In the fruit fly, evidence suggests that a pulse of light administered during constant darkness entrains the circadian cycle by stimulating degradation of TIM. The fall in levels of TIM then resets the mechanism shown in Figure 12.13B to the state in which CLK and BMAL1 are free to interact with the *tim* and *per* regulatory regions to drive a new cycle of PER and TIM expression.

In the mammalian SCN, resetting of the clock by a pulse of light in darkness is mediated by the release of glutamate from the synaptic terminals of retinal ganglion cells, which project to the SCN via the retinohypothalamic tract. Experiments show that glutamate may influence the clock by activating a transcription factor called **CREB (Ca^{2+}/cAMP response element–binding protein)**. CREB is phosphorylated in response to increased intracellular Ca^{2+} or cyclic adenosine monophosphate (cAMP). Phosphorylated CREB enters the nucleus and alters gene expression by binding to a particular DNA sequence (the **Ca^{2+}/cAMP response element, or CRE**) found within the regulatory regions of a variety of neuronal genes. The regulatory regions of genes involved in the clock mechanism may include CREB binding elements, and so CREB activation by glutamate may influence the molecular oscillations underlying the clock. In the fruit fly, CREB is known to affect oscillations in PER, which also may be the link between CREB activation and clock resetting in the SCN.

The picture is less clear for clock-regulated output genes that mediate the effect of the master clock on physiological and behavioral systems. Among the candidate output mechanisms in the SCN is vasopressin, which we discussed earlier in this chapter as one of the substances released in the posterior lobe of the pituitary by magnocellular neurosecretory neurons. In addition to functioning as a pituitary hormone, vasopressin is synthesized and released by neurons of the SCN, and this synthesis undergoes a circadian oscillation produced by rhythmic expression of the vasopressin gene. Vasopressin released by SCN neurons acts both locally within the SCN to alter action potential firing by SCN neurons and at distant sites within the brain where axons of SCN neurons project. Circadian oscillation in the expression of vasopressin in SCN neurons is controlled by the clock transcription factors CLOCK and BMAL1, which provide a link between the basic clock mechanism and vasopressin as an output signal. Other genes, as yet unknown, will undoubtedly be found to be regulated in a similar manner and to contribute to output from the SCN master clock.

SUMMARY

The hypothalamus is a complex group of nuclei located at the base of the diencephalon. It controls many basic physiological functions of animals, including temperature regulation, feeding, drinking, and sexual behavior. Because many of these functions require the concerted action of many parts of the autonomic nervous system, the hypothalamus is sometimes referred to as the "head ganglion" of the autonomic nervous system. The hypothalamus is also an important part of the limbic system, which includes the neocortical and paleocortical regions. Another important role of the hypothalamus is to control the pituitary gland, the master gland of the endocrine system. In the posterior lobe of the pituitary, the hormones vasopressin and oxytocin are released directly into the circulatory system by hypothalamic neurosecretory neurons. In the anterior lobe of the pituitary, endocrine cells release a total of seven different hormones under the control of a different group of hypothalamic neurosecretory neurons. The release of anterior-pituitary hormones is controlled by release factors secreted into special portal capillaries by the neurosecretory neurons. A part of the hypothalamus called the suprachiasmatic nucleus is the master control center for circadian rhythms, which are daily cycles in numerous biochemical, physiological, and behavioral processes. Circadian rhythms are maintained under the control of an endogenous, biological clock that is normally entrained to the exogenous day-night cycle.

REVIEW QUESTIONS

1. Describe the set of brain regions and their connections making up the Papez circuit.
2. What are portal vessels, and why are they important for the regulation of the pituitary gland?
3. What substances are released by hypothalamic neurosecretory cells (both magnocellular and parvocellular), and what functions do the released substances play?
4. Discuss the role of the hypothalamus in the regulation of body temperature. Include a description of the effects of specific hypothalamic regions.
5. An animal with a lesion in the brain eats very little and loses body weight. What part of the brain is likely damaged by the lesion?
6. Describe the effects of water loss on the hypothalamus, taking into account both neural and chemical signals.
7. Oscillations in the levels of the proteins PERIOD and TIMELESS are responsible for the circadian pacemaker in single cells. What is the mechanism underlying the oscillation? Include other proteins that are required for the mechanism

INTERNET ASSIGNMENT   CHAPTER 12

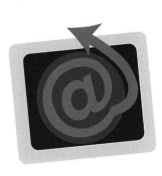

Search the Internet to find images illustrating the location of the limbic system and the interconnections among its components.

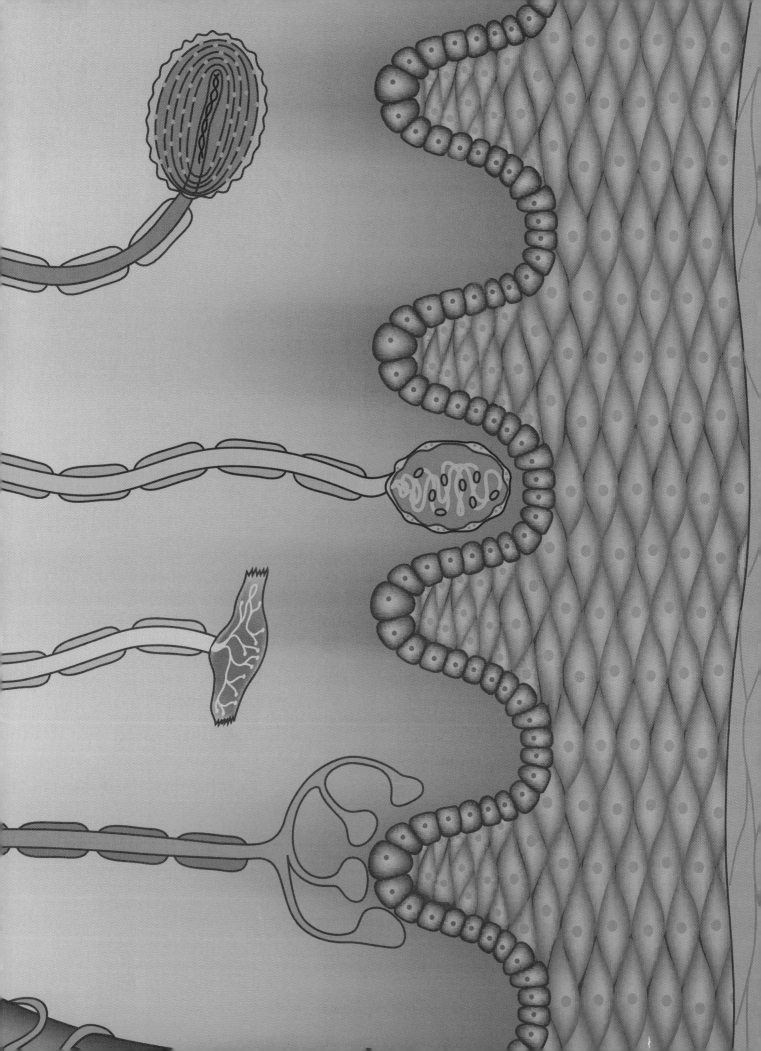

SENSORY SYSTEMS

In our description of motor systems in Part III, we frequently mentioned the role played by sensory information in initiating and modulating motor output. In some cases, such as the muscle-spindle sensory structure and the vestibular organ, we found it necessary to describe the sensory side of the control system in some detail. Sensory information about the environment and about the state of the organism's own body represents the starting point for much of the motor behavior of an animal. That is, much motor output is generated as a result of the receipt of a specific sensory stimulus. In this part of the book, we will examine in detail the portions of the nervous system devoted to obtaining and processing information about the environment—the sensory systems.

Chapter 13 introduces some general properties of sensory systems. The remainder of this part then examines the anatomical and physiological organization of specific sensory systems, with chapters devoted to each of the important sensory modalities. Chapter 14 explores the processing of information from the somatic senses, which arise from receptors located in the skin and musculature. The somatic senses include touch, pressure, pain, and temperature, as well as sensations related to muscle length, tension, and joint position. Chapters 15 and 16 discuss the visual system—one of the important ways that animals gather sensory information about the environment from a distance. Chapter 17 describes the auditory system and Chapter 18, the chemical senses (taste and olfaction).

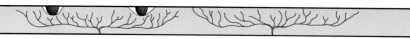

AN OVERVIEW OF SENSORY SYSTEMS

ESSENTIAL BACKGROUND

Excitatory and inhibitory synaptic transmission (Chapter 6)

Action potential (Chapter 4)

Evolution has equipped the nervous system with a great variety of specialized subsystems designed to gather information about the environment. This information is required for the nervous system as a whole to coordinate the actions of the organism in ways that make sense for survival. In subsequent chapters in Part IV, we will examine in detail the functional organization of some of these sensory systems. First, however, we will introduce some of the general principles of sensory systems that apply across the board, regardless of the type of sensory information being gathered from the environment.

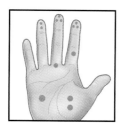

THE SENSORY RECEPTOR NEURON

Sensory Receptor Neurons Respond to Particular Types of Stimulus Energy

In order for the nervous system to react to an environmental stimulus, the energy form of that stimulus must be translated into an electrical signal, which can then be transmitted and processed in the nervous system. This task of translation is carried out by the **sensory receptor neurons** (also called **primary sensory receptors**), which sit at the interface between the nervous system and the outside world. The properties of our sensory receptors govern which aspects of the environment we are aware of and which aspects pass completely unnoticed. When we watch a bat flying at dusk, for example, it appears to flit silently across the sky. In reality, however, the bat is shrieking frequently and loudly as it flies. Because the bat's high-frequency cries are beyond the range of human hearing, they are not a part of our sensory world.

Even for the parts of the environment we can detect, the properties of our sensory receptors determine our level of sensitivity to stimuli, our ability to sense changes in intensity, and our adeptness at distinguishing qualitatively among different aspects of the stimulus. For example, humans normally perceive and identify colors based on the differential detection of light of a particular wavelength by the different visual pigment molecules found in the three classes of cone photoreceptors in the retina (see Chapter 15). If one class of visual pigment molecule is absent because of a genetic abnormality, the affected individual will confuse colors that normal humans can readily distinguish. Conversely, if a fourth pigment were added, a new and greater range of colors could be distinguished. Thus, everything the brain knows about the environment has been filtered through the sensory receptors, and the sensory world of an organism is determined by the sensory cells with which it is endowed.

If an organism is able to respond to a particular type of environmental stimulus, then it must possess sensory receptors that are sensitive to the form of physical energy that constitutes the stimulus. The nervous system encodes the qualitative properties of a stimulus based on the types of sensory neurons that are activated by it. Activity in neurons connected to photoreceptors will be interpreted by the nervous system as providing information about light, activity in neurons connected to muscle-spindle receptors will be interpreted as giving information about muscle stretch, and so on. The perceived **modality** of a stimulus (that is, whether it is perceived as light, touch, pain, or another sensation) is governed by the type of sensory neuron activated by the stimulus.

Coding of Stimulus Intensity

A generalized scheme for the processing of sensory information in the nervous system is summarized in Figure 13.1. When an event happens in the environment, an energy signal becomes available to interact with the sensory receptors that can detect that form of energy. The signal may be mechanical, as when the organism touches or is touched by an object in the environment (an "object" may include the molecules of air or water that transmit pressure waves leading to the sensation of sound). In the case of vision, the signal is electromagnetic (photons of light of particular wavelengths). The signal also may be chemical, as in olfaction, taste, or monitoring of the chemical state of the blood. These signals are transformed into electrical signals through the process of **sensory transduction**, which is the first event in the generation of a sensory signal. The electrical signal generated in the sensory receptor is called the **receptor potential**.

How do sensory receptor neurons translate a sensory stimulus into an electrical signal?

How does the nervous system encode the intensity of a sensory stimulus?

Figure 13.1.

A summary of the steps required in the processing of sensory information by the nervous system. Physical energy from the environment impinges on the organism and acts on specialized primary sensory receptor neurons. These specialized cells translate the physical energy of the stimulus into an electrical signal, a process termed sensory transduction. The electrical signal in the receptor neuron is then translated into action potentials in the intensity-coding stage. The action potentials pass through several stages of sensory analysis to extract information about the environment, which is then combined with motor commands to control the organism's motor output.

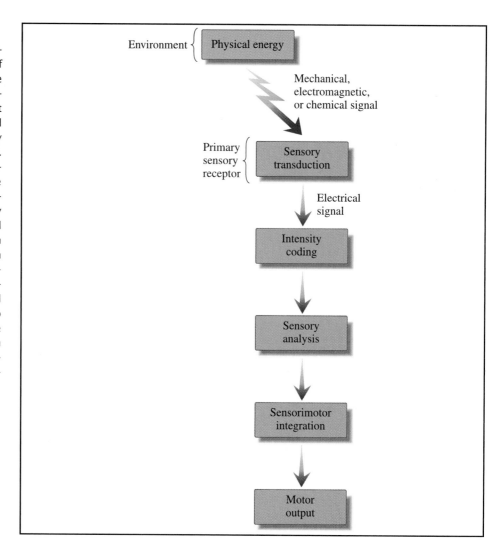

In most cases, mere detection of the presence of a stimulus is not sufficient. The nervous system also requires information about the strength of the stimulus. In most sensory receptors, the receptor potential is graded in size according to the intensity of the stimulus. For example, a strong light gives rise to a large change in the membrane potential of the photoreceptors in the eye, whereas a weak light produces a correspondingly smaller change in membrane potential (see Chapter 15). Figure 13.2A shows the relationship between the amplitude of a receptor potential and the strength of a sensory stimulus. As stimulus intensity progressively increases, the threshold intensity for the receptor is reached, and the receptor cell begins to respond. As intensity increases further, the amplitude of the receptor potential grows larger, until the maximum amplitude is reached. Thus, coding of stimulus strength is an inherent feature of the transduction process. This method of encoding stimulus strength is referred to as **amplitude coding**, to reflect the fact that the size of the electrical signal gives information about the strength of the stimulus that generated the signal.

Electrical signals are transmitted over long distances in the nervous system by action potentials, and so the graded receptor potential in the sensory receptor neuron must ultimately be translated into action potential activity. The action potentials may be triggered in the primary receptor neuron itself or in a secondary sensory neuron (a **second-order sensory neuron**) that receives synaptic input from the sensory cell. Because action potentials are all-or-none events (see Chapter 4), further increases in the receptor potential above the level necessary to trigger an

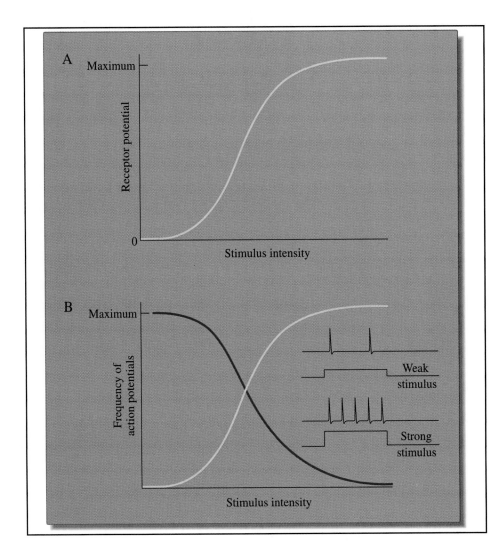

A

Maximum

Receptor potential

0

Stimulus intensity

B

Maximum

Frequency of
action potentials

Weak
stimulus

Strong
stimulus

Stimulus intensity

Figure 13.2.

The coding of stimulus intensity in the nervous system. **A.** In the primary sensory receptor neurons, the sensory stimulus produces a receptor potential whose amplitude increases with stimulus intensity. **B.** The receptor potential influences the rate of firing of action potentials, in either the primary receptor neuron or a secondary neuron that receives synaptic input from the primary receptor neuron. A weak stimulus produces action potentials at a low rate, while a strong stimulus produces action potentials at a rapid rate (see *inset*). The stimulus intensity can be encoded by either a decrease in action potential activity (*dark curve*) or an increase in action potential activity (*yellow curve*).

action potential will not be reflected in the amplitude of the action potential. Therefore, another intensity-coding mechanism besides amplitude coding is needed to signal the amplitude of the sensory stimulus. In many cases, the stimulus intensity is coded by the frequency of action potential firing in the sensory neuron, as shown in Figure 13.2B. A weak stimulus causes a small receptor potential and triggers action potentials only infrequently. A stronger stimulus produces a larger receptor potential and causes the sensory neurons to fire action potentials more frequently during the stimulus.

At stages of sensory processing after the generation of action potentials, the stimulus intensity is encoded by the frequency of action potentials during the stimulus. This method of encoding stimulus intensity is called **frequency coding**. The relationship between firing frequency and stimulus intensity is shown in Figure 13.2B. Figure 13.2B also demonstrates that stimulus intensity can be encoded by either a *decrease* in action potential activity or an *increase* in action potential activity. That is, cessation of firing can effectively signal the presence and intensity of a stimulus. In sensory systems, neurons that decrease their firing during a sensory stimulus (the "off" pathway) are frequently found in addition to neurons that increase their firing during a stimulus (the "on" pathway). The visual system is a good example of this principle (see Chapter 15). Neurons that receive inputs from both the on and off pathways can obtain a sensitive indication of stimulus intensity by comparing the level of action potential activity in the neurons of the on and off systems.

Figure 13.3.

Examples of responses of skin sensory receptor neurons. The traces show intracellular recordings of membrane potentials from a touch-sensitive neuron (**A**), a pressure-sensitive neuron (**B**), and a nociceptor neuron (**C**). Activity was stimulated by applying a blunt probe to the skin at the times indicated by the stimulus line below each trace. The pressure applied by the probe was very light for the touch receptor, moderate for the pressure receptor, and very strong for the nociceptor.

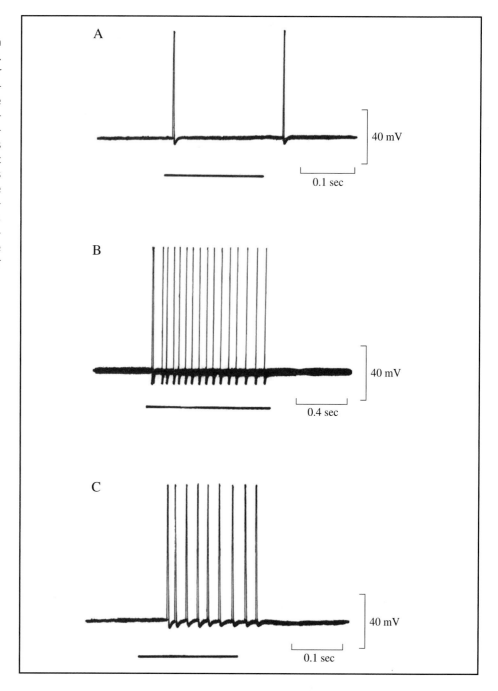

Stimulus intensity also is encoded by the population of sensory neurons activated by a stimulus. Strong stimuli activate more of the total population than do weak stimuli. Thus, neurons in a sensory system can obtain an indication of stimulus intensity by pooling activity across the population of sensory neurons sensitive to the stimulus. In addition, individual sensory receptors differ in their sensitivity to sensory stimuli, with some being activated by weaker stimuli and others only by stronger stimuli. For example, sensory receptor neurons that innervate the skin demonstrate widely varying threshold levels of mechanical stimulation for triggering action potentials. Some respond to light touch or brushing of the skin, others react to strong pressure on the skin, and still others respond only to stimuli sufficiently strong to damage the skin.

Figure 13.3 illustrates responses of skin sensory neurons to mechanical stimulation. The most sensitive cells, called touch receptors, respond to gentle pressure or stroking of the skin (see Fig. 13.3A). Pressure receptor cells (see Fig. 13.3B) require stronger pressure for activation. The least sensitive neurons (see Fig. 13.3C) do not respond to either touch or pressure but do react to a stimulus that damages or penetrates the skin. Because these latter cells respond only to damaging levels of stimulation, they are called nociceptors (the Latin verb *nocere* means "to hurt or injure"). Nociceptors produce the sensation of pain in humans. Thus, the nervous system can gauge the strength of mechanical stimulation of the skin, based on the particular populations of skin sensory neurons activated by the stimulus.

THE RECEPTIVE FIELD OF PRIMARY RECEPTOR NEURONS

Another common feature of sensory receptors is revealed by examining responses of individual skin sensory receptors. The pressure receptor cell whose response is shown in Figure 13.3B did not respond to pressure applied to all parts of the animal's body surface. Instead, the cell responded to pressure applied only to a small part of the skin, corresponding to the area where that particular neuron sends its peripheral processes. This portion of the skin where responses can be elicited in a particular sensory neuron is called the receptive field of the neuron.

Receptive fields for skin sensory neurons have different sizes and shapes in different parts of the body. In general, if a body part is particularly important for an organism's interactions with the external world, then many sensory neurons will be devoted to that part of the body, and the receptive fields for the individual neurons will be relatively small. For example, humans and other primates use their hands for many purposes in manipulating the environment. Consequently, the receptive fields of touch receptor neurons that innervate the palm and fingers are quite small, as shown in Figure 13.4. Because a primary sensory neuron signals touch anywhere within its receptive field, a second-order neuron receiving input from the sensory neuron cannot discern where within the receptive field the touch occurred. Having

What is the receptive field of a sensory neuron?

IN THE CLINIC

BOX 1

Sensory systems provide the nervous system with information about the body and the environment. This information arrives in the form of action potentials in the sensory neurons. The subjective sensation that results from these action potentials is determined by the identity of the sensory cell that is firing. This is the labeled line method of sensory coding, and it means that action potentials in a touch-sensitive mechanoreceptor will give rise to sensation of touch in the receptive field of that cell, action potentials in a nociceptor will give rise to sensation of pain in the appropriate receptive field, and so on. This will be true even if the receptive field for the sensory neuron no longer exists, as exemplified by the phenomenon of phantom limb sensation in amputees. When a limb is amputated, the nerves that innervate the limb are severed. Sometimes, however, the axons of the neurons in the cut nerve fire action potentials because of local inflammation or mechanical irritation of the cut end of the nerve. These action potentials are interpreted by the brain as sensations arising in the nonexistent limb. If action potentials arise in nociceptors that used to innervate the missing limb, chronic pain is the result, which can be severely debilitating.

Figure 13.4.

Representative receptive field sizes for light touch at different locations on the fingers, palm, and forearm.

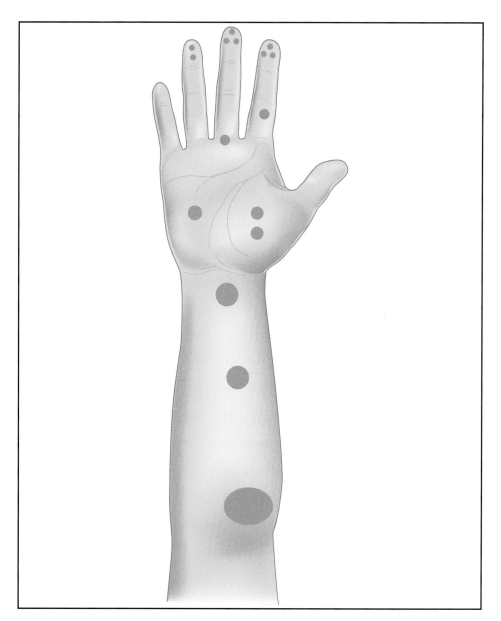

a large number of small receptive fields among the primary sensory neurons allows the population of second-order sensory neurons to construct a fine-grained map of an object being manipulated by the hand. In contrast, the receptive fields of the touch-sensitive sensory neurons are larger on the skin of the forearm, and even larger on the back and the trunk, than they are on the hand. For this reason, humans can easily distinguish two closely spaced objects with the fingertips but not with the forearm.

You can readily demonstrate this difference in receptive field size on yourself, using two blunt pencils (not sharp ones, please). Hold the two pencils together with their points in the same horizontal plane, as illustrated in Figure 13.5. If you touch the two pencils gently with your fingertip, you can readily perceive two distinct points of contact. The arrangement of receptive fields of the touch-sensitive sensory neurons in the fingertip makes this distinction possible, as illustrated in Figure 13.5A. Three sensory receptor neurons are shown for simplicity, but the fingertip is actually innervated by a large number of touch receptor neurons. The receptive fields are so small that sensory neuron A will be stimulated by the pressure of pencil 1, while sensory neuron C will be stimulated by pencil 2. Sensory neuron

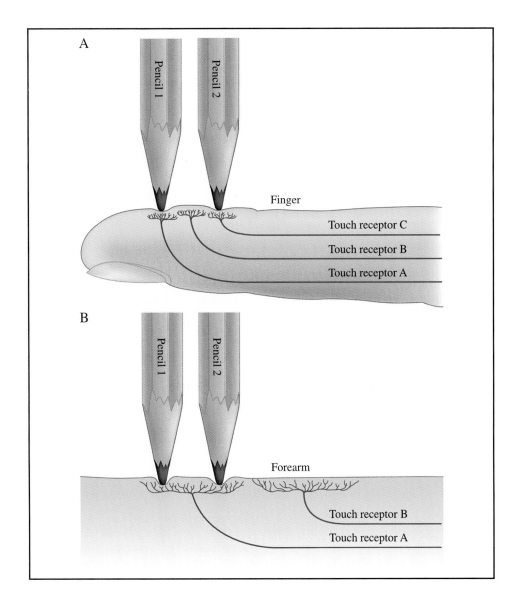

Figure 13.5.

Receptive field size determines the ability to discern closely spaced stimuli. In this experiment, two pencils are held together so that their points are in the same plane and are touched to the skin on the finger or the forearm. **A.** Using the fingertip, we can readily discern the two pencil tips. Each touch receptor neuron innervates a small patch of skin in the fingertip, giving rise to a small receptive field. **B.** In the forearm, the receptive fields of individual neurons are larger. The two pencil points fall within a single receptive field and thus cannot be distinguished.

B, on the other hand, will not be stimulated. When this pattern of action potentials reaches the brain, it gives rise to the perception of two points of contact, separated by an unstimulated region.

Now repeat the experiment, touching the pencils to the skin on the underside of the forearm (the underside works better because it is typically less hairy). This new situation is diagrammed in Figure 13.5B. In the forearm, the receptive fields of the skin sensory neurons are much larger, and both pencil tips fall within the receptive field of sensory neuron A. Sensory neuron B is not stimulated. The neurons of the brain sensory systems cannot discern that the action potentials in sensory neuron A were stimulated by two separate contact points, rather than a single contact point. Thus, the receptive field size of the primary sensory neurons limits the ability of a sensory system to discern small spatial variations in a stimulus object.

LATERAL INHIBITION

In reality, the arrangement of the receptive fields of adjacent sensory neurons on the skin is not as simple as that shown in Figure 13.5A, in which the fields of adjacent sensory neurons do not overlap. The receptive fields of sensory neurons actually overlap substantially. This overlap might be predicted to blur the localization

What is the role of lateral inhibition in the processing of sensory information?

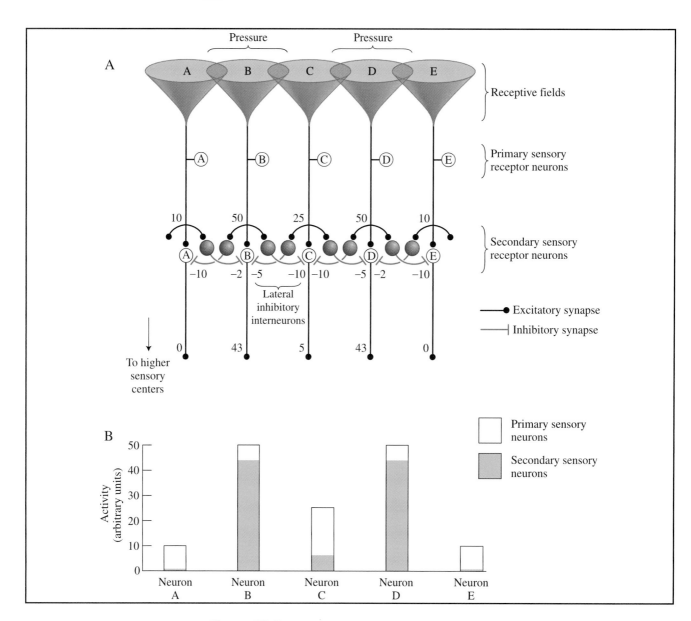

of a stimulus, because touch applied to any location would activate more than one receptor neuron. However, the synaptic interconnections among the higher-level neurons that receive inputs from the primary sensory receptors overcome this blurring action and enhance the discrimination of closely spaced stimuli.

Figure 13.6A shows that inhibitory interneurons at the second level of sensory processing are a key feature of the enhancement of spatial discrimination. Primary sensory neurons make excitatory synaptic connections with local inhibitory interneurons, as well as second-order neurons that send axons to higher sensory centers in the brain. The inhibitory interneurons extend lateral axons that make in-

Figure 13.6.

The effect of lateral inhibition on the ability to discriminate two closely spaced stimuli applied to the skin. **A.** A schematic diagram of the connections from five primary sensory receptor neurons (receptor neurons A to E) to their corresponding second-order sensory neurons in the central nervous system. The overlapping receptive fields of the neurons in the skin are shown above. The numbers next to each synaptic connection indicate the amount of excitatory activity (in arbitrary units) contributed by that synapse to the postsynaptic neuron. Negative numbers indicate an inhibitory influence. **B.** A bar graph showing the amount of activity in the primary receptor neurons (*unshaded*) and in the secondary neurons (*shaded tan*).

hibitory synaptic contact with the second-order neurons receiving connections from the *adjacent* primary sensory receptors. In this manner, the activity in a particular pathway (corresponding to a particular receptive field) feeds back to subtract from the activity in adjacent pathways. Because the inhibitory connections are made with the pathways to the side, this process is termed **lateral inhibition**. Lateral inhibitory interactions are a common feature of information processing in most sensory systems, not just in the skin sensory system.

Consider the specific example shown in Figure 13.6A. Two stimuli are applied that fill the receptive fields of two receptor neurons, neurons B and D in the figure. These two neurons fire action potentials corresponding to 50 arbitrary units of excitation arriving at the synapses with second-order neurons in the central nervous system.

Because of the overlapping receptive fields, the two stimuli also activate the three other receptor neurons, A, C, and E. The stimuli fall on only a portion of these receptive fields, however, so these three neurons have less activity than do neurons B and D. Primary receptor neurons A and E fire action potentials at a rate corresponding to 10 arbitrary units of excitation at their excitatory synapses with second-order neurons. The receptive field of sensory receptor neuron C is partially activated by both stimuli, so the activity in this neuron will be somewhat higher, corresponding to 25 arbitrary units of excitation in the example.

The outputs of the second-order neurons also depend on the effect of the lateral inhibitory connections. For purposes of illustration, we assume that the inhibitory connections in the lateral pathways produce sufficient inhibition to subtract 20% of the driving excitation from the primary sensory neuron of each pathway. For example, the lateral inhibitory interneurons driven by primary receptor B provide 10 units of inhibition (20% of 50, the amount of excitation in primary receptor B) to the neighboring secondary sensory neurons (A and C). Thus, second-order neurons A and E receive 10 units of excitation from their primary neurons and 10 units of inhibition from the neighboring, strongly stimulated pathways. Secondary neurons A and E remain silent, although their primary receptor neurons are mildly stimulated by the sensory stimuli. Second-order neuron C receives 25 units of excitation from its primary neuron but receives 10 units of inhibition from each side. The result is that second-order neuron C is minimally activated, even though its primary sensory neuron is moderately stimulated. Secondary sensory neurons B and D receive strong excitation from their primary sensory receptor neurons but only mild inhibition from their lateral inhibitory interneurons. Thus, these secondary neurons are maximally stimulated by the sensory stimuli.

The overall behavior of the network is shown graphically in Figure 13.6B for both the primary sensory neurons and the secondary neurons. The second-order neurons whose corresponding receptive fields are maximally stimulated (B and D) receive much excitation but little inhibition from their neighbors, whose corresponding receptive fields are not maximally stimulated. Conversely, the second-order neurons that are not maximally stimulated receive relatively little excitation but greater inhibition from their highly active neighbors. Thus, lateral inhibition enhances the contrast in activity between the second-order neurons receiving inputs from the maximally stimulated primary receptors and the neighboring pathways originating from adjacent receptive fields.

Notice that the bars in Figure 13.6B that correspond to the activity in the second-order neurons differ from one another more than the bars that correspond to the activity in the primary sensory neurons. In this way, the lateral inhibitory connections accentuate the differential activity present in the array of primary sensory receptors, enhancing the demarcation between stimulated and unstimulated regions. Lateral inhibition is also a prominent feature of synaptic processing in the visual system, where it serves to accentuate the boundary between light and dark portions of the visual world (see Chapter 15).

Another common feature of sensory systems is highlighted by our discussion of the circuitry of lateral inhibition. In Figure 13.6A, the primary sensory receptors connect in an orderly way with the second-order neurons, and the array of receptive fields of the primary receptors is retained in the spatial organization of the second-order neurons. The receptor surface (the skin, in our example) forms a map on the "surface" of the second-order neurons, which is retained as information is passed through subsequent sensory relay stations. This **somatotopic mapping** of the peripheral sensory system onto the neural systems involved in sensory processing in the brain is analogous to the somatotopic map of the body in the motor cortex (see Chapter 9). In Chapter 11, we saw a similar mapping of the retina surface onto the superior colliculus.

As in the motor map in the motor cortex, the representation of the skin in the internal sensory map in the brain does not depend on the actual surface area of the skin in different body regions. Instead, the representation in the map depends on the number of receptor neurons that innervate a particular region of the skin. As a result, body parts that have small receptive fields and thus large numbers of neurons per square centimeter of skin area receive a correspondingly larger representation in the sensory map in the central nervous system. The same principle applies for other sensory systems as well.

A related concept is the presence of information channels in the processing of sensory information in the central nervous system. In Figure 13.6A, neighboring touch receptive regions of the skin are segregated into neighboring pathways, or channels, in the subsequent processing of sensory information. These pathways form spatially coherent information channels, which simplify the wiring of the inhibitory connections underlying lateral inhibition. Local inhibitory interneurons can then form synaptic connections with all neighboring, through-conducting second-order neurons, creating the appropriate circuitry without elaborate identification schemes that would be required if the information channels were randomly intermixed.

Lateral Inhibition Alters the Receptive Fields of Higher-Order Sensory Neurons

How do synaptic connections among sensory neurons alter the receptive field of higher-order sensory neurons?

The receptive field of a neuron is defined as that portion of the sensory surface where stimuli affect the neuron's activity. For the primary sensory receptor neurons of the skin, this area corresponds to the portion of the skin contacted by the receptor endings of the neuron. The receptive field of higher-order neurons, however, differs from that of the primary receptor, because of the synaptic interactions mediated by lateral inhibitory interneurons.

Figure 13.7 illustrates the change in receptive field in a second-order sensory neuron. A stimulus is applied to the receptive field of a skin receptor neuron (receptor B), without activating the neighboring receptor (receptor A). The second-order neuron that receives a direct synaptic input from receptor B will be strongly excited. The second-order neuron that receives input from primary receptor A receives no excitation but does receive inhibitory input from the lateral inhibitory interneuron of pathway B. Even in the absence of a sensory stimulus, most higher-order sensory neurons typically fire action potentials at a moderate rate, providing a baseline level of spontaneous activity. Thus, the lateral inhibition from the active neighboring pathway causes second-order neuron A to cease firing during the stimulus.

The activity in second-order neuron A is influenced by stimulation in an area of the skin outside the receptive field of primary receptor A. By the definition of re-

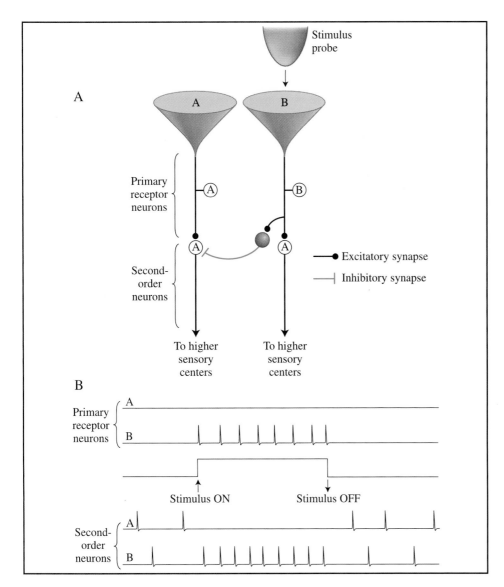

Figure 13.7.

Second-order sensory neurons respond to stimuli outside the receptive field of the primary sensory neuron to which they are directly connected. This response reflects the lateral inhibitory connections among second-order neurons. **A**. A schematic diagram of the synaptic circuitry. The stimulus is applied to the skin in the receptive field of primary sensory neuron B. **B**. Action potential activity during the stimulus in the primary sensory neurons (*above*) and in the second-order sensory neurons (*below*).

ceptive field then, the receptive field of the second-order neuron differs from the receptive field of the primary receptor. At each stage of synaptic processing, as the sensory information is relayed through the brain, the receptive fields of the neurons may change compared to the receptive fields of the neurons at the next lower stage.

If we moved the stimulus probe in Figure 13.7 from receptive field B to A, then the situation would be reversed. The activity in second-order neuron B would be reduced by the stimulus, and second-order neuron A would be excited. Thus, the receptive field of each second-order neuron is organized into an excitatory central region, surrounded by a concentric inhibitory region, as illustrated in Figure 13.8. If we move the stimulus progressively across the skin surface, we can map out the changes in action potential firing in the primary receptor and the second-order neuron, which are summarized in Figure 13.8A. The firing rate of the primary receptor neuron increases as the stimulus enters the receptive field and decreases again as the stimulus exits on the opposite side of the receptive field (see Fig. 13.8A).

When viewed from above, the receptive field of the primary receptor is uniformly excitatory and occupies an area delimited by the spread of the receptor's sensory processes in the skin (see Fig. 13.8B). In contrast, the firing rate of the sec-

Figure 13.8.

Receptive fields of primary and second-order sensory neurons differ because of lateral inhibition. **A**. The frequency of action potentials recorded in a primary sensory neuron (*yellow line*) and in the corresponding second-order neuron (*green line*) in response to a stimulus applied to various positions on the skin. The *dashed line* shows the frequency of "spontaneous" action potentials in the second-order neuron in the absence of stimulation. **B**. A top view of the receptive fields of the primary sensory neuron and the second-order neuron. A *plus sign* indicates that stimuli in that region excite the neuron; a *minus sign* indicates that stimuli in that region inhibit the neuron.

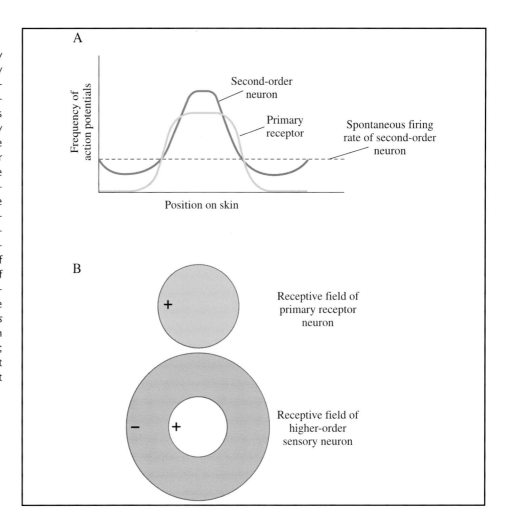

ond-order neuron initially decreases below the baseline rate as the stimulus moves across the skin because of the lateral inhibitory effect originating from the receptive fields of neighboring receptors. The firing rate then increases as the stimulus enters the receptive field of the receptor that makes a direct excitatory connection with the second-order neuron. Finally, the firing rate declines again when the stimulus passes out of this central portion of the receptive field and enters the inhibitory surrounding area on the other side. Figure 13.8B illustrates the inhibitory surround region and the excitatory central region of the receptive field of the second-order neuron.

The central excitatory portion of the receptive field of the second-order neuron is smaller than the purely excitatory receptive field of the primary receptor (see Fig. 13.8B). This size difference arises because of the spatial overlap of neighboring receptive fields of the primary receptors (see, for example, Fig. 13.6). A stimulus near the edge of the receptive field produces relatively weak excitation of the receptor but stronger excitation of the neighboring receptors. The net result will be inhibition of the second-order neuron. Only when the stimulus moves into the central portion of the receptive field will the direct excitatory connection from the primary receptor outweigh the inhibitory influence from the surrounding receptors. This sharpening of the excitatory portion of the receptive field is another important functional outcome of the lateral inhibitory connections—increasing the spatial resolution of the sensory system. Subsequent sensory centers in the brain that receive connections from the second-order neurons can then localize the stimulus on the skin more accurately than would be expected from the sizes of the receptive fields of the primary sensory receptors themselves.

ADAPTATION

Another general feature of sensory receptors is that they respond best to *changes* in stimuli. During a sustained stimulus, the response of the receptor typically diminishes or ceases altogether—a phenomenon known as sensory **adaptation**. In the touch receptor neuron shown in Figure 13.3A, for instance, the touch receptor fired only a single action potential at the onset of the stimulus and did not fire again, even though the stimulus probe remained in contact with the skin for some time. This example illustrates the behavior of a rapidly adapting sensory receptor. The touch receptor also fired another action potential when the probe was removed from the skin. This response to stimulus removal is commonly seen in touch receptor neurons, which might more properly be called skin-disturbance detectors that respond to a *change* in skin indentation within their receptive fields.

Unlike the touch receptor, the pressure receptor neuron fired a train of action potentials during indentation of the skin (see Figure 13.3B). Thus, the pressure receptor adapts more slowly than the touch receptor. If you look carefully at Figure 13.3B, however, you can see that the interval between successive action potentials lengthened during the pressure stimulus. In other words, the frequency of firing declined progressively, indicating that the pressure receptor also adapts during sustained stimulation.

The sensory receptors are our windows on the external world, and everything we know about the external world is governed by the outputs of these receptors. If the frequency of action potentials in the receptors declines during a sustained stimulus, the perceived magnitude of the stimulus diminishes in tandem. For example, you can readily feel the pressure exerted by a watchband when you first put on a wristwatch, but your perception of the pressure disappears within seconds because of receptor adaptation. Sensory adaptation is also readily apparent in the visual system. If you go from a dark movie theater to bright sunlight, you are initially dazzled by the brightness. Within minutes, however, your visual system adapts to the new conditions and the brightness of the light no longer seems overwhelming.

Sensory adaptation stems from two sources. First, adaptation occurs during the sensory transduction process in the primary receptors themselves. During a sustained stimulus, the amplitude of the receptor potential declines, which is then reflected in a reduced action potential frequency in the primary receptors or in the second-order neurons receiving synaptic input from the receptors. Second, adaptation results from changes in the synaptic interactions among neurons in the sensory system. For instance, the amount of neurotransmitter released from presynaptic terminals by an action potential may decline during a sustained train of action potentials, a phenomenon called **synaptic depression**. Even in the absence of synaptic depression, the postsynaptic response may decline during sustained activity because of postsynaptic changes mediated by a slow accumulation of internal second messengers or by synaptic feedback from other neurons. Collectively, these nonreceptor forms of adaptation are termed **neural adaptation**.

CLASSIFICATION OF SENSORY RECEPTOR TYPE

Sensory receptors can be classified into broad categories based on the source of the sensory stimulus. Sensory receptor cells that receive stimuli from the world outside of the organism are called **exteroceptive receptors** (or exteroceptors). These receptors that monitor the external environment include the visual recep-

What classifications of sensory receptor neurons exist?

tors, hearing receptors, touch receptors, smell receptors, and so on. Other receptors, called **interoceptive receptors** (or interoceptors), monitor the internal environment of the organism; they include the blood pressure sensors of the carotid sinus (see Chapter 11). Finally, **proprioceptive receptors** (proprioceptors) monitor the position of the body in space or the position of joints and muscles. Examples include the muscle-spindle stretch receptors, which form the sensory input to the patellar stretch reflex, and the gravity sensors of the vestibular apparatus (see Chapter 10).

Receptor neurons also can be classified based on the type of sensory stimulus to which they respond. In this chapter, we focused on receptors that respond to mechanical displacement, known as **mechanoreceptors**. The muscle-spindle receptors, the Golgi tendon organs, the touch and pressure receptors, and vestibular hair cells are all examples of mechanoreceptors. The sensory cells of the visual system that translate light energy into electrical signals are called **photoreceptors**. **Chemoreceptors** are cells that detect and respond to chemical substances from outside the body (for example, olfactory receptors) or inside the body (for example, oxygen sensors in the circulatory system). As described earlier, **nociceptors** respond to tissue damage and give rise to the sensation of pain. Nociceptors may actually be a class of chemoreceptors that detect substances released by damaged cells or as part of local inflammatory responses to damage. Other skin receptors, called **thermoreceptors**, respond to skin temperature (either hot or cold). Some species of fish can detect the weak electrical fields generated in the water by the activity of the muscles of other fish. This information is used to locate prey or mates and in some instances is used for communication. The receptor cells that detect the electrical fields are called **electroreceptors**.

SUMMARY

Sensory systems are the parts of the nervous system that detect and analyze stimuli from the external and the internal environment of the organism. Primary receptor neurons are the cells at the interface between the environment and the nervous system. Through the process of sensory transduction, the primary receptor neurons translate mechanical, chemical, or light energy from the environment into an electrical signal that can be passed along and analyzed in the nervous system.

Sensory stimuli generate electrical signals called receptor potentials in the primary receptor neurons. The receptor potential, which is graded in size according to the stimulus intensity, stimulates action potentials in either the primary sensory neurons or the second-order neurons that receive synaptic input from the primary receptors. The intensity of the stimulus is encoded by the frequency of action potentials, with more intense stimuli causing a higher rate of firing.

The receptive field of a sensory neuron is defined as the portion of the relevant sensory surface where receipt of a stimulus affects the activity of the neuron. The receptive fields of second-order and higher neurons are determined by the set of sensory receptors from which they receive synapses and by lateral inhibitory interactions. Lateral inhibition improves the spatial resolution of the sensory system. Receptive fields of second-order and higher neurons commonly have a concentric organization, with a central excitatory region surrounded by a ring-shaped inhibitory region. Sensory receptors typically show adaptation during sustained stimuli, with the response of the sensory cell diminishing even though the stimulus remains the same.

1. Describe why you agree or disagree with the following statement: The intensity of a sensory stimulus is encoded by the amplitude of the action potential generated by the stimulus in the primary receptor neuron.

2. What is the difference between "on" pathways and "off" pathways in a sensory system?

3. What is the definition of the receptive field of a sensory neuron?

4. Compare the receptive fields of a primary touch-sensitive receptor neuron and a second-order touch-sensitive neuron. Explain the differences between the two.

5. Discuss the following: Lateral inhibition enhances the contrast between regions of a sensory surface receiving stimuli of different intensities.

6. Define the following: exteroceptor, interoceptor, proprioceptor.

7. What is sensory adaptation, and how does it influence the perceived intensity of a sensory stimulus?

8. Why is it more difficult to discriminate two closely spaced touch stimuli on the forearm than on the hand?

INTERNET ASSIGNMENT   CHAPTER 13

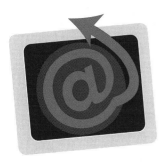

A fundamental aspect of sensory function is lateral inhibition, which was first described in studies of the compound eye of the horseshoe crab, genus *Limulus*. Research the work of Haldan K. Hartline and describe his contributions to the concept of lateral inhibition and its role in sensory processing.

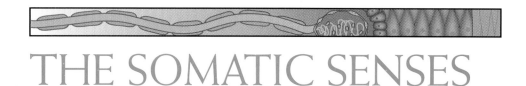

THE SOMATIC SENSES

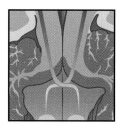

In Chapter 13, we described some of the properties of the sensory receptor neurons that innervate the skin. In Chapter 8 we discussed the response properties of muscle-spindle organs and Golgi tendon organs. In this chapter, we will consider how the sensory information arising from the skin and muscle receptors is analyzed by neural systems in the spinal cord and brain.

SOMATOSENSORY RECEPTORS

Skin Receptors

Collectively, the neural pathways concerned with the processing of signals arising from the receptors of the skin, muscles, and joints are called the **somatosensory** pathways. Several types of sensory receptors contribute to the somatosensory system. Figures 14.1 and 14.2 summarize the receptor types found in the human somatosensory system. When activated, each receptor type gives rise to a specific sensation, called the **sensory modality**. Some receptors give rise to the sensation of touch, some to the sensation of pressure, and still others to pain. The skin receptors can be distinguished based on the strength of stimulation required to excite them and on their adaptation characteristics.

In addition to these functional differences, there are anatomical differences in the types of sensory endings formed by the receptor neurons within the skin (see Fig. 14.1). The touch- and pressure-sensitive mechanoreceptors form specialized structures within the skin that help to determine the response properties of the receptor neuron. Three types of mechanoreceptors have nerve endings that terminate within fibrous capsules, called **corpuscles**. The **Pacinian corpuscle** and the **Meissner corpuscle** are very sensitive to touch and pressure, and both adapt rapidly during a sustained stimulus. Thus, these mechanoreceptors predominantly signal changes in stimulus intensity. Because of their rapid adaptation, both Pacinian and Meissner corpuscles are particularly sensitive to vibrating stimuli. A third type of encapsulated mechanoreceptor, the **Ruffini corpuscle**, is also sensitive to touch and pressure but adapts slowly during sustained stimuli. Another type of slowly adapting mechanoreceptor is the **Merkel receptor**, whose endings are not encapsulated but instead are a spray of endings that contact special epidermal cells (Merkel cells; the combination of the sensory ending and the epidermal cell is called a Merkel disk; see Fig. 14.1). Because of their slow adaptation, Merkel receptors and Ruffini corpuscles are well suited for encoding the intensity of a maintained pressure applied to the skin. A fifth type of mechanoreceptor, the **hair follicle receptor**, is found in hairy skin. These nerve endings spiral around single hair follicles and fire a rapidly adapting burst of action potentials when the hair originating from that follicle is deflected.

All skin mechanoreceptor neurons have moderately large-diameter axons that are myelinated. The conduction velocity of these axons is in the range of 30 to 70 m/sec, which is a bit slower than the larger-diameter axons of the muscle spindles (**group Ia**, 75 to 120 m/sec) and the Golgi tendon organs (**group Ib**, 50 to 100 m/sec; see Chapter 8). The medium-sized myelinated axons of the mechanoreceptors are called **group II**. (An alternative terminology for this group is **group Aβ**, with the faster-conducting muscle receptor axons being **group Aα**.)

The transduction mechanism that couples mechanical stimulation to a change in membrane potential is not completely understood in skin mechanoreceptors. Mechanical deformation of the membrane causes depolarization (the **receptor potential**), which in turn activates action potentials in the nerve fiber of the sensory neuron. The receptor potential arises when mechanosensitive nonspecific cation channels open in the sensory nerve ending. As with the opening of acetylcholine-gated nonspecific cation channels at the neuromuscular junction (see Chapter 5), the resulting increase in sodium and potassium permeability generates a depolarization. Exactly how deformation of the membrane induces the channels to open remains unclear. Ion channels that are activated by membrane stretch have been recorded in a variety of cell types, including neurons. The channel protein is thought to be physically connected to the cytoskeleton, so that movement of the

What types of sensory receptor neurons are found in the skin?

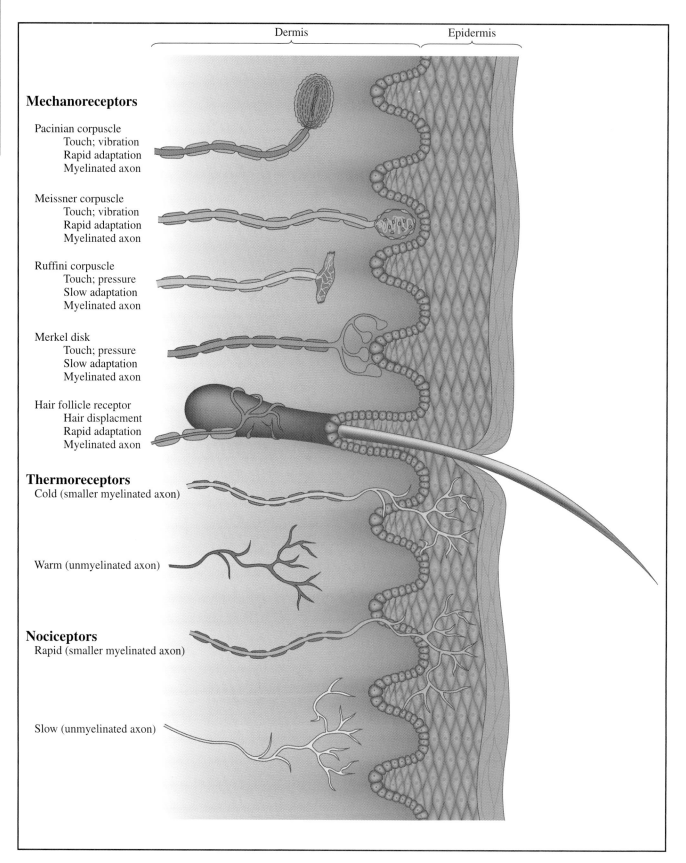

Mechanoreceptors

Pacinian corpuscle
Touch; vibration
Rapid adaptation
Myelinated axon

Meissner corpuscle
Touch; vibration
Rapid adaptation
Myelinated axon

Ruffini corpuscle
Touch; pressure
Slow adaptation
Myelinated axon

Merkel disk
Touch; pressure
Slow adaptation
Myelinated axon

Hair follicle receptor
Hair displacment
Rapid adaptation
Myelinated axon

Thermoreceptors
Cold (smaller myelinated axon)

Warm (unmyelinated axon)

Nociceptors
Rapid (smaller myelinated axon)

Slow (unmyelinated axon)

Dermis   Epidermis

Figure 14.1.

A summary of the sensory receptor types found in human skin. Not all parts of the skin contain all of the receptor types depicted. The density of receptors also varies in different regions of the skin.

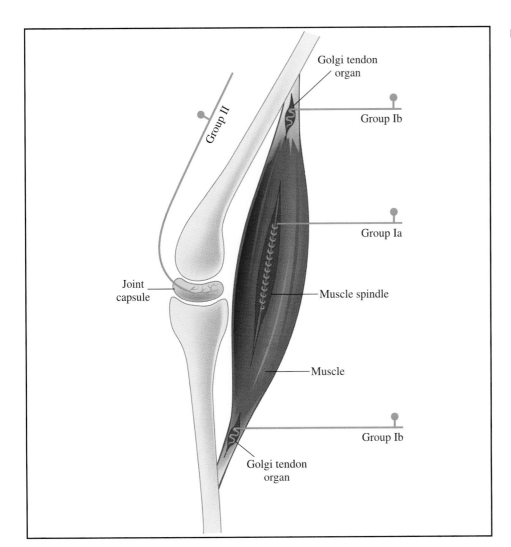

Figure 14.2.

A summary of receptor types involved in proprioception. The muscle spindle and the Golgi tendon organ of skeletal muscles were discussed in Chapter 8. The joint capsule receives sensory innervation from sensory neurons that respond to changes in joint angle.

membrane relative to the cytoskeleton either increases or decreases tension applied to the channel molecule. The change in tension presumably induces a conformational change in the channel, causing it to open and conduct ions.

Mammalian skin also is innervated by **thermoreceptor neurons** whose endings are particularly sensitive to the temperature of the skin (relative to body temperature). As shown in Figure 14.1, there are two types of thermoreceptors. **Cold receptors** are stimulated when the skin is cooled below the resting body temperature and have myelinated axons of **group III** (or **group Aδ**), which conduct more slowly than the mechanoreceptor axons. **Warm receptors** become active when the skin is warmed above the resting body temperature. The axons of warm receptors are unmyelinated and thus conduct action potentials relatively slowly (less than 1 m/sec) compared with myelinated fibers. The unmyelinated axons form conduction **group IV**, the slowest class of conduction speed. The unmyelinated axons also are called **C-fibers**, a term derived from the alternative name **group C** for the slowest-conducting axons in peripheral nerves. The thermoreceptors have no specialized sensory structures in the skin; instead, their axons form numerous fine branches called **free endings**. The process by which changes in skin temperature give rise to receptor potentials in the free endings of thermoreceptor neurons is unknown.

The **nociceptors** are the final class of sensory receptors found in the skin. These neurons fire when the skin is damaged in some way, such as pinching or puncture of the skin, or damaging levels of heat (skin temperatures higher than 45°C). Nociceptors produce the sensation of pain in humans. Nociceptors have either unmyelinated or small-diameter myelinated axons. The faster-conducting, myelinated nociceptors (group III or group Aδ) provide the sensory stimulus for activation of the withdrawal reflex (see Chapter 8) and give rise to the flash of searing pain we perceive immediately when a wound occurs. The unmyelinated nociceptors produce the long-lasting burning pain that persists after the damage is done (the pain we feel from a sunburn is a mild example of this sensation). The axons of the nociceptors form free endings in the skin. The free endings are thought to detect chemical substances released from damaged tissue. Thus, nociceptors may represent a type of chemoreceptor.

Proprioceptive Receptors

What types of sensory receptor neurons innervate the muscles and joints?

In addition to the sensory information arising from the receptors in the skin, the somatosensory pathways of the spinal cord and brain also transmit sensory information related to joint and limb position. Collectively, this type of sensory information is called **proprioception**. Proprioceptive information arises from the sensory receptors shown in Figure 14.2. The **muscle spindle** and the **Golgi tendon organ** give information about muscle length and muscle tension, respectively, as described in Chapter 8. In addition, mechanoreceptors that innervate the **joint capsule** give information about the angle of the skeletal elements at each point of articulation. The intrafusal muscle fibers of the muscle spindle are innervated by group Ia sensory fibers, the Golgi tendon organs are innervated by group Ib sensory fibers, and the joint capsules are innervated by sensory axons of group II.

In mammals, the muscle spindle contains two different types of intrafusal muscle fibers, called **nuclear bag** and **nuclear chain** fibers. The group Ia sensory axon innervating the muscle spindle makes annulospiral endings (called **primary endings**) on both types of muscle fiber within the spindle. In addition, the nuclear chain fibers receive a second spiral ending (called a **secondary ending**) from a smaller-diameter sensory axon of group II. The primary and secondary sensory neurons respond differently to stretch of the muscle. The secondary ending provides a steady discharge that reflects the steady-state stretch of the nuclear chain fibers (and thus the overall length of the muscle). The primary ending also has a steady discharge that signals the steady-state length, but its discharge increases dramatically when the length changes. Thus, the secondary sensory neuron signals the static length of the muscle, while the primary sensory neuron signals the change in length during stretch. To reflect these functional differences, the primary sensory fiber is also called the **dynamic** fiber and the secondary sensory fiber is called the **static** fiber.

SPINAL ORGANIZATION OF SOMATOSENSORY PATHWAYS

What parts of the white matter in the spinal cord contain axons carrying somatosensory information?

The cell bodies of the sensory neurons that provide the sensory information described earlier are located just outside the spinal cord in the dorsal root ganglia. The sensory axons enter the spinal cord via the dorsal roots and make synaptic connections that mediate the various spinal reflexes (see Chapter 8). In addition, the sensory information is transmitted to higher centers in the brain, where it is further analyzed and integrated with other sensory and motor information.

The ascending sensory axons on their way to the brain are located in the white matter of the spinal cord. Axons representing the different sensory modalities are located in different parts of the white matter. Axons that carry information about touch, pressure, and vibration are found mostly in the **dorsal columns**, whose location is show in Figure 14.3. Information from proprioceptors is also carried by dor-

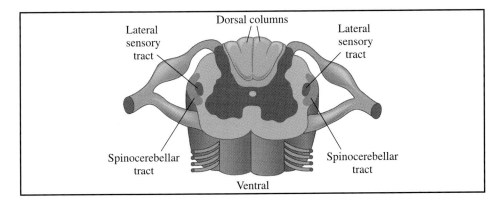

Figure 14.3.

A cross section through the spinal cord at the cervical level, showing the locations of ascending sensory pathways in the white matter. The major pathways are the dorsal columns, the spinocerebellar tracts, and the lateral sensory tracts.

sal column axons. Most myelinated sensory axons in the dorsal columns are branches of the primary sensory neurons themselves. As the axons of the sensory neurons innervating the touch and pressure receptors of the skin enter the spinal cord, they branch as shown in Figure 14.4. One branch enters the gray matter and makes local synaptic connections with spinal interneurons and motor neurons. The other branch enters the dorsal columns on the same side of the spinal cord and ascends into the brain. Thus, skin mechanoreceptor neurons in the dorsal root ganglia can have extraordinarily long axons that reach all the way from the receptive field in the skin (at the tip of the toe, for example) to the brain. In addition, the dorsal columns contain axons of interneurons in the dorsal part of the gray matter that receive direct synaptic connections from the primary sensory neurons. These second-order neurons also carry information from the touch, pressure, and vibration receptors, as well as proprioceptive information (see Fig. 14.4).

Another important group of ascending sensory axons is found in the **lateral sensory tract** of the spinal cord, whose location is shown in Figure 14.3. Unlike the sensory projections in the dorsal column, which mainly consist of axon branches of primary sensory neurons, the axons in the lateral sensory tract are predominantly those of interneurons found in the dorsal part of the gray matter in the spinal cord. These interneurons receive synaptic inputs from pain-sensitive and tempera-

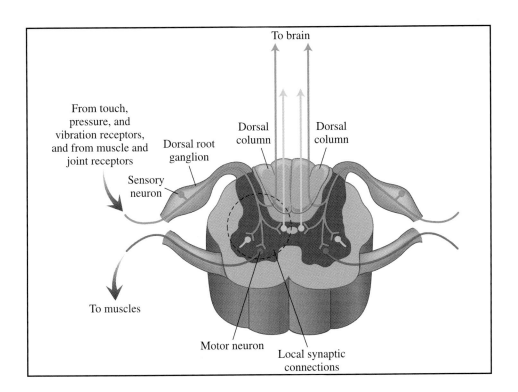

Figure 14.4.

The projection pattern of sensory information in the dorsal columns of the spinal cord. Tactile and proprioceptive sensory neurons (*red*) in the dorsal root ganglia send axons into the gray matter of the spinal cord. There, synaptic connections are made directly onto motor neurons (*blue;* as in the patellar reflex, for example) and onto a variety of spinal cord interneurons (*yellow*). In addition, the axon of the sensory neuron sends a branch into the white matter of the dorsal column on the same side of the spinal cord. This axon ascends in the ipsilateral side of the spinal cord to the brain. A smaller fraction of the ascending axons in the dorsal columns (*yellow*) originate from the interneurons contacted by the primary sensory neurons.

Figure 14.5.

The projection pattern of sensory information in the lateral sensory tracts. Pain-sensitive and temperature-sensitive sensory neurons (*red*) in the dorsal root ganglia send axons into the spinal cord via the dorsal roots. The sensory axons make synaptic connections with interneurons (*yellow*) in the gray matter, whose axons then cross the midline and ascend in the contralateral lateral column. The figure shows only the projections for one side of the spinal cord, but the same projections are present on both sides.

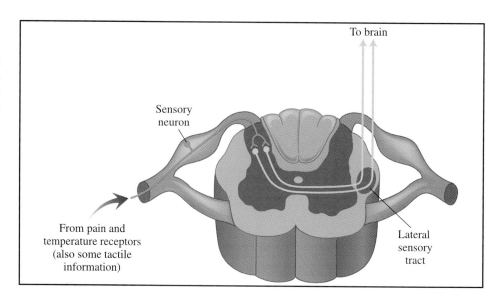

Figure 14.6.

The projection pattern of sensory information in the spinocerebellar tracts. Information to the cerebellum is provided by primary sensory neurons of joint and muscle receptors and tactile receptors (*red*). The sensory neurons are located in the dorsal root ganglia and send axons into the spinal cord via the dorsal roots. Synaptic contacts are made with interneurons in the gray matter of the spinal cord. The interneurons (*yellow*) project to the cerebellum via the spinocerebellar tracts in the lateral columns on either the contralateral or the ipsilateral side of the spinal cord. Note that one of the interneurons illustrated receives inputs from two different sensory neurons. The figure shows only the projections for one side of the spinal cord, but the same projections are present on both sides.

ture-sensitive sensory neurons. Figure 14.5 shows that the axons of the interneurons cross the midline of the spinal cord before entering the lateral sensory tract in the lateral column on the opposite side. Thus, the ascending lateral sensory tract on one side of the spinal cord carries pain and temperature information from the opposite side of the body. In the dorsal columns, the tactile and proprioceptive information on each side of the spinal cord originates from the same side of the body (compare the projection patterns shown in Figs. 14.4 and 14.5). In addition, some interneurons that receive synapses from tactile sensory neurons also send axons into the ascending lateral sensory tract. Thus, tactile and proprioceptive information can reach the brain via either the lateral sensory tract or the dorsal columns, although the latter is the dominant path.

As we discussed in Chapter 9, the cerebellum modifies motor performance based on proprioceptive information about joint and muscle position and tactile information about the contact of the body with the environment. Much of this sensory information is provided by sensory receptor neurons of the dorsal root ganglia. The ascending axons that carry sensory information from the spinal cord to the cerebellum are found in the **spinocerebellar tracts**, located in the lateral portions of the lateral columns (see Fig. 14.3). As with the lateral sensory tract, the axons in the spinocerebellar tract originate from interneurons in the gray matter of the spinal cord. Figure 14.6 shows that some of these interneurons send their axons

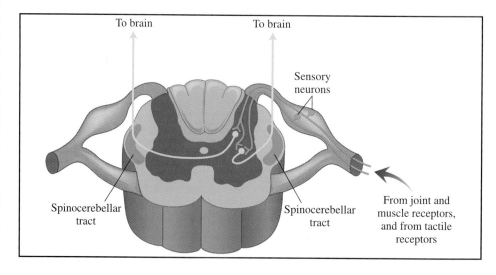

across the midline of the spinal cord to ascend in the contralateral spinocerebellar tract, while others remain on the same side and ascend in the ipsilateral tract.

Some interneurons that give rise to the spinocerebellar tract receive synaptic inputs from more than one type of sensory neuron (see Fig. 14.6). These interneurons can provide information about a confluence of sensory events. For example, limb contact with the ground during locomotion might produce both tactile stimulation (contact with the environment) and muscle stretch, as load from the body weight is transferred to the limb. Combined sensory information of this sort may be useful in the cerebellum's task of modulating motor output based on the sensory outcomes of motor acts.

BRAINSTEM RELAY STATIONS

During the evolution of the vertebrate brain, the brainstem was originally the sole "cerebral ganglion" responsible for modulating the responses of spinal reflex circuits and central pattern generators on the basis of sensory information. In primitive living vertebrates, such as the lamprey, the integrating centers of the reticular formation in the brainstem continue to be the principal targets of ascending sensory information from the spinal cord. As the cerebellum, midbrain, and forebrain became larger and more functionally complex during brain evolution, the older brainstem circuits were retained and modified. Thus, the sensory axons ascending from the spinal cord make a variety of synaptic connections in the brainstem, before the information is passed on to sensory processing centers in the newer parts of the brain.

The principal ascending paths for tactile and proprioceptive information are the dorsal columns, which consist predominantly of axon branches of primary sensory neurons. These ascending axons terminate in the **dorsal column nuclei** near the dorsal surface of the lower medulla, as shown in Figure 14.7. On each side of the medulla, the two dorsal column nuclei are the **gracile nucleus**, which is found nearer to the midline, and the **cuneate nucleus**, which is located more laterally. The gracile nucleus on each side receives axons from the medial portions of the ipsilateral dorsal column, while the cuneate nucleus receives axons from the lateral

What nuclei in the brainstem receive ascending somatosensory information from the spinal cord?

BOX 1

IN THE CLINIC

The spatial segregation of various sensory pathways in the spinal cord can provide important clues to the diagnosis of spinal cord disease or damage. For example, tingling or numbness, or both, in the arms and legs on both sides of the body would suggest a possible problem in the dorsal part of the upper region of the spinal cord, interfering with the transmission of signals in the dorsal columns on both sides of the cord. Symptoms restricted to one side of the body would suggest localization of the lesion to the same side of the spinal cord, because the dorsal column projections are ipsilateral within the cord. Sensory disturbance in pain and temperature sensation on the contralateral side of the body might result if the lateral part of the spinal cord is damaged instead of the dorsal part and if transmission in the lateral sensory tract is disrupted. Combined with a more complete neurological examination to test for possible reflex and other motor disturbances, careful analysis of sensory deficits can help guide more direct diagnostic tools such as magnetic resonance imaging.

Figure 14.7.

The projections of the dorsal columns into the dorsal column nuclei of the lower medulla. The more medial portions of the dorsal columns, containing axons originating at the sacral and lumbar spinal levels, send axons to the gracile nucleus on the same side of the brain. The lateral portions of the dorsal columns, containing axons of sensory neurons at the thoracic and cervical spinal levels, project to the cuneate nucleus on the same side of the brain.

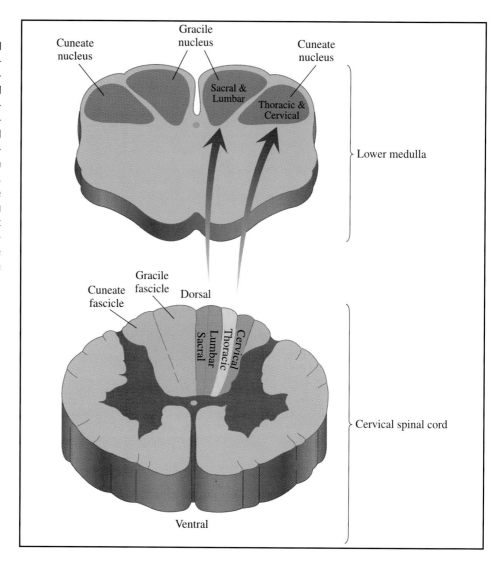

portions of the ipsilateral dorsal column (see Fig. 14.7). Ascending the spinal cord from the sacral end, sensory axons are added successively at the lateral edge of the dorsal columns at each vertebral segment. Thus, at the cervical end of the spinal cord, we find a medial-lateral organization of sensory axons in the dorsal columns, based on the spinal segment of origin (see Fig. 14.7).

Because sensory axons of the lower limbs, trunk, upper limbs, and neck enter the spinal cord at successively higher vertebral segments, the medial-lateral organization shown in Figure 14.7 translates into a sensory map of the body surface. The lower parts of the body are represented at medial positions in the map, and the upper parts of the body are mapped to more lateral positions. This **somatotopic map** is carried over into the dorsal column nuclei, with the lower portion of the body represented in the gracile nucleus and the upper portion in the cuneate nucleus.

As discussed in Chapter 13, lateral inhibitory synaptic interactions form the basis for sharpening the spatial resolution of skin sensory information. Because the axons of the dorsal columns are predominantly those of primary sensory neurons, the dorsal column nuclei offer the first opportunity for lateral synaptic interactions to establish center-surround receptive fields in this sensory pathway.

The ascending axons of the lateral sensory tract terminate primarily in the reticular formation of the medulla, pons, and midbrain. Axons of the lateral tract originate from interneurons in the dorsal part of the spinal gray matter that receive temperature and pain information. In organisms that lack a well-developed forebrain, the brainstem reticular system is the main integrating center for sensory and motor information, and the projection of the lateral sensory tract provides the information about temperature and pain required for coordinated motor responses to these stimuli. Thus, the sensory signals from the lateral sensory tract modulate the motor systems of the spinal cord, via the descending reticulospinal connections described in Chapter 9. In more complex brains, the neurons in the reticular formation that receive temperature and pain signals relay this information to higher brain centers, such as the thalamus. The reticular formation also sends widespread connections to the midbrain and forebrain, controlling the overall level of arousal and activity of the animal. Painful stimuli arouse the animal via these reticular formation connections.

In mammals, some of the ascending axons of the lateral sensory tract bypass the brainstem and project directly from the spinal cord to the thalamus (see Fig. 14.8). This direct projection stems from spinal cord interneurons that receive inputs from the fast-conducting pain-sensitive neurons (Aδ fibers, see Fig. 14.1). By contrast, the slow-conducting pain fibers (C-fibers) synapse on interneurons that project to the reticular formation via the lateral sensory tract. Thus, information from the fast-conducting pain system in the peripheral receptors is relayed most directly and rapidly to the thalamus, producing the immediate perception of searing pain felt immediately upon injury. The slow-conducting C-fiber system underlies the prolonged burning sensation that accompanies an injury.

Collectively, the projection system of pain and temperature pathways is called the **anterolateral system**, reflecting the position of the ascending axons in the lateral columns of the spinal cord. The anterolateral system also includes some tactile and proprioceptive information, although most of these mechanosensory projections reach the brain via the dorsal column pathway.

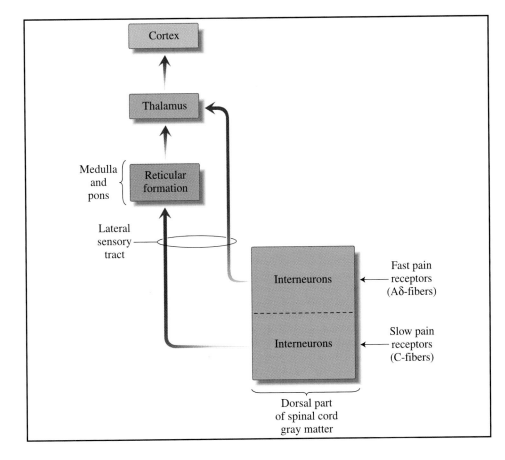

Figure 14.8.

The organization of the anterolateral system. Interneurons in the dorsal part of the gray matter in the spinal cord receive synaptic input from primary nociceptor neurons. The axons of the interneurons ascend in the contralateral lateral sensory tract in the lateral columns. The pathway originating from the C-fibers connects diffusely to the reticular formation in the brainstem, while the pathway originating from the faster-conducting Aδ-fibers projects directly to the thalamus.

THE THALAMUS

Which nucleus of the thalamus receives somatosensory information?

The anterolateral system carries information on pain and temperature from the spinal cord to the thalamus, either directly or indirectly via the reticular formation. The thalamus is also the next relay stage for the tactile and proprioceptive information carried via the dorsal columns to the dorsal column nuclei in the brainstem. The axons of neurons in the gracile and cuneate nuclei cross the midline and form bilaterally symmetrical axon bundles near the ventral midline of the medulla (Fig. 14.9). These bundles, called the **medial lemniscus**, move progressively dorsally and laterally as they ascend through the midbrain. When the axons of the medial lemniscus reach the diencephalon, they enter the ventral posterior nucleus of the thalamus and make synaptic contact with thalamic relay neurons.

As a result of the crossing (decussation) of the axons leaving the dorsal column nuclei in the medulla, the medial lemniscus on each side of the brain carries tactile and proprioceptive sensory information from the opposite side of the body. Thus, just as in the anterolateral system, the information reaching the thalamus on the right side of the brain in the dorsal column–medial lemniscus system comes from the left side of the body, and vice versa. In the anterolateral system, the crossover of axons occurs in the spinal cord; in the lemniscal system, the crossover occurs in the medulla. In both systems, decussation is accomplished by the axons of the first

Figure 14.9.

The projections from the dorsal column nuclei to the thalamus, in the diencephalon. The axons from the gracile and cuneate nuclei cross the midline and enter the medial lemniscus on the contralateral side of the medulla. This tract projects to the ipsilateral thalamus, where synaptic connections are made with neurons in the ventral posterior nucleus of the thalamus.

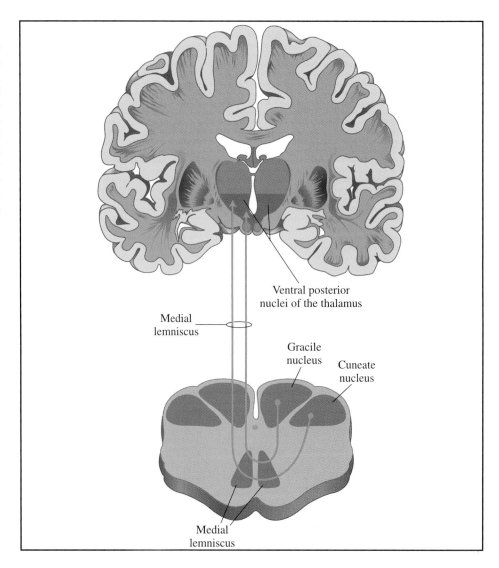

Ventral posterior
nuclei of the thalamus

Medial
lemniscus

Gracile
nucleus

Cuneate
nucleus

Medial
lemniscus

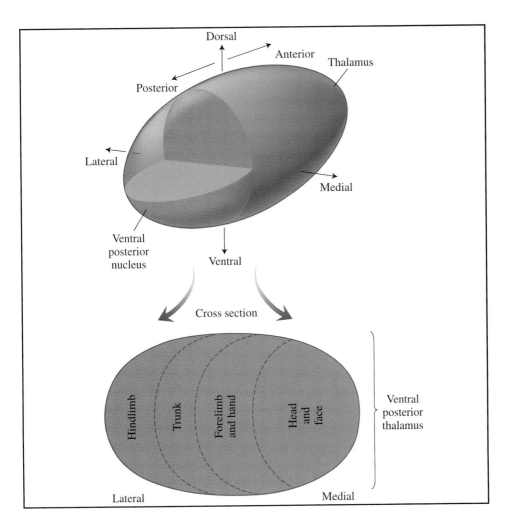

Figure 14.10.

The somatotopic organization of the tactile sensory information in the ventral posterior thalamus.

set of interneurons in the path—that is, the interneurons that receive synapses from the primary sensory neurons.

The lateral-medial somatotopic map observed in the dorsal column nuclei is evident in the ventral posterior nucleus of the thalamus as well. In the thalamus, however, the direction of the map is reversed. Tactile information from the hindlimbs projects to thalamic neurons in the most lateral portion of the ventral posterior nucleus, followed by information from the trunk and then the forelimbs as we move medially in the nucleus. This arrangement is illustrated in Figure 14.10. In the gracile and cuneate nuclei, on the other hand, the hindlimb sensory projection is the most medial, with forelimb information represented in a more lateral position.

The most medial portion the ventral posterior nucleus of the thalamus also receives tactile inputs from the face, which enter the brain via the trigeminal nerve (cranial nerve V). Like the sensory inputs from the dorsal column nuclei, the trigeminal sensory information reaches the thalamus in the medial lemniscus.

SOMATOSENSORY CORTEX

From the ventral posterior thalamus, the somatosensory information is relayed to the cortex. The main target in the cortex is the **postcentral gyrus**, which is located just behind the central sulcus approximately at the anterior-posterior midpoint of the brain (Fig. 14.11). Recall from Chapter 9 that the primary motor cortex is located just in front of the central sulcus, in the precentral gyrus. Therefore, the primary motor cortex and the primary somatosensory cortex parallel one

Where is the primary somatosensory cortex located?

another, separated only by the central sulcus. The somatosensory cortex corresponds to Brodmann's areas 1, 2, and 3, while the primary motor cortex corresponds to Brodmann's area 4 (see Chapter 9). Because of the decussation of the axons in the medial lemniscus in the medulla, the sensory cortex on the right side of the brain receives sensory information from the left side of the body, and vice versa. The same arrangement is found in the motor system, where the right motor cortex controls the left half of the body.

The body surface is represented in a orderly way in the primary somatosensory cortex, just as it is in the dorsal columns, the dorsal column nuclei, and the ventral posterior nucleus of the thalamus. Figure 14.11 shows the somatotopic map found in the somatosensory cortex. The sensory innervation from the toes, foot, and lower limb projects to the most medial parts of the postcentral cortex, the trunk and upper limb are represented at intermediate positions, and the face, lips,

What somatotopic map of the body is observed in the primary somatosensory cortex?

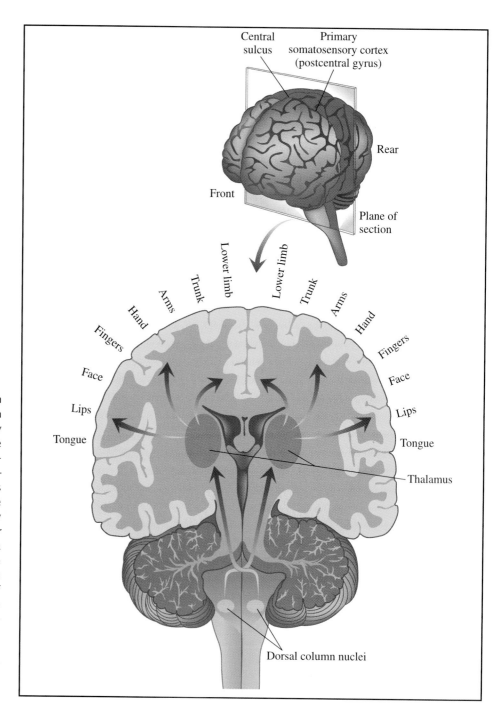

Figure 14.11.

The somatotopic organization of somatosensory information in the primary somatosensory cortex, which is located in the postcentral gyrus, just posterior to the central sulcus (*upper diagram*). The projections from the various parts of the body onto the somatosensory cortex are shown in the *lower diagram*, which depicts a cross section through the brain in the plane illustrated in the *upper diagram*. Because of the decussation of the ascending axons from the dorsal column nuclei in the brainstem, the sensory information on one side of the cortex originates from the contralateral side of the body.

and tongue are represented in the most lateral portions of the primary somato-sensory cortex. Thus, the somatotopic map of sensory information in the postcentral gyrus parallels the motor somatosensory map in the precentral gyrus (see Chapter 9).

The amount of somatosensory cortex devoted to a particular part of the body's surface does not correspond to the relative size of the body part. Instead, the amount of cortex devoted to a body region corresponds to the number of sensory neurons that innervate that region. In other words, the density of sensory innervation determines the size of the corresponding cortical representation. As we saw in Chapter 13, human fingers are innervated by large numbers of touch-sensitive sensory neurons, each having a small receptive field, while the arm and trunk receive relatively few sensory neurons, each having a large receptive field. Consequently, in the somatosensory cortex of the human brain, the fingers are represented by a large area, while sensory information from the arm and trunk is represented by a relatively small area.

Like other parts of the cortex, the somatosensory cortex is organized into six layers extending from the surface of the cortex to the underlying white matter. The basic cellular organization of these layers is described in Chapter 9 (see Fig. 9.6). As shown in Figure 14.12, the incoming axons from the ventral posterior thalamus make synaptic connections in layer IV—the cortical layer dominated by stellate cells. The stellate cells are interneurons that make local synaptic connections with

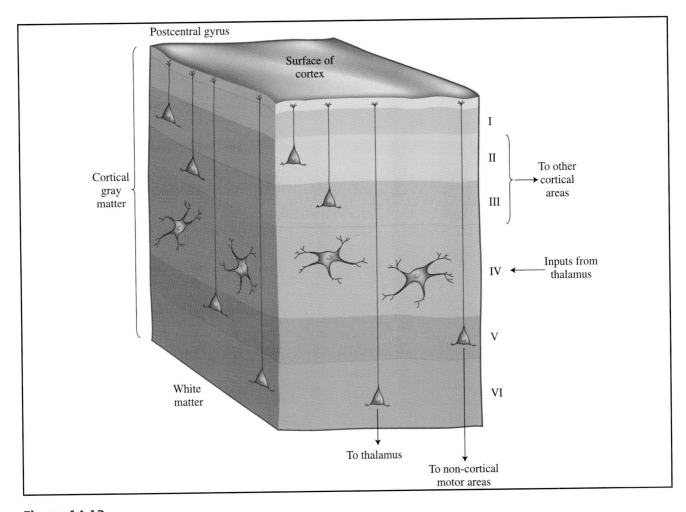

Figure 14.12.

The layers of the somatosensory cortex. Inputs to the cortex and outputs to particular brain regions are located in specific layers of the cortex.

pyramidal neurons in other layers of the cortex. The sensory parts of the cortex, such as the primary somatosensory cortex, receive large numbers of axons from the thalamus. Thus, layer IV is relatively thick in the sensory regions of cerebral cortex but comparatively thin in motor regions such as the primary motor cortex. The pyramidal neurons in layer VI of the somatosensory cortex send axons back to the thalamus, as they do in the motor cortex. This corticothalamic projection provides a feedback pathway by which the sensory cortex can influence the thalamic relay nucleus that supplies sensory information to the cortex.

Sensory information is required for proper motor function (see Chapters 9 and 10). For this purpose, the somatosensory cortex sends outputs to motor regions of the brain. The large pyramidal neurons of layer V in primary somatosensory cortex send axons to noncortical motor areas, including the basal ganglia. Connections to cortical motor areas are made by pyramidal neurons in layers II and III of the somatosensory cortex. These connections from the somatosensory cortex to cortical and noncortical motor areas supply the motor system with necessary information about limb position and contact with the environment.

Receptive Fields of Cortical Somatosensory Neurons

The receptive fields of neurons in the somatosensory cortex differ in important ways from the receptive fields of primary sensory neurons. As discussed in Chapter 13, lateral inhibitory interactions mediated by interneurons alter the receptive field properties of the neurons receiving synaptic input from the primary receptors. In the touch system, these lateral interactions occur at all synaptic relay stations: in the dorsal column nuclei, in the thalamus, and in the cortex itself. Because of lateral inhibition, the receptive fields of second-order and higher neurons have a center-surround organization, which is illustrated for a cortical neuron in Figure 14.13. Tactile stimulation in the center of the receptive field excites the neuron, and stimulation applied to the surrounding region inhibits it.. The lateral inhibitory interactions facilitate the discrimination of two nearby points of stimulation, increasing the spatial resolution of the sensory system.

In addition, cortical neurons can have more complicated receptive fields. For example, in the neuron illustrated in Figure 14.14, the receptive field is long and narrow, rather than circular. A touch applied to a single location within the receptive field produces little effect. In contrast, a stimulus brushed along the receptive field from right to left produces a sustained increase in action potential activity. This type of cortical neuron prefers a moving stimulus to a stationary stimulus. If we reverse the direction of the stimulus so that it moves from left to right, little response is observed. Not only must the stimulus move, but also it must move in a particular direction. Other neurons in the somatosensory cortex exhibit preference for movement in the opposite direction, and still others have a preference for a different orientation. Within the population of cells in the somatosensory cortex, all directional preferences for moving stimuli would be represented, covering all points of the compass.

Complex receptive fields like that illustrated in Figure 14.14 could arise from relatively simple combinations of synaptic connections from lower-level neurons in the sensory pathway. For example, the circuitry shown in Figure 14.15 could produce directional selectivity for moving stimuli. In a simple variation on the general lateral inhibitory scheme, inhibitory interneurons send connections to one side only.

Consider a stimulus moving across the receptive fields of the primary sensory neurons on the skin surface in the preferred direction, from right to left. The stimulus first encounters the receptive field of primary neuron 1, which responds by firing a burst of action potentials. This burst of activity in turn excites relay cell 1 and higher-order interneuron 1. The higher-order interneuron ultimately makes an ex-

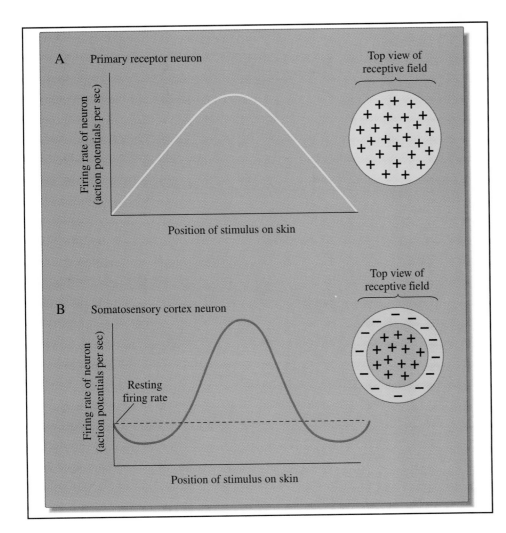

Figure 14.13.

The receptive fields of neurons in the somatosensory cortex differ from the receptive fields of primary sensory neurons. **A.** The rate of firing action potentials in the primary sensory neuron in response to a touch stimulus applied to various positions along the surface of the skin. A top view of the receptive field is also shown. **B.** The comparable behavior for a cortical neuron and a top view of the center-surround receptive field observed for some cortical neurons. The *plus signs* indicate that the neuron is excited by a stimulus in that region of the receptive field, and the *minus signs* indicate that the neuron is inhibited by stimuli in that region.

citatory connection with the directionally selective cortical neuron, which initiates the burst of action potentials in the cortical neuron. As the stimulus leaves the receptive field of primary neuron 1, it moves into the receptive field of primary neuron 2, stimulating a burst of action potentials in the path leading from that primary neuron to the cortical neuron. This activity provides excitation that continues the action potential activity in the cortical neuron. Action potentials in relay cell 2 also excite a lateral inhibitory interneuron that inhibits the higher-order interneuron in pathway 1. However, because the stimulus has left the receptive field of primary neuron 1, activity in that pathway has already ceased, and the inhibition has no functional effect on the relay of information.

As the stimulus continues to move, it successively encounters the receptive fields of primary sensory neurons 3, 4, and 5, each of which relays excitation to the directionally selective cortical neuron. Thus, the excitation that produces the burst of action potentials in the cortical neuron is sustained as the stimulus moves from right to left, producing a prolonged burst of activity during the moving stimulus, as shown in Figure 14.14.

Now consider what happens when the stimulus moves from left to right, in the nonpreferred direction. The stimulus first encounters the receptive field of primary sensory neuron 5, which is excited by the stimulus. The burst of action potentials is relayed through to the directionally selective cortical neuron, producing one or two action potentials at the onset of the stimulus. The activity in this pathway is also relayed to the higher-order interneuron in the neighboring pathway (pathway 4) via the lateral inhibitory interneuron. The stimulus next enters the receptive

Figure 14.14.

The response of a directionally selective cortical neuron. The receptive field on the skin is an elongated strip of skin. When a touch stimulus is applied to the skin and moved across the receptive field, the response of the neuron depends on the direction of movement. In this case, a stimulus moving from right to left produces a large increase in firing of the cortical neuron. A stimulus moving from left to right produces only a weak response.

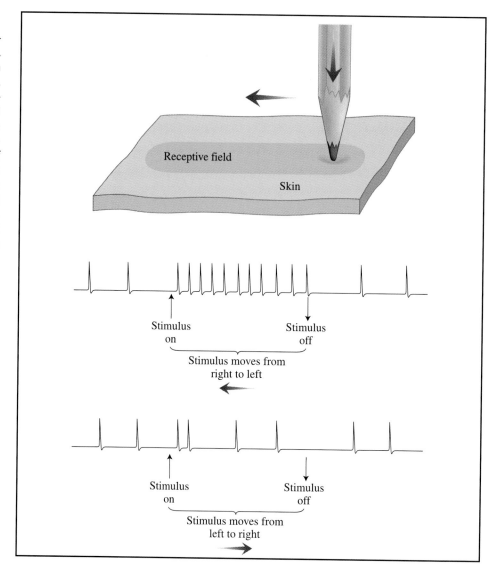

field of primary sensory neuron 4, and the excitation is relayed from the primary sensory neuron to relay cell 4. However, this excitation in pathway 4 sums with the preexisting inhibition from the inhibitory interneuron of pathway 5. If the inhibition is sufficiently strong and long-lasting, then it may completely prevent higher-order neuron 4 from firing. The directionally selective cortical neuron would then receive no excitation and would cease firing.

The activation of the relay cell in pathway 4 excites the lateral inhibitory interneuron of that pathway, feeding inhibition to the higher-order interneuron of pathway 3. That interneuron is then pre-inhibited when excitation arrives from the stimulation of receptive field 3 by the moving stimulus. Because of the lateral inhibition, the directionally selective cortical neuron is less likely to be stimulated when the stimulus moves from left to right. The result is the weak response of the cortical cell to movement in the nonpreferred direction, shown in Figure 14.14.

The circuit shown in Figure 14.15 provides a simple example of how synaptic interconnections can give rise to individual neurons that extract particular information about the environment. In general, receptive fields of cortical neurons are more complex than those of lower-order neurons in the sensory pathways. Because of the elaborate interconnections among the neurons of the cerebral cortex, ample opportunity exists for neural circuits that are tuned to detect complex combinations of sensory events.

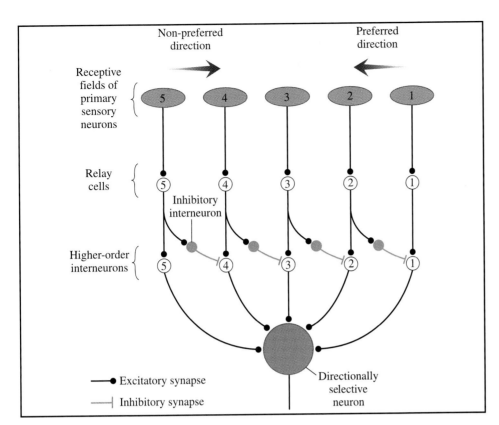

Figure 14.15.

Hypothetical synaptic circuitry that could produce a directionally sensitive response in a cortical somatosensory neuron. The circuit begins with five primary sensory neurons with receptive fields arrayed linearly along the skin (top level). The primary sensory neurons make excitatory synaptic connections onto a group of relay cells (second level). The relay cells excite higher-order interneurons (third level) whose outputs converge on a cortical neuron. The relay cells also excite inhibitory interneurons (*red*) that make inhibitory synaptic connections with the higher-order neurons of the neighboring pathway, but only to one side. (See text for a description of how this arrangement gives rise to a directionally selective response in the cortical neuron.)

The somatic senses provide information about the interaction of the skin with the environment and about the positions of joints and muscles. The skin contains several types of sensory receptor structures, each specialized for the reception of a particular type of sensory information. Each sensory modality (such as touch, pressure, and pain) is mediated via a specific class of sensory receptor. Receptors that are sensitive to touch or pressure are called mechanoreceptors. Some mechanoreceptors consist of nerve endings encapsulated within fibrous capsules called corpuscles. In human skin, the corpuscle receptors are the Pacinian corpuscle, the Meissner corpuscle, and the Ruffini corpuscle. Other mechanoreceptors are the Merkel receptors and the hair follicle receptors. The mechanoreceptors also can be distinguished by their adaptation properties, with some adapting rapidly and others slowly during a sustained mechanical stimulus. The skin also contains thermoreceptors that are stimulated by cooling of the skin below normal body temperature (cold receptors) or by warming the skin above the normal body temperature (warm receptors). Nociceptors are another class of receptor activated by stimuli that injure the skin (such as burns or punctures).

Proprioception (joint position, muscle length, and muscle tension) is also signaled within the somatosensory system. Muscle length is encoded by the sensory neurons that innervate the muscle spindles. Muscle tension is signaled by the Golgi tendon organs. Information about the angle of the joint is provided by joint receptors, which are sensory neurons that innervate the joint capsule.

The sensory receptors also can be classified according to the conduction velocity of their axons in the peripheral nerves. The fastest-conducting axons are those of the muscle spindles (group Ia), followed closely by the Golgi tendon organ axons (group Ib). These fast-conducting group I axons are also known as group Aα. The mechanoreceptors of the skin are innervated by sensory neurons with medium-size myelinated axons (group II, also known as group Aβ) that conduct more slowly than the muscle receptors. The joint receptor neurons also have group II axons. The smallest-diameter myelinated axons (group III, also known as group Aδ) are those of the cold receptors and the rapid, searing-pain nociceptors. Group IV, the slowest-conducting group of axons in peripheral nerves (also called group C, or C-fibers), includes warm receptors and nociceptors that underlie the sensation of slow, burning pain.

In the spinal cord, somatosensory information is carried to the brain by ascending axons found in the dorsal columns, lateral sensory tract, and spinocerebellar tract. The dorsal column projection consists predominantly of collateral branches of the axons of primary mechanoreceptor and proprioceptor neurons. The lateral sensory tract consists of axons of interneurons in the spinal gray matter that receive synaptic inputs from thermoreceptors and nociceptors, plus some mechanoreceptors and proprioceptors. The spinocerebellar tract, which is located in the lateral columns of the spinal white matter, carries somatosensory information to the cerebellum. The dorsal column axons project to the brainstem, where they terminate in the dorsal column nuclei, the gracile nucleus and the cuneate nucleus. The axons of the lateral sensory tract project to the reticular formation of the brainstem and (in some species) directly to the thalamus.

A major target of ascending somatosensory information is the thalamus. The dorsal column nuclei project to the thalamus via the medial lemniscus, which crosses the midline in the medulla and projects to the contralateral part of the thalamus. The axons of the lateral sensory tract cross the midline in the spinal cord and also project to the contralateral side of the brain. Thus, sensory information from the left side of the body is sent to the thalamus on the right side of the brain. The neurons of the thalamus relay the somatosensory information to the motor control areas of the brain and to the somatosensory cortex, which is located in the postcentral gyrus. At each relay nucleus, including the thalamus, lateral interactions mediated by local interneurons modify and sharpen the receptive field properties of the neurons, giving rise to center-surround receptive fields and more complex kinds of receptive fields. In the somatosensory cortex, for example, some neurons respond only to an object moving across the skin in a particular location and in a particular direction. Neurons with such complex response requirements are able to extract information about patterns of sensory stimulation.

1. List five different types of mechanoreceptors found in human skin and describe their responses to mechanical stimuli.
2. What features distinguish the two types of nociceptors?
3. Give an example of a sensory receptor type whose axons are categorized in group I, group II, group III, and group IV.
4. A sensory receptor neuron fires action potentials when pressure is applied to the skin, and the frequency of firing declines only slightly during maintained pressure. What kind of sensory receptor neuron could this be?
5. Describe the main projection pathway for touch information to reach the somatosensory cortex.

6. What somatotopic map of sensory information is found in the dorsal column nuclei, in the ventral posterior nucleus of the thalamus, and in the postcentral gyrus?

7. Describe the anterolateral pathway. What kind of sensory information does it carry?

8. Identify the following: lateral sensory tract, gracile nucleus, medial lemniscus, dorsal columns.

9. What role does lateral inhibition play in the generation of direction selectivity in receptive fields that require moving stimuli?

INTERNET ASSIGNMENT   CHAPTER 14

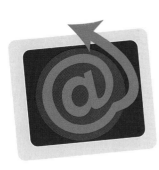

1 The following sensory structures are associated with skin somatosensory function: Pacinian corpuscle, Meissner corpuscle, and Ruffini corpuscle. Search the Internet to find histological images that illustrate the anatomy of these structures.

2 Use anatomical resources on the Internet, such as brain atlases, to locate the following structures in the brain: dorsal column nuclei (gracile and cuneate nuclei), medial lemniscus, and primary somatosensory cortex.

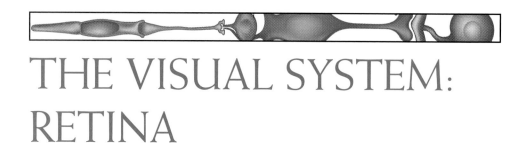

THE VISUAL SYSTEM: RETINA

For humans, the sense of vision is a dominant sense, playing a central role in our interaction with the environment. Unlike the mechanoreceptors and the somatosensory pathways described in Chapter 14, visual sensory receptors allow us to gather information about the environment from afar, without having to come into direct contact with the object giving rise to the sensation. In this chapter, we will consider this important sensory system. We begin 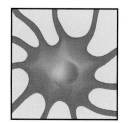 with the sensory organ of vision, the eye, paying special attention to the neural part of the eye, the retina. In Chapter 16, we will consider how the visual parts of the brain analyze and modify the information passed on from the retina to form a representation of objects and their relationships in the visual world.

STRUCTURE OF THE VERTEBRATE EYE

Light-sensitive sense organs are found in a wide variety of organisms. Indeed, even single-cell organisms have light-sensing organelles (in addition to the light-gathering photosynthetic organelles found in bacteria and plants). For example, single-cell algae have a light-sensitive "eyespot" that is used to sense the direction of illumination, providing information that allows the organism to move toward light (positive phototaxis). A somewhat more complex example of a photosensitive organ in multicellular organisms is found in the flatworm, *Planaria*, whose eyespot provides sensory information enabling negative phototaxis. Beyond these simple light-gathering organs, most invertebrate and vertebrate animals have developed more complicated light-sensing organs—true eyes—that optically focus the light onto the sensory surface of the organ to form an image of outside world.

Figure 15.1 shows a cross section of a human eye. Light enters the eye through the transparent covering at the front of the eye, the **cornea**. It then passes into the posterior portion of the eye through an aperture, the **pupil**, whose diameter is controlled by the muscles of the colored part of the front of the eye, the **iris**. Behind the iris is the lens, which acts in concert with the cornea to focus the incoming light onto the retina at the back of the eye.

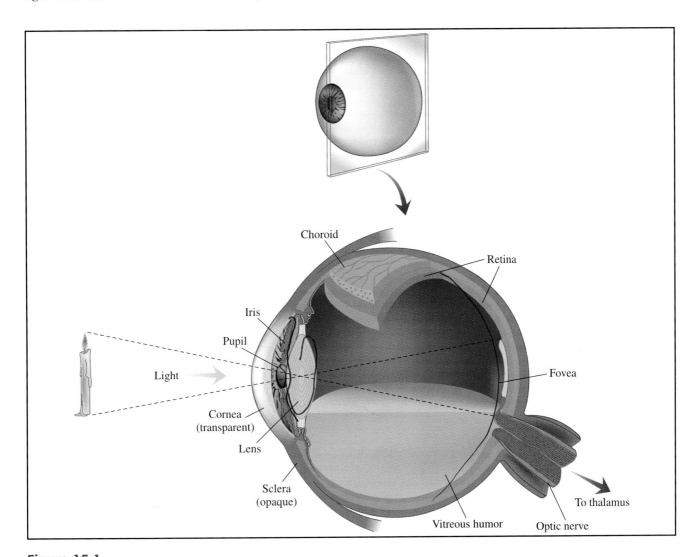

Figure 15.1.

The structure of the human eye. The retina is shown in *dark pink* at the rear of the inside of the eye.

All sensory organs must convert the energy of a sensory stimulus into an electrical signal that can be passed along and analyzed by the cells of the nervous system. In the eye, this sensory transduction process is accomplished in the retina. Because the sensory stimulus consists of photons of light, the visual transduction process is called **phototransduction**, and it is carried out in the primary receptor neurons of the retina, the **photoreceptors**. The organization of a retina in a typical vertebrate is shown in Figure 15.2. The photoreceptors are found at the rearmost part of the eye, facing the back of the eye. To reach the cells that absorb the light and translate it into electrical signals, the light must first traverse all the other cells of the retina.

Figure 15.2.

The neurons of the retina. The photoreceptors are located at the rear of the retina and make synaptic connections with horizontal cells and bipolar cells. The bipolar cells then connect with the amacrine cells and ganglion cells in the inner portion of the retina. The axons of the ganglion cells make up the optic nerve.

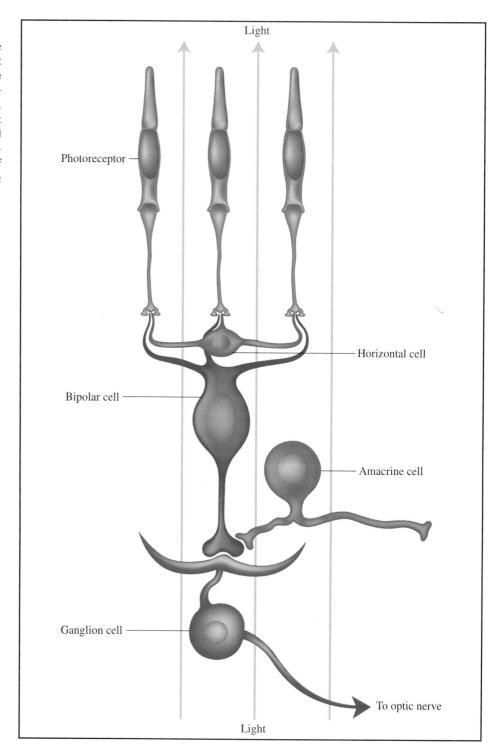

Including the photoreceptors, five general classes of neurons make up the retina. The photoreceptors make synaptic connections with second-order neurons called **bipolar cells**, which in turn make synaptic contact with retinal **ganglion cells**. The axons of the ganglion cells form the optic nerve, which carries the visual information to the thalamus in the diencephalon. In addition to this through-conducting pathway, two types of lateral interneurons are found in the retina. The **horizontal cells** receive synaptic inputs from the photoreceptors and then make synaptic connections with bipolar neurons or (in some species) with the synaptic terminals of the photoreceptors. The **amacrine cells** receive inputs from the bipolar cells and make synaptic connections back onto the synaptic terminals of the bipolar cells and onto the dendrites of ganglion cells. For both amacrine cells and horizontal cells, one synaptic target of the lateral interneuron is the synaptic terminal of the cell that provides synaptic input to the lateral interneuron (photoreceptors, in the case of horizontal cells; bipolar cells, for the amacrine cells). This type of feedback synapse, in which a cell makes a synapse back onto the synaptic terminal that is presynaptic to it, is quite common in the retina.

What types of neurons are found in the retina?

THE LIGHT RESPONSE OF THE PHOTORECEPTORS

In this section, we will examine the conversion of electromagnetic energy of light into an electrical signal in photoreceptors. Most vertebrate retinas include two classes of photoreceptors: **rods** and **cones**. The structural organization of rod and cone photoreceptors is shown in Figure 15.3. The light-sensitive portion of the cell, where light is absorbed and phototransduction occurs, is called the **outer segment**. In rods, the outer segment is long and cylindrical (rod-shaped, hence the name). In cones, the outer segment is typically tapered toward the distal end (cone-shaped). In vertebrate photoreceptors, the outer segment is actually a highly modified cilium, shaped by evolution to carry out the light-sensing function of the cell. The outer segment is connected to the rest of the photoreceptor cell via a thin ciliary neck that contains a vestigial ciliary apparatus. The non-light-sensitive part of the cell, which contains the nucleus and the usual cellular machinery of neurons, is called the **inner segment** (see Fig. 15.3). At the other end of the photoreceptor inner segment is the **synaptic terminal** of the photoreceptor, where synaptic connections are made with the second-order horizontal and bipolar neurons of the retina.

From the point of view of electrical signaling, the spatial compactness of photoreceptors is an important feature. The total length of the photoreceptor (less

What is the structure of photoreceptor cells?

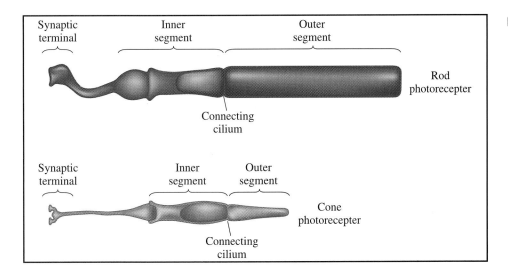

Figure 15.3.

The structural organization of rod photoreceptors (*top*) and cone photoreceptors (*bottom*). The outer segment is the light-sensitive portion of the photoreceptor.

than 100 µm) is sufficiently short that the receptor potential produced by light in the outer segment can easily spread to the synaptic terminal without requiring an action potential. Indeed, the photoreceptors do not express voltage-dependent sodium channels and hence do not generate action potentials.

The Electrical Response of the Photoreceptors to Light

In what way does light affect the membrane potential of photoreceptors?

If we record the membrane potential of a vertebrate photoreceptor in darkness, we find that the resting membrane potential is unusually positive, with a value of –30 to –40 mV being typical (Fig. 15.4). If we then turn on a bright light, the membrane potential of the photoreceptor shifts to approximately –70 mV (see Fig. 15.4). In the light, the photoreceptor membrane potential is similar to the resting potential of typical neurons; in darkness, however, the photoreceptor is depolarized. Thus, the receptor potential of the photoreceptor is a hyperpolarization. If we use a dim light instead of a bright light, a smaller hyperpolarization results, as shown in Figure 15.4. The degree of hyperpolarization depends on the light intensity, with brighter lights producing a more negative membrane potential than dimmer lights. The relationship between light intensity and membrane potential is

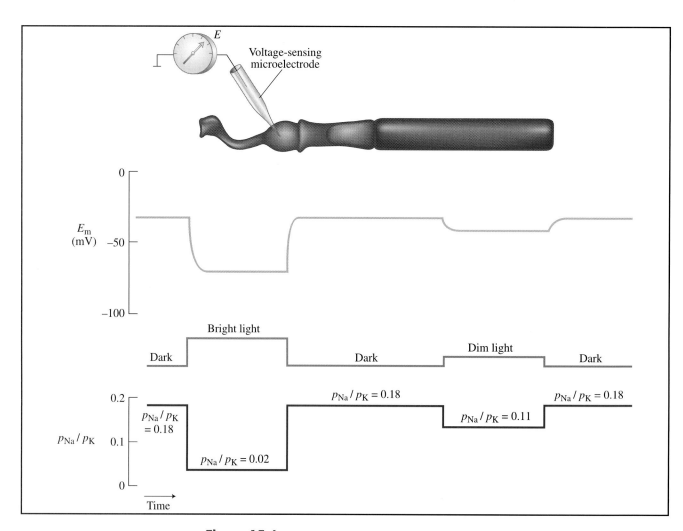

Figure 15.4.

The effect of light on the membrane potential of the photoreceptor. In darkness, the relative sodium permeability is high and the cell is depolarized. Light reduces the sodium permeability and makes the membrane potential (E_m) more negative. $p_\mathrm{Na}/p_\mathrm{K}$ = ratio of sodium permeability to potassium permeability.

summarized in Figure 15.5. Like other receptor potentials, the receptor potential of the photoreceptor is a graded potential, with an amplitude that depends on the magnitude of the sensory stimulus. Unlike other sensory receptors, however, the receptor potential of the photoreceptor is a hyperpolarization, rather than a depolarization. (You can think of *darkness* as the "stimulus" that depolarizes the photoreceptor, so that illumination acts by *removing* the "stimulus.")

As with other cells, a change in ionic permeability underlies the hyperpolarizing receptor potential of the photoreceptor cell. Recall from Chapter 3 that the resting membrane potential of a neuron is governed by the ratio of sodium to potassium permeability, p_{Na}/p_K, according to the Goldman equation:

$$E_m = 58 \text{ mV } \log\left(\frac{[K^+]_o + b[Na^+]_o}{[K^+]_i + b[Na^+]_i}\right) \tag{16.1}$$

where the scaling factor b is p_{Na}/p_K. The usual resting value of b in a neuron is approximately 0.02, which yields a resting potential near −70 mV under the usual ionic conditions (see Chapter 3). If the ratio p_{Na}/p_K were 0.18 instead of 0.02, however, the Goldman equation indicates that the resting potential would be near −40 mV, which is the approximate membrane potential of the photoreceptor in darkness. Thus, a shift of p_{Na}/p_K from 0.18 to 0.02 can account for the shift in membrane potential of the photoreceptor in bright light. Figure 15.4 summarizes the changes in p_{Na}/p_K associated with light-induced hyperpolarization of the photoreceptor.

The changes in p_{Na}/p_K upon illumination are produced by a *reduction* in ionic permeability of the outer segment of the photoreceptor. In darkness, nonspecific cation channels in the plasma membrane of the outer segment are open. As we saw with synaptic transmission at the neuromuscular junction (see Chapter 5), nonspecific cation channels produce a depolarization when they are open. Thus, the open cation channels maintain the photoreceptor in a depolarized state in darkness. Light closes these cation channels, and the fraction of channels closed depends on the light intensity (Fig. 15.6). When the light is sufficiently bright to close all of the channels, the membrane potential reaches its most negative value, and further

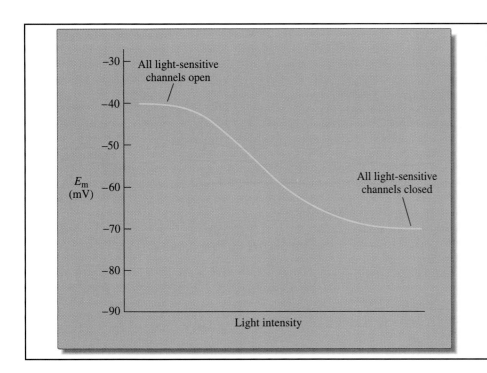

Figure 15.5.

The relationship between light intensity and membrane potential (E_m) in a photoreceptor.

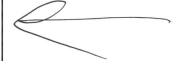

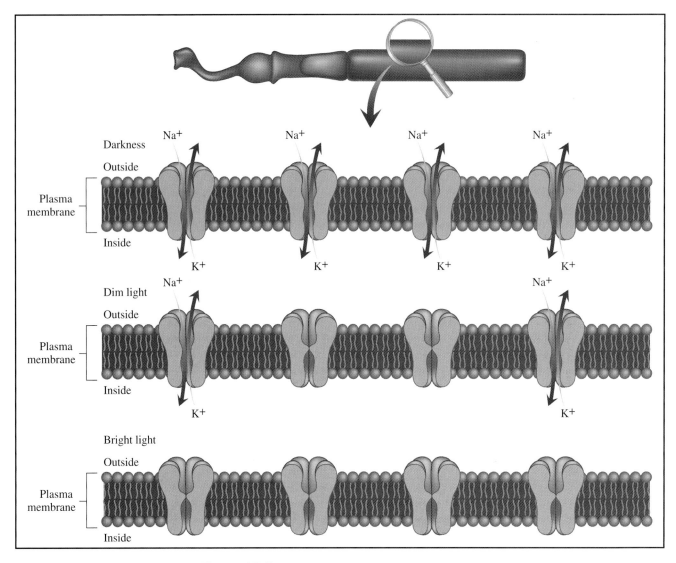

Figure 15.6.

Light closes nonspecific cation channels in the plasma membrane of the photoreceptor outer segment. The percentage of channels closed depends on the intensity of the light.

increases in light intensity fail to produce any further change in membrane potential (see Fig. 15.5).

We now turn our attention to the linkage between the absorption of light in the outer segment and the closure of the nonspecific cation channels. Two steps are required in this linkage. First, the light must be detected, which requires a detector molecule that absorbs light. Second, the detector molecule must then generate a cellular signal that ultimately leads to the closing of the ion channels. We will first describe the detector molecule and then return to the cellular signaling system triggered by the detector molecule.

The Light-Absorbing Molecules in the Photoreceptor Outer Segment

How is light absorbed by the photoreceptor cells?

The absorption of light in the photoreceptor is carried out by the visual pigment molecules, membrane proteins that are present at high density in the outer segment. To increase the chances that light will be absorbed in the outer segment, the membranes containing the pigment molecules are arranged in multiple layers perpendicular to the long axis of the outer segment, as illustrated in Figure 15.7. In

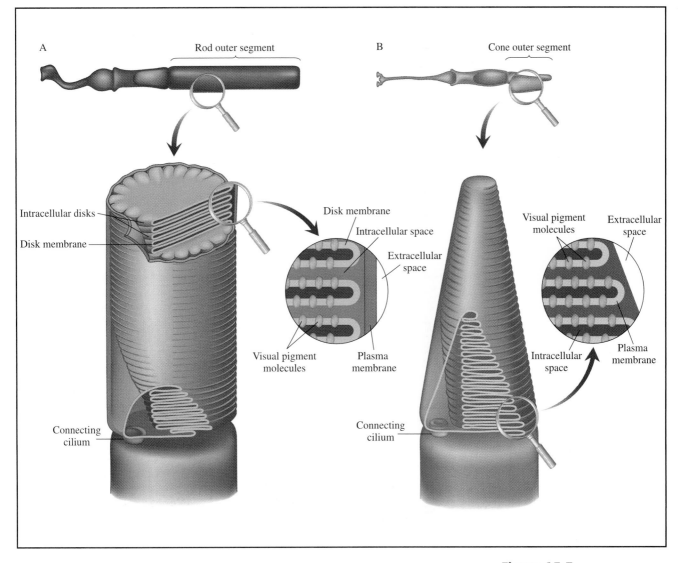

Figure 15.7.

Location of visual pigment molecules in rod photoreceptors (**A**) and in cone photoreceptors (**B**).

the rods, the pigment molecules are located in intracellular **disks**, whose membranes are not continuous with the plasma membrane of the outer segment. The intracellular disks are arranged in a tightly packed stack along the outer segment, like a stack of dimes inside a test tube (see Fig. 15.7A). A similar arrangement is seen in cones, although the stack of membranes is formed by infoldings of the plasma membrane (see Fig. 15.7B). In both cases, the functional effect is the same: to pass through the outer segment without being absorbed, a photon of light must pass through a series of about 2000 membranes, each studded with a high density of light-absorbing molecules. As a result, photons reaching the outer segment will usually be absorbed and detected by the photoreceptor.

Each type of photoreceptor expresses a particular type of visual pigment molecule. Humans have four types of photoreceptors (three types of cones and one type of rod) and thus four classes of visual pigment molecules. Each of the four classes absorbs light in the visible part of the electromagnetic spectrum, in the range of wavelengths from approximately 400 nm to 700 nm. Each class is maximally sensitive to light in a different range of wavelength, however. The best-studied visual pigment molecule is **rhodopsin**, which is found in rod photoreceptors and is most sensitive to light at a wavelength of approximately 500 nm. The three cone visual pigments absorb light best at wavelengths of 420 nm, 530 nm, or 560 nm.

Each pigment molecule is formed by a combination of a large protein molecule—opsin—with a special molecule that actually absorbs the light—the **chromophore**. The chromophore is the same for all the visual pigment molecules: the aldehyde of vitamin A_1, which is called **retinal** (the "-al" is pronounced like the "Al-" in "Albert" because it derives from the word "aldehyde"). Therefore, the different light-absorbing properties of the four classes of pigment molecules must arise from differences in opsin proteins of the rods and of the three cone types. Both retinal and opsin are colorless when separated from each other—that is, neither absorbs light in the visible wavelengths (both opsin and retinal absorb light in the ultraviolet region, at wavelengths shorter than those the human eye can sense). When retinal is chemically attached to opsin, its absorption shifts toward longer wavelengths, into the visible region. The amount of the shift, and thus the sensitivity to different parts of the visible spectrum, depends on the properties of the opsin protein. Because each class of pigment molecule has its own type of opsin, each class absorbs light differently.

The structure of the light-absorbing chromophore group, retinal, is shown in Figure 15.8. Retinal consists of a carbon ring with a long chain of carbon atoms attached to one side. The point of attachment to the opsin protein is at the end of a carbon chain, where an oxygen atom is attached via an aldehyde linkage. Retinal can assume two biologically important alternative shapes (called **isomers**). The chain of carbon atoms can be either straight (**all-*trans* retinal**) or bent by rotation around the double bond between carbon atoms 11 and 12 in the molecule (**11-*cis* retinal**). Retinal is in the 11-*cis* conformation in darkness but undergoes a conformational change to the all-*trans* isomer when it absorbs a photon of light. This **photoisomerization** of 11-*cis* retinal to all-*trans* retinal is the only light-dependent process in all of vision, and it forms the basis of the sense of sight.

Each visual pigment molecule consists of a single retinal chromophore group attached via a covalent chemical bond to a particular amino acid in the opsin protein. The protein forms a pocket in which the folded, 11-*cis* isomer of retinal fits snugly.

Figure 15.8.

The structure of the chromophore group of visual pigment molecules. The chromophore is the aldehyde of vitamin A (retinal). In the dark, the chromophore is in a folded configuration (11-*cis* retinal). Upon absorption of a photon, the chromophore straightens to the all-*trans* isomer.

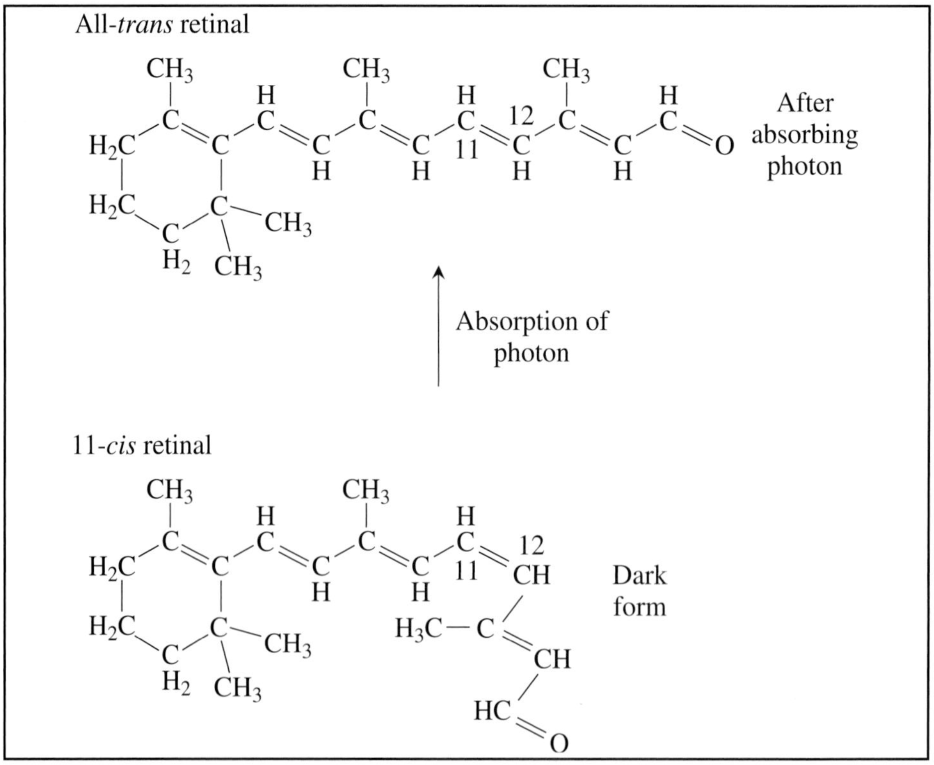

All-*trans* retinal

11-*cis* retinal

Absorption of photon

After absorbing photon

Dark form

Figure 15.9 shows the structure of the rhodopsin molecule. Opsin is a membrane protein that snakes its way through the membrane seven times. The seven transmembrane segments are arranged approximately in a circle (see Fig. 15.9), with parts of several transmembrane segments in close proximity to 11-*cis* retinal, which is chemically linked to the seventh segment. When the chromophore absorbs a photon, it isomerizes to the all-*trans* isomer. Straightening of the side chain alters the position of the chromophore in its protein pocket, which in turn induces a conformational change in opsin (see Fig. 15.9). When the transmembrane segments shift position with respect to each other, the cytoplasmic tail of the molecule uncoils to reveal reactive sites at which the photoactivated rhodopsin can interact with other proteins in the outer segment. These interactions form the basis of the signal that ultimately culminates in the closing of the nonspecific cation channels, which produces the hyperpolarizing light response of the photoreceptor. The linkage between photoactivated rhodopsin and membrane conductance is discussed in the next section.

Rhodopsin Activates G-proteins

In our description of synaptic transmission (see Chapters 6 and 11), we introduced the family of neurotransmitter receptor molecules that act via guanosine triphosphate (GTP)–binding proteins (G-proteins). When neurotransmitter binds to the receptor, the activated receptor molecule stimulates G-proteins inside the

How is absorption of light coupled to a change in membrane potential of the photoreceptor?

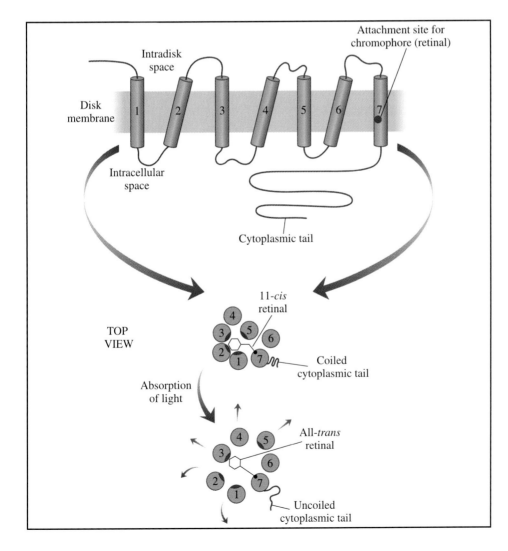

Figure 15.9.

The structure of the visual pigment molecule rhodopsin. The molecule threads through the membrane seven times. When the 11-*cis* retinal chromophore group absorbs a photon and isomerizes to the all-*trans* form, a conformational change is induced in the opsin protein.

cell by catalyzing the binding of GTP to G-protein. The G-proteins then carry out the changes in cellular properties induced by the neurotransmitter.

Rhodopsin is actually a member of the family of G-protein–coupled neurotransmitter receptors. Structurally, all the members of this family resemble rhodopsin, having seven transmembrane segments and a cytoplasmic loop that interacts with intracellular G-proteins. When rhodopsin is activated by absorption of a photon of light, a binding site for G-proteins is revealed in the cytoplasmic tail, allowing rhodopsin to trigger the signaling cascade of phototransduction. In essence, rhodopsin acts as a neurotransmitter-activated receptor molecule, except that the "neurotransmitter" (retinal) is covalently linked to its binding site. In the dark, the "neurotransmitter" is in an inactive form (the folded isomer, 11-*cis* retinal), and so the rhodopsin is inactive. Light converts the "neurotransmitter" to an active form (the unfolded isomer, all-*trans* retinal) and thus activates the rhodopsin molecule. All subsequent signaling events are analogous to those of other G-protein–coupled receptor molecules.

The G-protein activated by photoisomerized rhodopsin, called **transducin**, is associated with the cytoplasmic surface of the rhodopsin-containing intracellular disks in the outer segments of the rod photoreceptors. Transducin is a **heterotrimeric G-protein**, consisting of three separate protein subunits. GTP binds to the **alpha-subunit** to activate the G-protein, and the alpha-subunit with GTP bound then stimulates the next phase of phototransduction. The **beta-subunit** and the **gamma-subunit** form an inhibitory duplex that binds to the inactive, guanosine diphosphate (GDP)–bound form of the alpha-subunit. (In some cases, the beta-gamma complex is also a cellular signal acting in parallel with the alpha-subunit when the triplex is dissociated; see Chapter 11.) Thus, activation of the G-protein involves the replacement of GDP on the alpha-subunit with GTP, and dissociation of the beta-gamma-subunit complex from the alpha-subunit. This activating reaction is catalyzed by photoisomerized rhodopsin during phototransduction, as shown schematically in Figure 15.10. The activated transducin alpha-subunit, with GTP bound, is released by photoactivated rhodopsin, which

Figure 15.10.

The linkage between photo-activated rhodopsin and the hydrolysis of cyclic guanosine monophosphate (cGMP). The activated form of a molecule is indicated by an *asterisk*. See the text for a description of all the steps in the process. Rh = the rod photopigment rhodopsin; T = the G-protein transducin; PDE = phosphodiesterase; GDP = guanosine diphosphate; GTP = guanosine triphosphate; GMP = guanosine monophosphate; P_i = inorganic phosphate.

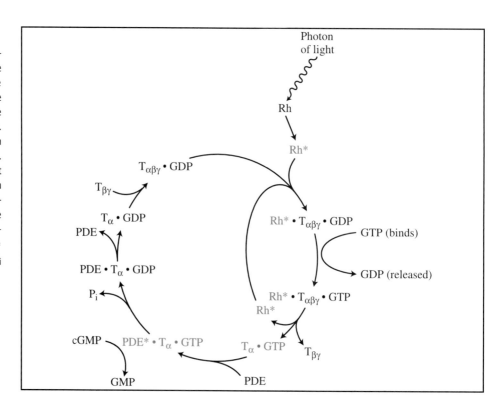

can then interact with another molecule of inactive transducin and convert it to the active form.

As with other G-proteins in neurotransmitter-mediated signaling systems, the transducin alpha-subunit stimulates an enzyme that controls the levels of an intracellular second messenger. In phototransduction, the target is **phosphodiesterase**, an enzyme that also is associated with the cytoplasmic face of the intracellular disks. Phosphodiesterase inactivates cyclic nucleotides (a common internal second messenger in cells) by breaking the cyclic phosphate bond and converting the molecule to nucleoside monophosphate. The noncyclic form of the nucleotide molecule is not effective as an internal second messenger in cells. In photoreceptors, phosphodiesterase inactivates **cyclic guanosine monophosphate (cyclic GMP)**.

The hydrolytic reaction catalyzed by phosphodiesterase is shown in Figure 15.11. The phosphodiesterase in the outer segment of the rod is inactive in darkness but becomes activated upon illumination by forming a complex with the GTP-bound form of the transducin alpha-subunit (see Fig. 15.10). The activated phosphodiesterase then cleaves cyclic GMP at a rapid rate, reducing the cytoplasmic concentration of cyclic GMP in the photoreceptor outer segment. This reduction in cyclic GMP concentration causes the nonspecific cation channels in the plasma membrane of the outer segment to close.

The Light-Dependent Ion Channels Are Directly Gated by Cyclic GMP

Cyclic nucleotides, such as cyclic GMP and cyclic adenosine monophosphate (cyclic AMP), commonly affect cellular functions indirectly, by activating cyclic nucleotide–dependent protein kinases, which in turn phosphorylate proteins (see, for example, the effect of norepinephrine on cardiac-muscle cells in Chapter 11). In the case of phototransduction, however, cyclic GMP affects the ion channels of the outer segment more directly. Cyclic GMP directly binds to the cation channel, causing the channel to open. Thus, the light-dependent ion channels are actually

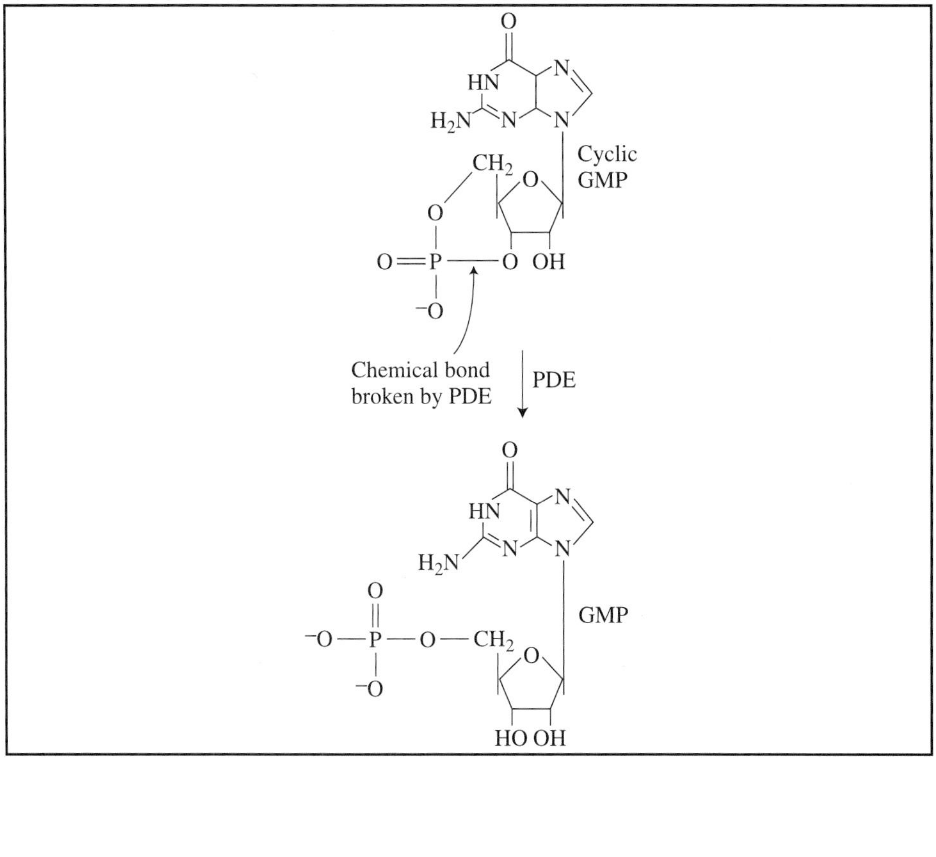

Figure 15.11.

The chemical structure of the internal messenger cyclic guanosine monophosphate (cGMP) (*top*), which is hydrolyzed to GMP (*bottom*) by the enzyme phosphodiesterase (PDE).

ligand-gated ion channels, similar in this regard to neurotransmitter-gated ion channels. Unlike neurotransmitter-gated channels, however, the ligand binding site of the cyclic GMP–gated channel faces the cell interior, where cyclic GMP is located.

The cyclic GMP–gated channel is formed by the combination of four protein subunits, each with a cyclic GMP binding site on the cytoplasmic side of the subunit. For the channel to be open, all four cyclic GMP binding sites must be occupied. The cyclic GMP level is higher in the outer segment in darkness than in light, when phosphodiesterase is active. Thus, the probability that all four binding sites are occupied by cyclic GMP is higher in darkness, and more channels are open. When the cyclic GMP level decreases upon illumination, cyclic GMP is released from the binding sites, the channels close, and the photoreceptor hyperpolarizes.

Turn-off Mechanisms: Restoring the Dark State When Illumination Ceases

Because the photoreceptor cell must be able to signal that light has been turned off as well as on, mechanisms must exist to turn off the activated rhodopsin, transducin, and phosphodiesterase molecules. The transducin alpha-subunit is a GTPase, and when the bound GTP is hydrolyzed to GDP, the transducin alpha-subunit becomes inactive. Therefore, transducin has an inherent lifetime in the activated state, governed by the GTPase activity of the alpha-subunit. In the GDP-bound form, the transducin alpha-subunit cannot stimulate the phosphodiesterase molecule to which it is bound, and the phosphodiesterase stops cleaving cyclic GMP (see Fig. 15.10). The inactive phosphodiesterase then dissociates from the transducin alpha-subunit, which recombines with the beta- and gamma-subunits to re-form the inactive form of the heterotrimeric G-protein (returning to the top of the cycle in Fig. 15.10).

If photoactivated rhodopsin is still present, transducin can be reactivated and enter the cycle for another round. In addition, the inactive phosphodiesterase can combine with a new activated alpha-subunit of transducin and become active again, as long as rhodopsin continues to supply new GTP-bound alpha-subunits. Thus, some mechanism is needed to inactivate rhodopsin and restore the dark state. Otherwise, each molecule of rhodopsin that has undergone photoisomerization would continue to activate transducin long after the light stimulus has disappeared.

Inactivation of rhodopsin involves the cytoplasmic tail of the molecule, where the interaction with transducin occurs. The conformational change induced by photoactivation reveals a number of **phosphorylation sites** in the cytoplasmic end of rhodopsin. **Rhodopsin kinase** begins to phosphorylate these sites when the cytoplasmic tail becomes accessible after the light-induced conformational change. Phosphorylated rhodopsin can re-enter the transducin activation cycle and produce a new molecule of activated transducin, or it can encounter another protein called **arrestin**, which binds to the cytoplasmic tail of phosphorylated rhodopsin. The greater the number of phosphate groups attached to rhodopsin, the higher the probability of arrestin binding. When arrestin attaches to rhodopsin, rhodopsin can no longer bind transducin and the cycle stops. This inactivation mechanism for photoisomerized rhodopsin is shown schematically in Figure 15.12.

Ultimately, the all-*trans* retinal of photoisomerized rhodopsin must be replaced with a new molecule of 11-*cis* retinal to regenerate the dark form of rhodopsin and to recycle the pigment molecule for future use in detecting light. Within minutes after photoisomerization, all-*trans* retinal dissociates from opsin, freeing the retinal binding site on opsin for chemical combination with another molecule of 11-*cis* retinal. The free all-*trans* retinal is converted back to the 11-*cis* form, a reaction cat-

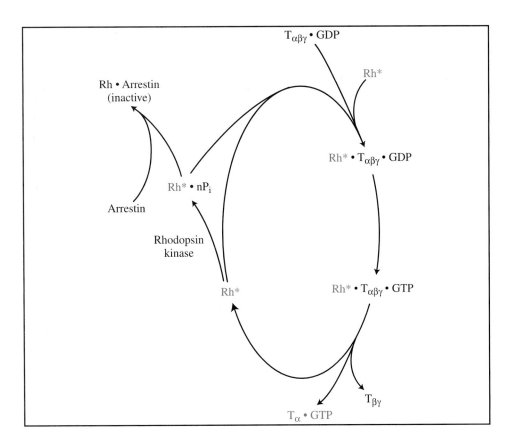

Figure 15.12.

The mechanism of inactivation of photoactivated rhodopsin (Rh). *Red lettering* indicates the activated form of a molecule. T = transducin; GDP = guanosine diphosphate; GTP = guanosine triphosphate.

alyzed by an isomerase enzyme. The conversion of all-*trans* to 11-*cis* retinal mostly takes place in specialized epithelial cells that surround the outer segments of the photoreceptors and provide the photoreceptors with a continuous supply of 11-*cis* retinal for the regeneration of used rhodopsin. Thus, the all-*trans* retinal is shuttled through the extracellular space to the epithelial cells, which take it up and enzymatically convert it to the 11-*cis* isomer. The 11-*cis* retinal is then shuttled back through the extracellular space to the outer segment of the photoreceptor. Specialized extracellular retinal-binding proteins act as molecular chaperones during the shuttling of retinal between the photoreceptors and the epithelial cells.

To restore the dark state of the photoreceptor after illumination has been turned off, the cyclic GMP level must be restored from the low level reached in light to the higher level in darkness. As cyclic GMP levels rise, cyclic GMP–gated channels reopen and the cell depolarizes to its resting potential in dark. Cyclic nucleotides are produced by enzymes called **nucleotide cyclases**, which convert nucleoside triphosphate molecules to the corresponding cyclic nucleoside monophosphate. The enzyme that manufactures cyclic GMP in the photoreceptor outer segment is **guanylyl cyclase**. The concentration of cyclic GMP in the outer segment—and thus the fraction of cyclic GMP–gated ion channels that are open—depends on the balance between the production of cyclic GMP by guanylyl cyclase and the degradation of cyclic GMP by phosphodiesterase. In light, phosphodiesterase is activated, the degradation rate of cyclic GMP is high, and the level of cyclic GMP is low in the outer segment. When illumination ceases, the activity of phosphodiesterase falls and the level of cyclic GMP rises as the cyclase restores the resting concentration in darkness.

The rate at which guanylyl cyclase produces cyclic GMP is also regulated by light, albeit in an indirect way. In the presence of light, the cyclase activity is higher than in darkness. This change in enzyme activity with lighting conditions is mediated by changes in the intracellular calcium concentration that accompany the transition from dark to light. In darkness, an influx of calcium ions represents a significant portion of the ion flux through the open cation channels in the outer segment. Thus, the calcium concentration inside the outer segment is higher in the dark, when the nonspecific cation channels are open, than in the light, when the channels are closed.

The rate of production of cyclic GMP is increased by a modulatory protein that binds to guanylyl cyclase and increases its catalytic rate. The modulatory protein is a calcium-binding protein, which can interact with and stimulate guanylyl cyclase only in its calcium-free form. The calcium-free form prevails in the presence of illumination, when the calcium concentration inside the outer segment is low. In the dark, when internal calcium levels are higher, calcium binds to the modulatory protein, preventing the interaction between the modulatory protein and cyclase and ensuring that cyclase activity is not enhanced. In this way, the calcium level in the outer segment provides feedback regulation of the cyclic GMP production rate, based on the number of open cyclic GMP–gated channels.

LIGHT RESPONSES OF SECOND-ORDER RETINAL NEURONS

Horizontal Cells

How does light affect the membrane potential of horizontal cells?

The photoreceptors make synaptic connections with two types of interneurons: bipolar cells and horizontal cells (see Fig. 15.2). The synaptic terminals of the photoreceptors release the neurotransmitter glutamate. Because the photoreceptors are depolarized in darkness and hyperpolarized in light, the rate of glutamate release is high in darkness and reduced by illumination. Therefore, the response to light of the neurons that receive inputs from the photoreceptors represents a reaction to the *removal* of glutamate. In the horizontal cells, glutamate opens nonspecific cation channels. Thus, like the photoreceptors, the horizontal cells are

BOX 1

IN THE CLINIC

A variety of diseases affect the visual system, and the neurons of the visual system are the targets for many of these diseases. Because the retina can be observed directly through the pupil of the eye, many diseases that affect the retina can be diagnosed during routine eye examinations by observing any change in appearance of the retina. Of course, vision requires functional photoreceptor cells, and a number of hereditary ailments produce blindness by causing degeneration of these cells. In many of the hereditary diseases, the mutated genes that underlie the disease have been identified, and the molecules of phototransduction are frequently the products encoded by the genes. For example, photoreceptor degeneration is known to result from mutations in the genes for the visual pigment molecule, the phosphodiesterase enzyme, and the cyclic GMP–gated ion channel. Exactly how mutations affecting the proteins of the phototransduction machinery produce degeneration of the photoreceptors is not known. Other diseases (for example, glaucoma) affect vision by causing a loss of retinal ganglion cells, whose axons form the only way for visual information from the retina to reach the rest of the brain.

depolarized in darkness—when glutamate is being released by the photo-receptors—and are hyperpolarized upon illumination.

The horizontal cells have widely spreading dendrites that receive inputs from the photoreceptors in a correspondingly large area of the retina, as shown in Figure 15.13. Light falling within this area—the receptive field of the horizontal cell—causes hyperpolarization of the horizontal cell. If a cell receives synaptic inputs originating from a group of photoreceptors, its receptive field is the region of the retinal surface encompassed by that group of photoreceptor cells. In the case of horizontal cells, the situation is somewhat more complicated. Horizontal cells are electrically coupled via gap junctions to their neighbors, forming an electrically coupled lateral network. When light falls on the photoreceptors that make synaptic contacts directly onto a particular horizontal cell, some of the resulting hyperpolarization in that horizontal cell will spread laterally via the electrical junctions into the neighboring horizontal cells, which do not receive direct synaptic inputs from that set of photoreceptors. Thus, the neighboring horizontal cells undergo hyperpolarization as well, even though their own directly connected photoreceptors were not exposed to a light stimulus. For this reason, the receptive field of a horizontal cell is actually larger than would be expected if its membrane po-

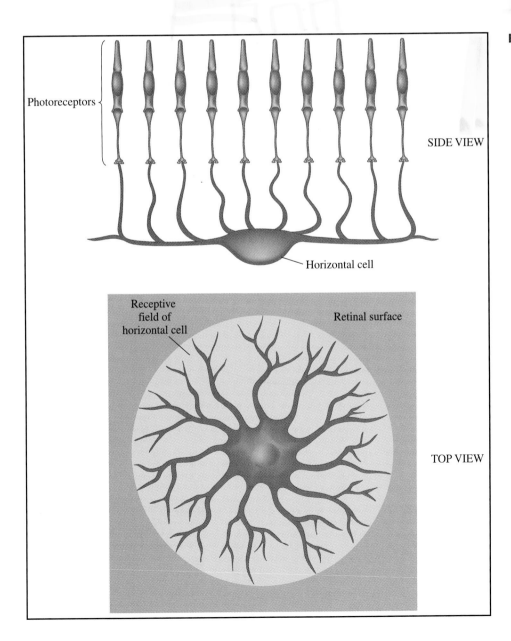

Figure 15.13.

The receptive field of a horizontal cell.

333

tential were affected only by light falling on the directly connected group of photoreceptors.

Two Classes of Bipolar Neurons: Off-Type and On-Type

Why do some bipolar cells depolarize in response to light, whereas other bipolar cells hyperpolarize?

The other type of second-order neuron in the retina is the bipolar cell. Like the horizontal cells, bipolar cells receive direct synaptic inputs from a group of photoreceptors, as shown in Figure 15.14. Thus, light falling on this group of photoreceptors influences the membrane potential of the bipolar neuron. Two classes of bipolar neurons are distinguished on the basis of the change in membrane potential elicited by illumination of the directly connected photoreceptors. **Off-type** or **hyperpolarizing bipolar cells** respond in the same way as the horizontal cells to illumination: these bipolar neurons are depolarized in the dark and are hyperpolarized in response to light (see Fig. 15.14). Glutamate released by the photoreceptors in darkness opens glutamate-gated nonspecific cation channels in off-type bipolar neurons, which depolarizes the bipolar cell. In contrast, **on-type** or **depolarizing bipolar cells** have the opposite response to light: they undergo hyperpolarization in darkness and depolarization upon illumination (see Fig. 15.14).

The depolarizing light response of the on-type bipolar cells arises because glutamate *closes* nonspecific cation channels in this type of bipolar neuron. When light reduces the release of glutamate from the synaptic terminals of the photoreceptors, the cation channels open, and the cell depolarizes. The linkage between the glutamate receptor molecule and the nonspecific cation channel is indirect. The glutamate receptor in on-type bipolar cells activates G-proteins when glutamate binds. The target for the activated G-protein is phosphodiesterase, just as in phototransduction. Figure 15.15 summarizes the action of glutamate in on-type bipolar neurons. Activated phosphodiesterase hydrolyzes cyclic GMP, which is thought to open cyclic GMP–gated ion channels. The number of open cyclic GMP–gated channels—and hence the amount of depolarization—depends on the balance between the degradation of cyclic GMP by phosphodiesterase and the production of cyclic GMP by guanylyl cyclase.

Figure 15.14.

Light responses of off-type and on-type bipolar neurons. E_m = membrane potential.

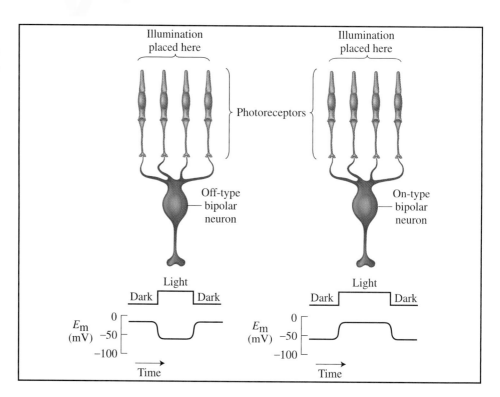

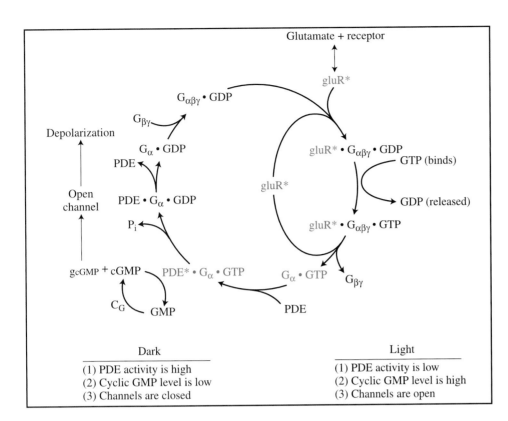

Figure 15.15.

The postsynaptic response to glutamate in on-type bipolar neurons. The activated form of a molecule is indicated by an *asterisk*. gluR = the glutamate receptor molecule; G = G-protein; PDE = phosphodiesterase; C_G = guanylyl cyclase; cGMP = cyclic guanosine monophosphate; g_{cGMP} = cyclic GMP–gated channel.

In the dark, the synaptic terminals of the photoreceptors release glutamate at a high rate, and phosphodiesterase is strongly activated (see Fig. 15.15). The level of cyclic GMP in the bipolar neuron is low, most of the cyclic GMP–gated channels are closed, and the membrane potential is relatively negative. In the light, the photoreceptors stop releasing glutamate, phosphodiesterase is reduced, and the balance between the degradation and the synthesis of cyclic GMP favors synthesis. As cyclic GMP levels rise, more cyclic GMP–gated channels open, and the on-type bipolar neuron depolarizes.

Receptive Field of Bipolar Neurons

As we have just discussed, light falling on the photoreceptors that make synaptic connections with bipolar cell dendrites causes depolarization of on-type bipolar cells and hyperpolarization of off-type bipolar cells. The indirect effects of illumination falling outside this region of directly connected photoreceptors must also be considered, however. These indirect effects are mediated via the connections of the lateral interneurons, the horizontal cells. Recall that horizontal cells have widely spreading dendrites that cover a large area of the retina. Bipolar cell dendrites typically cover a much smaller region of the retina, as illustrated in Figure 15.16. Thus, the receptive field of the horizontal cell is larger than the region contacted by the bipolar cell dendrites.

Like the photoreceptors, the horizontal cells depolarize in darkness and hyperpolarize in response to illumination. Neurotransmitter release from the horizontal cells is highest in darkness and is reduced by illumination. The decreased release of neurotransmitter by horizontal cells (that is, the effect produced by light) produces a synaptic response in bipolar cells that *opposes* the effect of illuminating the photoreceptors that are directly connected to the bipolar cell. Thus, an off-type bipolar cell depolarizes when the horizontal cells hyperpolarize, while on-type bipolar cells hyperpolarize when the horizontal cells hyperpolarize. In other words, the horizontal cells produce negative feedback onto bipolar neurons.

How do synaptic interactions among photoreceptors, horizontal cells, and bipolar cells explain the center-surround organization of receptive fields of bipolar cells?

Figure 15.16.

The receptive field of an off-type bipolar neuron. **A.** When a spot of light is moved across the receptive field in the direction of the *arrow*, the light first stimulates photoreceptors in the surround region of the receptive field and then stimulates the group of photoreceptors that make direct synaptic connections with the bipolar cell. **B.** When light falls on the central region of the receptive field, the bipolar neuron hyperpolarizes. **C.** Light falling within the receptive field of the horizontal cell produces the opposite effect. **D.** The response of the photoreceptor as a function of the light position is the sum of these two influences.

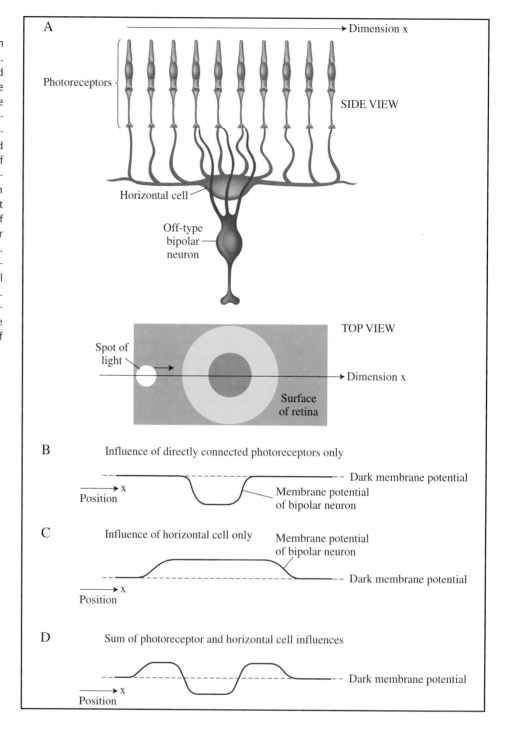

Figure 15.17 illustrates a simple mechanism for negative feedback from the horizontal cells to bipolar neurons. The synaptic terminals of the photoreceptors receive inputs from the horizontal cells, which are themselves the synaptic targets of the photoreceptors. Feedback synapses of this type are a common feature of neuronal information processing in the nervous system.

Let's examine how the feedback synapse from horizontal cells to photoreceptors can produce negative feedback in bipolar neurons, even in the absence of a direct connection between the horizontal cells and the bipolar neurons. In many species, at least some horizontal cells release γ-aminobutyric acid (GABA) as their neurotransmitter at the synaptic connection onto the synaptic terminal of photoreceptors. GABA directly binds to and opens GABA-gated chloride channels in the

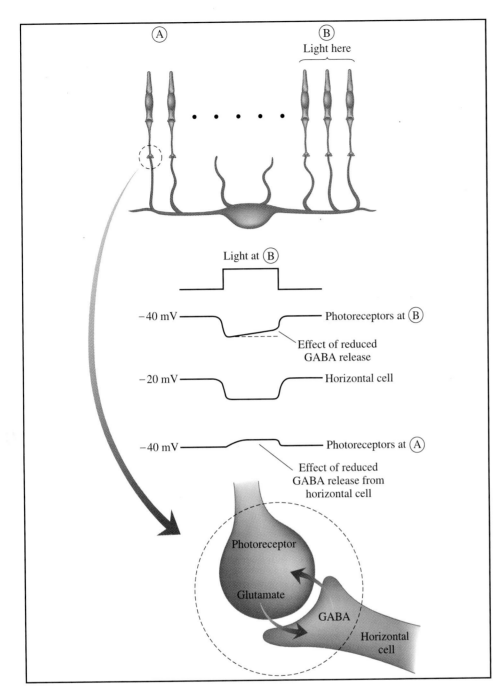

Figure 15.17.
The contribution of the synaptic input of horizontal cells to the response of photoreceptors to light. GABA = γ-aminobutyric acid.

photoreceptor terminal. When horizontal cells depolarize in darkness, more GABA is released at the feedback synapse, increasing the chloride permeability of the photoreceptor. In darkness then, the membrane potential of the photoreceptor is less positive than it would be in the absence of the GABA released by the horizontal cells. Upon illumination, both the photoreceptors and the horizontal cells hyperpolarize, reducing the release of GABA from the horizontal cells and removing the hyperpolarizing influence on the photoreceptor. Thus, during sustained illumination, the membrane potential of the photoreceptor first hyperpolarizes, because the cyclic GMP–gated channels of the outer segment close, and then depolarizes a bit, as the release of GABA from the horizontal cells declines (see Fig. 15.17).

Now consider what happens if light is placed to the side of a particular photoreceptor (rather than directly on it) but still within the receptive fields of nearby horizontal cells. Because the light does not fall directly onto the photoreceptor in question, no hyperpolarization of the photoreceptor is produced by direct illumination (see position A in Fig. 15.17). Nevertheless, the horizontal cell will still hyperpolarize because of the light falling on other nearby photoreceptors (see position B in Fig. 15.17). Thus, less GABA will be released by the horizontal cell onto the synaptic terminals of the photoreceptors at position A, even though no illumination strikes that location. The photoreceptors at position A *depolarize* in response to light displaced to the side, at position B. In other words, light falling on the surrounding portion of the retina produces the opposite effect of light falling directly on the photoreceptors.

Now return to Figure 15.16, which shows how the synaptic arrangement illustrated in Figure 15.17 affects the bipolar neurons. Consider first an off-type bipolar cell. If a small spot of light is directed onto the photoreceptors from which the bipolar cell receives direct synaptic inputs, the off-type bipolar cell will hyperpolarize because less glutamate is released onto its dendrites by the directly connected photoreceptors. If the light is moved to the side so that it no longer falls onto the directly connected group of photoreceptors, its hyperpolarizing influence on the bipolar neuron disappears. This effect of the directly connected photoreceptors on the membrane potential of the bipolar neuron is shown in Figure 15.16B as a function of the position of the illuminating spot on the retinal surface. When the light falls outside the region of the directly connected photoreceptors but still within the receptive field of the horizontal cell (see Fig. 15.16A), the photoreceptors that are directly connected to the off-type bipolar neuron in question will depolarize in response to illumination, as described in Figure 15.17. The depolarized photoreceptors will then release more glutamate from their synaptic terminals. As a result, the off-type bipolar neuron will depolarize in response to illumination. This depolarizing influence, produced by the indirect action of the horizontal cell, is shown as a function of the position of illumination in Figure 15.16C. The effect on the bipolar neuron of illumination at any particular position on the retina will then consist of the sum of the competing influences of the photoreceptors and horizontal cells (see Fig. 15.16D).

The receptive field of off-type bipolar neurons therefore will consist of two regions: a central region where light causes the cell to hyperpolarize (because of decreased glutamate release from the directly connected photoreceptors) and a concentric surrounding region where light causes the cell to depolarize (because of increased glutamate release from the directly connected photoreceptors). This type of receptive field is called a **center-surround receptive field**. Figure 15.18A shows a top view of the receptive field that would be mapped by placing a small spot of light at different positions on the retina and noting the effect on the membrane potential of the bipolar neuron. The most effective stimulus for producing hyperpolarization of an off-type bipolar neuron would be a central bright region, covering the directly connected photoreceptors, surrounded by a region of darkness. Diffuse illumination across the entire receptive field would not be as effective, because it would activate both of the competing influences shown in Figure 15.16. In other words, bipolar neurons signal information about **brightness contrast** on the retinal surface.

The receptive fields of on-type bipolar neurons also have a center-surround organization, but the signs of the responses in the center and surround regions are reversed (see Fig. 15.18B). For both on-type and off-type bipolar cells, light placed in the central region decreases the release of glutamate from the photoreceptor synaptic terminals that contact the bipolar cell, while light placed in the surround region increases glutamate release. Because the lateral inhibitory effect mediated by the horizontal cells targets the synaptic terminal of the photoreceptor and affects the release of glutamate, illumination in the surround region of the receptive field

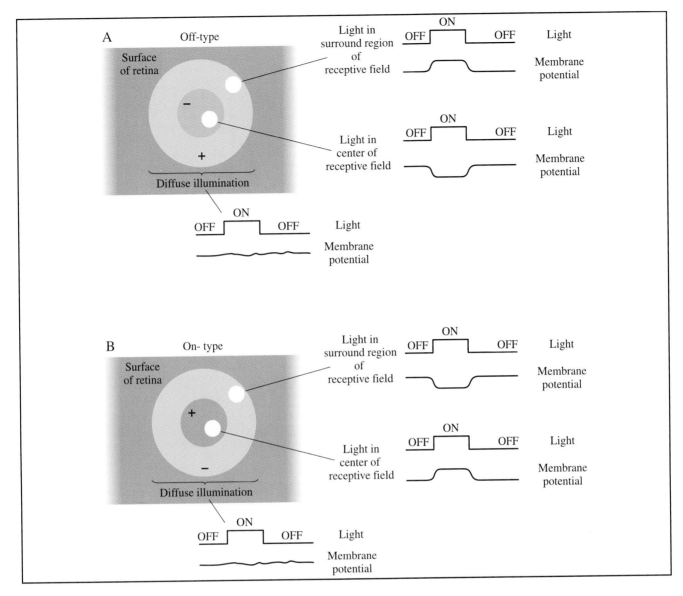

Figure 15.18.

Receptive fields and light responses of off-type and on-type bipolar neurons. **A.** Light placed in the central portion of the receptive field produces hyperpolarization of the off-type bipolar cell. Conversely, light placed in the surround portion of the receptive field produces depolarization of the off-type bipolar cell. Diffuse illumination that covers the entire receptive field has little effect on the bipolar cell. **B.** Light placed in the central portion of the receptive field produces depolarization of the on-type bipolar cell, whereas light in the surround portion produces hyperpolarization of the cell. The membrane potential does not change in response to diffuse illumination that covers both the center and the surround regions of the receptive field.

always opposes the action of illumination in the center, regardless of whether glutamate depolarizes or hyperpolarizes the bipolar cell.

This mechanism is thought to account for the center-surround organization of the receptive fields for the bipolar cells in the retinas of some species, but it is not universally true of all species. In some cases, the postsynaptic targets of the horizontal cells are the bipolar neurons themselves, rather than the photoreceptor synaptic terminal. In addition, not all horizontal cells release GABA as their neurotransmitter. In these cases, the exact mechanism responsible for the antagonism between the center and the surround of the receptive field remains uncertain.

Presumably, however, the horizontal cell transmitter must hyperpolarize off-type bipolar neurons and depolarize on-type bipolar cells, which in both instances would produce responses from the surround that oppose responses from the center of the receptive field.

LIGHT RESPONSES OF AMACRINE CELLS

In what ways do amacrine cells respond to illumination?

Just as lateral interconnections mediated by horizontal cells are found at the synapses of the photoreceptors, lateral interconnections also occur at the synapses of the bipolar cells. In this case, amacrine cells mediate the lateral interconnections (see Fig. 15.2). Amacrine cells receive inputs from bipolar cells and make feedback synaptic connections with the terminals of the bipolar neurons. Like horizontal cells, at least some amacrine cells use GABA as their neurotransmitter, and the synaptic terminals of the bipolar cells have GABA-gated chloride channels like those found in the terminals of photoreceptors. Thus, the amacrine cells are lateral inhibitory interneurons whose actions on bipolar cells are analogous to the actions of horizontal cells on photoreceptors.

Amacrine cells depolarize in response to changes in light intensity within their receptive fields. The dendrites of amacrine cells commonly extend for a considerable distance in the retina, receiving synaptic inputs from bipolar cells in a large area. Consequently, the receptive fields of amacrine cells are typically quite large, corresponding to the region covered by all of the photoreceptors that are connected to the entire set of bipolar neurons sampled by the amacrine cell. Glutamate released by bipolar cells opens nonspecific cation channels and depolarizes amacrine cells. Some amacrine cells, called **on-type amacrine cells**, receive inputs only from on-type bipolar cells. On-type amacrine cells depolarize at the onset of illumination, when on-type bipolar cells depolarize and release transmitter. In contrast, **off-type amacrine cells** receive synaptic inputs only from off-type bipolar cells and therefore depolarize at the termination of illumination. Still other amacrine cells, called **on-off amacrine cells**, receive synaptic inputs from both on-type and off-type bipolar cells and depolarize at both the onset and the termination of illumination. The different light responses of amacrine cells are shown in Figure 15.19.

Figure 15.19 also illustrates that amacrine cells depolarize only briefly following a change in illumination level. Most amacrine cells, then, respond transiently to illumination. If the depolarization produced by a change in illumination is sufficiently large, amacrine cells produce action potentials in response to the synaptic

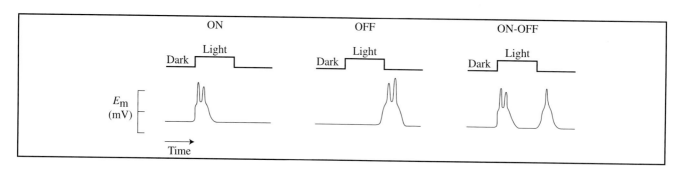

Figure 15.19.

Light responses of three types of amacrine cells. The on-type cell produces a transient depolarization when the light is turned on, the off-type cell produces a depolarization when the light is turned off, and the on-off cell produces transient depolarizations at both the onset and termination of illumination. Amacrine cells also fire action potentials when the depolarizing synaptic response is sufficiently large.

depolarization (see Fig. 15.19). Thus, the amacrine cells represent the first occurrence of action potentials in the responses of the retinal neurons to light. In photoreceptors, horizontal cells, and bipolar cells, the changes in membrane potential produced by illumination spread electrically throughout the cell without requiring action potentials.

LIGHT RESPONSES OF RETINAL GANGLION CELLS

The output from the eye is carried to the rest of the brain by the axons of the retinal ganglion cells, which come together to form the optic nerve (cranial nerve II). Because the information carried by the ganglion cells must be transmitted over long distances, action potentials are necessary to carry the signal. In the optic nerve, therefore, information about light falling on the retina must be coded in the frequency of action potentials fired by the retinal ganglion cells. In the output cells of the retina, the light responses are represented by changes in action potential activity, rather than the depolarizing and hyperpolarizing synaptic potentials characteristic of light responses in the bipolar cells and horizontal cells. Keep in mind, however, that the changes in the firing of action potentials in ganglion cells reflect the combined excitatory and inhibitory synaptic interactions from the bipolar cells and amacrine cells that make synaptic connections with the ganglion cells.

The responses of ganglion cells to light fall into the same general categories as those of amacrine cells, based on whether a cell is excited by an increase in light intensity, a decrease in light intensity, or both. In addition, the responses in ganglion cells can be either sustained for the duration of the stimulus or transient. These response characteristics are summarized in Figure 15.20. Ganglion cells can have complex response properties as well. For instance, some ganglion cells respond only to light moving in a particular direction across the retina. These motion-sensitive ganglion cells are analogous to the motion-sensitive cortical neurons in the somatosensory system discussed in Chapter 14. Motion selectivity in the visual system probably arises via synaptic arrangements like those that produce the motion-selective cells in the touch sensory pathway—that is, via lateral inhibitory connections made selectively to one side (see Fig. 14.15). Other ganglion cells respond to light by firing action potentials at a rate proportional to the overall average level of illumination falling on a wide area of retina, which suggests that these cells inform the brain about the average light intensity, or luminance, of the visual world.

The receptive fields of ganglion cells vary widely in size. Some ganglion cells receive inputs from only a single bipolar neuron, while others receive inputs from thousands of bipolar cells. The receptive fields of ganglion cells commonly have the concentric center-surround organization described previously for bipolar neurons. Examples of the receptive fields of ganglion cells are shown in Figure 15.20. Light in the center of the receptive field of an **on-type ganglion cell** increases the action potential activity, while light in the surround region inhibits the cell. Conversely, light in the center of the receptive field of an **off-type ganglion cell** inhibits the cell, while light in the surround region excites the cell. For both types of ganglion cells, a diffuse light across the entire receptive field has little effect. For an on-type ganglion cell, the stimulus that best excites the cell would be a spot of light that fills the central part of the receptive field, surrounded by darkness. For an off-type ganglion cell, the greatest excitation would result from a dark spot on a bright background. In both cases, the ganglion cell signals the brain about the spatial contrast in light intensity at the position of the ganglion cell's receptive field. In the visual world, a change in light intensity typically defines the edge of an object,

In what ways do ganglion cells respond to illumination?

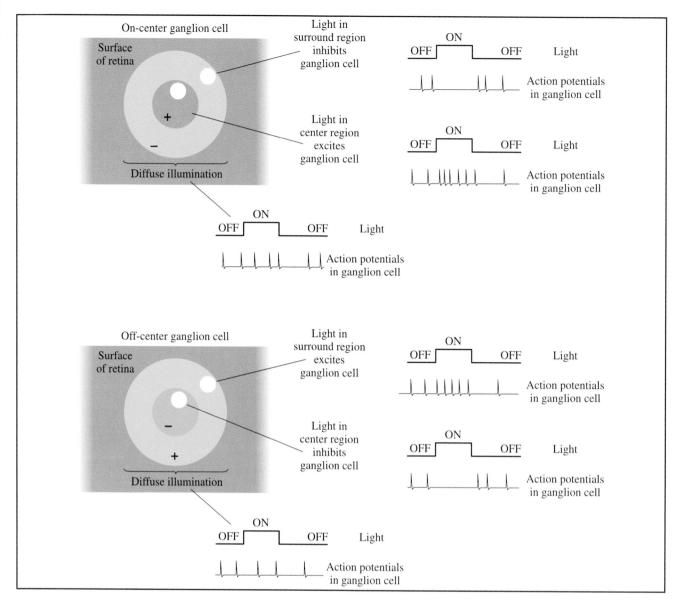

Figure 15.20.

Receptive fields of on-center and off-center ganglion cells. Light placed in the center of the receptive field increases the rate of action potential firing in on-center cells and decreases the rate of action potential firing in off-center cells. Light in the surround region of the receptive field has the opposite effect, exciting off-center cells and inhibiting on-center cells. In both cases, the ganglion cells fire action potentials at a slow rate even in the absence of illumination. This "spontaneous" firing allows the nervous system to distinguish both increases and decreases in firing rate. Diffuse illumination applied to the entire receptive field produces only a weak response to light in the ganglion cells.

and so information about spatial contrast in intensity is important to the visual system in defining the shape and location of an object.

In extracting information about the spatial pattern of light intensity, the visual system sometimes perceives differences in light intensity when no such difference actually exists in the stimulus. The center-surround organization of the receptive fields of the ganglion cells produces some of these illusory perceptions, including the one illustrated in Figure 15.21. In the figure, black rectangles are separated by uniform white lines. If you gaze at the center of one of the black rectangles, you will notice a dim gray spot at each intersection of the surrounding white lines. These gray spots are not present in the stimulus but are "created" in the retina by

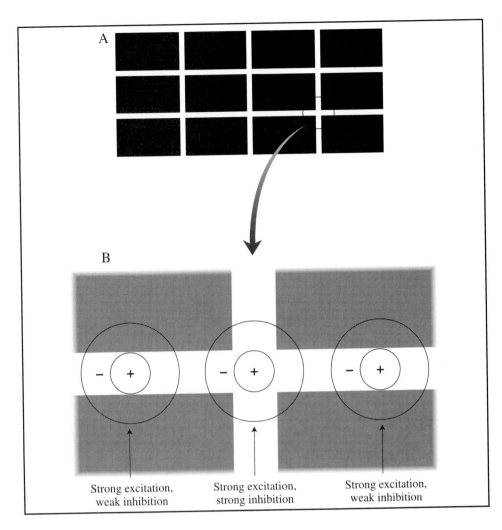

A

B

Strong excitation,
weak inhibition

Strong excitation,
strong inhibition

Strong excitation,
weak inhibition

Figure 15.21.

A visual illusion that arises from the center-surround organization of the ganglion cells in the human retina. **A.** When you look at the center of a black rectangle, you observe a gray spot at each intersection of the white lines defined by the spaces between adjacent rectangles. Note that gray spot disappears when you gaze directly at an intersection, although you can still see the spots at other intersections in your peripheral vision. **B.** This perception of reduced light intensity is produced when your brain interprets the outputs of retinal ganglion cells whose receptive fields are arranged as shown. The reason the perceived gray spot disappears when you gaze directly at an intersection is that the receptive fields of ganglion cells are much smaller in the central part of the visual field, so that both the center and surround portions of a single field fall entirely within the white area without overlapping the black zones.

the center-surround receptive fields of the retinal ganglion cells. The basis of the illusion is illustrated in Figure 15.21B, which shows receptive fields for three on-center ganglion cells. The receptive fields of the two cells on each side, away from the corners of the rectangles, receive full illumination, but the surround areas are mostly in darkness. As a result, these ganglion cells are strongly excited but only weakly inhibited, giving rise to a relatively high firing rate. In the receptive field of the ganglion cell at the intersection of the two white lines, however, the center is fully illuminated, but the surround area is also strongly illuminated. Thus, this cell fires action potentials at a lower rate than the two other ganglion cells to each side. The visual system interprets the lower firing rate of the central cell as a lower light intensity, causing us to perceive a gray area at the intersection.

Lateral inhibition in the retina aids in the detection of borders between regions of differing light intensity on the surface of the retina (that is, the edge of an object in the visual world). Figure 15.22 illustrates how lateral interactions enhance the perceived brightness contrast at an edge. An array of ganglion cells receives excitatory inputs from a set of on-type bipolar neurons, which also excite lateral inhibitory neurons that inhibit the ganglion cells on each side. On the left portion of the array, each bipolar neuron receives 100 units of excitation, while the bipolar cells on the right receive 50 units of excitation (the "excitation units" are arbitrary and are used only to illustrate the neuronal calculations performed at the synaptic connections). Each excitatory synapse transmits 100% of the incoming excitation to the postsynaptic cell, while each inhibitory synapse subtracts 20% of the incoming excitation from the total amount of excitation in the postsynaptic cell. Thus, each

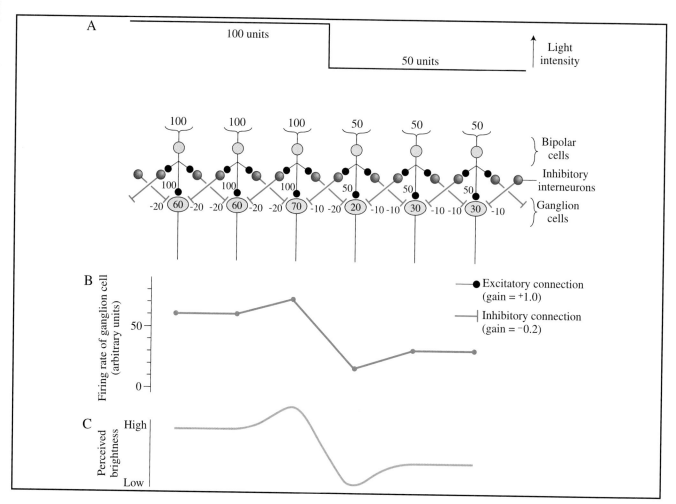

Figure 15.22.

Lateral inhibitory connections enhance the perceived brightness contrast at a border between a lighter and a darker region. **A.** The spatial arrangement of light intensity falling on the retina is shown on the *top*, with an array of bipolar cells and ganglion cells shown *below*. In this schematic example, the excitatory connections from the bipolar neurons are assumed to transmit to the postsynaptic cell 100% of the "excitation units" produced in the bipolar neuron by the illumination. The inhibitory connections from the inhibitory interneurons (*red*) are assumed to subtract from the postsynaptic ganglion cell 20% of the "excitation units" in the inhibitory interneuron. **B.** The resulting rates of action potential firing in the ganglion cells. **C.** The visual system then interprets the firing rates of the ganglion cell to give rise to the perceived pattern of brightness.

ganglion cell within the brighter region receives 100 units of excitation from the bipolar neuron while having 20 units subtracted by each of the two inhibitory inputs, for a total of 60 units of excitation. Within the dimmer region, each ganglion cell receives 50 units of excitation, while inhibition subtracts 20 units (10 units from each side), for a total of 30 units of excitation.

Now consider the two ganglion cells in the array whose receptive fields are located at the border between the brighter and dimmer regions. For the ganglion cell on the bright side of the border, the bipolar cell provides 100 units of excitation, while the inhibitory interneuron from the left subtracts 20 units. The inhibitory interneuron from the right receives its excitation from the dim side of the border and so subtracts only 10 units (20% of 50). Consequently, the ganglion cell on the bright side of the border receives a total of 70 units of excitation. For the ganglion cell on the dim side of the border, the bipolar cell provides 50 units of excitation, while the two inhibitory connections subtract a total of 30 units (20 from the left and 10 from the right). Thus, the two ganglion cells at the border differ from their neighbors in the uniformly illuminated regions on each side, with the ganglion cell on the bright side of the edge being more strongly excited and the ganglion cell on the dim side being less strongly excited. Figure 15.22B shows the resulting spatial distribution of firing rate in the ganglion cells.

The visual system in the brain interprets the firing rate of each ganglion cell in the array as an indication of the light intensity at that point in the visual field. Thus, the perceived brightness of the stimulus (see Fig. 15.22C) parallels the pattern of neural activity shown in Figure 15.22B. Because the ganglion cell on the brighter side of the edge is more active than its neighbors to the left and the ganglion cell on the dimmer side is less active than its neighbors to the right, a human looking at a step change in light intensity perceives a brighter band on the bright side of the edge and a darker band on the dim side. In other words, the lateral inhibitory synaptic connections within the retina enhance the perceived contrast between the bright and the dim side of the edge.

COLOR VISION

To this point, we have focused on the detection of light, the determination of relative light intensity, and the processing of information about spatial patterns of illumination reaching the retina. In addition, however, information about the *color* of an object is also important in discerning and identifying parts of the environment. The physical characteristic of the stimulus that gives rise to the perceived color is the wavelength composition of the light that is reflected from or transmitted by an object. To understand how neurons of the retina distinguish different wavelengths of light, we will need to examine the properties of the cone photoreceptors.

How is color information encoded in the retina?

Cone Photoreceptors

Cone photoreceptors differ from the rod photoreceptors not only morphologically (see Fig. 15.3) but also in the types of photopigment molecules they contain. In the human retina, three different cone types are distinguished, each containing a unique type of photopigment. In all three types of cone photopigments, the light-absorbing chromophore molecule is the same as in rhodopsin: 11-*cis* retinal. However, the opsin protein portion of the photopigment differs.

Because the interaction between the opsin protein and the chromophore group determines the wavelength of light that is absorbed best by the chromophore, the different opsin proteins produce different **spectral sensitivities** for each of the three cone photopigments. The sensitivity of the three pigments of human cones to light of different wavelengths is illustrated in Figure 15.23. One type of photopigment absorbs light best at about 420 nm, one type has highest sensitivity at approximately 530 nm, and the third is most sensitive to light at a wavelength near 560 nm. The cones that contain the 420-nm pigment are called **S-cones** (for short-wavelength cones; "short" refers to their sensitivity to short wavelengths, not their size). The cones containing the 530-nm pigment are called **M-cones** (for middle-wavelength cones). The cones that have the 560-nm pigment are called **L-cones** (for, you guessed it, long-wavelength cones). The three cone classes are also called **blue cones**, **green cones**, and **red cones**, respectively, because the S-cone pigment is most sensitive in the blue portion of the visible spectrum (at short wavelengths), the M-cone pigment is most sensitive in the green portion of the spectrum, and the L-cone photopigment is the most sensitive in the red portion of the spectrum (at longer wavelengths). Most visual neuroscientists prefer the

How do the three types of cones differ in their sensitivity to lights of different wavelengths?

Figure 15.23.

The sensitivity of the photo-pigments in the three different cones to lights of different wavelengths in the visual spectrum. The cones sensitive to short-wavelength light (S-cones) have a photopigment that absorbs light best in the violet and blue portion of the visual spectrum (*blue curve*). The cones sensitive to long-wavelength light (L-cones) have a pigment that absorbs best in the yellow and red part of the spectrum (*red curve*). The cones sensitive to middle-wavelength light (M-cones) have a photopigment that absorbs best in the green and yellow portion of the spectrum (*green curve*).

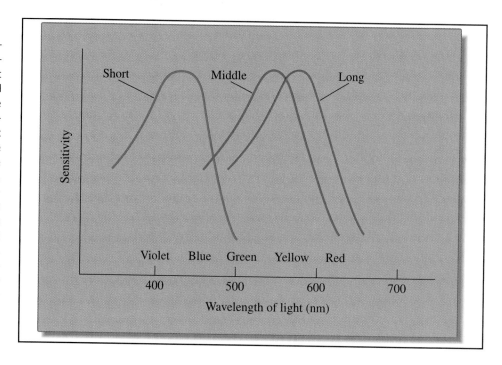

"short," "middle," and "long" terminology, however. By comparison, the photopigment of the rods (rhodopsin) is most sensitive to light at a wavelength of 500 nm.

Rod and cone photoreceptors also differ in their absolute sensitivity to light. The rods are responsible for vision at dim light levels (for example, starlight and moonlight), while the cones respond to light only at higher levels (for example, normal room light and daylight).

The three types of cones account for the ability of humans to distinguish lights of different wavelengths and thus to perceive colors. To understand why multiple photopigments with different spectral sensitivities are required for color discrimination, we must first consider the response of a single class of photoreceptor (rods) with only a single type of photopigment (rhodopsin) to lights of different wavelengths, as shown in Figure 15.24. A rod photoreceptor gives a large response to even a dim 500-nm light, the optimal wavelength for rhodopsin. To produce a response of the same size in the rod, however, light of either a shorter or longer wavelength must be brighter than the 500-nm light. Rhodopsin is less likely to absorb photons of light at wavelengths other than 500 nm (see Fig. 15.24A), and so a more intense light is required to obtain the same number of photoisomerizations in the rod outer segment. The size of the light response in the rod is the same at all three wavelengths, however. Cells receiving synaptic input from the rod cannot determine whether the response was produced by a dim 500-nm light or by brighter lights of other wavelengths. In other words, brightness and wavelength are inherently confused if the visual system receives the output of a single type of photoreceptor having a single type of photopigment. For this reason, humans cannot perceive color when the level of illumination is sufficiently dim that only the rod photoreceptors are active (for example, in moonlight or starlight).

Now consider the response of the cone photoreceptor system to a similar set of light stimuli at three different wavelengths. Figure 15.25A shows the spectral sensitivity curves of the three types of cone photoreceptors. At the intermediate wavelength (wavelength A), M-cones are most sensitive, followed by the L-cones, and then the S-cones. Thus, the response to this wavelength will be greatest in the M-cones, intermediate in the L-cones, and smallest in the S-cones (see Fig. 15.25B). At the shorter wavelength (wavelength B), the S-cones have the highest

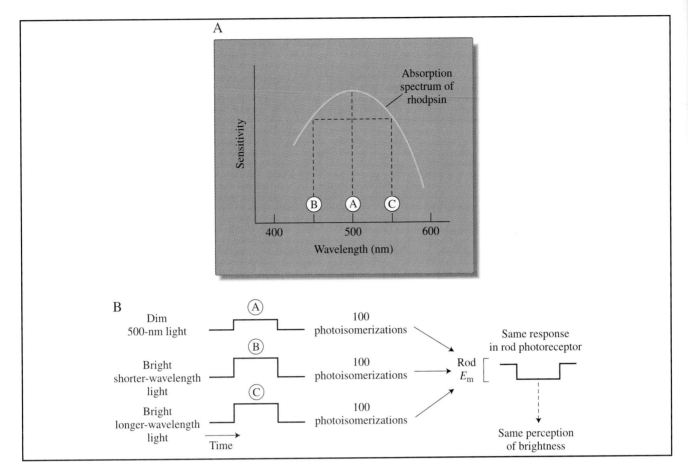

Figure 15.24.

The response of a rod photoreceptor to light of various wavelengths. **A.** The sensitivity of the rod photopigment, rhodopsin, to light of different wavelengths. Rhodopsin absorbs light best at 500 nm (letter A); at shorter wavelengths (letter B) and longer wavelengths (letter C), it absorbs light less effectively. **B.** The hyperpolarization produced in the rod by 100 photoisomerizations is shown on the *right*. This number of photoisomerizations of rhodopsin could be produced by a dim light at a wavelength of 500 nm (letter A) or by brighter lights at wavelength B or C. All of these lights produce the same perception of brightness because they generate responses of the same size in the rod. Thus, with a single photopigment, there is no basis for distinguishing lights of different wavelengths from lights of different intensities.

sensitivity and the largest light response, the M-cones have a smaller response, and the L-cones do not respond. Conversely, at the longer wavelength (wavelength C), the S-cones are insensitive, while the L-cones show the largest response.

There is a unique pattern of responses to light for the three cone types at each wavelength. By comparing the responses originating from the cones, cells of the visual system can distinguish which wavelength of light was presented to the retina. This comparison forms the basis for the perception of color in the visual system. Normally, the light arriving at the eyes is a mixture of different wavelengths, rather than a single wavelength. The visual system can then determine the relative contribution of light from different wavelengths by analyzing the strength of the neural signals originating from each type of cone photoreceptor.

Color-Sensitive Ganglion Cells

In part, the comparison of the three different cone signals occurs within the retina itself. Some types of ganglion cells do not respond well to white light (which

Figure 15.25.

The pattern of responses in the three types of cone photoreceptors provides the information necessary to distinguish lights of different wavelengths. **A.** The absorption spectra of the three cone photopigments. Lights of wavelengths A, B, and C are absorbed to different extents by the three photopigments. **B.** Examples of responses of three cones to the wavelengths illustrated in **A**. At the middle wavelength, all three cones respond to the light, but the response is largest in the M-cone. At the shorter wavelength, the largest response occurs in the S-cone. At the longer wavelength, the L-cone generates the largest response.

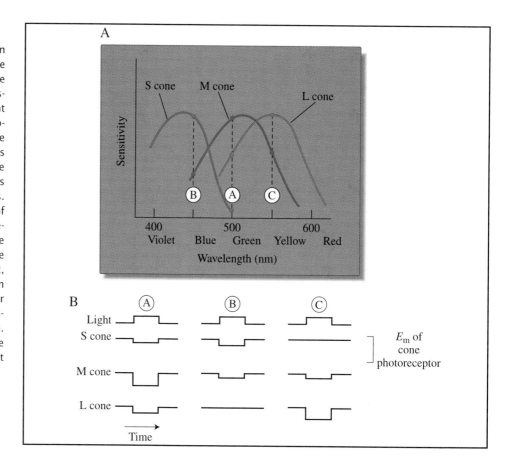

consists of all wavelengths in the visual part of the spectrum). Instead, these cells respond best to light of a specific color. Like many other ganglion cells, the color-sensitive ganglion cells have center-surround receptive fields, as illustrated in Figure 15.26. Illumination in the center and surround regions of the receptive field produces opposing effects, as in other ganglion cells. In the color-sensitive cells, however, the center and surround responses originate from different types of cone photoreceptors. Thus, the responses depend on the wavelength of light falling on the central region and the surround region of the receptive field.

Consider, for example, the receptive field of the ganglion cell shown in Figure 15.26. In this example, the excitatory center of the receptive field is mediated via L-cones, while the inhibitory surround region originates from M-cones. If a red light covers the entire receptive field of this neuron, the cell will be strongly excited (see Fig. 15.26A). The L-cones in the excitatory center of the receptive field are more sensitive to the red light than the M-cones in the inhibitory surround region, producing excitation of the ganglion cell. Conversely, if a green light covers the receptive field (see Fig. 15.26B), the M-cones of the inhibitory surround will be preferentially stimulated, resulting in inhibition of the ganglion cell. Therefore, this ganglion cell will be excited by red light and inhibited by green light.

There are many different varieties of such color-sensitive ganglion cells. Some ganglion cells have receptive fields with an organization opposite of that illustrated in Figure 15.26—that is, the surround portion of the receptive field originates from L-cones and the center of the receptive field originates from M-cones. These ganglion cells will be inhibited by a diffuse red light and excited by a diffuse green light. The ganglion cells that have opposing responses to red and green lights are called **red/green opponent ganglion cells**. The two varieties of red/green cells are red excitatory center, green inhibitory surround (as shown in Fig. 15.26) and green excitatory center, red inhibitory surround. Other ganglion cells have re-

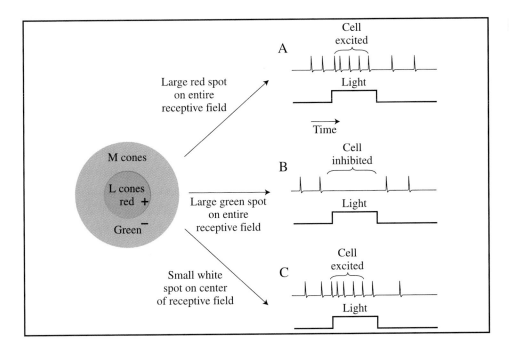

Figure 15.26.

An example of the receptive field of a color-sensitive ganglion cell. A top view of the concentric receptive field on the surface of the retina is shown on the *left*. In this case, the excitatory center of the receptive field is formed by synaptic connections to L-cones, while the inhibitory surround region originates from M-cones. **A.** A red spot that covers the receptive field will preferentially stimulate the L-cones and excite the ganglion cell. **B.** A green spot that covers the receptive field preferentially affects the M-cones and inhibits the ganglion cell. **C.** A white spot placed on the center of the receptive field also excites the ganglion cell and cannot be distinguished from a red stimulus.

ceptive fields whose centers originate from S-cones and whose surrounds originate from M-cones or vice versa. These **blue/yellow opponent ganglion cells** produce opposing responses to blue lights (affecting primarily S-cones) and yellow lights (affecting primarily M-cones). The two varieties of blue/yellow cells are blue excitatory center, yellow inhibitory surround and yellow excitatory center, blue inhibitory surround. Because both the center and the surround of all such ganglion cells derive from a single type of cone photoreceptor, color-sensitive cells of this group are called **single-opponent cells**.

Although the responses of these ganglion cells are sensitive to the wavelength of the illuminating light, they do not provide unambiguous information about the color of a stimulus. Figure 15.26C shows that the output of the red-center ganglion cell fails to distinguish between a red stimulus and a white-light stimulus that covers only the center of the receptive field. White light, which consists of photons of all visible wavelengths, stimulates the L-cones in the excitatory center of the receptive field of the ganglion cell. Consequently, a small spot of white light on the center of the receptive field excites the ganglion cell in the same manner as a diffuse red light. By examining only the output of this type of single-opponent ganglion cell, the nervous system cannot distinguish between the two types of stimuli. Clearly, information coming from other types of ganglion cells must be combined with information from single-opponent color-sensitive cells to resolve the ambiguity. In Chapter 16, we will discuss the further processing of color information in the parts of the brain devoted to vision.

SUMMARY

The translation of light energy into electrical signals takes place through the process of phototransduction, which occurs in specialized neurons called photoreceptors. The photoreceptors are located in the retina at the back of the vertebrate eye. The two general classes of photoreceptors are the rods, which function in dim light, and the cones, which function in brighter light. Photons of light are absorbed by visual pigment molecules located in the photoreceptor cells. The pigment molecule of the rods is called rhodopsin. The pigment molecule is formed from the covalent linkage of the light-absorbing chromophore group, retinal (or vitamin A aldehyde), and a large membrane protein, opsin.

When retinal absorbs a photon of light, it undergoes photoisomerization from a folded form (11-*cis* retinal) to a straight form (all-*trans* retinal). The isomerization triggers a conformational change in the opsin protein, revealing a cytoplasmic binding site for a GTP binding protein called transducin. The activated rhodopsin catalyzes the replacement of GDP by GTP on transducin, thereby activating the G-protein. Transducin in turn activates a phosphodiesterase enzyme, which hydrolyzes cyclic GMP to GMP. Thus, absorption of light decreases the intracellular concentration of cyclic GMP in the photoreceptor. Cyclic GMP is an internal messenger that binds to and opens nonspecific cation channels in the plasma membrane of the outer segment. In darkness—when cyclic GMP levels are high—the channels are open and the photoreceptor is depolarized. In light—when cyclic GMP levels are low—the channels close and the photoreceptor membrane potential is more negative. Thus, light causes the hyperpolarization of photoreceptor cells.

The photoreceptors release glutamate from synapses onto bipolar cells and horizontal cells. The release of glutamate is increased in darkness, when the photoreceptors are depolarized. Horizontal cells are depolarized by glutamate, which opens nonspecific cation channels. As a result, horizontal cells hyperpolarize in response to illumination. The horizontal cells are lateral inhibitory interneurons, some of which release the neurotransmitter GABA.

Bipolar neurons exhibit two types of postsynaptic responses to glutamate. In off-type bipolar neurons, glutamate opens nonspecific cation channels, causing the cells to depolarize in darkness and hyperpolarize in response to light. In on-type bipolar neurons, glutamate closes cyclic GMP–gated channels, and as a result the cells hyperpolarize in darkness and depolarize in response to illumination. Glutamate reduces the cyclic GMP concentration in on-type bipolar neurons, via GTP–binding proteins and phosphodiesterase in a manner analogous to the phototransduction process in the photoreceptors. Receptive fields of bipolar neurons have a center-surround organization, with a central region where light either produces depolarization of the cell (on-type bipolar cells) or hyperpolarization of the cell (off-type bipolar cells) and a larger concentric region where light produces the opposite effect. This opposing effect from the surrounding portion of the receptive field is mediated via the lateral synapses made by the horizontal cells.

The bipolar cells carry light signals to the third-order neurons in the retina, the amacrine cells, and the ganglion cells. Amacrine cells are lateral inhibitory interneurons that mediate lateral interactions analogous to those of the horizontal cells. The ganglion cells are the output cells of the retina, and their outgoing axons form the optic nerve. Electrical signals in the ganglion cells are carried by action potentials, and amacrine cells also make action potentials in response to depolarization. In the other retinal neurons (photoreceptors, horizontal cells, and bipolar cells), electrical signals are carried passively, and action potentials are not involved.

Information about the color of incoming light originates in the cone photoreceptors, which contain photopigments that are sensitive to different parts of the visible spectrum. Humans have three types of cones: the S-cones are most sensitive to short wavelengths (perceived as blue), the M-cones are sensitive to the middle wavelengths (perceived as green and yellow), and the L-cones are most sensitive to long wavelengths (the red part of the visible spectrum). Some ganglion cells have receptive fields that originate from particular types of cones, making these ganglion cells sensitive to the wavelength of illumination. Color-sensitive ganglion cells have center-surround receptive fields, but the center and surround regions originate from different types of cones. For this reason, lights in different parts of the visible spectrum produce opposing effects on the color-sensitive ganglion cell. For example, a red light might excite the cell, while a green light inhibits it.

1. Identify each of the following: outer segment, rhodopsin, 11-*cis* retinal.
2. What protein is stimulated by photoactivated rhodopsin, and how does rhodopsin convert the protein to its active form?
3. Describe the role of cyclic GMP in phototransduction.
4. Name five classes of neurons in the retina and describe the functional role of each class.
5. Describe the two different types of bipolar cells and their responses to glutamate.
6. What is the organization of the receptive field of bipolar cells, and how does this organization arise from synaptic connections among retinal neurons?
7. What classes of cone photoreceptors are present in the human retina, and how are the classes distinguished?
8. Why are we unable to distinguish the colors of objects in moonlight?
9. What is a single-opponent ganglion cell, and how is its receptive field organized?

INTERNET ASSIGNMENT CHAPTER 15

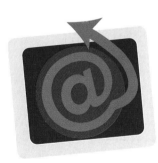

1 Rhodopsin is the photopigment of rod photoreceptors. Locate information about the molecular structure of rhodopsin. Find images that illustrate the three-dimensional structure of the opsin protein.

2 Search the Internet to find information about the anatomy of the retina. Identify the cellular layers that contain the cell bodies of the different types of neurons found in the retina.

THE VISUAL SYSTEM: HIGHER VISUAL PROCESSING

ESSENTIAL BACKGROUND

Excitatory and inhibitory synaptic transmission (Chapter 6)

Action potential (Chapter 4)

Anatomy of the forebrain (Chapter 2, Chapter 9)

In Chapter 15, we learned how light is absorbed in the retina and converted into electrical signals. We also saw that the synaptic connections among the neurons in the retina are arranged to extract particular kinds of information about the patterns of illumination falling on the array of photoreceptors. This visual information is carried from the retina to the rest of the nervous system by the

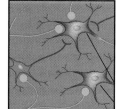

temporal patterns of action potentials in the axons of retinal ganglion cells, which make up the optic nerve. The ganglion cells do not report a simple point-by-point representation of the outputs of the photoreceptors. Instead, each ganglion cell is sensitive to a particular aspect of a visual stimulus, such as the spatial pattern of illumination, the direction of motion of an object, the color of the light, and so on. In other words, the ganglion cells are specialized to extract particular kinds of information about the visual world, which they then pass on to the other parts of the visual system for analysis and construction of visual perceptions. The ganglion cells of various types form multiple, parallel information channels into the brain. In this chapter, we will turn our attention to the parts of the visual brain that are specialized to analyze object form, location, motion, and color based on the information provided by the retina in these parallel channels.

TARGETS OF THE RETINAL GANGLION CELLS IN THE BRAIN

The axons of the retinal ganglion cells project to multiple targets in the brain. In animals without a well-developed forebrain, the principal target is a part of the dorsal midbrain called the **optic tectum**. In mammals, the equivalent part of the brain is the **superior colliculus**, which integrates visual information with motor output in the neural systems that control eye movements (see Chapter 10). Some retinal ganglion cells also send axons to the **suprachiasmatic nucleus**, which controls the entrainment of biological rhythms by the diurnal light cycle (see Chapter 12). As the large cerebral cortex emerged during mammalian evolution, these older visual areas of the brain were supplemented by the **geniculostriate pathway**, in which visual information is relayed from the retina to the **thalamus** and then from the thalamus to the **striate cortex** (see Fig. 16.1). In primates, the geniculostriate pathway has come to dominate the processing of visual information, and large por-

What parts of the brain comprise the geniculostriate pathway?

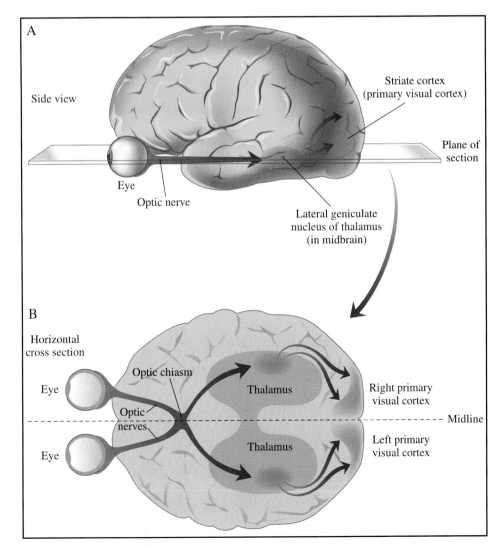

Figure 16.1.

The anatomical organization of the geniculostriate visual pathway. **A**. Side view. **B**. Horizontal cross section in the plane shown in **A**.

tions of the cerebral cortex are devoted to the analysis of the neural outputs of the geniculostriate pathway.

The geniculostriate pathway is named after its two components: the visual relay station in the thalamus (the **lateral geniculate nucleus**) and the striate cortex. The striate cortex is an alternative term for the **primary visual cortex**, and it receives its name from a conspicuous stripe (or striation) in the middle of the cortical layers. This stripe arises because the unusually large number of thalamic synaptic inputs to layer IV (the cortical layer that receives thalamic inputs; see Chapter 9) makes this layer particularly prominent in the primary visual cortex. Under Brodmann's cortical numbering scheme (see Chapter 9), the primary visual cortex is known as **area 17**.

The optic nerves from the two eyes merge at the base of the brain, forming a structure called the **optic chiasm**. The axons of the retinal ganglion cells then separate again to form the two **optic tracts**, which terminate in the lateral geniculate nucleus on each side of the brain. The thalamic neurons that receive synaptic inputs from the retinal ganglion cells in turn send their axons to the primary visual cortex, in the occipital lobe at the back of the brain.

Most of the primary visual cortex is hidden from view on the medial surface of the occipital lobe, within the midline infolding where the two cerebral hemispheres face each other. In addition, the primary visual cortex in each of the two occipital lobes forms a deep infolding at the rearmost pole of the brain, called the **calcarine fissure**.

Another name for the primary visual cortex is **area V1**, which stands for visual cortical area number one. As we will see later, many other cortical areas in the primate brain also are concerned with further processing of visual information that first reaches the cortex in area V1.

Organization of Retinal Inputs to the Lateral Geniculate Nucleus

How are the left and right halves of the visual field spatially segregated in the projection from the retina to the thalamus?

In many vertebrates, including fish and amphibians, the two eyes are located on the sides of the head and take in light from nonoverlapping parts of the visual world, as shown in Figure 16.2A. The part of the visual world seen by the left eye is called the left **visual field**, and the part seen by the right eye is called the right visual field. In these animals, the axons of the ganglion cells from the two eyes cross completely at the optic chiasm, so that the right visual field projects to the left tectum and the left visual field to the right tectum (see Fig. 16.2A). In animals whose eyes are located in the front of the head, such as primates, the eyes overlap in their coverage of the visual world, so that the same visual stimulus appears simultaneously on both retinas (see Fig. 16.2B). This overlap provides the basis for **binocular vision**.

In animals with binocular vision, the visual world is still divided into two visual fields, but the left and right halves are defined with respect to the point of fixation of the two eyes. Images of objects in the left and right visual fields appear on both retinas, but the optics of the eye dictate that light from the left visual field is focused onto the **temporal retina** (toward the temples) of the right eye and onto the **nasal retina** (toward the nose) of the left eye (see Fig. 16.2B). Conversely, light from the right visual field falls on the nasal retina of the right eye and the temporal retina of the left eye. The fixation point at the center of the visual field is represented at the **fovea**, the area of the retina with the highest density of photoreceptor cells and the best visual acuity. As with vertebrates that have the eyes placed laterally, the left visual field projects to the right side of the brain and the right visual field to the left side of the brain.

Figure 16.2B shows that the projection pattern of the optic nerve axons required to separate the two visual fields is a bit more complicated in animals with binocular vision than in vertebrates with laterally placed eyes. The axons of the retinal gan-

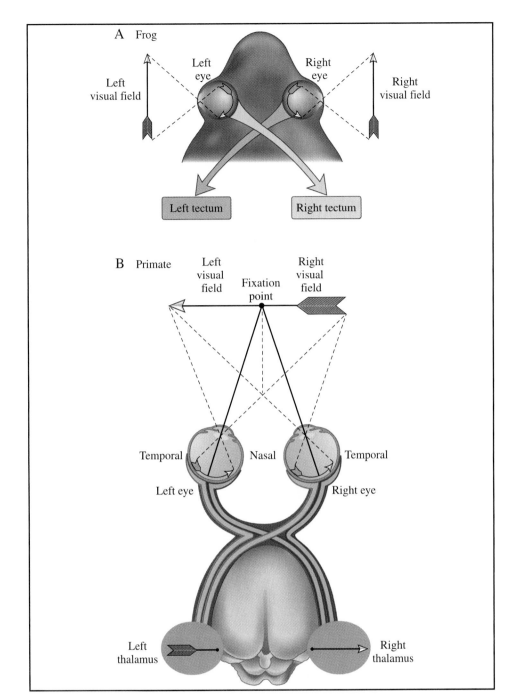

A Frog

Left
eye

Right
eye

Left
visual field

Right
visual field

Left visual field

Right visual field

Left tectum

Right tectum

B Primate

Left
visual
field

Fixation
point

Right
visual
field

Temporal

Nasal

Temporal

Left eye

Right eye

Left
thalamus

Right
thalamus

Figure 16.2.

Each half of the visual field projects to the opposite side of the brain. **A.** In animals with laterally placed eyes, the left and right visual fields do not overlap, and the optic nerves from the two eyes cross completely at the midline. **B.** In animals with frontally placed eyes, the left and right visual fields are represented in both eyes. To produce the correct separation of the two visual fields, the axons of ganglion cells in the nasal part of both retinas cross to the opposite side of the brain at the optic chiasm. The axons from the temporal part of the retinas of both eyes remain on the same side of the brain.

glion cells sort themselves at the optic chiasm according to the location of the ganglion cell in the retina. Ganglion cells in the temporal part of each retina send their axons to the same side of the brain, while the ganglion cells in the nasal part of each retina send their axons to the opposite side of the brain. As shown in Figure 16.2B, this projection pattern allows the left half of the visual field to be represented in the right thalamus and the right half of the visual field to be represented in the left thalamus. In reality, the dividing line between the temporal and the nasal regions of the retina is not as sharp as that shown in the figure. There is a narrow strip of retina, centered on the fovea, where ganglion cells sort their axons randomly to either the ipsilateral or the contralateral side of the brain. That is, some ganglion cells in this central region behave as though they are "nasal" and some behave as though they are "temporal." Thus, the foveal region of the retina is actually represented on both sides of the brain.

In addition to the contralateral-ipsilateral sorting of ganglion cell axons, there is also a specific ordering of the projections of optic nerve axons within each lateral geniculate nucleus. As shown schematically in Figure 16.3, each lateral geniculate nucleus is a laminated structure with distinct cellular layers. The number of layers varies somewhat in different species of mammal. In primates, six layers, numbered 1 through 6 from bottom (ventral) to top (dorsal), are present. The two most ventral layers are further distinguished from the top four layers on the basis of the size of the neurons they contain. Neuronal cell bodies are larger in the bottom two layers, which are called the **magnocellular layers** (*magno* means "large"). The top four layers are called the **parvocellular layers** because their neurons have smaller cell bodies (*parvo* means "small"). As we will discuss shortly, the parvocellular and magnocellular layers differ in the type of visual information they relay.

Each layer in the lateral geniculate nucleus receives input from a particular eye. In other words, all of the thalamic neurons within a layer are **monocular**, even though the nucleus as a whole receives inputs from both eyes. As shown in Figure 16.3, layers 2, 3, and 5 receive inputs from ganglion cells of the ipsilateral eye, while layers 1, 4, and 6 receive inputs from the contralateral eye. Thus, the inputs from the two eyes remain segregated and do not merge at the level of the thalamus. The receptive fields of the lateral geniculate neurons are thus confined to one eye or the other, depending on the layer of the nucleus in which the cell is found.

Synaptic Circuitry of the Lateral Geniculate Nucleus

What synaptic interactions occur in the parts of the thalamus that are concerned with visual information?

The lateral geniculate nucleus contains two general types of neurons, both of which receive direct synaptic inputs from retinal ganglion cells. Approximately 75% of the neurons in the lateral geniculate nucleus are **projection neurons** (also called **relay neurons**), whose axons leave the thalamus and terminate in the pri-

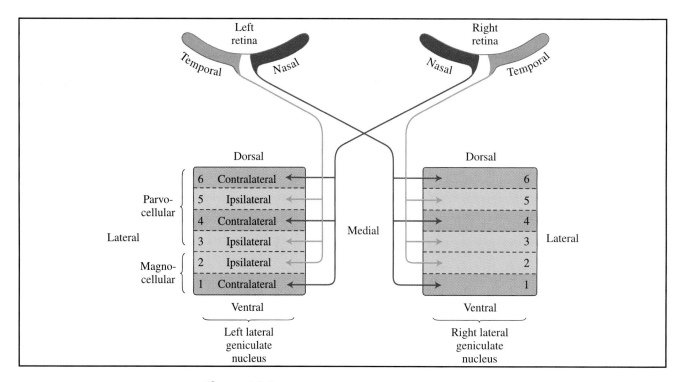

Figure 16.3.

The lateral geniculate nucleus is organized into layers, each dedicated to a particular eye. Inputs from the contralateral eye are shown in *purple*, and the contralateral-eye layers in the lateral geniculate nucleus are shaded *purple*.

mary visual cortex, at the rearmost pole of the occipital lobe. These axons remain on the same side of the brain. As a result, the left half of the visual field is represented in the right primary visual cortex, and the right half of the visual field is represented in the left primary visual cortex.

The remaining 25% of the lateral geniculate neurons are **local interneurons**, which use the neurotransmitter γ-aminobutyric acid (GABA) and make inhibitory synaptic connections onto nearby projection neurons within the lateral geniculate nucleus (Fig. 16.4A). The local interneurons provide lateral inhibition, which

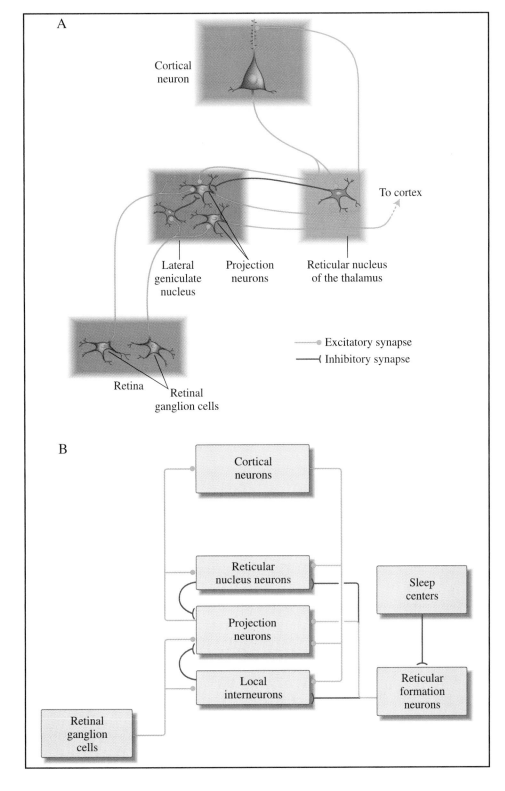

Figure 16.4.

The synaptic circuitry of the lateral geniculate nucleus of the thalamus. **A.** The axons of retinal ganglion cells make excitatory synaptic connections within the lateral geniculate nucleus on projection neurons and local inhibitory interneurons (*red*). The projection neurons send their axons to the primary visual cortex and also send axon branches to inhibitory feedback neurons in the reticular nucleus of the thalamus. Cortical neurons make feedback synaptic connections on both the reticular nucleus neurons and the projection neurons of the lateral geniculate nucleus. **B.** The synaptic circuitry shown in **A** is also influenced by neurons in the reticular formation that generate arousal. These reticular formation neurons are in turn inhibited by brain centers that induce sleep.

enhances the antagonism between the center region and the surround region of the receptive fields of projection neurons in the lateral geniculate nucleus. The receptive fields of the projection neurons in the lateral geniculate nucleus have a center-surround organization, with either on-centers or off-centers, as in ganglion cells.

In addition to the local interneurons, additional inhibitory interneurons are located just outside the thalamus in the **reticular nucleus of the thalamus**, which forms a shell surrounding the thalamic nuclei themselves. As the axons of the projection neurons pass through the reticular nucleus on the way to the visual cortex, they branch and make excitatory synaptic contacts with the inhibitory interneurons in the reticular nucleus (see Fig. 16.4A). These interneurons send axons back to the projection neurons, where they make inhibitory feedback synaptic connections that decrease the activity in the projection neurons and suppress the relay of information through the lateral geniculate nucleus.

Another important feedback loop that affects the activity of the projection neurons is also shown in Figure 16.4A. Neurons in the primary visual cortex—the target for the thalamic projection neurons—send axons back to the lateral geniculate nucleus, where they make excitatory synapses onto the projection neurons. These excitatory connections enhance the activity of the projection neurons, providing positive feedback for on-type light responses. In the off-pathway, in which illumination produces an inhibition of action potential activity, the level of activity in darkness is enhanced by the corticothalamic excitatory synapses. In addition, as the axons descending from the cortex pass through the reticular nucleus of the thalamus, they send branches that make excitatory synaptic connections with the inhibitory interneurons of the reticular nucleus. By exciting the reticular nucleus neurons, this synaptic connection indirectly inhibits the activity of the projection neurons. Therefore, the net effect of the descending cortical axons on the projection neurons may be either excitation or inhibition, depending on the relative strength of the excitation applied to the projection neurons and to the reticular nucleus neurons.

The cortical axons also target the local inhibitory interneurons in the lateral geniculate nucleus (not shown in Fig. 16.4A). This synaptic pathway provides another mechanism for the cortex to influence both inhibitory light responses and excitatory light responses of projection neurons.

The balance between excitatory and inhibitory influences in the lateral geniculate nucleus is under the control of the brain mechanisms involved in arousal and sleep (see Fig. 16.4B). Neurons in the **reticular formation** of the midbrain and brainstem send axons to the thalamus, where they make synaptic contact with projection neurons, local interneurons, and neurons in the reticular nucleus of the thalamus. (Be careful to distinguish the reticular *nucleus* of the thalamus from the reticular *formation* of the midbrain and brainstem.) Recall that the reticular formation receives inputs from a variety of sensory sources and modulates spinal motor circuitry. The reticular formation also controls the organism's overall level of arousal. During sleep, when the arousal level is at a minimum, the neurons of the reticular formation are inhibited (see Fig. 16.4B). In the thalamus, the projection neurons are excited by inputs from the reticular formation while the local interneurons within the lateral geniculate nucleus and the inhibitory neurons in the reticular nucleus of the thalamus are inhibited. Through direct excitation of the projection neurons and inhibition of the inhibitors of the projection neurons, the overall level of excitation in the projection neurons is greatly enhanced. Thus, when the reticular formation is active, the relay of visual information from the thalamus to the cortex is enhanced. Conversely, during sleep, the inhibitory influences within the thalamus are maximal because the reticular formation is inactive, and the relay of sensory information to the cortex is not favored.

The inhibitory and the excitatory synapses onto the three different types of thalamic neurons arise from branches of the axons of the same group of reticular formation neurons. The neurotransmitter released at both the inhibitory and the excitatory synapses is acetylcholine. Thus, as we saw in Chapter 6, a neurotransmitter can be either excitatory or inhibitory, depending on the characteristics of the postsynaptic receptor. At excitatory synapses connecting the reticular formation neurons to the lateral geniculate projection neurons, acetylcholine directly binds to and activates a ligand-gated ion channel that increases the sodium permeability of the postsynaptic neuron. At inhibitory synapses connecting the reticular formation neurons to the local inhibitory interneurons and the reticular nucleus neurons, acetylcholine binds to a receptor that acts via G-proteins, indirectly opening potassium channels in the postsynaptic cell.

Different Types of Retinal Ganglion Cells Project to Different Targets in the Brain

In mammals, retinal ganglion cells can be classified into three general categories: **X cells**, **Y cells**, and **W cells**. These categories are defined in part by the size of the soma of the ganglion cell and by the dendritic branching pattern in the retina, as shown in Figure 16.5. Y cells have the largest cell bodies and large dendritic

What functional and anatomical differences distinguish the three categories of retinal ganglion cells?

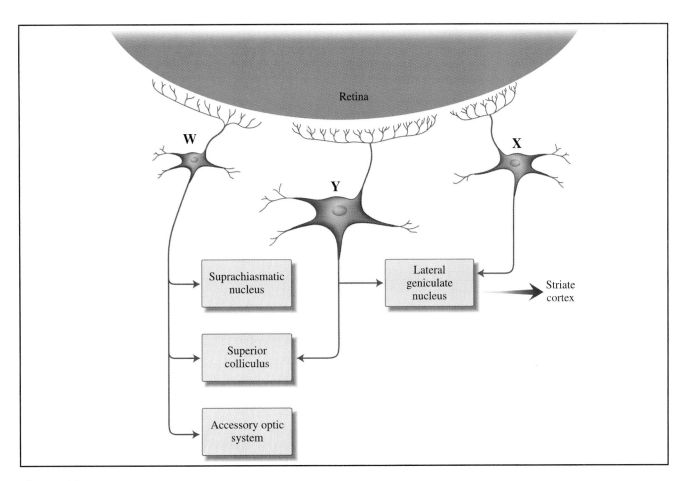

Figure 16.5.

The three general classes of ganglion cells in the mammalian retina. The W cells represent a phylogenetically older class of ganglion cells whose axons project to the more primitive visual centers. The geniculostriate pathway originates from the X and Y cells. X cells are smaller than Y cells and have smaller dendritic fields and receptive fields.

fields; X cells have medium-size cell bodies and small, dense dendritic arbors; W cells have the smallest somata with widely spreading dendrites.

In addition, important functional differences distinguish the three ganglion cell categories. W cells are thought to represent a phylogenetically more ancient class of ganglion cells. In keeping with this notion, W cells send axons to the "older" parts of the visual nervous system, including the superior colliculus, the suprachiasmatic nucleus, and parts of the brainstem involved in controlling eye movements (the accessory optic system discussed in Chapter 10). The W cells do not seem to participate in the "newer" geniculostriate pathway. The projection pattern for the W cells is summarized in Figure 16.5. W cells are functionally diverse and exhibit a variety of different light responses. Some W cells are selectively sensitive to moving stimuli, whereas others are not; some W cells have center-surround receptive fields, whereas others do not; and so on.

Both X cells and Y cells have center-surround receptive fields. In keeping with the relative sizes of their dendritic trees, however, Y cells have receptive fields that are three to four times larger than those of X cells. As a result, X cells are better suited for distinguishing closely spaced stimuli. X cells project exclusively to the lateral geniculate nucleus, whereas Y cells send axons to both the lateral geniculate nucleus and the superior colliculus. In addition, Y cells typically respond transiently to illumination and tend to prefer moving targets, whereas X cells produce a sustained response. In species in which color vision is highly developed (for example, in primates), X cells are sensitive to color, and Y cells are not. Both categories include on-center and off-center ganglion cells.

It is important to recognize that each point in the retina is sampled in parallel by several different types of ganglion cells, each of which is able to detect a different aspect of the visual stimulus. These parallel information paths are maintained at higher levels of analysis in the visual system, as the information passes from one stage to another.

The X, Y, and W categories of ganglion cells were first described in the visual system of the cat, but functionally equivalent categories have been found in the retinas of other mammals as well. In primates, the X cells are termed **P cells** (for *parvocellular*), and the Y cells are called **M cells** (for *magnocellular*). For simplicity, we will use the X and Y terminology in this book, but you should be aware that you may encounter a different terminology (and some functional differences) in original research papers on the primate visual pathways.

Perhaps the most compelling reason for splitting X and Y cells into different categories is that the projections from these two types of ganglion cells are segregated and connect with different sets of neurons in the lateral geniculate nucleus and the primary visual cortex. Thus, the visual system makes distinctions between these two pathways and the information they carry. In the lateral geniculate nucleus, each projection neuron receives input from either X cells or Y cells, but not both. Furthermore, Y cells send inputs only to layers 1 and 2 in the primate lateral geniculate nucleus. Recall that these layers are the magnocellular layers in primates. Thus, the largest ganglion cells (Y cells) project to the largest lateral geniculate neurons. Layer 1 receives inputs from the contralateral eye, whereas layer 2 receives inputs from the ipsilateral eye (see Fig. 16.3). Thus, for the lateral geniculate nucleus on each side of the brain, Y cells from the nasal part of the retina of the contralateral eye project to layer 1, while Y cells from the ipsilateral temporal part of the retina project to layer 2. The parvocellular layers of the primate lateral geniculate nucleus receive inputs only from X cells (parvocellular ganglion cells to parvocellular lateral geniculate neurons). In this way, the layers of the lateral geniculate nucleus segregate not only the inputs from the two eyes but also the X and Y pathways for visual information.

ORGANIZATION OF THE PRIMARY VISUAL CORTEX

The inputs to the striate cortex (Brodmann's area 17) from the lateral geniculate nucleus are also spatially organized with respect to the contralateral and ipsilateral eyes and with respect to the X and Y pathways. Recall from the discussion of the motor cortex in Chapter 9 that the cerebral cortex is divided into six layers. As in the motor cortex, the arriving inputs from the thalamus terminate predominantly in layer IV of the primary visual cortex, as shown in Figure 16.6. The unusually large thalamic input in the primary visual cortex makes layer IV thicker and more prominent than in other parts of the cerebral cortex. Indeed, layer IV is sufficiently thick in the primary visual cortex to warrant further subdivision into four sublayers: IVa, IVb, IVcα, and IVcβ. These subdivisions and the origin of their inputs from the lateral geniculate nucleus are illustrated in Figure 16.6.

The inputs from the ipsilateral and contralateral eyes are segregated into specific dorsal-ventral layers in the lateral geniculate nucleus. In the cortex, the inputs from these geniculate layers remain segregated, so that inputs coming from the contralateral and ipsilateral eyes do not overlap. The cortical neurons receiving inputs from a particular eye are arranged in vertically oriented columns, called **ocular**

What functional organization is found in the primary visual cortex?

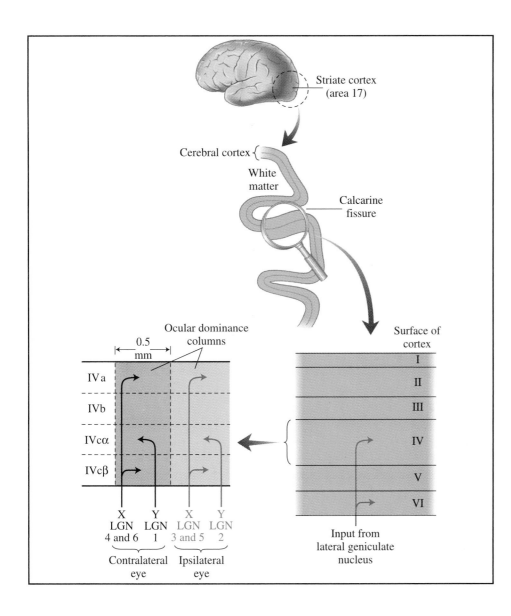

Figure 16.6.

The location and laminar organization of the primary visual cortex. Like other areas of the cerebral cortex, the primary visual cortex has six layers. Layer IV is further divided into four sublayers. The inputs derived from the ipsilateral and contralateral eyes are spatially separated into vertically oriented columns, called the ocular dominance columns. The inputs from the X-cell and Y-cell pathways in the lateral geniculate nucleus are spatially segregated within each ocular dominance column.

dominance columns, that are approximately 0.5 mm wide (see Fig. 16.6). The contralateral and ipsilateral columns alternate throughout the primary visual cortex. Thus, on each side of the brain, the ipsilateral-eye columns receive inputs from layers 2, 3, and 5 of the lateral geniculate nucleus on that side of the brain, while the contralateral-eye columns receive inputs from layers 1, 4, and 6 (see Fig. 16.6).

The X and Y pathways of the lateral geniculate nucleus terminate in different sublayers of cortical layer IV, as illustrated in Figure 16.6. The incoming Y axons make synaptic connections in sublayer IVcα, and the incoming X axons project to sublayers IVa and IVcβ. This arrangement holds for both the axons carrying information from the contralateral eye and the axons from the ipsilateral eye, in their respective ocular dominance columns. The incoming axons from the lateral geniculate nucleus make synaptic connections onto stellate cells (see Chapter 9) in layer IV. In addition, the axons of both the X and the Y pathway branch as they pass through layer VI of the primary visual cortex and make synapses with pyramidal neurons in layer VI. These pyramidal neurons are the source of the feedback axons that return to the lateral geniculate nucleus from the cortex (see Fig. 16.4).

Receptive Fields of Cortical Neurons

How do the receptive fields of neurons in the primary visual cortex differ from those of retinal ganglion cells and thalamic neurons?

Like the retinal ganglion cells and the neurons of the lateral geniculate nucleus, the stellate cells in layer IV of the primary visual cortex have concentric center-surround receptive fields with either excitatory or inhibitory centers. Above and below layer IV, however, most of the neurons have receptive fields that differ substantially from those with the center-surround organization.

Figure 16.7 shows the properties of a commonly observed receptive field for neurons in the primary visual cortex. In this example, a central excitatory region is surrounded by an inhibitory region, but both are elongated rather than circular, as in retinal ganglion cells and lateral geniculate neurons. The best stimulus for this neuron would be a bar of light just wide enough to cover the central excitatory region and oriented parallel to the long axis of the receptive field. If the bar is rotated so that it is perpendicular to the long axis of the receptive field, it fails to excite the neuron (see Fig. 16.7A). Similarly a circular spot of light would not be a particularly effective stimulus for this cell. Thus, cortical neurons of this type are most sensitive to a bright line or bar of light with a particular orientation.

A receptive field of this type can be constructed if an appropriate series of on-center stellate cells from layer IV (or similar cells in the lateral geniculate nucleus) make excitatory synapses onto the cortical neuron in the manner shown in Figure 16.7B. If off-center cells were used as building blocks instead of on-center cells, the resulting cortical cell would be most sensitive to a dark line of a particular orientation on a bright background. The receptive fields of the retinal ganglion cells form the building blocks for construction of more complex receptive fields, after the outputs of the ganglion cells are relayed through the thalamus and the stellate cells of layer IV of the cortex. Several variations of rectangular receptive fields are observed in the primary visual cortex, involving different receptive field sizes, or antagonistic regions flanking only one side of the excitatory region, or other arrangements. As a group, these orientation-sensitive cortical neurons were called **simple cells** by their discoverers, David Hubel and Torsten Wiesel, who won the Nobel Prize for their studies of visual cortical neurons and their response properties.

Like the inputs from the two eyes, the orientation-sensitive cortical neurons are arranged into vertical columns in the primary visual cortex. The arrangement of these orientation columns is shown in Figure 16.8. Within an orientation column, all simple cells have a similar orientation preference but cover slightly different retinal locations. In the adjacent ocular dominance column from the opposite eye, the

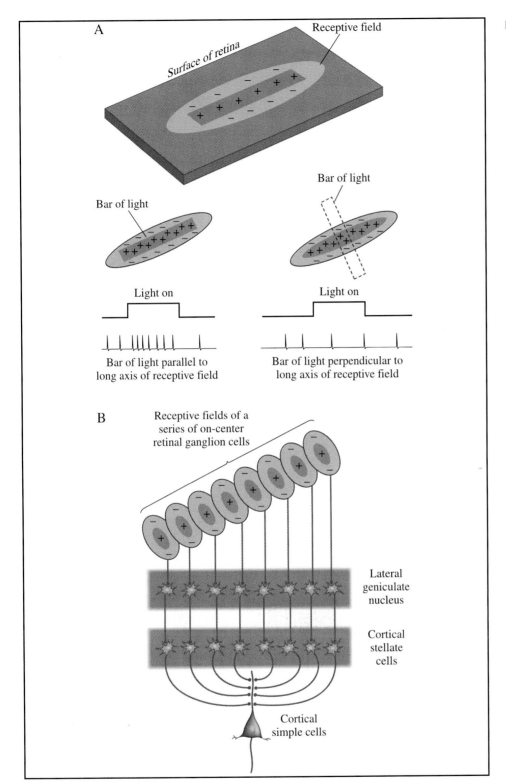

Figure 16.7.

The receptive field of a cortical neuron that is most sensitive to a long bar or line of light with a particular orientation. **A.** The shape of the receptive field on the surface of the retina. If a bar of light is oriented so that it coincides with the long, narrow excitatory center of the receptive field, the cell is strongly excited. If the bar of light is rotated so that its long axis does not coincide with the long axis of the receptive field, the cell fails to respond. **B.** A receptive field of this type can be constructed from the combination of an appropriate set of center-surround receptive fields. *Plus signs* indicate that the cell is excited by illumination within that region of the receptive field, whereas *minus signs* indicate that the cell is inhibited by light falling in that region.

simple cells have a similar orientation preference but are driven more strongly by the other eye. The simple cells within an ocular dominance column are driven more strongly by the eye of that column but are also typically sensitive to illumination placed in the other eye. The locations of the receptive fields on the two retinas precisely coincide so that each simple cell that receives input from the two eyes is driven binocularly by correctly oriented bars of light (or dark) at a particular position in the visual field. Because the incoming lateral geniculate axons project exclusively to a single ocular dominance column, the binocular responses of the simple cells must arise from cortico-cortical connections within the primary visual cortex.

Figure 16.8 shows that the cortical surface in the primary visual cortex consists of a two-dimensional array of columns, with the ocular dominance columns forming one axis of the array and the orientation columns forming the other axis. Neighboring orientation columns have slightly different preferred orientations, which vary progressively along the axis formed by the orientation columns (see Fig. 16.8). Thus, the map of the retinal surface consisting of the circular receptive fields of the retinal ganglion cells is transformed into a map of **orientation-selective line detectors** in the primary visual cortex. Each point in the visual field is covered by simple cells of all directions of orientation; similarly, among the simple cells of a particular orientation, all positions in the visual field are covered.

In addition to the simple cells, Hubel and Wiesel described cortical cells with more complex response properties, which they called **complex cells** and **hypercomplex cells**. Like simple cells, complex cells are sensitive to the orientation of edges and lines. They have much larger receptive fields than simple cells and show more variation in their response characteristics. Complex cells are commonly excited by a dark or light bar or by an edge between light and dark regions placed anywhere in the receptive field, provided the stimulus has the correct orientation. Cells of this type signal stimulus *orientation*, independent of stimulus *location*, within broad limits. The orientation-sensitive complex cells constitute the building blocks of a cortical system that analyzes the form or shape of a visual stimulus.

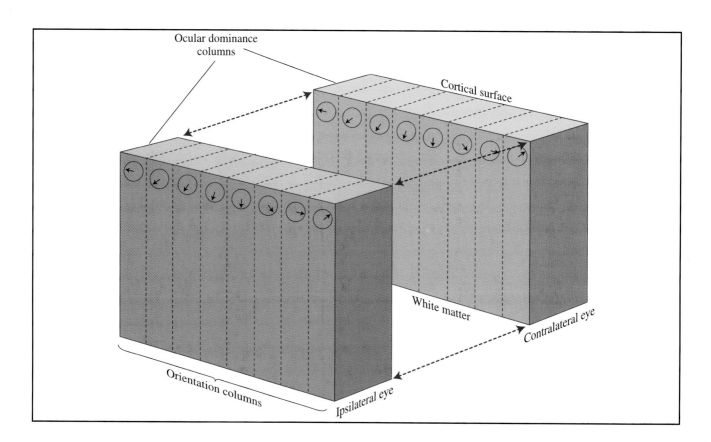

Figure 16.8.

Cells with a similar orientation preference form vertical columns in the primary visual cortex. The successive orientation columns within an ocular dominance column have slightly different preferred orientations, indicated by the *arrows* on the clock faces in each column. The differences in the directions of the *arrow* in successive columns are exaggerated for illustrative purposes.

In some cases, the response of complex cells is greatest when an edge of the correct orientation moves through the receptive field in one direction, while movement of an edge in the opposite direction produces inhibition. These motion-sensitive neurons likely represent a separate analysis system, concerned with visual motion. Hubel and Wiesel suggested that the response properties of complex cells could be produced by a synaptic combination of inputs from an appropriate group of orientation-sensitive simple cells, just as the response properties of simple cells could be constructed from the combination of appropriate center-surround receptive fields of stellate cells.

Hypercomplex cells resemble complex cells, except that the bar or edge must not extend beyond the boundaries of the receptive field. In other words, hypercomplex cells are stimulated best by lines of a particular orientation and particular *length*. According to Hubel and Wiesel's theory, receptive fields of hypercomplex cells could result if the neuron receives excitatory and inhibitory connections from groups of complex cells.

These studies of the receptive field properties of cortical neurons suggest how information about orientation and length of the borders that define objects in the visual world might be extracted from lower-level data provided by retinal ganglion cells and lateral geniculate neurons. Two important and mutually complementary principles of cortical information processing emerge from Hubel and Wiesel's work. First, features of the visual stimulus are extracted by a **hierarchical arrangement** of neurons whose receptive fields are constructed by combinations of receptive fields of lower-level neurons in the hierarchy. Second, at each position on the retina, the "testing" of the visual stimulus for lines of particular orientation and length occurs **in parallel** for all of the possible orientations and lengths that the visual system can distinguish. Each position on the retina is represented many times in the visual cortex, so that many different simple cells (and hence, complex and hypercomplex cells) are simultaneously examining the same part of the visual world. *Thus, information processing in the visual cortex is both hierarchical and parallel: hierarchical within an orientation system, and parallel across orientation systems.* This principle is likely to apply not only in the visual cortex but also in all parts of the cortex, including other sensory systems, motor systems, and cortical areas involved in more complex processes.

Color-Sensitive Cells in the Primary Visual Cortex

Another parallel information-processing pathway in the primary visual cortex is concerned with the color of visual stimuli. In Chapter 15, we discussed the responses of single-opponent, color-sensitive retinal ganglion cells. In the receptive fields of these ganglion cells, the center and surround regions originate from different types of cone photoreceptors. However, the single-opponent ganglion cells cannot distinguish unambiguously between colored lights and white light that covers only part of the receptive field (see Fig. 15.26).

In the lateral geniculate nucleus, color-sensitive projection neurons have the same receptive field organization as single-opponent ganglion cells. At the level of the cortex, however, the color-sensitive cells have receptive fields that differ in a subtle but important way from the receptive fields of the single-opponent cells. The response of a color-sensitive cortical neuron to various combinations of illumination is shown in Figure 16.9A. Unlike the single-opponent cells, color opponency is observed *within* the center and surround of the receptive field, as well as *between* the center and surround. Cells with receptive fields of this type are called **double-opponent, color-sensitive cells**. The example in Figure 16.9 illustrates a red/green double-opponent cell.

Opponent responses within both the center and the surround of the receptive field allow the cortical cells to respond in a specific way to colored stimuli, without

How do neurons in the visual cortex respond to colored stimuli?

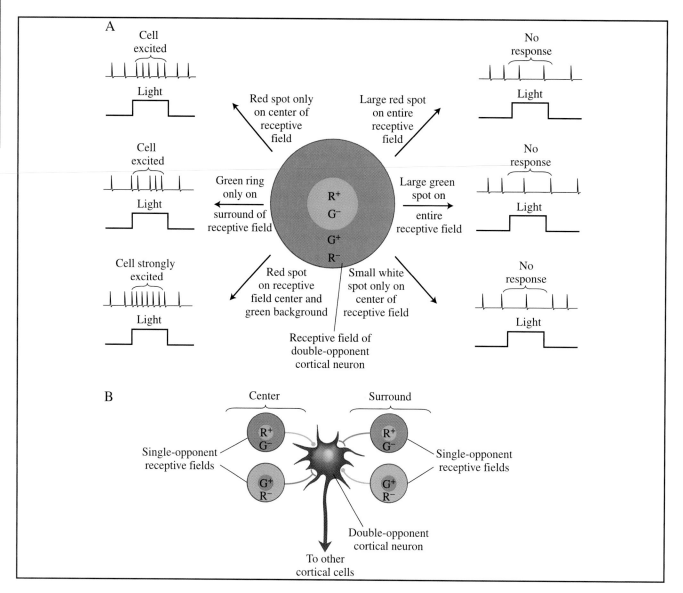

Figure 16.9.

The response properties of a double-opponent, color-sensitive neuron in the primary visual cortex. In this example, red light (R) in the center of the receptive or green light (G) in the surround of the receptive field excites the cell (*plus sign*), whereas red light in the surround or green light in the center inhibits the neuron (*minus sign*). **A.** The receptive field is shown in the center, with responses to various types of stimuli arrayed around the outside. (See the text for a full description of the responses.) The best excitatory response is observed with a red spot of light on a green background (*lower left*). **B.** Synaptic circuitry that could produce a double-opponent, color-sensitive neuron from appropriate combinations of single-opponent neurons.

being confused by white lights. A large red spot that covers the receptive field of the cortical cell produces no response, because the superimposed excitation from the center and the inhibition from the surround cancel each other. By contrast, this stimulus would strongly excite a red/green single-opponent cell (see Fig. 15.26). Similarly, a large green spot that covers the receptive field would inhibit a red/green single-opponent cell but has no effect on the double-opponent cell in Figure 16.9A because the green light simultaneously produces inhibition from the center and excitation from the surround of the receptive field. A white light is also not an effective stimulus for the double-opponent cell. White light affects the red-sensitive and the green-sensitive mechanisms equally, producing both excitation and inhibition of the double-opponent cell, even when the white light is restricted to the center of the receptive field. In a single-opponent cell, a white light in the excitatory part of the receptive field produces strong excitation, causing the cell to confuse white and colored lights.

Now consider the response of a double-opponent cell to combinations of red and green lights (see Fig. 16.9A). The cell is excited by a red spot of light restricted to the center of the receptive field or a green ring of light falling only on the surround of the receptive field. The strongest excitatory response would occur with the combination of these two stimuli: a red spot on a green background. The strongest inhibition of this double-opponent cell would be produced by a green spot on a red background.

Several varieties of double-opponent, color-sensitive neurons are found in the visual cortex. Some are red/green cells (as in Fig. 16.9) but with the opposite effects of red and green lights in the center and surround of the receptive field (that is, green excitation and red inhibition in the center, red excitation and green inhibition in the surround). Other double-opponent neurons are sensitive to yellow and blue lights, rather than red and green.

Double-opponent, color-sensitive neurons can be created in the visual cortex by simple synaptic connections from single-opponent, color-sensitive cells of the lateral geniculate nucleus. A cell with receptive field properties shown in Figure 16.9A could arise from the synaptic arrangement illustrated in Figure 16.9B. The central portion of the double-opponent cell's receptive field is formed by the combination of excitatory connections from red on-center single-opponent cells and inhibitory connections from green on-center single-opponent cells. In the surround portion of the receptive field, the connections are reversed (excitatory from green on-center and inhibitory from red on-center single-opponent cells). With this synaptic arrangement, red light on the receptive field center and green light on the receptive field surround would produce the strongest excitation, in keeping with the response properties shown in Figure 16.9A.

The color-sensitive cortical cells form a functionally distinct pathway in the cortex, operating in parallel with the orientation pathway discussed previously. Color-sensitive cortical cells are also spatially segregated from the orientation-sensitive cells. Groups of color-sensitive neurons are interspersed among the orientation columns in a semiregular array of vertically oriented columns called **blobs**. Figure 16.10 shows the array of blobs when the primary visual cortex is sliced parallel to the cortical surface and then viewed from the top. The blobs are found above and below layer IV but are excluded from layer IV itself. The overall arrangement of the ocular dominance columns, the orientation columns, and the color-sensitive blobs is shown in Figure 16.11.

The blobs in the primary visual cortex were first identified by anatomical characteristics rather than on functional grounds. When the cortex is stained to reveal cells rich in the mitochondrial enzyme cytochrome oxidase, the blobs are selectively stained. Therefore, the neurons in the blobs are capable of sustaining high metabolic activity. Subsequently, physiological experiments revealed that the cells within the blobs are color-sensitive cells. The relative importance of color in visual information processing in primates is reflected in the increased action potential activity in the color-sensitive cells and thus a greater requirement for metabolic energy to sustain the transmembrane ionic gradients.

The color-sensitive cells within the blobs receive direct inputs from the lateral geniculate nucleus, independent of the primary lateral geniculate projection to layer IV of the cortex. In primates, the color-sensitive retinal ganglion cells are X cells that project to the parvocellular layers of the lateral geniculate nucleus. Therefore, the color pathway in the primary visual cortex receives its inputs from the parvocellular layers (layers 3 to 6) of the lateral geniculate nucleus. In animals

Figure 16.10.

Color-sensitive neurons are localized in the primary visual cortex within blobs revealed by staining for the mitochondrial enzyme cytochrome oxidase. The plane of a section parallel to the cortical surface is shown on the *left*, and a top view of the resulting section is shown on the *right*.

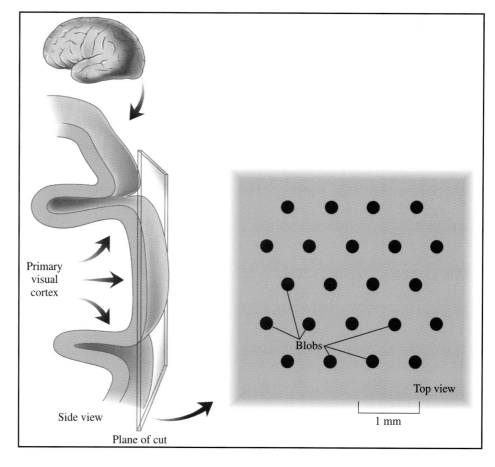

Primary visual cortex

Blobs

Top view

1 mm

Side view

Plane of cut

with well-developed color vision, the color-sensitive blob system is one of the principal cortical targets of the parvocellular pathway from the lateral geniculate nucleus.

HIGHER-ORDER VISUAL CORTICAL REGIONS

What kinds of visual information are processed in the higher visual cortical areas (areas V2 to V5)?

The primary visual cortex (area V1) contains multiple pathways, operating in parallel, that analyze each point on the retina for different stimulus properties, including line length and orientation, object color, and motion. These functionally distinct pathways are also anatomically distinct. From area V1, outputs from each of these parallel analysis systems are passed to selected higher-order cortical areas for further processing of specific stimulus attributes. Ultimately, these separate stimulus attributes must be merged to form an integrated view of the visual world. Neurobiologists do not yet understand how these integrated perceptions arise, but clues about the higher-order cortical circuitry involved in analyzing specific aspects of visual stimuli are beginning to emerge.

In primates, large portions of the cerebral cortex are devoted to visual tasks, including parts of the cortex that were once classified as "association" cortex because no clearly defined sensory or motor function could be ascribed to them. It is now clear that a great deal of this association cortex is actually part of the visual system in the primate brain. In keeping with the principles of combined hierarchical and parallel processing found in the primary visual cortex, these higher-order cortical regions show a hierarchical arrangement, but different types of visual analyses are carried out in parallel in several cortical regions. We will begin by examining the anatomical layout and the interconnections of these higher-order visual areas, be-

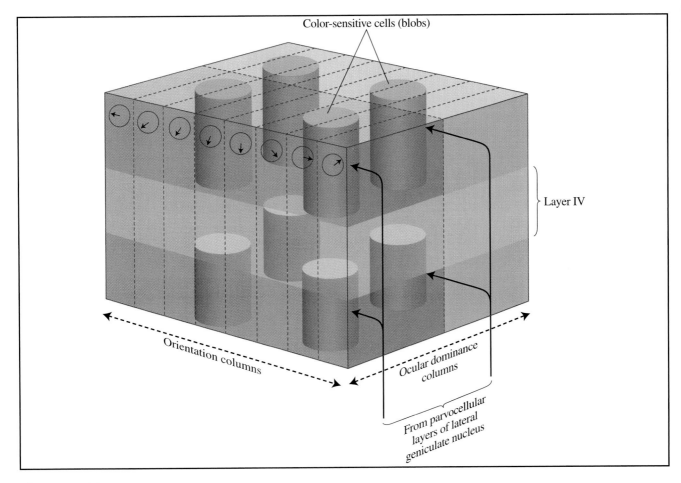

Figure 16.11.

The blobs form columns interspersed among the orientation columns and ocular dominance columns of the primary visual cortex. The blobs are found in all layers except layer IV. The inputs to the blobs originate from the parvocellular layers of the lateral geniculate nucleus.

fore turning to the visual responses of the neurons in some of the best-studied higher centers.

Anatomical Arrangement of Nonstriate Visual Cortical Regions

The primary visual cortex is located at the rearmost pole of the occipital cortex. The higher-order visual regions in the cortex form a series of progressive rings, anteriorly through the occipital lobe into the posterior part of the temporal lobe. This is illustrated for the primate brain in Figure 16.12. The higher-order areas are numbered V2 through V5 successively in a posterior to anterior direction. In addition, area V3 is subdivided into areas V3 and V3A, and area V5 is subdivided into areas V5 and V5A. With the exception of area V4, the higher-order areas are buried mostly or entirely within the deep infoldings (sulci) of the cortical surface and are not directly visible on the external surface of the brain. The three-dimensional relationship among the areas and their positions within the infoldings can be better appreciated by examining a horizontal cut through the visual cortical areas, which is illustrated in Figure 16.13.

Area V2 receives extensive inputs from the cortical neurons of area V1. Consequently, the multiple maps of the retinal surface represented in area V1 are also

Figure 16.12.

The location of the higher-order visual cortical areas in the occipital and temporal lobes of the primate brain. Many of the visual cortical areas are hidden from external view within infoldings of the cortical surface (see Figure 16.13).

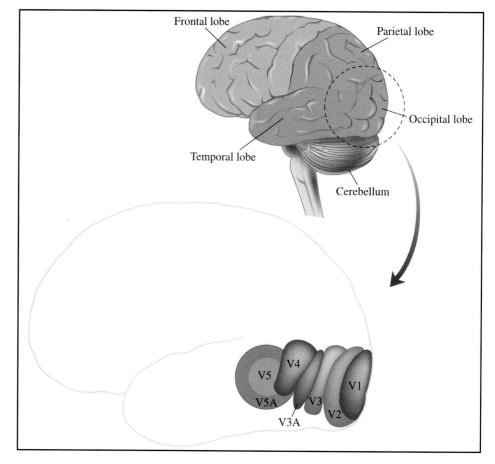

found in area V2. Area V2 is organized into spatially segregated functional subdivisions that handle different aspects of visual stimuli, in a manner analogous to the organization of area V1. Also like area V1, the functional subdivisions of area V2 are revealed anatomically by cytochrome oxidase staining. In area V2, there is a regularly repeating pattern of **stripes** of neurons rich in cytochrome oxidase, corresponding to groups of neurons with high metabolic activity resulting from high neuronal activity during visual analysis. The stripes run vertically from the cortical surface to the underlying white matter, as shown in Figure 16.14. The stripes are separated from each other by regions where the neurons have relatively little cytochrome oxidase, called the **interstripe** region. The stripes come in two different thicknesses and so are called **thin stripes** and **thick stripes**. These bands occur in strict order—thin stripe, interstripe, thick stripe, interstripe, and so on—in a repeating pattern throughout area V2 (see Fig. 16.14).

Functional Connections from Area V1 to Area V2

Figure 16.15 summarizes the functional connections between area V1 and the different portions of area V2. The thin stripes in area V2 receive inputs from the cells in the blobs of area V1—that is, from the color-sensitive cells in the primary visual cortex. In turn, the cells in the thin stripes send axons to area V4, which is involved in color vision. Therefore, the pathway from the blobs of V1 to the thin stripes of V2 to area V4 can be thought of as a neural system specialized for the analysis of color of visual stimuli. The thick stripes in area V2 receive synaptic connections from orientation-selective neurons in area V1. The thick stripes also receive inputs from the motion-sensitive neurons of area V1. Thus, the neurons in the thick stripes analyze both object shape and motion. The orientation-selective neurons in the thick stripes

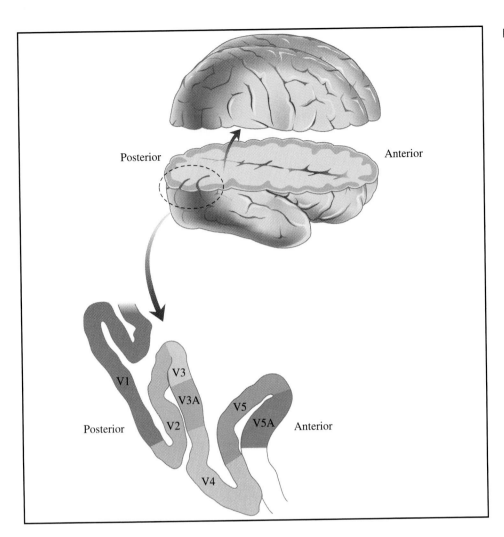

Posterior

Anterior

V3
V3A
V5
V1
V5A
Posterior
V2
Anterior

V4

Figure 16.13.

The locations of the higher-order visual cortical areas as revealed by a horizontal section through the primate brain.

send axons to area V3, which further analyzes object shape. The motion-sensitive neurons of the thick stripes project to area V5, which analyzes object motion independent of object form, as we will describe in the next section.

The interstripe regions of area V2 receive inputs from orientation-selective neurons of the primary visual cortex, as do the thick stripes (see Fig. 16.15). The thick stripes receive their orientation-sensitive connections from V1 regions that are part of the magnocellular (or Y-cell) pathway, while the interstripes receive their orientation-sensitive connections from V1 regions that are part of the parvocellular (or X-cell) pathway. Recall that in the retina, the Y ganglion cells (the origin of the primate magnocellular pathway) have large receptive fields and thus low spatial resolution. Conversely, the X cells (the origin of the primate parvocellular pathway) have small receptive fields and thus high spatial resolution. As a result, the shape-analysis pathway that passes through the thick stripes in area V2 is best suited to crude recognition and approximate spatial localization of objects within the visual field. The pathway through the interstripes in area V2 is more likely involved with fine form analysis.

In keeping with the separation of the magnocellular and parvocellular pathways through area V1 and into area V2, the interstripe regions and the thick stripes project to different higher-order targets: area V4 for the interstripe neurons and area V3 for the thick-stripe neurons. As might be expected given that area V4 receives inputs from both the color-sensitive cells in the thin stripes and the orientation-sensitive cells of the interstripe regions (see Fig. 16.15), some neurons in area V4 are sensitive to the orientation of lines or bars of a particular color.

Figure 16.14.

In area V2, staining for cytochrome oxidase reveals thick
and thin stripes oriented perpendicular to the cortical surface.

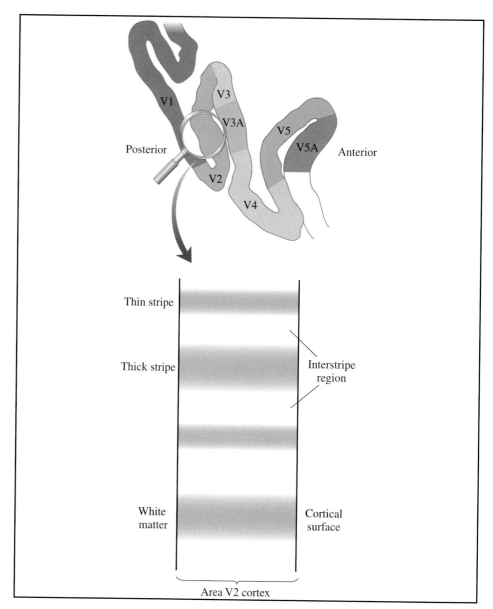

It is tempting to think that the cortical visual areas form a linear hierarchy, with
V1 projecting to V2 and V2 feeding the specialized higher areas. In reality, however, the pattern of interconnections is more complex. Area V1 sends outputs directly to the cortical regions specialized for motion and form, bypassing area V2;
area V1 also makes indirect connections to those areas via area V2. In addition,
intracortical connections from areas V3, V4, and V5 feed back to the "lower-order"
areas V1 and V2. The precise function of these complex interconnections has not
yet been established.

Area V2 mirrors in many respects the organization observed in area V1. The orientation-sensitive and color-sensitive cells are spatially segregated, and the magnocellular and parvocellular subsystems are separately represented. Thus, the scheme
of multiple, parallel subsystems—each concerned with a different aspect of the visual world—is observed in area V2, as it was in area V1. The principal difference is
that the proportion of cells with hypercomplex receptive field properties is higher
in area V2 than in area V1.

At the next level of cortical processing, however, cells have receptive fields that
differ in fundamental ways from those encountered in area V1 and area V2. As an

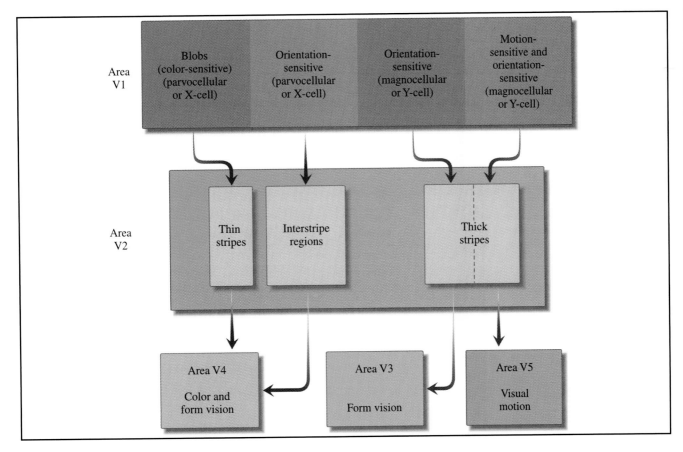

Figure 16.15.

The organization of connections from area V1 to area V2 and from area V2 to the specialized cortical visual areas.

example, we will consider the properties of cells in area V5, which are specialized for processing information about the motion of visual stimuli.

Detection and Analysis of Visual Motion: Area V5

One of the most important tasks of the visual system is to detect moving objects and determine their direction of motion. A moving object may represent food or an approaching predator, both of which are visual stimuli with obvious implications for survival. The analysis of movement also provides an excellent example of how different aspects of visual information processing are carried out in spatially distinct cortical areas, each specialized for a particular type of information. In the case of motion, the specialized cortical area is area V5, which is also known as **area MT** (*middle temporal area*). Area V5 is buried within a sulcus in the posterior and superior part of the temporal lobe (see Figs. 16.12 and 16.13). The cells in this area commonly have large receptive fields, but they do not respond well to steady illumination. However, a spot of light moved anywhere within the receptive field does generate a brisk response. An example of the response of a cortical neuron in area V5 to a moving stimulus is shown in Figure 16.16. Each cell has a strong preference for movement in a particular direction. Movement in other directions produces weaker excitation, while movement in the opposite direction produces inhibition. For each cell in area V5, it is possible to construct a direction preference curve like that shown in Figure 16.16. Among the population of motion-sensitive cells in area V5, all possible direction preferences and all possible receptive field locations are

Figure 16.16.

Responses of a motion-sensitive neuron in area V5. **A.** The preferred direction of motion for this example is from left to right in the horizontal plane, which corresponds to 90° on the circular direction diagram. When a spot of light moves through the receptive field in this direction, it strongly excites the cell. Movement in the opposite direction inhibits the cell. **B.** The relationship between direction of movement and firing rate of the cell in this example.

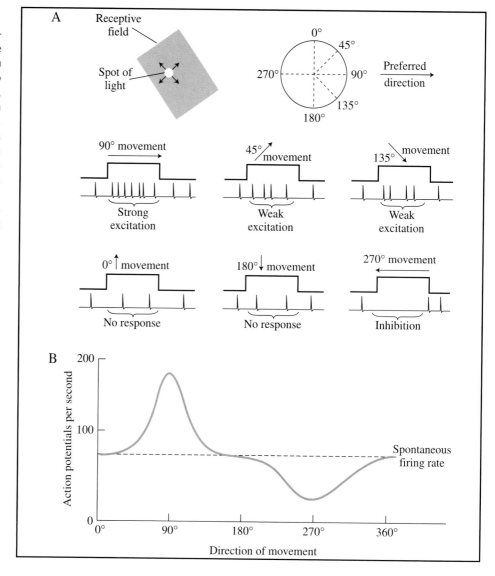

represented. The cells in area V5 respond equally well to lights of different wavelengths—that is, the cells are not color-sensitive.

Interestingly, the neurons in area V5 are specialized to signal *movement*, independent of the *shape* of the moving stimulus. Under normal conditions, movement will be associated with a particular form or shape, because the stimulus arises from a particular object moving in the visual world. Thus, movement and shape will not normally be separable traits of an object. Nevertheless, the cells in area V5 are able to respond briskly to a moving stimulus, even when it has no shape.

To see how experimenters produce a shapeless but moving stimulus, consider the diagrams in Figure 16.17. The stimulus consists of a large number of dots of light, which remain on for a brief time and then are turned off again (only a small number of dots are shown in the figure for the sake of clarity). At the next instant, the dots are turned on again at a new, randomly determined position within the field of view. The result is a randomly scintillating field, similar to the "snow" on a TV screen that is tuned to an empty channel. If all of the dots are moved to a random position (see Fig. 16.17A), a human observer does not perceive any coherent direction of movement in the stimulus. Perception of motion can be induced, however, if a small percentage of the dots are moved in a particular direction, rather than to a random position (see Fig. 16.17B). Thus, at each point in time, a small

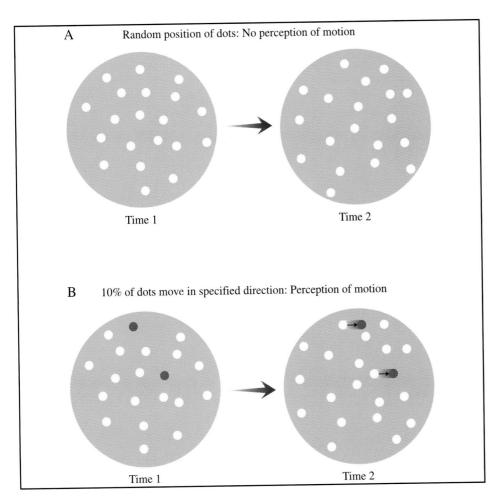

A
Random position of dots: No perception of motion

Time 1 → Time 2

B
10% of dots move in specified direction: Perception of motion

Time 1 → Time 2

Figure 16.17.
A random-dot stimulus can be used to produce a perception of movement, without an accompanying object shape or form. **A.** White dots are illuminated on a dark background at time 1. At time 2 the dots are extinguished and reappear at new, random positions. This stimulus produces no overall perception of motion in a particular direction. **B.** In this case, most of the dots reappear at random positions, but 10% of the dots (*red*) undergo a shift in a specified direction. This stimulus produces a perception of drifting motion from left to right.

fraction of the dots undergoes a correlated shift in direction. At the next instant, a different subset of dots undergoes a correlated shift in the same direction. This process is repeated at each successive instant for the duration of the stimulation. Although the stimulus still lacks a discernible overall pattern and human observers report that it has no "shape," the dots nevertheless produce a strong perception of "movement" in the direction of the correlated shift. In other words, this laboratory-generated stimulus has effectively separated motion and shape. The larger the fraction of dots undergoing the correlated shift, the easier a human observer can detect the direction of motion and report it reliably. When the percentage of correlated dots falls below approximately 4%, human and monkey observers can no longer detect the direction of motion.

The movement-sensitive cells in area V5 also respond strongly to the random-dot stimulus illustrated in Figure 16.17B, provided that the direction of correlated movement agrees with the cell's preferred direction. Area V5, then, contains neurons that respond to motion, even when the moving stimulus is "shapeless." Furthermore, the properties of the responses of neurons in area V5 to the random-dot stimuli can account quantitatively for the animal's motion perceptions. For example, the neurons fail to detect motion if the percentage of correlated dots is lower than 4%—the same percentage necessary to produce a behavioral response in the observer. This similarity suggests that the output of the motion-sensitive neurons in area V5 determines the animal's perceptual performance in detecting motion.

Neurobiologists also have tested the role of area V5 in motion perception by placing a small stimulating electrode in area V5 in an awake monkey. Weak electrical stimulation then was applied to artificially activate a small group of neurons that have a particular directional preference, while the monkey viewed a random-dot stimulus. Electrical stimulation biased the monkey's perceptual performance toward the direction of motion favored by the stimulated neurons. In other words, the monkey behaved as though it saw a moving stimulus when area V5 was electrically stimulated. This finding provided further evidence that the neurons of area V5 are uniquely responsible for determining the perception of visual motion.

It is interesting that one cortical target for the outputs of the motion-sensitive cells of area V5 is the **lateral intraparietal area**, which we encountered in our discussion of the oculomotor system in Chapter 10. An important goal of the oculomotor system is to move the eyes so that the fovea coincides with the position of a moving object, and then to track the moving target by means of appropriate eye movements. The information provided by the motion analysis system in area V5 is likely to be an important aspect of the sensorimotor integration carried out in the lateral intraparietal area, which correctly positions the eyes to bring the moving object to the foveal region of the retina.

IN THE CLINIC

Damage to the striate cortex (area V1) in human patients produces cortical blindness in the corresponding portion of the visual field. For example, destruction of the entire left occipital lobe results in a lack of awareness of visual stimuli presented in the right half of the visual field. Although patients are not consciously aware of stimuli in the affected portion of the visual field, damage to area V1 does not completely eliminate visual function. For instance, cortically blind patients are often able to correctly determine when a visual stimulus has been presented, even though they report no awareness of the stimulus. Emotional responses to visual objects may also be intact in patients with cortical blindness, which suggests that some form of perceptual identification of objects occurs in the absence of cortical visual processing. This phenomenon of blindsight may reflect the operation of noncortical visual pathways, such as the accessory optic system, which remain intact when area V1 is damaged. Nevertheless, an intact geniculostriate system appears to be required for conscious perception of visual stimuli.

In some cases, more specific forms of visual impairment arise from strokes or accidents that damage visual areas of the occipital and temporal lobes. Central achromatopsia is the loss of conscious color vision produced by lesions in the cortex, without interference with the discrimination of object shape. As with other forms of cortical blindness, however, color information can still be used in other visual tasks such as the detection of motion, albeit without awareness of the color of the stimulus. In keeping with the role of area V5 in detecting moving stimuli, damage to area V5 produces selective impairment of motion perception. The selectivity of these deficits emphasizes that the visual system processes visual information in parallel, using spatially distinct parts of the cortex to analyze particular aspects of the visual world. However, because strokes or accidents rarely respect anatomical boundaries between functionally distinct cortical areas, cortical damage in human patients most often involves a mixture of visual impairments affecting various aspects of visual information processing.

The axons of the retinal ganglion cells form the optic nerves, which merge at the base of the brain at the optic chiasm. At the chiasm, the axons coming from ganglion cells in the nasal half of each retina cross to the opposite side of the brain; axons coming from ganglion cells in the temporal half of each retina remain on the same side of the brain. As a result, the left half of the visual field (nasal retina from the ipsilateral eye, temporal retina from the contralateral eye) is represented in the right half of the brain, while the right half of the visual field is represented in the left half of the brain.

The synaptic targets of the retinal ganglion cells in the brain include the optic tectum and, in mammals, the lateral geniculate nucleus of the thalamus. From the thalamus, visual information is relayed to the primary visual cortex (also called area V1 or the striate cortex). The lateral geniculate nucleus acts as a gate that controls the access of visual information from the retina to the visual cortex. The ability of the thalamic relay cells to transmit visual information is governed by neurons in the reticular formation that are activated when the animal is aroused.

In the lateral geniculate nucleus, the projection neurons that send their axons to the cortex have receptive fields that resemble those of retinal ganglion cells—that is, they have a center-surround organization. In the primary visual cortex, however, a variety of different receptive fields are encountered. Many neurons in area V1 are best stimulated by a bar or line of light of a particular orientation. These orientation-selective cortical neurons detect the edges that define the borders of objects in the visual world. Some cortical neurons are motion-sensitive, requiring that the stimulus must be moving in a particular direction. Other cortical neurons are color-sensitive, responding best to light of a particular wavelength.

The primary visual cortex is organized into a two-dimensional array of functionally defined columns of cells that extend from the cortical surface to the underlying white matter. Ocular dominance columns form one dimension of the array; these columns receive inputs preferentially from either the contralateral or the ipsilateral eye. Orientation columns make up the other dimension of the array. Within an orientation column, the neurons have the same preferred orientation, but their receptive fields are located at slightly different retinal positions. In the primary visual cortex, each point on the retinal surface is examined in parallel by a group of orientation-selective neurons whose preferred orientations cover all directions. Similarly, each point on the retina is examined simultaneously by motion-sensitive neurons whose preferred directions of movement cover all possibilities. The primary visual cortex thus carries out in parallel an analysis of the visual field for a wide variety of aspects of visual stimuli, including line orientation, direction of movement, and object color.

Information processing also is arranged hierarchically within the cortical visual system. For example, the orientation-selective neurons in the primary visual cortex are used as building blocks to construct cells with more complex receptive fields. Some of these more complex cells require that lines of light must have a specific length and a particular orientation. In this way, cortical neurons with more complex properties are constructed by various combinations of synaptic inputs from cells with simpler receptive field properties.

In addition, the information from the primary visual cortex is passed on to higher-order cortical areas for further processing of specialized information. Area V2 is found just anterior to the primary visual cortex (area V1)

SUMMARY

SUMMARY

and receives inputs from area V1. Area V2 contains subdivisions devoted to the further processing of the form, color, and motion of objects. Both area V1 and area V2 also project to more specialized areas that are found in progressively more anterior portions of the occipital lobe and the posterior part of the temporal lobe of the cortex. Area V4 is specialized for color vision; area V3, for analysis of object shape; and area V5, for detection of motion.

REVIEW QUESTIONS

1. Describe the connections of retinal ganglion cells that lead to the left visual field being represented in the right primary visual cortex.
2. What layers are present in the lateral geniculate nucleus of the primate brain, and what functional differences exist in the inputs from the retina to each layer?
3. Describe the differences between X cells, Y cells, and W cells in the mammalian retina.
4. What are the two dimensions of columnar organization in area V1, and how do the neurons within each type of column respond to visual stimuli?
5. What is a blob, and what kind of visual information is processed by the cells in a blob?
6. What is the difference between a single-opponent and a double-opponent, color-sensitive neuron?
7. What is the structural organization of area V2, and what kinds of visual information are processed in each subdivision?
8. Draw a picture of a horizontal section through the cortex of the primate brain, and indicate the locations of areas V1, V2, V3, V4, and V5.
9. Why is the primary visual cortex also called the striate cortex?

INTERNET ASSIGNMENT   CHAPTER 16

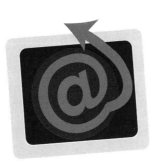

1 Use anatomical resources on the Internet, such as brain atlases, to locate the following structures in the brain: lateral geniculate nucleus, primary visual cortex, and area V2.

2 Find a histological section that shows the layers of the primary visual cortex. Point out the histological feature that gives rise to the alternative name "striate cortex" for the primary visual cortex.

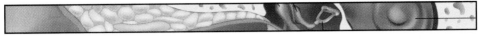

HEARING AND OTHER VIBRATION SENSES

ESSENTIAL BACKGROUND

Vestibular system
(Chapter 10)

General anatomy of the brain (Chapter 2)

Ionic permeability and the ionic basis of membrane potential (Chapter 3)

Synaptic transmission (Chapter 5, Chapter 6)

Action potential (Chapter 4)

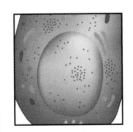

Chapters 15 and 16 focused on vision, one of the important senses used by organisms to detect objects in the environment from afar. In this chapter, we will examine another major sensory mechanism that allows animals to gather information about the environment without having to come into direct contact with objects. In this case, the physical energy used by the sensory system is mechanical vibration of the medium in which the organism is immersed. For terrestrial animals, that medium is the air; for aquatic animals, it is water. The human sensation produced by vibration of the air is called **hearing**. We will begin by examining the properties of the sensory receptors that are sensitive to mechanical vibrations. We then describe the brain mechanisms that analyze the information provided by those sensory receptors, concentrating on the sense of hearing in mammals.

MECHANORECEPTORS OF VIBRATION SENSES: HAIR CELLS

How do hair cells transduce mechanical vibration into an electrical signal?

Movements of both animate and inanimate objects in either air or water produce vibrations that propagate through the medium. The distance that these vibrations travel depends on their strength and frequency, as well as on the physical properties of the medium. When each vibration reaches the relevant sensory organ of the receiving animal, the mechanical energy of the vibration must be translated into an electrical signal, as in any sensory transduction process.

The mechanoreceptors for the vibration senses are **hair cells**, which we encountered in our discussion of the vestibular system in Chapter 10. As an example of a vibration receptor organ, we will consider the **lateral line organ**, which is illustrated in Figure 17.1. Many aquatic vertebrates possess some variant of this organ, which is used to detect the motion of water around the animal's body. The sensory hair cells are located within pits or tubes in the skin, through which water flows. The moving water displaces a gelatinous body (called the **cupula**, just as in the vestibular apparatus) that projects into the pit or tube (see Fig. 17.1). The hair-like cilia of the hair cells in the organ are embedded in the cupula, whose motions produce deflections of the cilia. As with the vestibular hair cells (see Chapter 10), these deflections change the membrane potential of the hair cell. In the next section, we will consider the mechanism by which the movements of the cilia are translated into electrical signals, a process called **mechanosensory transduction**.

Figure 17.1.

The structure of a lateral line organ. Within the lateral line, fluid movements deflect the cupula. The ciliary bundles of the sensory hair cells are embedded in the cupula.

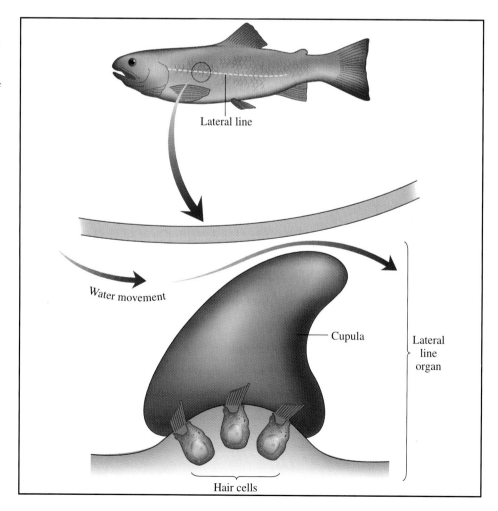

Lateral line

Water movement

Cupula

Lateral line organ

Hair cells

Mechanosensory Transduction in Hair Cells

The cilia of each hair cell form a bundle at the top of the cell, which is shown in cross section in Figure 17.2. The lengths of the cilia are not all the same, however, but increase progressively from one side of the bundle to the other. When the bundle is deflected toward the longest cilium, the hair cell depolarizes (see Fig. 17.2A). Depolarization increases the release of excitatory neurotransmitter at the synaptic connection between the hair cell and the sensory neuron that contacts it. As a result, the rate of action potential firing in the sensory neuron increases for this direction of movement. When the bundle is deflected in the opposite direction, away from the longest cilium, the hair cell hyperpolarizes (see Fig. 17.2B). The release of excitatory transmitter from the hair cell decreases in response to hyperpolarization, and the rate of action potential firing in the sensory neuron decreases below the resting level. Thus, in response to movements of the cilia, the hair cell produces graded changes in membrane potential, which are then translated into changes in the firing frequency of action potentials in the sensory neuron.

Vibration caused by water flowing over the cupula produces oscillating stimulation during which the cilia move back and forth, first toward and then away from the longest cilium. This situation is depicted in Figure 17.3. The membrane poten-

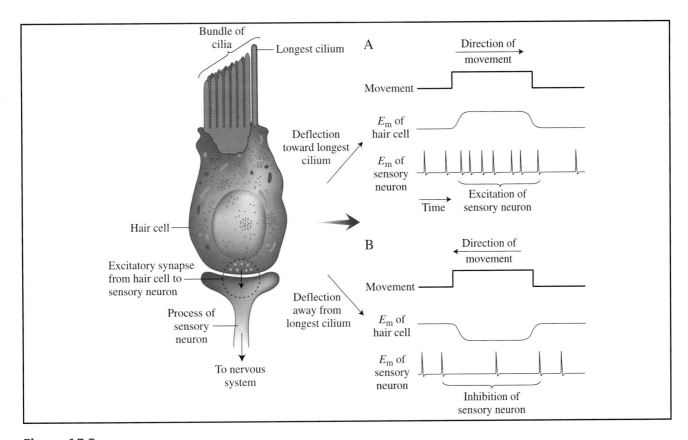

Figure 17.2.

The electrical response of a hair cell and its sensory neuron to deflections of the bundle of cilia. The hair cell produces graded changes in the membrane potential in response to movement of the cilia and makes an excitatory synaptic connection onto the process of the sensory neuron. **A.** When the ciliary bundle is deflected toward the longest cilium (to the right in the diagram), the hair cell depolarizes, and the excitation of the sensory neuron increases. **B.** When the ciliary bundle is deflected away from the longest cilium (to the left), the hair cell hyperpolarizes, less excitatory transmitter is released, and the sensory neuron fires action potentials less frequently.

Figure 17.3.

Oscillatory motion of the ciliary bundle produces oscillating changes in the membrane potential of the hair cell. The oscillatory changes in the hair cell are reflected in bursts of action potentials in the sensory neuron, which occur with the same periodicity as the oscillating stimulus.

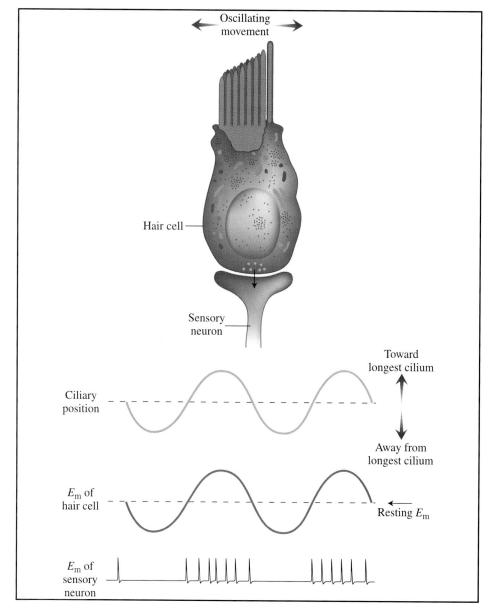

tial of the hair cell oscillates as the cilia move back and forth, tracking the position of the ciliary bundle. Coinciding with each depolarizing phase in the hair cell, the sensory neuron fires a burst of action potentials. During each hyperpolarizing phase in the hair cell, the sensory neuron ceases firing. Thus, the nervous system receives a series of repetitive bursts of action potentials from the sensory neuron, with the interval between bursts being determined by the frequency of the vibrating stimulus. If the frequency of the vibration increases, the duration of each burst of action potentials and the interval between successive bursts becomes shorter. The nervous system therefore can obtain information about the frequency of a vibrating stimulus applied to the lateral line organ by analyzing the temporal pattern of action potential activity in the sensory neuron. This encoding mechanism works best, however, for low-frequency vibrations like those produced by the motions of a fish (predator, prey, or mate) swimming nearby. In the case of sound perception in mammals, the relevant frequencies of oscillation are often much higher, and other mechanisms for encoding the frequency of a stimulus are required. We will describe these mechanisms later in this chapter, when we discuss the mammalian auditory organ.

Mechanically Sensitive Ion Channels in Hair Cell Cilia

The changes in the hair cell's membrane potential in response to ciliary movements are caused by changes in the ionic permeability of the hair cell membrane induced by deflection of the cilia. The mechanism thought to underlie the change in permeability is illustrated in Figure 17.4. The cilia in the bundle are tethered together near their tips by fine filaments that extend from each cilium to the next taller one in the bundle. These filaments behave like little springs. In the resting state (see Fig. 17.4A), the springs are slightly stretched, transmitting tension to each anchor point on adjacent cilia. This tension influences the opening of mechanosensitive ion channels in the cilia. Because of the resting tension, some of the channels open even when the bundle is in the neutral, upright position. The

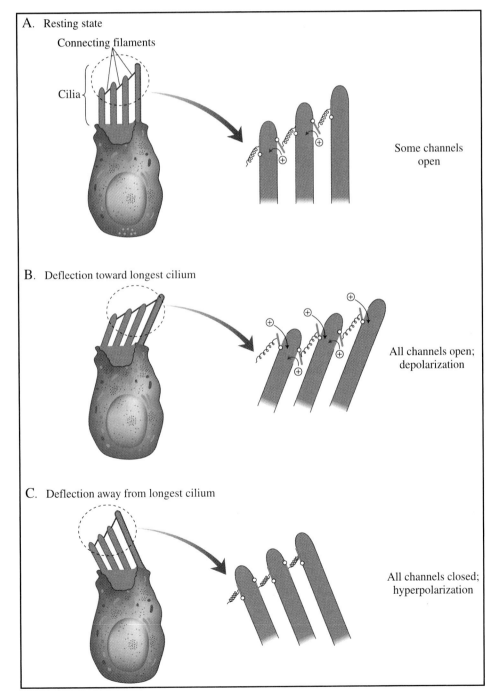

A. Resting state
Connecting filaments
Cilia
Some channels open

B. Deflection toward longest cilium
All channels open; depolarization

C. Deflection away from longest cilium
All channels closed; hyperpolarization

Figure 17.4.

A schematic representation of the mechanotransduction process in hair cell cilia. Connecting filaments extend from one cilium to the next near the tips of the cilia. **A**. In the resting state, there is some tension on the filaments (shown as *black springs*) connecting the tips of adjacent cilia. Some mechanosensitive cation channels therefore open, and the hair cell is partially depolarized because of the influx of positive charge. **B**. When the cilia are deflected toward the longest cilium, the distance between the filament attachment points increases, all the cation channels open, and the hair cell depolarizes more strongly. **C**. When the cilia are deflected away from the longest cilium, the tension exerted by the connecting filaments is lessened, all channels close, and the hair cell hyperpolarizes.

mechanically sensitive channels are cation channels that allow positive charge to enter the cilia, depolarizing the hair cell.

Consider what happens when the bundle is deflected. Despite the name "hair cell," which implies flexibility, the cilia are stiff and rigid (resembling the wires of a wire brush rather than the bristles of a paint brush). Therefore, the length of each cilium remains fixed during deflection, and the cilia slide past each other. You can easily construct a simple mechanical analogy of the cilia. Hold two pencils of slightly different lengths together vertically, with their eraser ends contacting a flat surface, such as a tabletop. While maintaining the contact point with the tabletop, move the tips of the pencils (still keeping them together) first toward the longer pencil, then toward the shorter pencil. Note that the pencils slide past each other during the movement and that the distance between the tips gets longer and shorter as you move them back and forth. This behavior is illustrated for the cilia of the hair cell in Figure 17.4B and C.

In hair cell cilia, deflection of the bundle toward the longest cilium causes the distance between the tips of successive cilia to become greater, and the connecting filaments are stretched more than at rest (see Fig. 17.4B). More of the mechanosensitive channels open, more positive charge enters the cell, and the hair cell depolarizes. Conversely, when the direction of deflection is away from the longest cilium, the distance between tips of adjacent cilia becomes smaller (see Fig. 17.4C). The connecting filaments are less stretched, and the reduced tension causes mechanosensitive cation channels to close. For this direction of movement, the hair cell hyperpolarizes because the cation conductance is smaller than it is in the resting state.

THE MAMMALIAN EAR

How are sound vibrations transferred from the tympanic membrane to the basilar membrane?

The ear is the specialized organ for sensing airborne vibrations in mammals. Figure 17.5 shows the basic structure of the mammalian ear. The mechanosensory cells that transduce mechanical vibration into electrical signals in the ear are also hair cells. In the mammalian ear, however, the cells are located within a spiral-shaped bony enclosure within the inner ear, called the **cochlea**. The cochlea can be thought of as an outgrowth of the vestibular labyrinth, whose function in the perception of head motion was discussed in Chapter 10. Indeed, during the course of evolution the cochlea developed as an additional chamber of the phylogenetically older vestibular apparatus.

Like the labyrinth and the lateral line system, the hair cells of the cochlea are bathed in fluid. Vibrations in the air reaching the ear of a terrestrial mammal must be transferred to this fluid. This coupling of airborne vibrations to the fluid within the cochlea is carried out by the middle ear (see Fig. 17.5). The eardrum, or **tympanic membrane**, is stretched across the ear canal like the head of a drum and separates the middle ear from the external world. Air vibrations set the eardrum in motion, and this motion is transferred to the cochlea via the small bones of the middle ear (the hammer, the anvil, and the stirrup). Because the walls of the cochlea are rigid, the movement of the bones is transferred to the interior of the cochlea via a flexible membrane, called the **oval window**, located at the point where the bones of the middle ear contact the cochlea.

The cochlea is divided into two compartments by another membrane, the **basilar membrane**. (As we will see later, the anatomical arrangement is actually more complicated than this description of two compartments, but this representation will suffice for understanding the mechanical coupling within the cochlea.) If a wave of increased pressure arrives at the eardrum, the oval window is pushed inward, increasing the pressure above the basilar membrane. For this increased

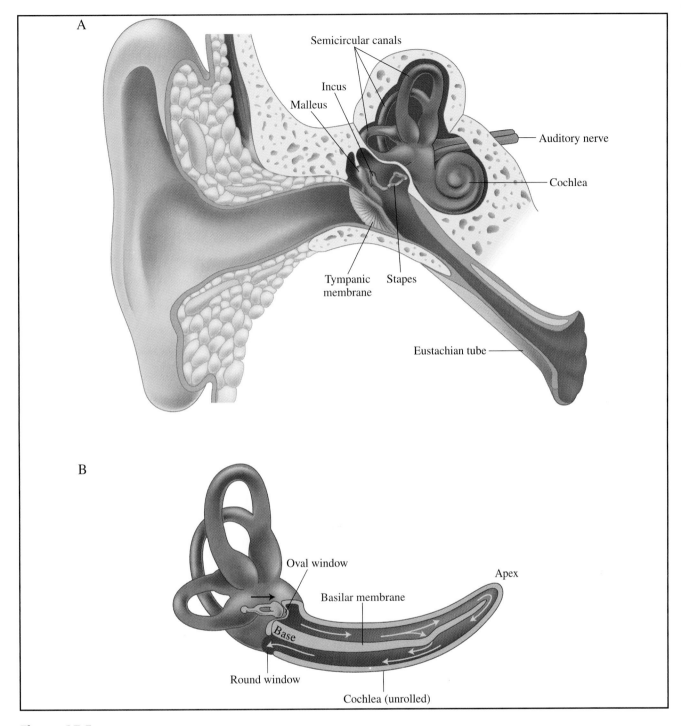

Figure 17.5.

An overview of the structure of the human ear. **A**. The outer ear is separated from the middle ear by the tympanic membrane, whose vibrations are transmitted to the cochlea by the bones of the inner ear. **B**. The cochlea is represented here in a straightened form, to clarify its internal structure. In this diagram, the separation between the upper and lower compartments of the cochlea is simplified, in that the separation is represented solely by the basilar membrane. (See Fig. 17.12 for a more complete view of the internal structure of the cochlea.)

pressure to deflect the basilar membrane, another flexible membrane is required within the cochlear compartment below the basilar membrane. This flexible membrane, called the **round window**, bulges outward, allowing the pressure increase in the upper compartment to move the basilar membrane downward. If a wave of decreased pressure reaches the eardrum, the oval window is pulled outward, the round window bulges inward, and the basilar membrane moves upward. Therefore, an oscillation of the tympanic membrane produces an oscillatory movement of the basilar membrane inside the cochlea (see Fig. 17.5B).

The sensory hair cells ride on top of the basilar membrane, and the hair bundles of the hair cells are deflected in response to vibrations of this membrane. The cell bodies of the sensory neurons that receive synaptic inputs from the hair cells are located within the cochlea, in the **spiral ganglion**. Each spiral ganglion cell sends an axon into the central nervous system via the **auditory nerve**. Together with the axons coming from the vestibular apparatus (the vestibular nerve), these axons make up **cranial nerve VIII**.

Response of Single Auditory Nerve Fibers: Tuning Curves

Natural sounds consist of complex combinations of vibrations at many different frequencies. However, the responses of neurons in the auditory system can be characterized using simple sinusoidal sound stimuli. If a loudspeaker is driven by a sinusoidal voltage (Fig. 17.6A), the movement of the speaker cone produces a sine wave sound stimulus, which a human will experience as a pure tone whose pitch depends on the frequency of the sine wave. The listener's sensitivity to stimuli of different frequencies can be determined by varying the intensity of the stimulus. Normal humans can detect sounds in the frequency range of 20 cycles/sec (hertz, or Hz) to approximately 20,000 Hz, with the greatest sensitivity being in the range of 1000 to 4000 Hz.

The same type of experiment can be performed while recording the action potential activity of a single auditory nerve fiber. Each nerve fiber is most sensitive to a particular frequency, and it will respond less well to stimuli of both higher and lower frequencies. The relationship between the sensitivity of the nerve fiber and the frequency of the stimulus defines the **tuning curve** for the fiber, as shown in Figure 17.6B. The tuning curve for an individual auditory nerve fiber is much sharper than the overall curve measured for the organism as a whole. For example, fiber A in Figure 17.6B does not respond well to stimuli below 100 Hz or above 2000 Hz, although a human can readily detect such tones. Different auditory nerve fibers are most sensitive to different portions of the audible frequency spectrum. Fi-

Figure 17.6.

Tuning curves of single auditory nerve fibers. **A**. A loudspeaker can produce a pure tone stimulus, whose sinusoidal frequency and amplitude can be controlled independently. **B**. The sensitivity of two auditory nerve fibers to sinusoidal stimuli of different frequencies. High sensitivity means that the nerve fiber responds to very quiet tones; low sensitivity means that loud tones are required to elicit a response. The frequency of the sine wave stimulus is shown on a logarithmic scale. **C**. Examples of action potential activity elicited in the two fibers of **B** by stimuli at 500 Hz (*left*) and at 5000 Hz (*right*).

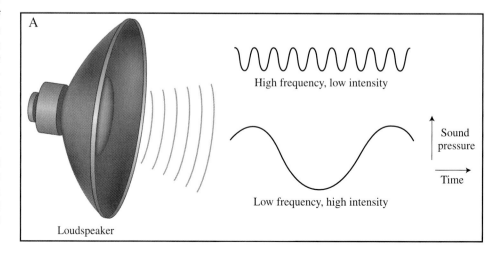

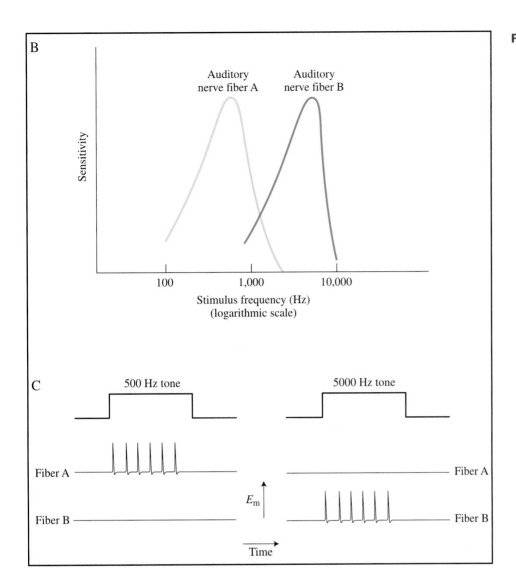

Figure 17.6.

(continued)

ber B, for instance, responds to tones in the range of 1000 to 10,000 Hz and is most sensitive at 5000 Hz. The patterns of action potentials triggered in fibers A and B by brief tone bursts at 500 Hz and 5000 Hz are shown in Figure 17.6C.

In humans, each cochlea gives rise to approximately 25,000 auditory nerve fibers. As a group, this population defines the entire audible spectrum that humans can perceive. In other species, the auditory system can respond to stimulus frequencies that humans find inaudible. A "silent," ultrasonic dog whistle is certainly not silent to your dog, for example. Bats use even higher-frequency sounds as the basis for their echolocation system.

Cochlear Mechanics Contribute to Frequency Tuning in the Auditory System

Multiple mechanisms underlie the narrow frequency tuning of the individual auditory nerve fibers. The first mechanism we will consider is mechanical and is based on the construction of the basilar membrane. Vibrations of the tympanic membrane are translated into pressure fluctuations within the fluid-filled compartments of the cochlea, producing vertical movements of the basilar membrane (see Fig. 17.5). The basilar membrane is not uniform from the base to the apex of the cochlea, however. This nonuniformity is illustrated in Figure 17.7. When viewed

How does the structure of the basilar membrane account in part for the differential response of auditory nerve fibers to different sound frequencies?

from above, the basilar membrane is tapered, with the width being narrowest at the basal end and broadest at the apex. Like the strings of a harp, the narrow end of the membrane vibrates best at high frequencies, and the wide end vibrates best at lower frequencies. In addition to being narrower, the basal end of the basilar membrane is stiffer than the apical end. As a result, low-frequency sound stimuli preferentially vibrate the apical end of the basilar member, while high-frequency sounds preferentially vibrate the basal end.

When the ear receives a sinusoidal sound stimulus, the greatest up-down movement of the basilar membrane occurs at a particular location along the length of the cochlea, depending on the frequency of the stimulus (see Fig. 17.7). This mecha-

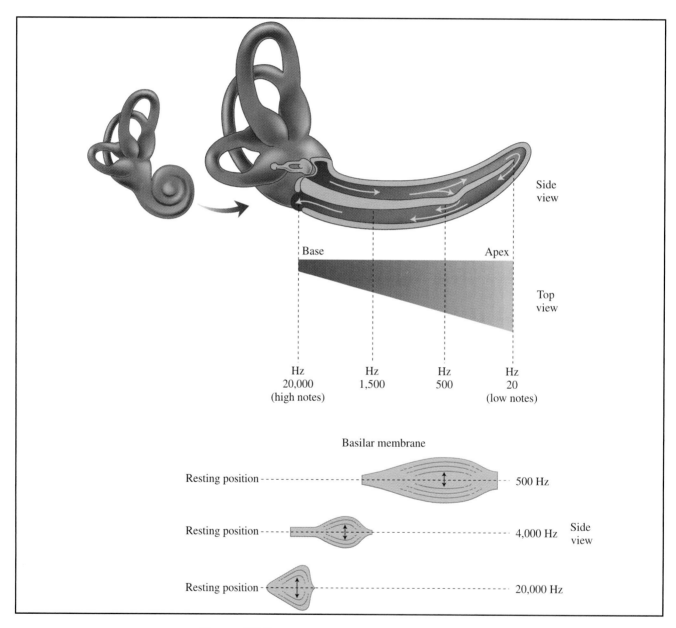

Figure 17.7.

The basilar membrane vibrates most strongly at different locations in response to tones of different frequencies. The cochlea is shown in coiled and uncoiled representations at the *top*. When viewed from above, the uncoiled basilar membrane is wider at the apex (low-frequency end) than at the high-frequency end (base). In the side views, the *tan shading* shows the maximal up-down extent of the vibrations of the basilar membrane produced by three different stimulus frequencies. The *dashed line* indicates the resting, unstimulated position of the basilar membrane.

nism accounts for part of the frequency tuning of the auditory nerve fibers. Spiral ganglion neurons that receive inputs from hair cells at the apex of the cochlea will be stimulated best by low-frequency stimuli, while those that receive inputs from basal hair cells will be stimulated best by high-frequency stimuli. The frequency tuning that would be expected from the mechanical properties of the cochlea is rather broad, however, compared with the sharp tuning curves actually observed in single auditory nerve fibers. As shown in Figure 17.7, the amplitude envelope for low- and middle-frequency stimuli includes most of the basilar membrane. Consequently, a broad range of stimulus frequencies would excite the nerve fibers connected to hair cells at the middle of the basilar membrane. Therefore, additional tuning mechanisms are required to explain the behavior of the auditory nerve fibers.

Hair Cell Electrical Properties Also Contribute to Frequency Tuning

Hair cells respond to oscillatory movements of their hair bundles with an oscillatory change in membrane potential (see Fig. 17.3). However, individual hair cells respond differently to hair bundle movements at different frequencies. Some hair cells give larger responses to low-frequency stimuli, while others produce larger responses to high-frequency stimuli. Figure 17.8 illustrates this behavior. When the hair bundle is moved back and forth slowly, a low-frequency cell follows the stimulus

How do ion channels in hair cells determine the frequency tuning of individual cells?

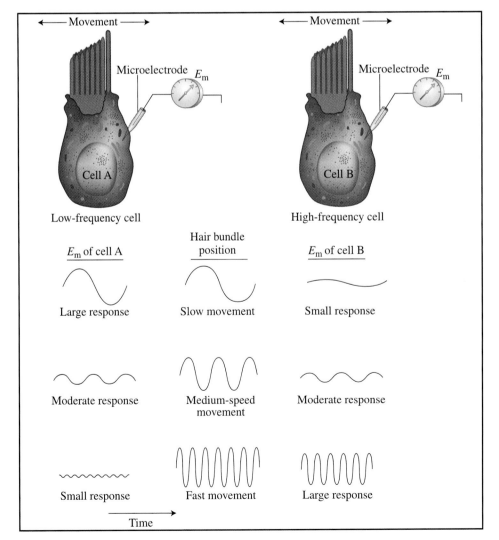

Figure 17.8.

Frequency tuning in single hair cells. Hair cells have a preferred frequency of stimulation that matches the maximal vibration frequency of their location on the basilar membrane. The *left column* shows responses of a hair cell from a low-frequency position along the basilar membrane (toward the apex). The *right column* shows the responses of a hair cell from a high-frequency position (toward the base). The *middle column* shows the oscillatory motion applied to the hair bundles in each case.

with a matching, large-amplitude change in membrane potential at the same frequency. A high-frequency cell also responds to the low-frequency stimulus, but the response amplitude is much smaller. When the hair bundle is moved rapidly, both cells respond, but the high-frequency cell has a large response and the low-frequency cell shows a small response. Both cells give an intermediate response to a moderate-speed movement. Thus, individual hair cells respond best to a particular preferred frequency of stimulation.

The characteristic tuning frequency of an individual hair cell is also reflected in the cell's response to electrical stimulation, as shown in Figure 17.9. Even in the absence of a mechanical stimulus, the resting potential of an isolated hair cell oscillates at a frequency that matches the cell's characteristic frequency. Thus, low-frequency cells exhibit a low-frequency oscillation (see Fig. 17.9A), whereas high-frequency cells oscillate at a high frequency (see Fig. 17.9B). When a positive current is injected into the cell, the cell depolarizes, and the amplitude of the oscillation increases. In both high-frequency and low-frequency cells, the speed of the oscillation during depolarization matches the frequency preference of the cell for mechanical stimuli.

These oscillations of membrane potential result from the interplay of two different types of ion channels in the plasma membrane of the hair cell: voltage-activated calcium channels and calcium-activated potassium channels. Figure 17.10

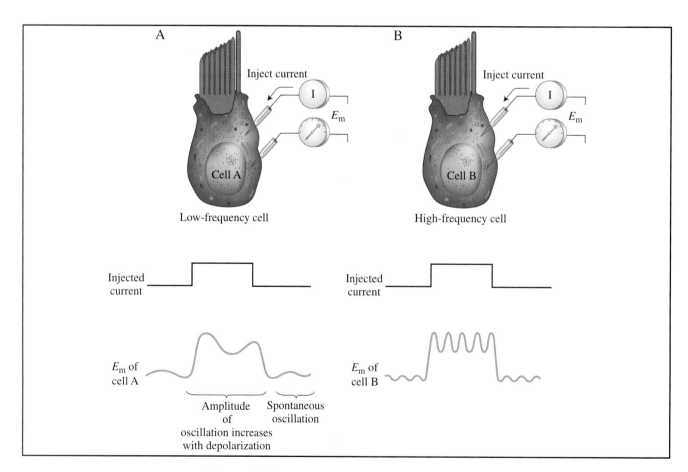

Figure 17.9.

Hair cells have endogenous electrical tuning. Even in the absence of an applied stimulus, the membrane potential of hair cells oscillates. The frequency of the oscillation matches the preferred mechanical stimulation frequency of the cell. A low-frequency hair cell generates slow oscillations (*left*), while a high-frequency hair cell produces fast oscillations (*right*). The amplitude of the oscillation increases when depolarizing electrical current is injected into the hair cell.

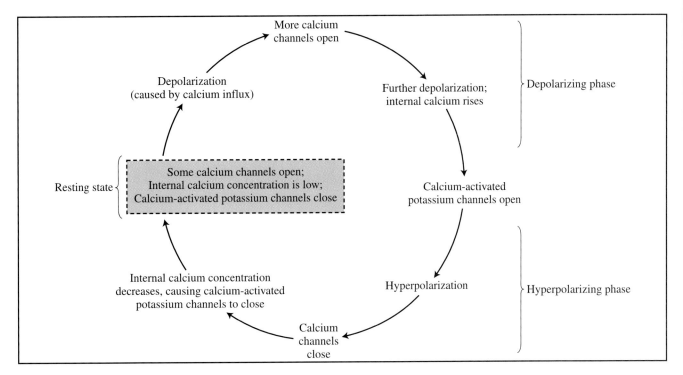

Figure 17.10.

The proposed mechanism for endogenous electrical tuning of hair cells. The resting state is indicated by the *dashed box*. The depolarizing phase is represented in the upper part of the cycle, while the hyperpolarizing phase is represented in the lower part.

summarizes how these channels interact to produce cyclical depolarization and hyperpolarization. In the resting state, the hair cell is slightly depolarized, which causes some voltage-activated calcium channels to open. The resulting influx of calcium ions tends to further depolarize the cell, opening more calcium channels. As more calcium enters through the open channels, however, the internal calcium concentration rises, resulting in the opening of calcium-activated potassium channels. Hyperpolarization produced by the potassium channels causes the voltage-activated calcium channels to close, which in turn decreases calcium influx. As the internal calcium concentration falls again—because of calcium pumps and cellular uptake mechanisms—the calcium-activated potassium channels close, and the cycle begins again. In this way, repetitive cycles of depolarization and hyperpolarization are produced, as shown in the cyclic diagram in Figure 17.10.

The depolarizing phase of the oscillation represents the opening of voltage-activated calcium channels, and the hyperpolarizing phase represents the opening of calcium-activated potassium channels. The frequency of oscillation depends on the time delay between the opening of the calcium channels and the opening of the calcium-activated potassium channels. This time delay is short in cells that have a high characteristic frequency and long in cells that have a low characteristic frequency. One possible mechanism that determines the length of the delay involves the distance between the calcium channels and the potassium channels. If the distance is large, calcium entering through the calcium channels requires a longer time to reach the potassium channels and to accumulate the concentration necessary to open the potassium channels. Another possibility is that different types of potassium channels with different sensitivities to calcium are found in low-frequency and high-frequency cells.

The frequency tuning of an individual hair cell reflects the characteristics of the ion channels in the cell's membrane. Thus, an electrical mechanism underlies the tuning process. The hair cells at a particular location along the basilar membrane are thought to have a preferred frequency that matches the frequency tuning of the cochlea at that position. In this way, the broad mechanical tuning of the basilar membrane is sharpened by the electrical response of the hair cells. If a 4000-Hz stimulus is presented, for example, the hair cells at the 4000-Hz position on the basilar membrane (see Fig. 17.7) will be stimulated more than the hair cells at other positions: the motion of the membrane is largest at that location, and this stimulus frequency produces the largest electrical response in the hair cells at that position. Although the basilar membrane at other positions undergoes substantial motion during the 4000-Hz stimulus (see Fig. 17.7), the frequency of vibration does not match the preferred frequency of the hair cells at other positions, and so their response is smaller.

Hair Cells Also Produce Active Movements

What are the functional differences between inner and outer hair cells in the organ of Corti?

So far, we have discussed the electrical responses produced by hair cells when an external stimulus sets the bundle of cilia in motion. Hair cells also *produce* movements in response to electrical stimulation. Thus, hair cells can generate active movement as well as respond passively to imposed movement. Cilia are commonly used to produce movement in a variety of different cell types. For instance, many single-cell organisms use ciliary motions to locomote. In the air passages of vertebrate lungs, moving cilia of epithelial cells clear debris that enters from the outside world during breathing.

Hair cells can produce two types of motions, as shown in Figure 17.11. First, the ciliary bundle moves back and forth in response to oscillations in membrane potential. The molecular motor that drives this ciliary motion is based on the protein actin, which we encountered in our description of skeletal-muscle contraction (see

Figure 17.11.

Hair cells move in response to changes in membrane potential. Both the position of the ciliary bundle and the length of the hair cell change when the membrane potential is altered.

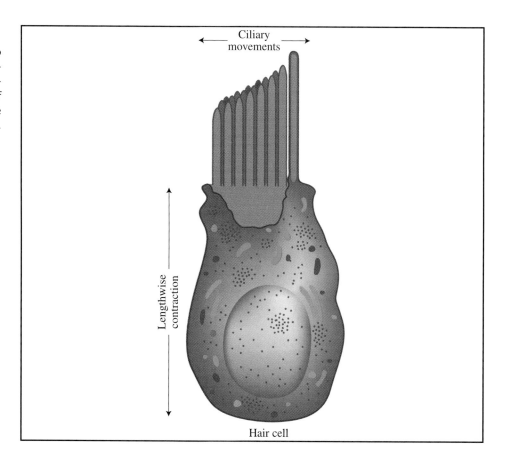

Chapter 7). Because the oscillatory change in membrane potential has a particular characteristic frequency for each hair cell, the oscillatory ciliary movements produced by a given cell also have the same characteristic frequency. Second, the length of the hair cell changes. Depolarization shortens the cell, while hyperpolarization causes the cell to lengthen. The molecular mechanisms for this longitudinal movement are not yet understood, but the motion appears to depend on a lattice of filaments located just under the plasma membrane.

The active movements of hair cells are thought to play an important role in amplifying small motions of the basilar membrane. Before examining this mechanical amplification, we must first describe additional structural details of the cochlea. Figure 17.12 shows a cross section through the cochlea to reveal its internal organization. As described earlier (see Fig. 17.5), the cochlea contains two fluid-filled compartments. The compartment connected to the oval window, where the incoming vibrations arrive, is called the **scala vestibuli**. The compartment connected to the round window is called the **scala tympani**. In Figure 17.12, note that these two compartments are separated by a third, smaller compartment that is bounded on one side by the basilar membrane and on the other side by the **vestibular membrane**. The third compartment is called the **scala media** (or the **cochlear duct**). The hair cells themselves are part of the **organ of Corti**, which rests on the basilar membrane and moves up and down when the membrane vibrates during acoustic stimulation.

The organ of Corti contains two groups of hair cells: the **inner hair cells** and the **outer hair cells** (see Fig. 17.12). The two types of hair cells differ in several ways. There are three rows of outer hair cells along the length of the cochlea but only a single row of inner hair cells. The entire cochlea contains about five times as many outer hair cells as inner hair cells (about 20,000 versus about 4000). In addition, the outer hair cells are larger than the inner hair cells and have larger hair bundles. Unlike the cilia of the inner hair cells, the cilia of the outer hair cells are embedded in an overlying membrane, the **tectorial membrane**. When the basilar membrane moves up and down, the shearing motion generated between the tectorial membrane and the underlying hair cells deflects the hair bundles of the outer hair cells. The inner hair cells, on the other hand, are coupled to the relative movements of the basilar and tectorial membranes indirectly via the motions of the intervening fluid.

These differences would seem to suggest that the outer hair cells are likely to play a more important role in auditory transduction than are the inner hair cells. A surprise awaits us, however, when we examine the pattern of innervation of the inner and outer hair cells by the sensory neurons of the spiral ganglion. Almost all of the sensory neurons make synaptic contact exclusively with the inner hair cells: for every sensory neuron that contacts outer hair cells, approximately 20 contact inner hair cells. Thus, the great majority of auditory nerve fibers reflect the responses of the inner hair cells. Because the outer hair cells are much more numerous, each of the few sensory axons that innervate the outer cells must contact a large number of cells (approximately 20). The opposite situation occurs for the inner hair cells, where innervating nerve fibers outnumber hair cells. Thus, each inner hair cell synapses onto several sensory neurons (5 to 10 per hair cell). So, the inner hair cells, not the more numerous outer hair cells, are largely responsible for generating the sensory signal in the cochlea.

The primary function of the outer hair cells may be to mechanically amplify the motions of the tectorial membrane. The outer hair cells move in response to depolarization and hyperpolarization, as described earlier (see Fig. 17.11). By adding a component of active motion, the cilia of the outer hair cells attached to the tectorial membrane reinforce vibrations at the preferred frequency. This hypothesis explains why the outer hair cells are so numerous and why their ciliary bundles

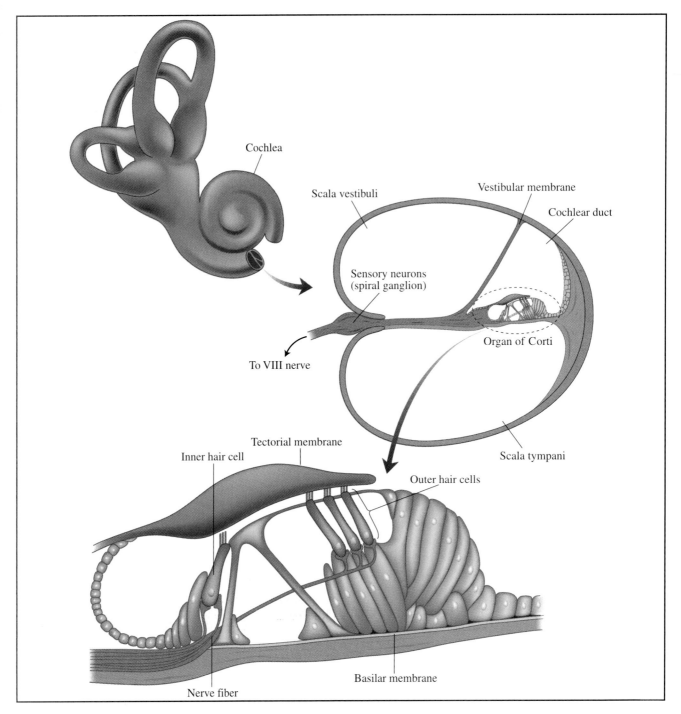

Figure 17.12.

The internal structure of the cochlea viewed in cross section.

are larger than those of inner hair cells. Longitudinal contractions of the hair cells (see Fig. 17.11) are also important in amplifying small motions of the basilar membrane. Because the outer hair cells are attached to the tectorial membrane via their cilia and are embedded in the organ of Corti, they pull up on the basilar membrane when they contract. Similarly, when the outer hair cells elongate during hyperpolarization, they push down on the basilar membrane. The electrical tuning of the outer hair cells guarantees that these motions will occur at the preferred frequency of each cell, which matches the preferred frequency of the basilar membrane at each position along the cochlea. Thus, the outer hair cells mechanically amplify the vibrations of the basilar membrane imposed by an auditory stimulus and do so preferentially at the location that is best stimulated by the stimulus.

Efferent Synapses onto Hair Cells

The nerve fibers of the spiral ganglion neurons receive excitatory synaptic input from the hair cells and carry the outgoing, or afferent, sensory information into the brain. The cochlea also receives incoming, efferent nerve fibers that originate from neurons in the brainstem. The efferent nerve fibers make synaptic connections predominantly onto outer hair cells. Activation of the efferent neurons reduces the sensitivity of the cochlea to sound and inhibits the sensory output from the ear. Thus, the efferent synaptic connections produce negative feedback on the auditory transduction system.

The neurotransmitter released by the efferent synaptic terminals is acetylcholine, which acts via muscarinic cholinergic receptors to open potassium channels in the hair cells. The increase in potassium permeability hyperpolarizes the outer hair cells, inhibits the oscillations in membrane potential, and inhibits the motor movements of the cilia. The fact that the outer hair cells are the principal target of the efferent input provides further evidence for the importance of the outer cells in regulating the sensitivity of the cochlear transduction mechanisms.

THE AUDITORY SYSTEM IN THE BRAIN

Cochlear Nucleus

After entering the central nervous system via the auditory nerve, the auditory information is distributed and processed in a pattern similar to that of other sensory systems. The first stop is the **cochlear nucleus** in the brainstem, where audi-

What parts of the brainstem receive and process auditory information on its way to the thalamus?

BOX 1 — IN THE CLINIC

Because the ear is a mechanical system, a common source of hearing loss is mechanical damage to the auditory apparatus. This is often produced by exposure to very loud sounds. When motions of the basilar membrane are too large, the hair cells can be damaged or destroyed, or the ciliary bundles of the outer hair cells can be dislodged from the tectorial membrane. If this happens, there is a loss of sensitivity to sound stimuli at the frequency corresponding to the damaged portion of the cochlea. In addition to the loss of sensitivity to external stimuli, the remaining hair cells in the damaged area may also become spontaneously active, in the absence of sound stimuli. This may occur because of the electrical tuning mechanisms of the hair cell, which can produce spontaneous oscillations in membrane potential at the preferred frequency of the hair cell even in the absence of stimulation. Because the spiral ganglion neurons that receive inputs from the spontaneously active hair cells fire action potentials just as they would in the presence of a sound stimulus, the rest of the auditory nervous system interprets the activity as a continuous sound at the corresponding pitch. The result is "ringing in the ears" or tinnitus, which can be much more debilitating for patients than the actual hearing loss itself.

tory nerve fibers terminate. The auditory nerve fibers originating from different parts of the cochlea are geometrically mapped onto specific regions within the cochlear nucleus. Recall that each position along the cochlea is most sensitive to a particular stimulus frequency. The spatial mapping of the cochlea onto the cochlear nucleus translates, therefore, into a map of preferred stimulus frequency within the cochlear nucleus. This **tonotopic map** is analogous to the retinotopic map found in the visual system.

By determining which part of the cochlea is activated, the auditory nervous system can determine the frequency composition of a sound stimulus. For tones above a few hundred hertz (which includes most of the audible frequency spectrum for humans), the auditory nerve fibers cannot follow the cycle-by-cycle pressure variations of the stimulus, and the temporal pattern of the action potentials carries no information about the frequency of the stimulus tone. Thus, each auditory nerve fiber can be thought of as a labeled line that signifies the presence of a particular auditory stimulus frequency. Only by keeping precise track of the labels on the lines—via the tonotopic spatial organization in the cochlear nucleus—can the nervous system analyze the overall frequency content of an auditory stimulus.

The neurons in the cochlear nucleus respond to other specific aspects of the auditory stimulus in addition to the stimulus frequency. Some cochlear nucleus neurons fire only a single action potential abruptly and reliably just at the onset of a tone at their preferred frequency. These neurons extract precise information about the time of onset of an arriving sound stimulus. Other neurons in the cochlear nucleus show the opposite pattern of response, remaining silent at the onset of a stimulus and then increasing their firing rate during a sustained tone. These transmit information about the ongoing intensity of a sound. Several other variants of these response patterns are observed in the cochlear nucleus. Thus, inputs from the cochlea are analyzed in parallel in the cochlear nucleus to extract particular kinds of information about the auditory stimulus. This approach to information processing is similar to the pattern observed in the visual system (see Chapters 15 and 16).

Superior Olivary Nucleus

The outputs of the cochlear nucleus illustrate a general principle of neural organization: both hierarchical and parallel organizations are observed in the anatomical connections made by the neurons of the cochlear nucleus. Figure 17.13 summarizes the projection pathways in the mammalian brain leading from the cochlear nucleus to the primary auditory cortex. The target for auditory information ascending from the brainstem is the **inferior colliculus**. Two parallel pathways lead from the cochlear nucleus to the inferior colliculus: a direct, bilateral projection of axons of cochlear nucleus neurons, and an indirect path via an intermediate brainstem nucleus, the **superior olivary nucleus** (also called the **superior olive**).

Neurons in the olivary nucleus give rise to the efferent axons that project back to the cochlea, where they make synaptic connections with the outer hair cells and control cochlear sensitivity. The main function of the neurons within the superior olivary nucleus, however, is to process aspects of auditory information related to the localization of sound sources in the external environment. The location of a sound source relative to the head can be ascertained in two ways.

First, if a sound source is located to the left of the head, the sound waves will reach the left ear sooner than the right ear. Although this time difference is very small (a few hundred microseconds), it is nevertheless detectable by specialized

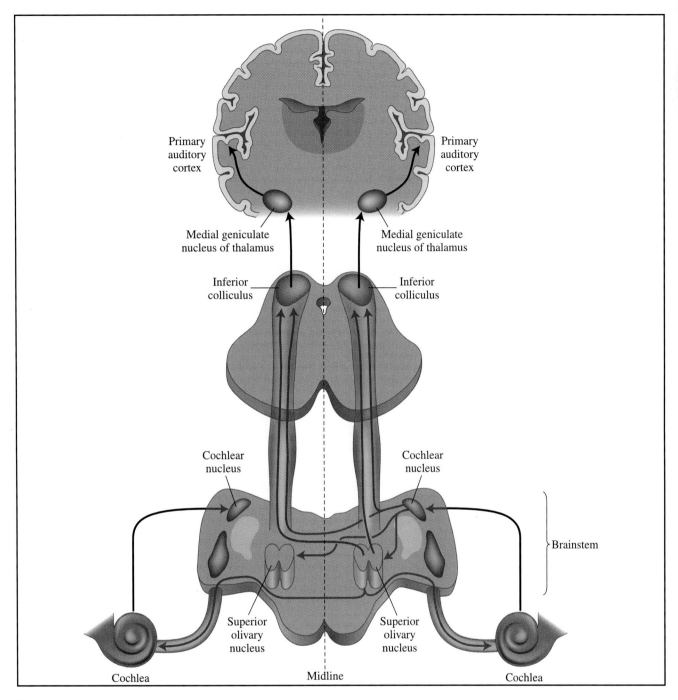

Figure 17.13.

The organization of the brain auditory pathways. In the brainstem, only the connections for the nuclei on the right side are illustrated (to make the pattern of connections easier to follow). Mirror-image connections are made on the left side.

neurons within a subdivision of the superior olivary nucleus. These neurons receive inputs from the cochlear nuclei on both sides of the brain (**binaural inputs**) and fire action potentials only when a slight time difference separates the activation of the inputs originating from the two ears.

Second, sounds can be localized by the small difference in intensity of the sound in the two ears. Sound arriving from a source to the left of the head will have a slightly higher intensity in the left ear than in the right ear because of the "shadowing" effect of the head. Once again, specialized neurons within a different subdivision of the superior olivary nucleus carry out a sensitive comparison of the sound intensities reported by the two ears.

Because of the subtlety of the cues involved, sound localization is not very precise in humans and in most other mammalian species. We (and other animals) often turn our heads from side to side as we attempt to locate the source of a sound, allowing our superior olive neurons to search for slight changes in arrival time and intensity as the head changes positions. Moveable external ears offer a major advantage in this regard. In addition, animals that have a highly developed ability to localize sounds—such as bats, owls, and coyotes—often have elaborate external ear structures that maximize the intensity and arrival-time cues to improve performance.

The Pathway to the Primary Auditory Cortex

What columnar organization of auditory information is observed in the primary auditory cortex?

The neurons of the superior olivary nucleus send projecting axons that join with the axons of cochlear nucleus neurons and ascend in a fiber tract called the **lateral lemniscus**. These axons terminate in the inferior colliculus. As shown in Figure 17.13, the outputs from both the cochlear nucleus and the superior olivary nucleus project bilaterally so that the inferior colliculus on each side of the brain receives information from both ears.

As with the other sensory systems we have studied, the thalamus is the gateway to the auditory cortex. For auditory information, the relevant thalamic nucleus is the **medial geniculate nucleus** (see Fig. 17.13). The projections from the inferior colliculus to the thalamus and from the thalamus to the cortex are primarily ipsilateral. Because the inputs from the two ears are thoroughly mixed at lower levels, however, the neurons in the thalamus and cortex receive binaural inputs. The primary auditory cortex is located in the superior part of the temporal lobe of the cerebral cortex (Brodmann's areas 41 and 42), as shown in Figure 17.14. A tonotopic map of the cochlea, similar to that found in the cochlear nucleus in the brainstem, is also present in the auditory cortex. As in the visual cortex, where the retinotopic map is repeated several times in subdivisions of the cortex specialized for different visual functions (see Chapter 16), the tonotopic map in the primary auditory cortex is represented multiple times.

The auditory cortex and visual cortex are structurally similar in additional ways. In both, the cortex is organized into a two-dimensional array of vertically oriented columns across the cortical surface. In the auditory cortex, one dimension of the array consists of **frequency columns**, in which cells have the same frequency preference for sound stimuli (see Fig. 17.14). Neighboring columns have a similar frequency preference, which varies in a consistent way from low frequency to high frequency across the surface of the cortex. The frequency columns are functionally analogous to the orientation columns of the visual cortex.

The other axis of the two-dimensional array in the auditory cortex consists of **binaural columns**, which are somewhat analogous to the ocular dominance columns encountered in the visual cortex. In one type of binaural column (called a **summation column**), cells respond best to sound stimuli presented simultaneously to both ears. In the other type of binaural column, cells respond best to a stimulus in only one ear, with the response being smaller when the stimulus is presented binaurally. This type of column is called a **suppression column**. The functional significance of these columns is not as well worked out in the auditory cortex as in the visual cortex. Nevertheless, columnar organization of cortical neurons into functionally related, vertically oriented units is a common feature of the cerebral cortex.

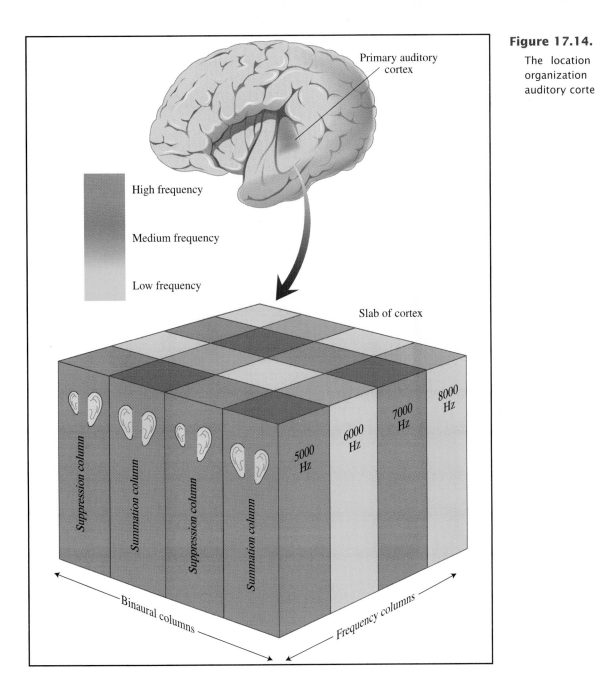

Figure 17.14.
The location and functional organization of the primary auditory cortex.

Vibrations of the air or water in which animals live are sensed by specialized hair cells that have a bundle of modified cilia at one end. The hair cells translate movements of the ciliary bundle into electrical signals, in a process called mechanotransduction. The cilia are tethered to one another via filamentous threads near their tips. When the bundle is deflected toward the longest cilium in the bundle, these filaments exert tension on cation channels in the cilia, causing the ion channels to open. Deflection in the opposite direction (away from the longest cilium) reduces tension and causes the channels to close. Because the open channels allow positively charged ions to enter the hair cell, the cell depolarizes when the bundle is moved toward the longest cilium and hyperpolarizes when the movement is in the opposite direction. If the hair bundle oscillates back and forth, the membrane potential of the hair cell oscillates in phase with the cilia. The

SUMMARY

hair cell makes excitatory synaptic contact onto a sensory neuron, which reports the activity of the hair cell to the nervous system.

In the mammalian ear, the hair cells that respond to sound stimuli are located within the cochlea, a spiral-shaped compartment in the inner ear. Vibrations in the air are transferred to the fluid inside the cochlea via the tympanic membrane (eardrum) and the bones of the middle ear. Vibrations within the cochlea move the basilar membrane, which has the hair cell–containing organ of Corti riding on top of it. The up-down motions of the basilar membrane stimulate the hair cells, which are located within the organ of Corti on top of the basilar membrane. The hair cells make excitatory synaptic connections with the sensory neurons of the spiral ganglion, whose axons form the auditory nerve and carry auditory information into the brain.

Each auditory nerve fiber is sensitive to sound stimuli only within a specific frequency range. The frequency to which the fiber responds depends on the part of the cochlea innervated by the nerve fiber. Low-frequency sounds are sensed at the apical end of the cochlea, while high-frequency sounds are sensed at the basal end. The frequency tuning of the cochlea is determined by the mechanical properties of the basilar membrane, the electrical tuning of individual hair cells, and the active motions produced by the hair cells in response to changes in membrane potential.

The auditory nerve fibers enter the brainstem and synapse on neurons of the cochlear nucleus. These neurons extract specific types of information about the auditory stimulus and relay their signals to the nearby superior olivary nucleus and to the inferior colliculus. The superior olivary nucleus is largely concerned with the localization of the sound source with respect to the head. Localization is determined by differences in the arrival time and intensity of the sound in the two ears. From the inferior colliculus, auditory information is sent to the medial geniculate nucleus of the thalamus, which in turn relays auditory signals to the primary auditory cortex in the superior portion of the temporal lobe.

Like the primary visual cortex, the primary auditory cortex is organized into a two-dimensional array of vertical cell columns. One dimension consists of frequency columns, within which the neurons have the same preferred stimulus frequency. The other dimension consists of binaural columns, in which the cells respond best to either binaural or monaural stimulation.

SUMMARY

REVIEW QUESTIONS

1. Why do hair cells depolarize when the cilia bundle is deflected toward the longest cilium and hyperpolarize when the cilia bundle is deflected away from the longest cilium?

2. Draw a cross section of the mammalian cochlea and label the following structures: scala vestibuli, scala media, scala tympani, organ of Corti, basilar membrane, vestibular membrane, tectorial membrane.

3. List at least four important functional differences between the inner and outer hair cells in the organ of Corti.

4. What ionic mechanisms account for the oscillations in membrane potential at a particular frequency in individual hair cells?

5. How do the movements of the hair cells contribute to frequency tuning in the cochlea?

6. List the synaptic relays from the spiral ganglion in the cochlea to the auditory cortex.

7. What sound cues are used to locate a sound source in relation to the head?

8. What two types of binaural columns are found in the primary auditory cortex?

9. Discuss the similarities between the visual and auditory cortex.

INTERNET ASSIGNMENT   CHAPTER 17

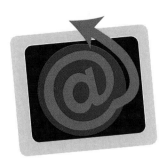

1 Part of the mechanism of frequency discrimination in the auditory system resides in the mechanical properties of the basilar membrane, which vibrates preferentially at different positions in response to tones of different frequencies. Find information about the mechanical response of the basilar membrane, including illustrations of the responses to different vibration frequencies.

2 Locate the following structures using a brain atlas: cochlear nucleus and superior olive.

CHEMICAL SENSES

ESSENTIAL BACKGROUND

Ionic permeability and the ionic basis of membrane potential (Chapter 3)

G-proteins (GTP binding proteins), second messengers, and receptors coupled to G-proteins (Chapter 6, Chapter 11)

General anatomy of the brain (Chapter 2)

Synaptic transmission (Chapter 5, Chapter 6)

Action potential (Chapter 4)

In this chapter, we will examine the reception of chemical signals that originate outside the organism. As with the other senses we have considered, specialized sensory cells detect the presence of the chemical signal and generate an electrical response that can be passed along and analyzed in the nervous system. The principal focus of this chapter will be the two major chemical senses in mammals: smell (**olfaction**) and taste (**gustation**).

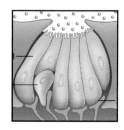

DISTINCTION BETWEEN OLFACTION AND GUSTATION

The ability to respond appropriately to the chemical composition of the environment is fundamental for life and must have developed early during evolution. Even single-cell organisms such as bacteria possess chemical senses. Bacteria exhibit **chemotaxis**, in which they will swim toward a source of nutrients (for example, sugar or amino acids; positive chemotaxis) and away from a noxious stimulus (for example, carbon dioxide or high pH; negative chemotaxis). More complex single-cell animals such as paramecium also demonstrate similar kinds of chemotaxic behavior. Among multicellular invertebrate animals, chemical senses are ubiquitous, and a wide variety of chemical sensory organs have evolved to provide the organism with information about its chemical environment.

We usually classify the sensory receptor organs of the chemical senses into two classes: those concerned with taste and those concerned with smell. In broad terms, the sensory modality we call *gustation* detects molecules associated with food, and the information provided by this sense is used to regulate ingestion. Gustation usually involves direct contact between the organism and the food material. Olfaction, on the other hand, involves the detection of molecules that originate at a distance from the animal. The distinction between smell and taste is rather fuzzy, however. From the point of view of the sensory receptor cells (**chemoreceptors**), the fundamental process is identical in the two cases: the detected molecule dissolves into the aqueous fluid at the cell's sensory surface and activates specific receptor molecules, which change the electrical properties of the cell. This sensory transduction process is called **chemotransduction**. As we know from our own experience, the sensations of taste and smell are closely related. Consider, for example, the impairment of your ability to taste food when your nose is congested from a cold.

Nevertheless, it is useful to draw a functional distinction between the sensory modalities of olfaction and gustation. In vertebrates—and particularly in mammals—the relevant sensory receptors for taste and smell are those associated with the tongue and nose, respectively. Although the sensory receptor cells in both are chemoreceptors, the mechanisms of sensory transduction differ in many respects. In addition, the neural pathways in the brain that process olfactory and gustatory information are quite distinct and are organized in different ways. For these reasons, we will treat the olfactory and taste systems separately. We will begin with a description of the chemoreceptor cells, comparing and contrasting the transduction processes in taste and olfaction. We will then move on to examine the brain mechanisms for the two systems.

CHEMOTRANSDUCTION IN OLFACTORY RECEPTOR CELLS

Structure of the Olfactory Epithelium

For terrestrial animals, odors are transmitted via the air from the source to the receptive organ. Air taken in through the nose passes over the sensory surface of the olfactory apparatus before continuing on into the air passages that lead to the lungs. Any odorant molecules carried by the air thus have a chance to interact with the **olfactory receptor cells**, which are illustrated in Figure 18.1. The receptor cells are specialized neurons located within the epithelial layer lining the upper part of the nasal passage. The peripheral process of the olfactory receptor cell extends to the outer surface of the epithelial sheet, where it gives rise to several long thin cilia.

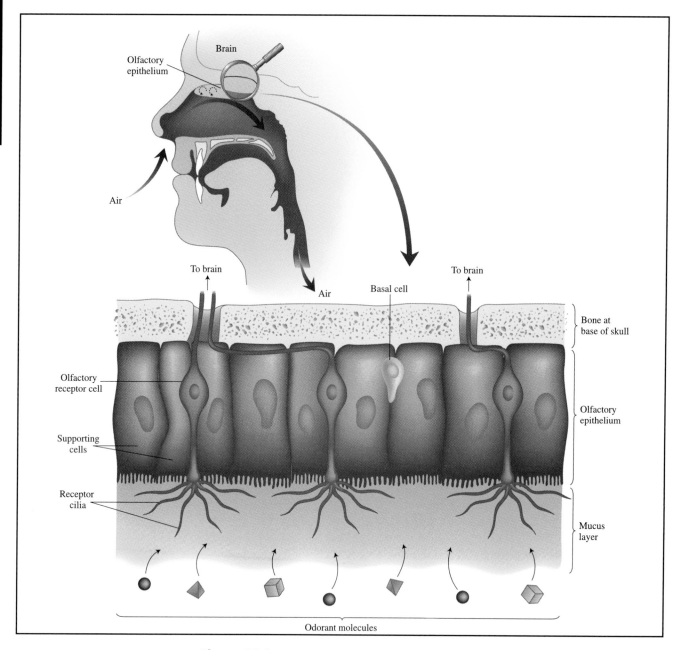

Figure 18.1.

The location and structure of the olfactory epithelium. The position of the epithelium within the nasal passage is shown in *orange* in the *upper figure*. The *drawing below* shows the cellular structure of the epithelial sheet. The olfactory receptor cells are indicated in *red*; the basal cells, in *yellow*; and the supporting cells, in *brown*. The axons of the olfactory receptor cells penetrate through the bone at the base of the cranium and enter the overlying brain.

The cilia form a dense net within the layer of mucus that covers the inside of the nasal passage. The receptor molecules that interact with arriving odorants are located in the membranes of these cilia. The axons of the olfactory receptor cells that arise from the other end of the cell project directly to the brain, forming the olfactory nerve (the first cranial nerve).

In addition to the receptor cells, two other cell types are found in the olfactory epithelium. The **supporting cells** are epithelial cells that provide structural support for the epithelium. The **basal cells** are undifferentiated neuronal precursor cells that continually give rise to new receptor cells. Unlike most other neurons, the receptor cells have a short life span (approximately 2 months) and must be replaced by newly developed cells as they degenerate.

Olfactory Transduction Cascade

The transduction process in the olfactory cilia shares a number of features with phototransduction in the retinal photoreceptors. In both processes, the receptor molecule that is activated by the stimulus is a member of the G-protein–coupled receptor family. In olfaction, an odorant molecule combines with and activates an **olfactory receptor molecule**, which in turn activates a specific type of G-protein. This transduction process is analogous to the activation of the photoreceptor G-protein called transducin by photoactivated rhodopsin, the receptor molecule in the rod photoreceptor (see Chapter 15). The olfactory and visual sensory transduction systems differ, however, in the number of different types of receptor molecules present in the receptor cells. The human retina contains only four different visual pigment molecules: rhodopsin in the rods and the three cone opsins. By contrast, there are 1000 or so different receptor molecules in the olfactory epithelium. This large variety of receptor molecules reflects the fact that each odorant binding site is designed specifically for the detection of a particular odor-producing molecule, and the system encounters many different odorant molecules with highly variable chemical structures.

The olfactory transduction mechanism is summarized in Figure 18.2. As with other G-proteins, the activation of the olfactory G-protein involves the replacement of guanosine diphosphate (GDP) bound to the G-protein by guanosine triphosphate (GTP), followed by the dissociation of the active G-protein alpha-subunit from the beta- and gamma-subunits. In olfactory transduction, the intracellular target of the active alpha-subunit is an enzyme that controls the internal concentration of a cyclic nucleotide. Unlike phototransduction, the enzyme activated by the G-protein in olfaction is a *synthetic* enzyme (**adenylyl cyclase**)

How do olfactory receptor cells transduce chemical signals into changes in membrane potential?

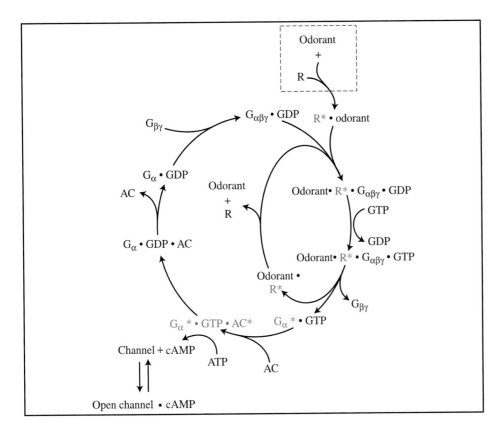

Figure 18.2.

The transduction cycle for olfactory receptor cells. The entry point for the cycle is the combination of an odorant molecule with a specific receptor molecule (*R*) in the cilia of the olfactory receptor neuron. Activated forms of molecules are indicated in *red*, with an *asterisk* (*). The cycle is described in detail in the text. ATP = adenosine triphosphate; G_α and $G_{\beta g}$ = alpha- and beta/gamma-subunits of the olfactory G-protein, respectively; AC = adenylyl cyclase; cAMP = cyclic AMP, which is synthesized from ATP by adenylyl cyclase; GDP = guanosine disphosphate; GTP = guanosine triphosphate.

rather than a *degradative* enzyme (phosphodiesterase). In addition, the cyclic nucle-otide involved in olfactory transduction is cyclic adenosine monophosphate (cAMP), rather than cyclic guanosine monophosphate (cGMP). Thus, in the presence of odorant molecules, the rate of synthesis of cyclic AMP increases (see Fig. 18.2). Inactivation of the activated G-protein occurs because of the endogenous GTPase activity of the alpha-subunit, which is analogous to the inactivation of transducin in photoreceptors. The olfactory receptor molecule—the initiator of the cascade—deactivates upon dissociation of the odorant molecule.

Electrical Response of Olfactory Receptor Cells

The chemotransduction process alters the membrane potential of the olfactory receptor by changing the ionic permeability of the plasma membrane. The increase in cyclic AMP in the cell is coupled to the ionic permeability in the same way as in photoreceptors. Cyclic AMP directly opens cyclic nucleotide–gated cation channels in the plasma membrane of the receptor cell. These ion channels closely resemble the cyclic GMP–gated ion channels in the outer segment of photoreceptors, except that they are opened by cyclic AMP rather than cyclic GMP. The cyclic AMP–gated channels are nonspecific cation channels that allow an influx of cations and thus depolarize the olfactory receptor cell in response to odorants.

The electrical response of an olfactory receptor neuron is illustrated in Figure 18.3. Upon receipt of an odor stimulus, the cell depolarizes because of the opening of cyclic AMP–gated cation channels in the cilia. This depolarization is the **receptor potential** of the olfactory receptor cell, and its size is graded with the intensity of the odor (that is, the number of odorant molecules that combine with receptor molecules in the cilia). Because the distance from the cilia to the soma of the receptor cell is quite short, the depolarizing receptor potential spreads to the cell body, where it stimulates action potentials (see Fig. 18.3).

The electrical response of the olfactory receptor cell is the opposite of the response to light in a retinal photoreceptor (see Chapter 15). The photoreceptor hyperpolarizes in response to light because cyclic nucleotide–gated channels *close;*

BOX 1

IN THE CLINIC

In humans, the ability to detect odors varies substantially from one individual to another. In some instances, individuals have a generalized reduction in sensitivity to odors, much like the reduced sensitivity that occurs in all of us when we catch a cold and experience nasal congestion. However, in some individuals, the overall sensitivity to odors is normal, but the ability to detect a particular substance or related group of substances is lacking. Such specific anosmia may result from mutations in the gene encoding a particular type of the many olfactory receptor molecules normally found in olfactory receptor cells, which prevents the expression of that receptor type. Without the receptor molecule, the presence of the odorant that binds to that particular receptor cannot be detected. Frequently, the affected person is not aware of any defect, probably because the absence of a single receptor type out of 1000 or so different types does not normally alter olfactory perception appreciably. A more generalized reduction in olfactory sensitivity (hyposmia) often occurs with aging. Because of the importance of olfaction in the "taste" of food (witness impairment of taste with nasal congestion), such hyposmia frequently leads to clinical complaints.

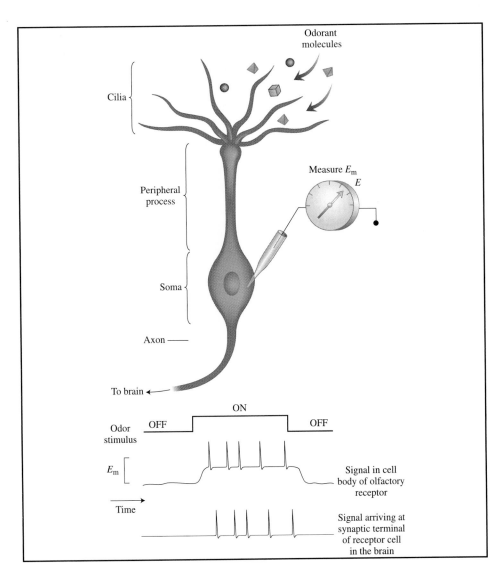

Cilia

Odorant
molecules

Peripheral
process

Measure E_m

E

Soma

Axon

To brain

ON

Odor
stimulus   OFF   OFF

E_m

Signal in cell
body of olfactory
receptor

Time

Signal arriving at
synaptic terminal
of receptor cell
in the brain

Figure 18.3.

The electrical response of an olfactory receptor neuron to an odor stimulus. The recording situation is diagrammed *above*, and the electrical response is shown *below*. When an odor stimulus is applied (*top trace*), both the receptor potential and the resulting action potentials are observed in the cell body of the olfactory receptor cell (*middle trace*). The action potentials propagate along the axon and arrive at the synaptic terminal of the receptor cell in the brain (*bottom trace*).

in the olfactory receptor cell, however, the stimulus *opens* cyclic nucleotide–gated channels.

The depolarizing receptor potential of olfactory receptor cells generates action potentials, which then propagate along the axon of the receptor into the brain. Action potentials do not occur in photoreceptors, whose synaptic terminals are located close to the cell body. As a result, the light-induced change in membrane potential spreads directly to the synaptic terminal without an intervening action potential. By contrast, the synaptic terminals of the olfactory receptor cells are located far from the cell body, and so action potentials are required to transmit the electrical signal from the cell body to the synaptic terminal.

CHEMOTRANSDUCTION IN TASTE RECEPTOR CELLS

Structure of the Taste Buds

Now we will turn our attention to the transduction mechanism in the other major type of chemoreceptor, the taste cells. These specialized sensory cells are found on body surfaces that come into direct contact with food. In mammals, the princi-

What different types of taste receptor cells are found in the taste buds of the tongue?

pal receptive surface for taste sensation is the tongue, although taste receptor cells are found in other parts of the mouth as well. The taste cells are not spread evenly over the epithelial surface of the tongue; instead, they are grouped together into structures called **taste buds** (because of their resemblance to the bud of a flower; see Fig. 18.4). Each taste bud contains about 100 taste receptor cells. The top surface of each taste cell is covered with microvilli, which detect chemicals dissolved in the saliva on the surface of the tongue. The taste buds are in turn grouped into **papillae** (see Fig. 18.4), which take the form of either protrusions or trenches on the surface of the tongue. Like the olfactory receptor cells, the taste receptor cells have a limited life span. Consequently, basal cells within the taste bud continually differentiate into new receptor cells to replace the old ones as they die off. Unlike the olfactory receptors, however, the taste cells have no axon. Information is carried into the central nervous system from the taste buds by the axons of sensory

Figure 18.4.

Location and structure of taste buds. Taste buds are embedded in the epithelial surface of the tongue, as shown in the *upper diagram*. The *lower diagram* shows the cellular organization of a taste bud. The taste receptor cells are shown in *pink*; the basal cells, in *yellow*; and the afferent nerve fibers that receive synaptic input from the taste cells, in *purple*. The taste cells make excitatory synaptic connections with afferent nerve fibers. Each taste cell synapses onto an afferent nerve fiber.

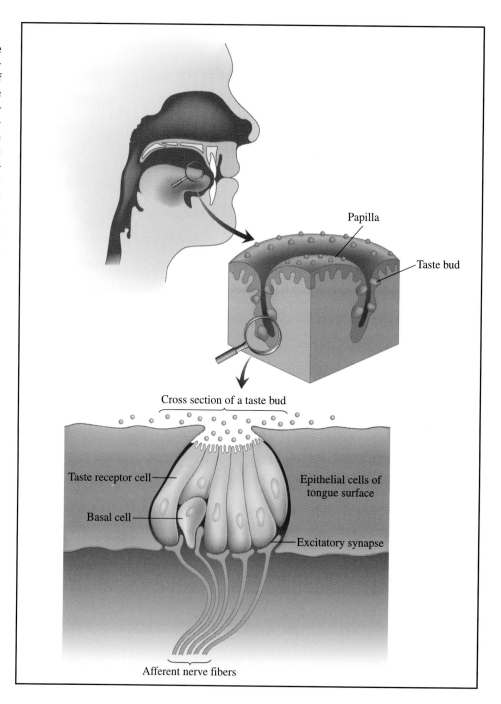

Papilla

Taste bud

Cross section of a taste bud

Taste receptor cell

Epithelial cells of tongue surface

Basal cell

Excitatory synapse

Afferent nerve fibers

neurons, which receive excitatory synaptic contacts from the taste receptor cells within the taste bud (see Fig. 18.4).

Transduction Mechanisms in Taste Receptor Cells: Salty and Sour Tastes

Naturally occurring taste stimuli are complex combinations of various chemical substances that give rise to complex subjective experiences of food flavor. Despite the variety of subjective flavors, there are only four underlying subgroups (or **submodalities**) of taste: **salty, sour, sweet,** and **bitter**. Combinations of these four dimensions account for the perceptions of complex tastes (together with the contribution to flavor perception from the olfactory system, which is stimulated by aromatic compounds in foods). Salty stimuli are those with a high concentration of sodium ions. Sour taste arises from the application of acidic solutions, which contain a high concentration of protons. The natural stimulus for sweet sensations is sugars of various kinds (such as sucrose), while bitter taste is stimulated by a variety of organic compounds, including some amino acids.

Each submodality of taste has a different transduction mechanism. Salty and sour stimuli have no true "receptor" molecule in the same sense as the olfactory receptor molecules described earlier. Instead, the ions (sodium and hydrogen ions for salt and sour, respectively) interact directly with ion channels to alter the membrane potential of the taste receptor cell. Because the sweet and bitter submodalities usually involve the detection of more complicated molecules that generally do not directly interact with ion channels, the transduction mechanisms for these tastes resemble olfactory and visual transduction. Specific receptor molecules in the membrane bind the substances perceived as sweet or bitter, and the occupied receptor in turn activates intracellular signals that indirectly affect ionic permeability of the taste receptor cell. Substances that are perceived as sweet have a wide variety of molecular structures, as do bitter substances. Thus, taste cells probably contain many different sweet and bitter receptor molecules in taste cells with binding sites sculpted to fit particular stimulus molecules. Because the salty and sour submodalities are less complex, we will consider these transduction mechanisms first, before examining the sweet and bitter submodalities.

The simplest sensory transduction scheme is that used by salt-sensitive taste receptor cells, shown in Figure 18.5A. Open sodium channels are located in the plasma membrane of the taste cell at the top surface, where the membrane is exposed to the fluid covering the tongue. Under resting conditions, this fluid is ordinary saliva, which contains a low concentration of sodium ions. Thus, even though the sodium channels are open, little sodium flows into the cell through the open channels, and the membrane potential remains at its normal negative resting value. If food with a high salt content is ingested, however, the sodium content of the saliva rises, sodium ions enter the taste receptor cell, and the cell depolarizes. This depolarizing receptor potential increases the release of excitatory transmitter from the receptor cell, causing the sensory neuron receiving synaptic input from the receptor cell to fire a train of action potentials (see Fig. 18.5A). In addition, at least in some species, voltage-dependent sodium and calcium channels in the taste receptor cell add to the depolarization produced by the receptor potential and amplify the response of the sensory cell. Thus, for a salty taste stimulus, the stimulus chemical itself is an ion whose influx into the cell directly produces the receptor potential.

For sour taste, the transduction mechanism is only slightly more complicated. The stimulus in this case is an increase in acidity of the saliva—that is, an increase in the concentration of hydrogen ions (protons) in the fluid bathing the top surface of the receptor cell. When the proton concentration rises, the sour taste receptor

How do the taste receptor cells transduce chemical signals into changes in membrane potential?

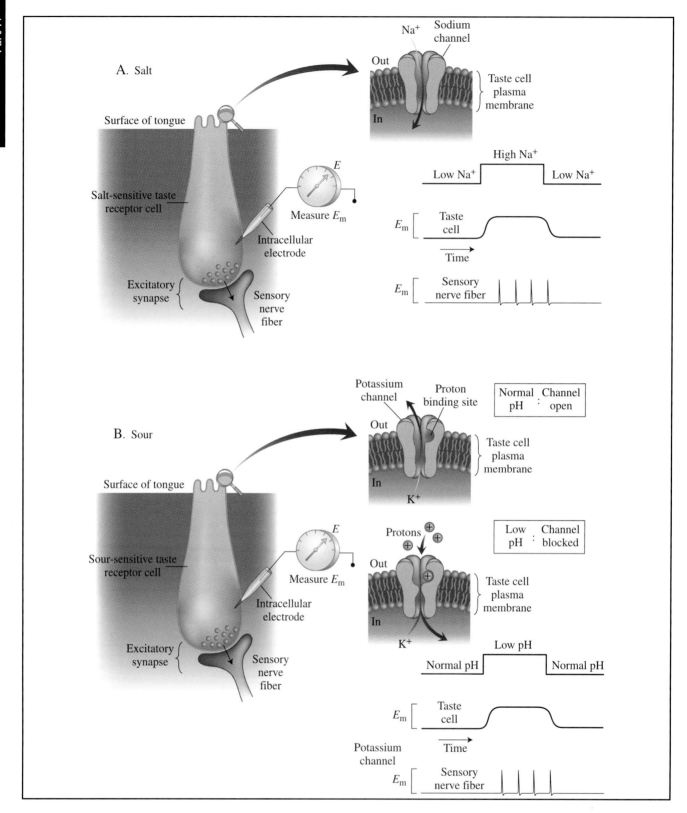

Figure 18.5.

Chemotransduction in salt-sensitive and sour-sensitive taste receptor cells. **A**. A salt stimulus depolarizes a salt-sensitive taste cell. The recording configuration is shown on the *left*, and the electrical responses on the *right*. The sodium ions in the saliva enter the taste cell via sodium channels, depolarizing the cell. The depolarization increases the release of excitatory neurotransmitter from the taste receptor cell, and the firing rate of the sensory neuron increases. **B**. A sour stimulus arises from an increase in the proton concentration of the saliva (low pH). The sour-sensitive taste cell has a particular type of potassium channel that remains open under resting conditions. Protons block this potassium channel, reducing the potassium permeability of the receptor cell and causing depolarization. The depolarization increases the release of excitatory neurotransmitter and accelerates the firing of action potentials by the sensory neuron.

cell depolarizes. Like sodium ions, hydrogen ions are cations. In this case, however, the depolarization does not result from direct permeation of protons through open cation channels. Instead, the protons act as channel *blockers*, in the manner illustrated in Figure 18.5B. External protons block potassium channels located in the upper part of the cell, exposed to the saliva. When a proton occupies the proton binding site of these potassium channels, potassium ions are unable to move through the channel pore. The resulting reduction in potassium permeability produces a depolarizing receptor potential, which increases the release of excitatory neurotransmitter and stimulates action potentials in the sensory neuron that receives input from the receptor cell. As with the salt-sensitive receptor cells, the generator potential in some species is amplified by voltage-dependent sodium and calcium channels that respond to the depolarization produced by closure of the pH-sensitive potassium channels.

Transduction Mechanisms in Taste Receptor Cells: Sweet and Bitter Tastes

The chemical substances that give rise to sweet and bitter sensations are detected by receptor molecules at the sensory surface of the taste cells. Although these receptor molecules have not yet been characterized, they are coupled to their intracellular actions via G-proteins. Thus, like the olfactory receptor molecules and the visual pigment molecules, the sweet and bitter receptor molecules are members of the family of G-protein–coupled receptors. Activated G-proteins stimulate enzymes that control the levels of cyclic nucleotides (either cyclic AMP or cyclic GMP) in sweet- and bitter-sensitive taste cells. Cyclic nucleotides in turn regulate the open state of ion channels, thereby affecting the membrane potential of the receptor cell.

The details of the transduction mechanism have not yet been completely worked out, but two possible schemes are illustrated in Figure 18.6. In scheme I, the activated taste receptor molecule is coupled through G-proteins to stimulation of the synthetic enzyme for cyclic AMP, adenylyl cyclase—just as in olfactory transduction. Thus, a taste stimulus causes an increase in the intracellular concentration of cyclic AMP. Instead of a direct effect on a cyclic nucleotide–gated ion channel (as in olfaction), cyclic AMP is thought to activate protein kinase A (cyclic AMP–dependent protein kinase), which in turn phosphorylates potassium channels. The phosphorylated potassium channels close, decreasing potassium permeability of the taste receptor. This decline in potassium permeability produces a depolarizing receptor potential, which is reflected in increased action potential activity in the sensory neuron that receives synaptic input from the taste receptor cell.

Scheme II for the coupling between the activated tastant receptor and membrane permeability is shown in Figure 18.6B. Once again, the first step in the sequence is activation of an intermediary G-protein. In this scheme, however, the G-protein targets phosphodiesterase—which cleaves cyclic nucleotides—rather than the synthetic enzyme. In this regard, the proposed scheme resembles phototransduction. In fact, the G-protein involved is quite similar to the G-protein of phototransduction, which is called transducin (see Chapter 15). Because of this similarity, the taste cell G-protein is called **gustducin** (for *gus*tatory trans*ducin*). In this scenario, a taste stimulus decreases the intracellular cyclic nucleotide level. In scheme II, cyclic nucleotides directly *close* cation channels in the membrane of the taste cell. Therefore, when the cyclic nucleotide concentration inside the taste receptor cell decreases in response to a taste stimulus, the cation channels open and the cell depolarizes.

The detection of sweet substances probably occurs via a G-protein pathway leading to activation of adenylyl cyclase, an increase in cyclic AMP, and subsequent closure of potassium channels (scheme I in Fig. 18.6A). Evidence suggests

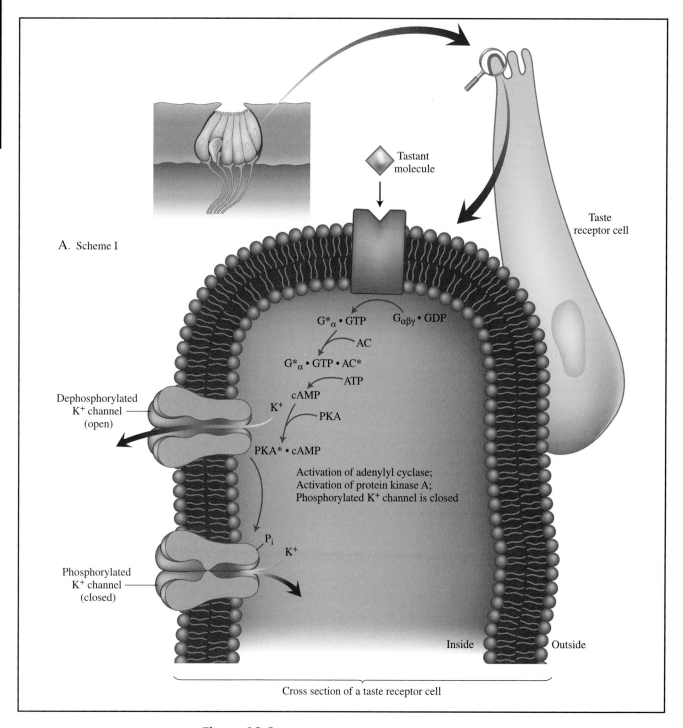

A. Scheme I

Tastant molecule

Taste receptor cell

G*$_\alpha$ • GTP   G$_{\alpha\beta\gamma}$ • GDP

AC

G*$_\alpha$ • GTP • AC*

ATP

cAMP

Dephosphorylated K$^+$ channel (open)

K$^+$

PKA

PKA* • cAMP

Activation of adenylyl cyclase;
Activation of protein kinase A;
Phosphorylated K$^+$ channel is closed

P$_i$ K$^+$

Phosphorylated K$^+$ channel (closed)

Inside   Outside

Cross section of a taste receptor cell

Figure 18.6.

Two schemes for taste transduction using indirect coupling between the activated receptor molecule and ionic permeability of the receptor cell. **A**. Scheme I: The molecules of the
taste stimulus activate a G-protein–coupled receptor molecule. The G-protein increases the
activity of adenylyl cyclase (AC), which in turn increases the internal concentration of cyclic adenosine monophosphate (AMP) (cAMP). Cyclic AMP activates protein kinase A (PKA),
which phosphorylates and closes potassium channels. **B**. Scheme II: The taste stimulus is
detected by a receptor molecule that activates a G-protein, which then stimulates a
phosphodiesterase enzyme (PDE). The phosphodiesterase enzyme hydrolyzes cyclic nucleotides (cNMP) and decreases the internal concentration of both cyclic AMP and cyclic
guanosine monophosphate. Because the cyclic nucleotides keep nonspecific cation channels closed, the fall in cyclic nucleotide concentration causes the channels to open and the
cell depolarizes. P$_i$ = inorganic phosphate; GTP = guanosine triphosphate; GDP =
guanosine diphosphate; G$_\alpha$ = G-protein alpha-subunit; G$_{\alpha\beta\gamma}$ = G-protein alpha-, beta-,
gamma-subunits; NMP = nucleotide monophosphate.

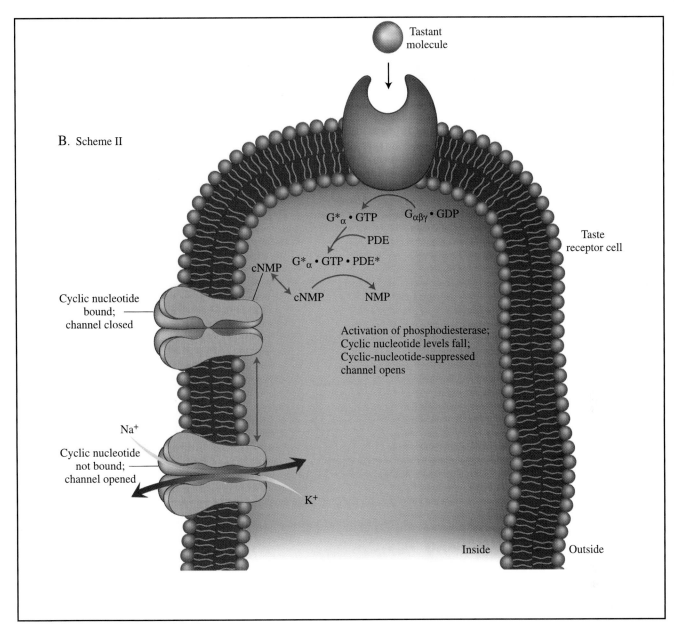

B. Scheme II

Tastant molecule

G*_α • GTP G_{αβγ} • GDP

$G*_\alpha \cdot GTP$ $G_{\alpha\beta\gamma} \cdot GDP$

PDE

$G*_\alpha \cdot GTP \cdot PDE*$

cNMP

cNMP   NMP

Activation of phosphodiesterase;
Cyclic nucleotide levels fall;
Cyclic-nucleotide-suppressed
channel opens

Cyclic nucleotide
bound;
channel closed

Cyclic nucleotide
not bound;
channel opened

Na^+

K^+

Taste
receptor cell

Inside   Outside

Figure 18.6.

(continued)

that bitter taste transduction involves scheme II in Figure 18.6B. It is not yet certain, however, that the two schemes are segregated into two different functional types of taste receptor cells.

PROCESSING OF TASTE INFORMATION IN THE BRAIN

Sensory Coding in the Taste System

We will now turn our attention to the processing of the sensory information after it leaves the receptor cells. In the taste system, we must first consider how the submodalities (salt, sour, sweet, and bitter) are encoded at the level of the receptors and at the level of the sensory neurons to which they are connected. One simple

What parts of the brain are involved in processing gustatory information?

way to separate the different types of taste stimuli would be to have different taste cells that are specific for each of the four submodalities. However, in reality, individual taste receptor cells respond to more than one type of chemical stimulus, although each cell responds best to one particular submodality. In the cells illustrated in Figure 18.7, for example, one cell depolarizes most strongly in response to a salt stimulus, and the other cell responds best to a sweet stimulus. The sensory neuron that receives synaptic input from the salt-preferring taste cell fires most rapidly during a salt stimulus but also is weakly excited by sour and bitter stimuli (see Fig. 18.7A). A different pattern of activity is found in the sensory neuron receiving input from the sweet-preferring taste cell (see Fig. 18.7B). In this case, the sensory neuron is strongly excited by a sweet stimulus but only weakly by sour and salt stimuli.

Although the sensory neurons respond preferentially to a particular submodality, the rate of action potentials reaching the brain in the axon of any indi-

Figure 18.7.

Encoding of sensory information in the taste system. The *upper traces* show the electrical responses of taste cells to stimuli of the four submodalities (salt, sour, sweet, and bitter). The *lower traces* show the resulting action potential activity in the sensory neurons receiving synaptic input from the taste cells. **A.** Responses originating in a taste receptor cell that responds best to salty stimuli. **B.** Responses originating in a sweet-preferring taste receptor cell. In each case, the taste cell and the sensory neuron respond to more than one submodality.

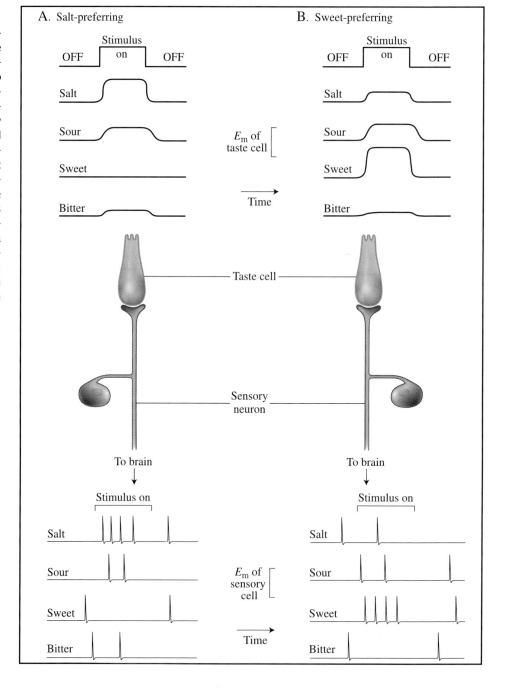

vidual sensory neuron does not provide an unambiguous indication of the taste stimulus. For example, increased firing of the sweet-preferring neuron in Figure 18.7B could result from a dilute sugar stimulus or a highly salty stimulus. Higher-order neurons receiving inputs from this single sensory cell would not be able to discriminate between the two very different taste stimuli. Only by comparing the response patterns from different types of sensory neurons can the stimulus characteristics be uniquely discerned.

In the case of the dilute sugar stimulus versus the strong salty stimulus, for example, the nervous system could distinguish the two stimuli by comparing the activity in the two neurons shown in Figure 18.7. If the sweet-preferring neuron fires at an elevated rate but the salt-preferring neuron does not, then the stimulus is sweet. If the salt-preferring neuron is more strongly excited than the sweet-preferring neuron, then the stimulus is salty.

The decoding of taste stimulus quality is analogous to the detection of color in the visual system, where the outputs from the three types of cone photoreceptors are compared at higher levels in the visual system in order to distinguish the color of a visual stimulus. In the visual system, however, the comparison is carried out among receptor signals along a single *physical dimension* of the stimulus (wavelength of light); in the taste system, the comparison is among four different *categories* of chemical stimuli (the four submodalities). Thus, the perception of a taste stimulus is governed by the representation of the stimulus on four internally generated, subjective dimensions, whereas the perception of color is based in large measure on a physical aspect of the stimulus itself.

Anatomical Organization of the Taste Sensory Pathway

The axons of the sensory neurons that innervate the taste buds are found in **cranial nerve VII** (the **facial nerve**) and **cranial nerve IX** (the **glossopharyngeal nerve**). The facial nerve carries the inputs from the anterior part of the tongue, and the glossopharyngeal nerve carries the inputs from the posterior part. In addition, these two nerves contain the sensory fibers of the somatosensory receptors of the tongue (touch, pressure, and temperature). The tongue sensory fibers enter the central nervous system in the medulla and make synaptic connections in the **nucleus of the solitary tract** (see Fig. 18.8), which we encountered previously in our discussion of the autonomic nervous system (see Chapter 11). In the nucleus of the solitary tract, the inputs from the taste buds are segregated from the somatosensory tongue inputs and make connections in a specific subdivision called the **gustatory nucleus**. The neurons in the nucleus of the solitary tract receive sensory inputs from a variety of body organs involved in homeostatic functions, including the gut, the lungs, and the cardiovascular system. Thus, taste sensory information is integrated with this other sensory information to regulate feeding behavior and the viscera. In organisms without a well-developed forebrain, this evolutionarily ancient control system in the medulla is the only target of taste sensory information.

From the solitary nucleus, taste sensory information is sent to two principal targets, which differ in importance in different species, depending on the prominence of the thalamocortical pathway in sensory information processing. The first, evolutionarily older target is the **pontine taste nucleus** in the dorsal part of the pons. This nucleus transmits taste sensory information to the hypothalamus and other parts of the limbic system, which is the subdivision of the vertebrate brain concerned with feeding behavior, homeostasis, and emotion. In the course of evolution, this pathway from the medulla through the pons to the limbic system probably represents a more primitive organizational scheme that was retained as other parts of the brain became more elaborate. In organisms with more highly

Figure 18.8.

A schematic diagram of the taste sensory pathway in the central nervous system. The *red arrows* indicate the pathway to the limbic system, and the *black arrows* indicate the pathway leading to the cerebral cortex.

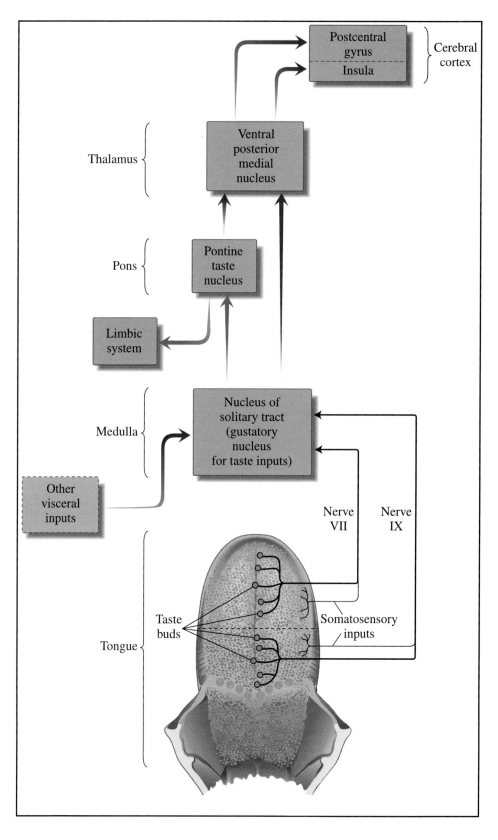

developed forebrains, the pontine taste nucleus also provides input to the thalamocortical pathway for taste perception.

In animals with the most highly developed thalamocortical sensory systems (such as primates), ascending axons from the nucleus of the solitary tract also project directly to the thalamic nucleus concerned with sensory signals from the tongue, the **ventral posterior medial nucleus** (see Fig. 18.8). Like the nucleus of the solitary tract, the ventral posterior medial nucleus receives both somatosensory inputs and taste inputs from the tongue, but the taste inputs are spatially segregated to a specific subdivision of the nucleus.

The thalamic neurons that receive information about touch, pressure, and temperature on the tongue send their axons to the primary somatosensory cortex in the postcentral gyrus (see Chapter 14). These inputs follow the general somatotopic map in the primary somatosensory cortex and project to the most lateral part of the postcentral gyrus, where the other inputs from the face and head are found (see Fig. 18.9). Once again, sensory information from the taste buds remains separate from the tongue somatosensory information in the cortex. Two cortical regions receive inputs from the thalamic neurons of the taste system: the gustatory cortex and the insula. The **gustatory cortex** is located in the postcentral gyrus, just below and slightly anterior to the region that receives the tongue somatosensory inputs (see Fig. 18.9). The **insula** is hidden from view within one of the deep infoldings of the cortical surface, the lateral sulcus (see Fig. 18.9).

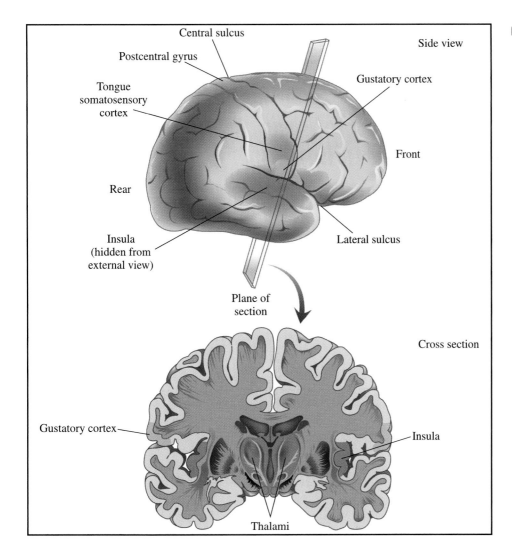

Figure 18.9.

The locations of the cortical areas concerned with processing taste sensory information in the human brain. A side view is shown *above*, and a cross section is shown *below*.

PROCESSING OF OLFACTORY INFORMATION IN THE BRAIN

Anatomical Organization of the Olfactory System

What parts of the brain are involved in processing olfactory information?

The olfactory epithelium is located at the upper surface of the nasal passage, separated from the overlying brain by only the bone at the base of the cranium. The primary olfactory receptor cells send their axons directly into the brain without any intervening synaptic connections. These axons terminate in the **olfactory bulbs**, which are finger-like projections of the telencephalon on each side of the brain, located immediately above the olfactory epithelium. The relative size of the olfactory bulbs is quite large in animals in which olfaction is a major sense, such as rodents. In humans, however, the olfactory bulbs are small compared with other parts of the telencephalon, reflecting humans' relatively poor olfactory abilities. Figure 18.10 compares relative sizes of the olfactory bulbs in human and rat brains.

The outputs of the olfactory bulbs project to a set of basal brain structures collectively called the **olfactory cortex**. These primitive cortical structures have pyramidal cells, like the other parts of the cortex, but the cells are organized into fewer layers than are found in the more complex cortical areas, such as the motor cortex (see Chapter 9) and the visual cortex (see Chapter 16). Because these simpler cortical areas arose earlier in the course of brain evolution, they are referred to as **paleocortex**. The newer cerebral cortical areas—what we normally mean when we

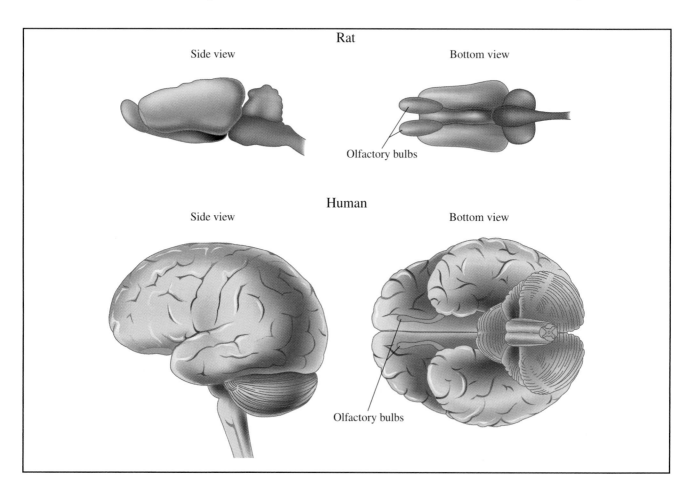

Figure 18.10.

The location and relative sizes of the olfactory bulbs in a rat brain (*above*) and a human brain (*below*). The olfactory bulbs are shown in *red*.

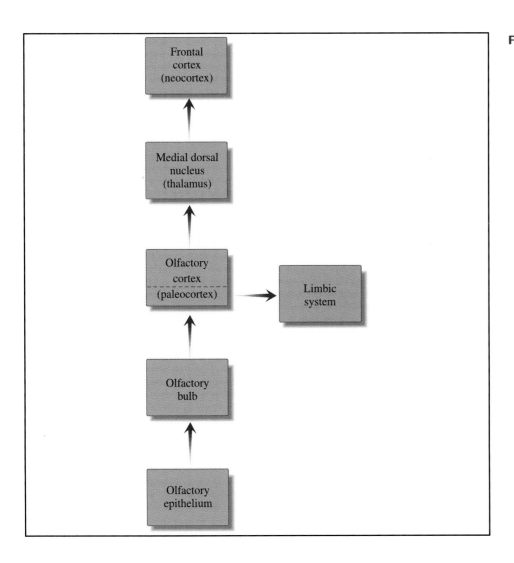

Figure 18.11.

A schematic diagram of the olfactory sensory pathway in the central nervous system.

use the word *cortex*—are called **neocortex**. The olfactory paleocortex is subdivided into several regions that are distributed along the lower portion of the brain: the **anterior olfactory nucleus**, the **piriform cortex**, the **olfactory tubercle**, the **amygdala**, and the **entorhinal cortex**. These subdivisions relay olfactory information to various brain regions, including the limbic system and a thalamocortical pathway to the neocortex. The thalamocortical projection involves the **medial dorsal nucleus** in the thalamus and transmits olfactory information to part of the frontal cortex.

Synaptic Organization of the Olfactory Bulb

Little is known about the processing of olfactory information in either the limbic system or the neocortex. However, more is known about the synaptic processing of olfactory information in the olfactory bulbs. Figure 18.12 summarizes the basic structural organization of the synaptic inputs from the olfactory receptor neurons in the olfactory bulb. The synaptic terminals of the receptor neurons cluster in spherical patches called **glomeruli** (singular: **glomerulus**), which form a regular array just below the surface of the olfactory bulb. Within each glomerulus, the axons of the receptor neurons make excitatory synaptic connections on the dendrites of **mitral cells** and **tufted cells**, which are the output neurons whose axons project to the olfactory cortex. Each olfactory receptor neuron sends its axon to a single glomerulus, and each glomerulus receives inputs from more than 1000 receptor neurons. Approximately 100 mitral and tufted cells send their dendrites into

What synaptic connections are made among neurons in the olfactory bulb?

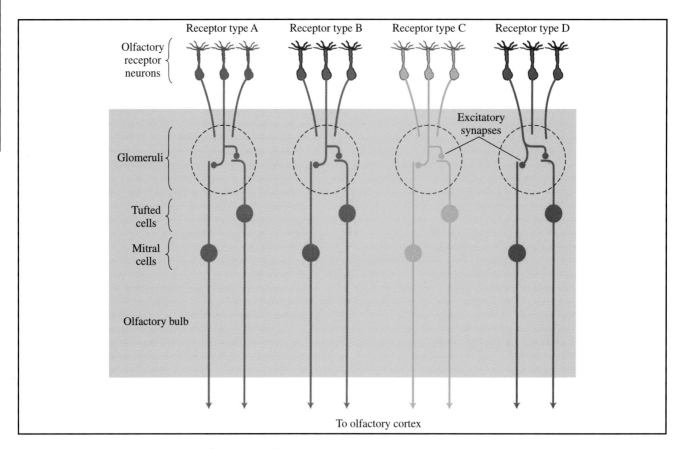

Figure 18.12.

The synaptic organization of the olfactory bulb. Four different types of olfactory receptor neurons are shown at the *top* (out of the approximately 1000 different types). Each type projects to a single glomerulus (*dashed circles*) within the olfactory bulb. Within the glomerulus, the receptor neurons make excitatory synaptic connections with the dendrites of mitral cells and tufted cells, whose axons project out of the olfactory bulb to the olfactory cortex.

a single glomerulus, so there is more than a 10-fold convergence of receptor neurons onto second-order neurons in the glomeruli.

In addition to serving as structural units, the glomeruli act as functional units of olfactory processing. Olfactory transduction involves approximately 1000 different receptor molecules, each tuned to detect a specific class of odorant molecule. Each olfactory receptor neuron is thought to possess a single type of the many possible odorant receptor molecules. In other words, the olfactory epithelium contains roughly 1000 different types of olfactory receptor neurons, each expressing a different class of odorant receptor molecule in its sensory cilia. Compare this situation, for example, with the human retina, which uses only four different types of photoreceptor cells (the rods and the three classes of cones). All of the receptor neurons of a particular type are thought to send their axons to a single glomerulus within the olfactory bulb, as illustrated in Figure 18.12. In the example shown in the figure, all receptor neurons of type A send their axons to one glomerulus, all the receptor cells of type B send their axons to another glomerulus, and so on. A single glomerulus apparently receives inputs from only one receptor neuron class. Thus, an individual glomerulus is activated by odor stimuli that activate a single type of olfactory receptor molecule.

Given the specificity of the connections between olfactory receptor types and glomeruli in the olfactory bulb, a particular odorant molecule might be expected to activate only one of the 1000 types of receptor neurons and thus only one glomerulus. Although each receptor neuron expresses only one type of receptor molecule, single receptor neurons and single glomeruli are actually activated by more than one type of odorant stimulus. Thus, each type of olfactory receptor molecule is broadly tuned to detect odorant molecules of a particular class, rather than only a single chemical. The receptor molecules in the olfactory cilia behave as though they are equipped with receptor sites that detect some special aspect of the molecular structure of an odorant molecule, rather than the entire molecule. This characteristic is illustrated schematically in Figure 18.13. If a given chemical compound has parts that can bind to two different receptor molecules, it will activate both olfactory receptor neurons bearing those receptor molecules. If a different chemical has only one of the relevant constituent parts, then only one of the two receptor neuron types will be activated. If an odorant molecule lacks both component parts, it will activate neither receptor neuron and must be detected by some other subtype of olfactory receptor neuron. The situation is similar to what we found in the taste sensory system, except that potentially hundreds of submodalities of olfaction are involved rather than the four submodalities of taste. Thus, to decipher the composition of an olfactory stimulus, the nervous system must compare the overall pattern of activity in the different types of olfactory receptor neurons—and hence in the different glomeruli in the olfactory bulb.

Lateral inhibitory interactions represent an important aspect of sensory information processing in the nervous system (see Chapter 13 for an overview). This holds true in the olfactory bulb as well. Two types of lateral inhibitory inter-

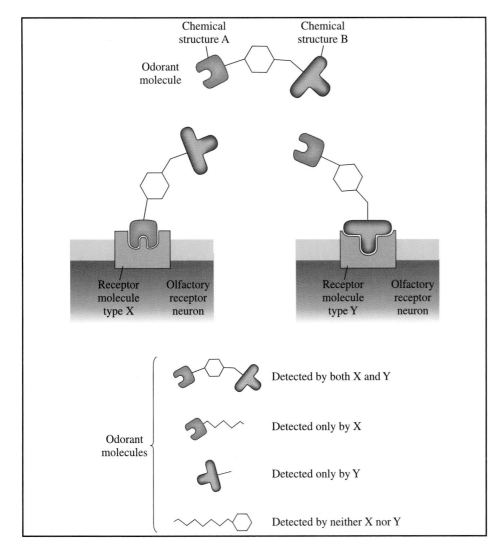

Figure 18.13.

Olfactory receptor molecules selectively bind particular structural parts of odorant molecules. The receptor molecule on the left (type X) can be activated by any odorant molecule that has chemical structure A (shown schematically at the *top*) as part of its molecular structure. The receptor molecule on the right (type Y) has a different binding site, which can be occupied selectively by chemical structure B. If an odorant molecule has both structures A and B, it can bind to and activate both types of receptor molecules. Other odorant molecules (shown *below*) that have only structure A or only structure B will bind to one or the other type of receptor molecule, but not both. Odorants that lack both structures will not interact with type X or type Y receptors and must be detected by others of the approximately 1000 types of receptor molecules.

neurons, the **periglomerular cells** and the **granule cells**, influence the activity of the output neurons of the bulb (the mitral and tufted cells). The synaptic connections of these inhibitory interneurons are summarized in Figure 18.14.

The cell bodies of the periglomerular cells, as the name implies, are located in the region around the glomeruli. Their dendrites receive excitatory synaptic inputs from the olfactory receptor neurons and from branches of the dendrites of the mitral and tufted cells within the glomerulus. In turn, the periglomerular cells make inhibitory feedback synapses with the mitral and tufted cell dendrites in the same glomerulus. The axon of the periglomerular cell extends laterally to the dendrites of mitral and tufted cells in neighboring glomeruli, where it also makes inhibitory synaptic con-

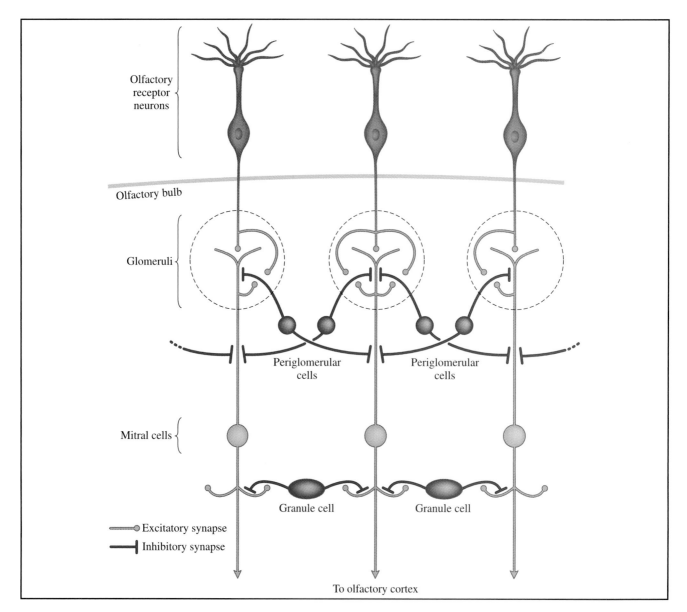

Figure 18.14.

Lateral inhibitory interactions in the olfactory bulb. The two types of inhibitory interneurons are the periglomerular cells and the granule cells. The periglomerular cells receive excitatory inputs within a glomerulus and make inhibitory synaptic connections both within that same glomerulus and on the output neurons of neighboring glomeruli. The granule cells receive excitatory inputs from collateral branches of the output fibers and make inhibitory feedback synaptic connections both locally and onto neighboring output cells. For simplicity, only the mitral cells are shown for the output pathways, but similar connections are made with the tufted cells, as well.

tact. Thus, if the receptor neurons feeding a particular glomerulus are active, the periglomerular cells within that glomerulus are excited, producing inhibition within the glomerulus and in neighboring glomeruli. This inhibitory feedback circuit resembles the synaptic circuit formed by the photoreceptor cells and the horizontal cells in the retina (Chapter 15)—a circuit that also produces lateral inhibition.

The granule cells are located deeper within the olfactory bulb, but they form similar inhibitory feedback connections, as shown in Figure 18.14. Granule cells receive excitatory synaptic input from output branches of mitral cells and tufted cells and make inhibitory synaptic contact back onto the same output cells and onto the output cells of neighboring glomeruli. These connections add a second level of lateral inhibition, analogous to the lateral inhibitory effect of the amacrine cells in the retina (see Chapter 15).

The lateral inhibitory connections in the olfactory bulb enhance the "contrast" between neighboring glomeruli, as reflected in the activity of mitral and tufted cells. If an olfactory stimulus activates one glomerulus more strongly than its neighbors, then the lateral connections shown in Figure 18.14 magnify the difference in activity of the output cells from those glomeruli (see descriptions of contrast enhancement in Chapters 13, 14, and 15).

SUMMARY

The translation of a chemical signal into an electrical signal in the nervous system is called chemotransduction. In mammals, the two important chemical senses are olfaction (smell) and gustation (taste). Chemotransduction is carried out by specialized olfactory receptor cells found in the olfactory epithelium and by taste receptor cells located predominantly in the taste buds of the tongue in mammals. Table 18.1 summarizes the transduction mechanisms in olfactory and taste receptor cells and compares them with phototransduction, which shares many features with chemotransduction.

In chemoreceptors and photoreceptors, the receptor molecules that detect the stimulus are coupled indirectly to changes in membrane potential, via intracellular G-proteins (for taste cells, this holds true for sweet and bitter tastes; salty and sour tastes act directly on ion channels). As in photoreceptors, ion channels that are directly gated by cyclic nucleotides are involved in the electrical responses of olfactory receptors and probably also in the responses of taste cells to bitter stimuli. In olfactory receptors, odor stimuli increase the intracellular levels of cyclic AMP, which results in the opening of nonspecific cation channels and depolarization of the receptor cell. By contrast, in photoreceptors, light decreases cyclic GMP levels, which causes channels to close and hyperpolarizes the cell.

In taste receptor cells, sweet, sour, and salty stimuli do not involve cyclic nucleotide–gated ion channels. Sweet stimuli depolarize taste cells by activating adenylyl cyclase and increasing internal cyclic AMP, which in turn promotes the phosphorylation of potassium channels. The phosphorylated potassium channels close, which reduces the permeability of the membrane to potassium ions and depolarizes the cell. In salt-sensitive taste cells, sodium ions directly enter the taste receptor cell through open sodium channels and depolarize the cell. Sour taste is elicited by increased acidity (increased proton concentration) in the saliva. The protons enter and block potassium channels, which depolarizes the taste cell.

In the mammalian brain, both the gustatory and olfactory sensory systems provide inputs to the limbic system, which is a primitive part of the brain controlling feeding, reproductive behavior, emotion, and homeostatic functions. In addition, neurons communicating both taste and olfac-

Table 18.1

Comparison of sensory characteristics in olfaction, taste, and vision

	Olfaction	**Taste**	**Photoreception**
Stimulus	Chemical	Chemical	Light
Direct linkage of stimulus to ion channels?	No	Yes (salt, sour) No (sweet, bitter)	No
Indirect linkage of stimulus to ion channels via G-proteins?	Yes	Yes (sweet, bitter) No (salt, sour)	Yes
Effect of stimulus on membrane potential	Depolarization	Depolarization	Hyperpolarization
Cyclic nucleotide–gated ion channels involved in change in membrane potential?	Yes	No (sweet, salt, sour) Yes[a] (bitter)	Yes
Axon of sensory cell projects to brain?	Yes	No	No[b]

[a]In bitter taste transduction, the cyclic nucleotide–gated channels *close* when cyclic nucleotides bind to the channel. In olfaction and phototransduction, the cyclic nucleotide–gated channels *open* when cyclic nucleotides bind to the channel.

[b]Because the retina is in reality part of the brain (the diencephalon), this entry is slightly inaccurate. The "No" here indicates that the synaptic output of the photoreceptor is near the site of transduction, not distant as with olfactory receptor neurons.

SUMMARY

tory information project via the thalamus to the cortex, where odors and flavors are consciously perceived and identified. Both systems encode the identity of a particular chemical stimulus by the overall pattern of activity in different subtypes of primary receptor cells, rather than by the specificity of the receptor cell for one particular type of chemical stimulus. In this regard, the chemical sensory systems are analogous to the processing of color in the visual system, in which outputs originating from the three types of cone photoreceptors are compared in the brain to establish the color of the stimulus.

REVIEW QUESTIONS

1. Describe the mechanism by which cyclic AMP influences the membrane potential of olfactory receptor neurons.

2. How does a chemical stimulus produce a change in the intracellular cyclic AMP level in olfactory receptor neurons?

3. Describe the synaptic interactions found in the olfactory bulb. Be sure to include inhibitory interneurons.

4. Compare and contrast the chemotransduction mechanisms found in taste receptor cells and olfactory receptor cells.

5. List the synaptic relays leading from the taste buds to the neocortex. Specify which parts of the cortex receive taste sensory information.

6. Identify the following: nucleus of the solitary tract, ventral posterior medial nucleus of the thalamus, glossopharyngeal nerve.

7. What are the four submodalities of taste? How many submodalities are found in the olfactory system?

8. Discuss some similarities between the synaptic interconnections found in the olfactory bulb and the retina.

9. Identify the following: glomerulus, medial dorsal nucleus of the thalamus, entorhinal cortex, paleocortex.

INTERNET ASSIGNMENT

CHAPTER 18

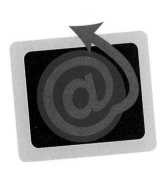

1 Use PubMed to investigate current information about taste receptor molecules that are coupled to G-proteins.

2 Use anatomical resources on the Internet, such as brain atlases, to locate the following structures in the brain: facial nerve, glossopharyngeal nerve, and nucleus of the solitary tract.

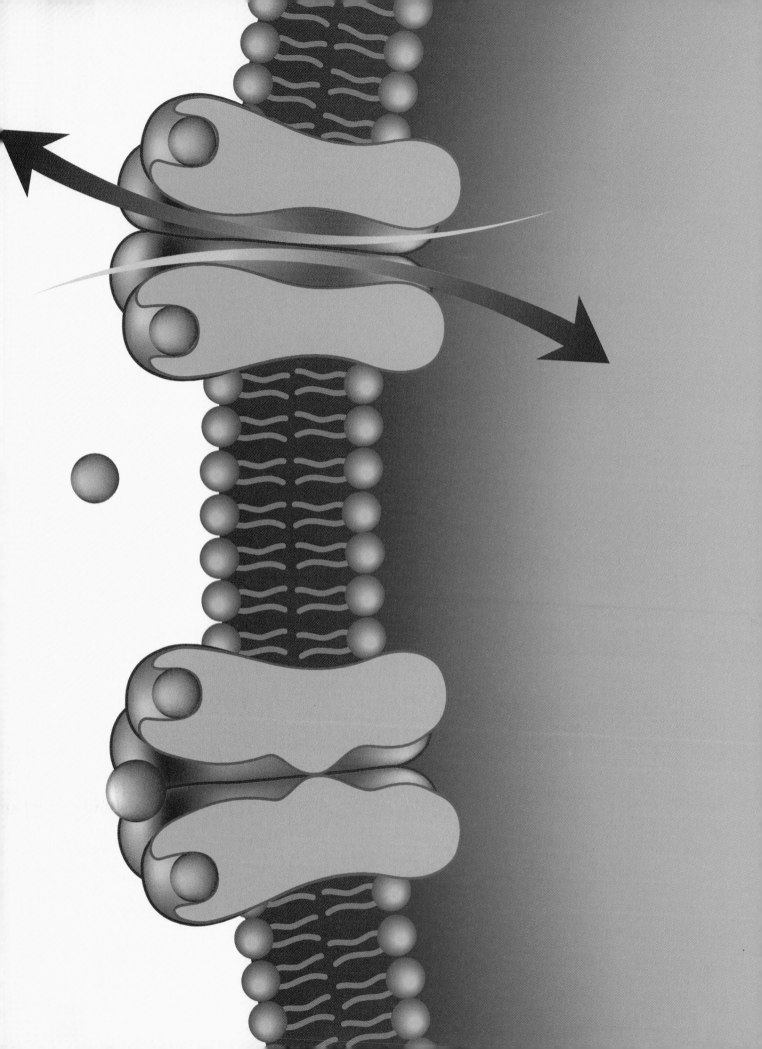

NEURONAL PLASTICITY AND HIGHER CORTICAL FUNCTION

In the first four parts of this book, we devoted our efforts to understanding the basic properties of nerve cells and neuronal circuits. For the most part, we have viewed neurons and the circuits into which they are organized as static objects whose properties remain fixed. One hallmark of the nervous system, however, is its ability to alter its own circuitry and to change the processing of information over time. In broad terms, this capability is referred to as **plasticity** in the nervous system. In Part V, we will turn our attention to neuronal plasticity.

Perhaps the ultimate neural plasticity is represented by the dramatic changes that occur during the embryonic development of the nervous system. From a few precursor cells, an entire nervous system arises, containing thousands of different kinds of neurons wired into a marvel of intricate detail. Although we know little about how this transformation occurs, increasing progress has been made in understanding the molecular mechanisms underlying important pieces of the process. Chapter 19 is devoted to a description of some of these mechanisms of neuronal genesis, growth, and differentiation. We will emphasize cellular communication systems used by neurons and non-neuronal cells to send signals that guide development.

The other major form of neuronal plasticity is more subtle because it is not associated with dramatic changes in structure like those that occur during the development of the nervous system. This form of plasticity underlies the day-to-day changes in behavior exhibited even by simple organisms, based on their experience with the environment. These behavioral events are usually referred to as "learning," and the retention of these changes is called "memory." One of the guiding principles in our approach to the nervous system is that changes in behavior must ultimately reflect changes in the cellular properties of the neuronal circuits that give rise to the behavior. In a sense, this guiding principle is the foundation for any cellular approach to the nervous system. Chapter 20 focuses on the cellular mechanisms of synaptic plasticity. In particular we will emphasize special examples that allow cellular principles to be applied to behavioral changes that accompany learning and memory.

In Part V, we also will consider some uniquely human aspects of brain function: language and cognition. The large size and complexity of the neocortex is one of the principal distinguishing features of the human brain. Substantial parts of the human neocortex are devoted to cognition, which refers to the complex functions of the brain having to do with language and thought. Although little is known about the cellular and molecular mechanisms of cognition, information about the parts of the cortex involved in language and thought is available from studies of brain-damaged patients and from noninvasive functional imaging studies. Chapter 20 focuses on these especially mysterious cortical functions.

In this part, you will find that the level of understanding of the underlying mechanisms is perhaps not as deep as for the topics encountered earlier in this book. Put simply, we know less about the genesis of the nervous system, learning and memory, and cognition. However, progress is rapid in these areas (perhaps because we know less), and you should view the material here as an introductory guide to learning more about neural plasticity and higher cortical function.

NEURAL DEVELOPMENT

Throughout this book, we have encountered numerous examples of neuronal circuits. They have ranged from the simplest spinal reflexes, such as the patellar stretch reflex, to more complicated synaptic interconnections involved in locomotor pattern generation or sensory information processing. If even the simplest neuronal circuit is to function properly, a precise set of cellular connections must be made among the cells in the circuit. Until now, we have

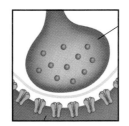

focused on the adult form of the wiring diagram, without considering how it reached this form. In this chapter, we will approach the fundamental question of how the circuit wiring was established during development of the nervous system. Although we are not yet able to completely answer this important question, much information is available about neuronal growth, differentiation, and the formation of appropriate synaptic connections.

The complex process of nervous system development can be divided into four broad stages. First, the precursor cells of neurons must divide and proliferate to produce the cellular raw material of the nervous system. This stage of neuronal specification and proliferation is called **neurogenesis**. Second, the newly produced neurons must move from their birthplace to their appropriate locations within the overall plan of the nervous system. This dispersal is called **neuronal migration**. Third, the cell body of the neuron must grow dendrites to receive inputs from other neurons and an axon to connect with the appropriate targets. This stage, known as **process outgrowth**, is related in some ways to the migration of the cell body in the second stage. Fourth, after the axon has reached the target site, it must recognize the desired target cells and form synaptic connections. This stage is called **synapse formation**. We will consider each of these stages in turn in this chapter.

NEUROGENESIS

Neuronal Determination

In Chapter 2, we briefly considered some of the early embryonic events in the generation of the nervous system. Viewed from the perspective of developmental biology, the production of a nervous system is just one example (albeit a particularly complex one) of the sequential steps of determination and differentiation that are required to generate any organ system. As a fertilized egg divides and gives rise to an embryo, some of the progeny cells are targeted to give rise to internal organs, some to muscles, and still others to the skin. Among the latter group, a subpopulation of cells becomes specified early on to give rise to the neurons and glial cells of the nervous system. This cellular targeting process is called **determination**.

Vertebrate embryos have three cellular layers: an inner layer called the **endoderm**, a middle layer called the **mesoderm**, and an outside layer called the **ectoderm**. These layers form via a complex infolding of the single-layer early embryo, a process called **gastrulation**, which is illustrated in Figure 19.1. The nervous system arises from a portion of the ectoderm called the **neuroectoderm**. The differentiation of the neuroectoderm from the surrounding ectoderm occurs during gastrulation, as the cells of the mesoderm migrate inward beneath the ectoderm. In a process known as **neural induction**, the mesodermal cells send a signal to the cells of the overlying ectoderm, inducing them to form the **neural plate**, which will give rise to the nervous system.

An important structure formed by the mesoderm is the **notochord**. This long, rod-shaped group of cells forms along what will become the midline of the organism. The notochord defines the longitudinal axis of the body (see Fig. 19.1). The neuroectoderm is induced in the part of the ectoderm lying above the forming notochord. The importance of the notochord in neural induction was established by experiments like that illustrated in Figure 19.2, in which a small piece is removed from the region of the dorsal lip that will give rise to the notochord during gastrulation. This piece is transplanted into another early embryo, where it develops into a second notochord at a position where no notochord is usually present. When the recipient embryo undergoes gastrulation, it produces its own notochord at the normal position, in addition to the transplanted notochord. In such an embryo, two neural plates will be induced, both of which will go on to form neural tubes (Fig. 19.3). Thus, under the influence of the transplanted notochord, ectodermal cells that would normally produce skin tissue can be induced to form neural tissue (see Fig. 19.2). The portion of the dorsal lip that is capable of inducing the development of neural tissue is called the **Spemann organizer**, in honor of the biologist who first performed transplantation experiments of this type.

How is the tissue that will give rise to the nervous system established during gastrulation?

431

Figure 19.1.

Early stages in the embryonic formation of the vertebrate nervous system. The diagrams show a time series during the process of gastrulation. At the *top*, gastrulation has just started; at the *bottom*, it is almost complete. Each drawing represents a section parallel to what will become the long axis of the body. In each case, the endoderm is shaded *pink*, the notochord is *red*, the ectoderm is *yellow*, and the developing neuroectoderm is *brown*. The direction of cell migration for various regions during gastrulation is indicated by the *arrows*.

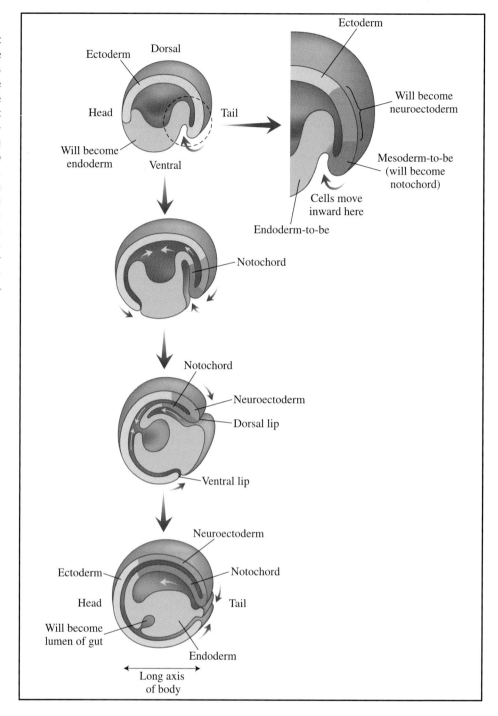

Neural induction does not require direct physical contact between the ectoderm and the underlying notochord, which indicates that a diffusible messenger molecule is responsible for neuronal determination. This diffusible message could be transmitted in either of two ways. First, the underlying mesoderm in the notochord region could release a molecule that diffuses to the ectoderm, where it stimulates the ectodermal cells to become neural cells. In such an **inducer mechanism**, the neuronal state is viewed as being actively stimulated in cells that would otherwise become other types of tissue. Second, the mesoderm under the neural plate could suppress a signal that causes the ectoderm to develop as non-neuronal tissue. In this **suppressor mechanism**, neuronal determination is considered to be the default state for ectodermal cells, which must be actively pushed down non-neuronal developmental paths by diffusible factors stemming from the endoderm. Experimen-

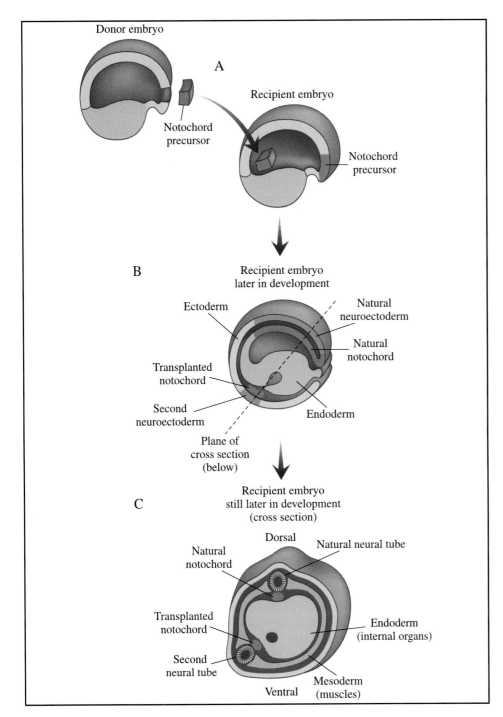

Figure 19.2.

A transplantation experiment demonstrating the importance of the notochord in the induction of the neuroectoderm in early vertebrate embryos. **A.** At the onset of gastrulation, a piece is removed from a donor embryo at the dorsal lip, which develops into the notochord during gastrulation. The piece is transplanted inside another embryo. **B.** As gastrulation proceeds in the recipient embryo, the transplanted piece of notochord tissue is carried to a part of the embryo that normally has no notochord. A second region of neuroectoderm is induced by the transplanted notochord in the recipient embryo. **C.** A cross section through the recipient embryo at a later stage of development shows the presence of two separate neural tubes.

tal evidence supports both views, and both could possibly come into play for different aspects of neural development or for different animal species. Also, multiple chemical messengers might be involved in either induction or suppression.

One specific version of the suppressor mechanism is hypothesized to work as follows. The endoderm releases a signal protein called **activin**, which induces the formation of mesoderm by the dorsal pole of the embryo prior to gastrulation. If ectodermal tissue is isolated from the dorsal pole before gastrulation and placed in culture, treatment with activin induces the ectodermal cells to transform into mesodermal cells. As the mesoderm develops and migrates inward during gastrulation in the embryo, cells of the notochord release a protein called **follistatin**, which binds to and inactivates activin. Therefore, in the vicinity of the notochord—where follistatin is released—the level of activin is reduced. The lack of

How are activin, follistatin, and noggin thought to regulate the induction of the nervous system?

433

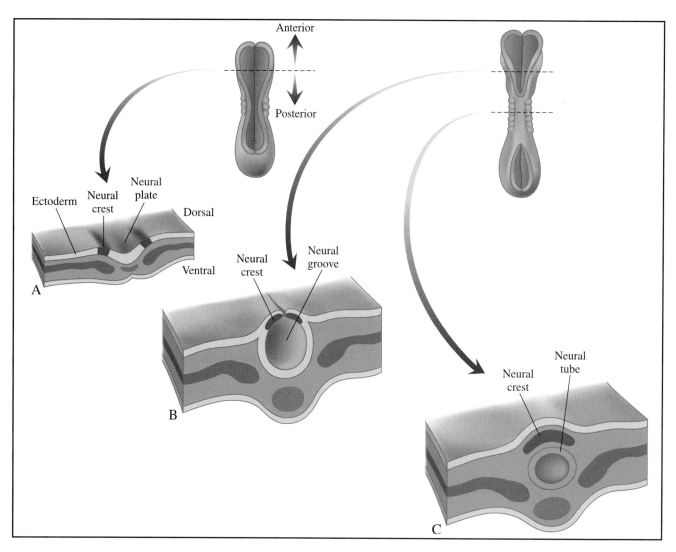

Figure 19.3.

Early differentiation of the nervous system in a vertebrate embryo. **A**. The nervous system begins as undifferentiated ectodermal cells along the dorsal midline, called the neural plate. At this stage, the cells that will form the neural crest (shown in *red*) lie along each side of the neural plate. **B**. At a later stage, the neural plate invaginates to form the neural groove, with the neural crest located along the lips of the groove. **C**. The neural groove eventually pinches off to form the neural tube, as the two opposing parts of the neural crest fuse.

activin causes cells in the ectoderm just above the notochord to revert to their default developmental state—that is, the neural developmental path. As a result, the neural plate develops in the ectodermal cells lying over the notochord, where follistatin is released.

The identification of inducing factors, which are required under the inducer hypothesis, is currently a topic of active research. One candidate for an inducing factor is the protein **noggin** (so-named because it can induce excessive brain and head development when injected into frog embryos). Like follistatin, this protein is manufactured and released by the cells of the notochord, and it can induce the expression of neuronal genes in ectodermal cells. Noggin also may be involved in directing the production of muscle tissue by mesodermal cells. Most likely, noggin is only one of several soluble inducing factors released at various times during development of the nervous system; it does seem to be involved in very early stages of neural induction, however.

Both suppressor and inducer mechanisms may be involved in normal neural development. It is possible that suppression of activin is required, together with release of an inducer, to properly form the nervous system during embryonic development.

As the cells of the neural plate proliferate, they invaginate to form the **neural groove**, which then pinches off to become the **neural tube**. This sequence is illustrated in Figure 19.3. The neural tube goes on to form the brain and spinal cord. At the margin of the neural groove lie the cells of the **neural crest**, which separates from the other neural plate cells when the neural tube forms (see Fig. 19.3). The neural crest gives rise to the cells of the dorsal root ganglia, the sympathetic ganglia, and other neurons whose cell bodies are located in the peripheral nervous system.

Neuronal Proliferation

The precursor cells of the neural tube ultimately give rise to all the cells of the central nervous system. Thus, the cells of the neural tube must divide prolifically to supply the large number of cells needed in the adult brain and spinal cord. The neural tube begins as a single layer of cells and develops into a structure many centimeters thick, in the human brain. The cells do not proliferate uniformly throughout the neural tube as it grows, however. Instead, new nerve cells are produced at the inner surface of the neural tube, at the edge of the internal lumen that will ultimately become the ventricles of the brain and the central canal of the spinal cord (see Chapter 2). For this reason, the region of the neural tube specialized for the production of new neural cells is known as the **ventricular zone**.

Figure 19.4 shows that at early stages of development, the neural tube consists of only two layers: the **ventricular zone** where dividing cells are found, and the relatively cell-free **marginal zone** toward the outer edge of the neural tube. As the neural precursor cells of the neural tube proliferate, they repetitively go through the movements shown in Figure 19.4 during the cell cycle. As DNA replication proceeds in preparation for division, the cell nucleus moves outward toward the marginal zone. After the replication of DNA is complete, the nucleus returns to the ventricular zone. At this point, the cell is anchored via long, thin processes to the two edges of the neural tube, and the nucleus moves along these processes (see Fig. 19.4). The reason for this migration of the nucleus along the length of the cell is unknown. After the nucleus reaches the ventricular zone on its return trip, the cell retracts its long processes and divides. The two daughter cells then take one of two avenues: they reenter the cell cycle and continue to produce more progeny cells, or they exit from the ventricular zone and migrate to form the developing nervous system. The departing cells become either neurons or glial cells. Those that become neurons lose the ability to divide, whereas the glial precursors retain the ability to proliferate.

Although the ventricular-zone neuron factory produces most neurons in the central nervous system, the neurons of the peripheral nervous system have a different origin. When the lips of the neural groove fuse to form the neural tube, the neuroectodermal cells at the lateral margin are left behind and become the neural crest. These cells generate the neurons of the dorsal root ganglia, the sympathetic ganglia, the peripheral ganglia of the parasympathetic nervous system, and the adrenal medulla. In this case, however, the precursor cells themselves move out to form the peripheral structures, generating the full complement of neural cells after they have reached their target sites in the developing body. By contrast, in the central nervous system, the dividing precursor cells generally remain in the ventricular zone, and the nondividing immature neurons leave the ventricular zone to occupy their positions in the brain and spinal cord.

Where in the developing nervous system are the nerve cells born?

435

Figure 19.4.

The early neural tube is subdivided into the ventricular zone, where cell division occurs, and the marginal zone. The *bottom diagram* shows the movements of the cell body during one cycle of cell division in a neuronal precursor cell. Moving from top to bottom, the cell is shown at different phases of the cell cycle, as indicated by the letters to the right of the cell. The daughter cells can either reenter the cycle or migrate out of the ventricular zone.

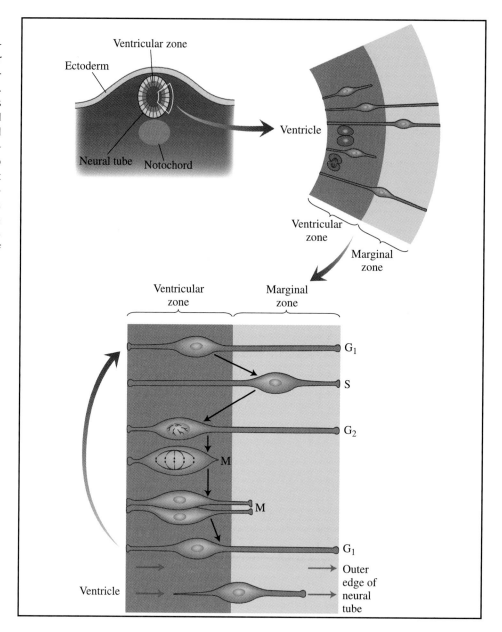

Cell Lineage

Even simple neuronal circuits consist of multiple types of neurons, each of which plays a particular functional role. The spinal cord, for example, contains motor neurons, excitatory interneurons, inhibitory interneurons, and sensory projection neurons. At a finer level of detail, neurons can be subdivided into flexor and extensor motor neurons, stretch-sensitive and touch-sensitive sensory cells, and so on. Each of these neuronal subtypes has characteristic synaptic connections and projection patterns. The heritage of each neuron can be traced back to an individual precursor cell, called a **stem cell**. Some stem cells give rise to a variety of different neuronal subtypes. In the retina, for example, a single precursor cell can have progeny among all of the different cell types of the retina, including neurons, glial cells, and retinal pigmented epithelium cells. In other cases, the stem cells are more restricted in scope, giving rise to only a restricted set of neuronal subtypes. In the cerebellum, for example, the output cells of the cerebellum (Purkinje cells) arise from one set of precursor cells, whereas interneurons within the cerebellum (granule cells) arise from a separate, distinct set of precursor cells. (We will discuss cerebellar development in more detail shortly.)

Typically, all of the cells that will become neurons of a particular type in a particular brain region arise at a specific time during the proliferation of the precursor cells. During neural development, the different neuron types are generated in a fixed sequence, which is thought to be genetically programmed. As the neuronal precursor cells divide, different **regulatory genes** switch on and off in a programmed sequence. Each regulatory gene specifies a particular neuronal subtype.

At each point in development, different regulatory genes are expressed in different parts of the nervous system. For example, in the prosencephalon, the precursor cells at a particular instant in development may produce immature neurons slated for the deep layers of the cerebral cortex. At the same time, parts of the rhombencephalon may produce immature neurons slated for the cerebellum. At the same point in development, cells in the prosencephalon and in the rhombencephalon express different regulatory genes that define cerebral cortical neurons and cerebellar neurons, respectively. This expression pattern is depicted schematically in Figure 19.5. Later in development, a different subset of regulatory genes becomes activated, driving further differentiation into specific cell types found in the adult brain (see Fig. 19.5).

The identities of the master regulatory genes that govern regional differentiation of the nervous system and guide the production of particular types of neural cells are mostly unknown. The search for such genes is currently a very active part of neurobiology. Much of this work is based on studies of genes that control the patterning of the body and nervous system in the fruit fly, genus *Drosophila*, which is a well-studied organism for genetic research. For example, homologues of a *Drosophila* gene called **Engrailed** are thought to control the development and differentiation of the mammalian cerebellum. Thus, "gene X" in Figure 19.5, which initiates the cerebellar lineage, may be a gene called *Engrailed-1*. The protein encoded by this gene is a transcription factor—that is, a protein that controls the expression of other genes. Another member of the *Engrailed* family of genes, *Engrailed-2*, may be involved in the further differentiation of cells in the cerebellum (for example, gene Y or Z in Fig. 19.5). The expression of *Engrailed-1* is spatially segregated to the part of the neural tube that gives rise to the cerebellum. This spatial segregation in turn is controlled by other regulatory genes, which probably encode transcription factors that control the expression of *Engrailed* genes.

Environment Also Affects Neuronal Differentiation

To this point, we have emphasized genetic mechanisms by which the basic pattern for the nervous system is determined early in neural development. In addition to these important genetic factors, however, environmental factors influence the development of the nervous system. After an early genetic switch commits a cell to a particular line of development, the cell usually retains the potential to differentiate into any of several different cell types within that lineage. The choice of a specific cell type frequently depends on environmental factors.

An example of plasticity in neuronal phenotype is found in the development of the sympathetic and parasympathetic neurons of the peripheral autonomic nervous system (see Chapter 11). The neurons of these two branches of the autonomic nervous system arise from precursor cells in the neural crest (see Fig. 19.3). As shown in Figure 19.6A, the anterior portion of the neural crest gives rise to parasympathetic neurons, which use acetylcholine as their neurotransmitter. The immature neurons from this part of the neural crest migrate to form the parasympathetic ganglia near their peripheral target tissues and make cholinergic synaptic connections with the proper targets. The neurons of the sympathetic chain ganglia, on the

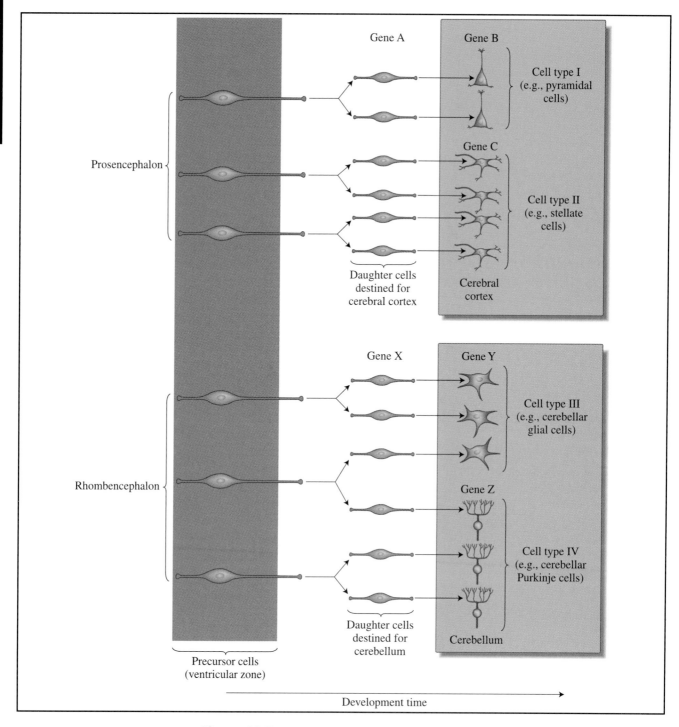

Figure 19.5.

A sequence of expression of particular neuronal genes leads to a progressively more restricted specification of cell type. This hypothetical diagram shows the fates of neuronal precursor cells generated in either the prosencephalon (*top*) or the rhombencephalon (*bottom*). The cells in the prosencephalon express one set of genes appropriate for cerebral cortical neurons. The cells in the rhombencephalon express a different set of genes appropriate for cerebellar neurons and glial cells.

other hand, arise from the middle portion of the neural crest (see Fig. 19.6A). These neurons remain near the spinal cord and give rise to the axons of the sympathetic nerves, which extend to the appropriate targets and make synaptic connections that release the neurotransmitter norepinephrine.

The parasympathetic and sympathetic portions of the neural crest can be removed from a developing embryo and transplanted into a recipient embryo with their positions reversed, as illustrated in Figure 19.6B. If the precursor cells from the anterior and middle parts of the neural crest were genetically programmed to become parasympathetic and sympathetic neurons, respectively, then the origins of the sympathetic and parasympathetic neurons would be reversed in the recipient embryo. That is, the anterior neural crest would give rise to sympathetic ganglia, while the middle neural crest would generate parasympathetic ganglia. Instead, the normal pattern is maintained in the embryo receiving the reversed transplants (see Fig. 19.6B). The anterior neural crest still generates parasympathetic neurons, even though the precursor cells at that location were originally slated to become sympathetic neurons. Conversely, sympathetic neurons arise from cells that would have produced parasympathetic ganglia if left in their normal positions. To achieve this result, the cells must alter their migration patterns and also switch on a different set of genes to synthesize the appropriate neurotransmitter substance. The precursor cells have the potential to become either sympathetic or parasympathetic neurons, and their location near the upper or middle portion of the spinal cord determines the choice. Thus, the environment of the precursor cells—not just their genetic programming—determines the migration patterns of the immature neurons, as well as the type of neurotransmitter (acetylcholine versus norepinephrine) produced by the cells.

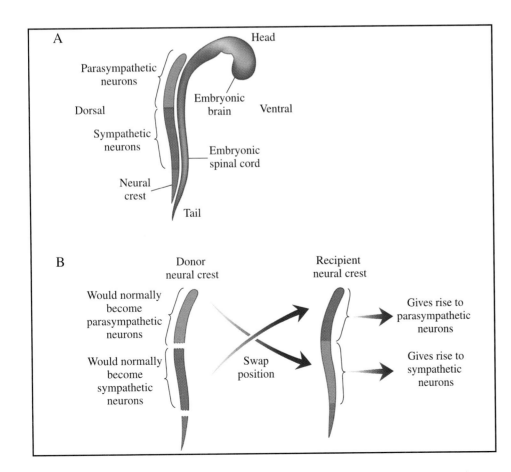

Figure 19.6.

A transplantation experiment illustrating developmental plasticity in neuronal precursor cells. **A.** The normal situation. The anterior part of the neural crest (*brown*) gives rise to parasympathetic neurons, and the middle part (*green*) gives rise to sympathetic neurons. **B.** If the positions are switched, the precursor cells behave appropriately for their new positions in the neural crest. The cells from the middle part now produce parasympathetic neurons when placed in the anterior part of the neural crest. The cells from the anterior part now give rise to sympathetic neurons when placed in the middle position.

NEURONAL MIGRATION

Movement of cells from one part of the developing nervous system to another is a crucial aspect of neural development. The movement of immature neurons from their place of birth to the correct position within the three-dimensional structure of the nervous system is referred to as **neuronal migration**. In this section, we will consider some aspects of the mechanisms that guide the migrating neurons.

Purkinje Cell Migration in the Cerebellum

How do neurons migrate from their birthplace to their correct position in the developing nervous system?

As an example of the mechanisms that guide the migrating neurons, consider the formation of cellular layers during the development of the cerebellar cortex. Like the cerebral cortex, the cortex of the cerebellum is a layered structure, with particular neuronal subtypes localized to specific layers. The cerebellum has three distinct layers, shown in Figure 19.7: the **molecular layer**, the **Purkinje cell layer**, and the **granule cell layer**. The innermost granule cell layer consists largely of small, excitatory interneurons called **granule cells**, which receive synaptic input from incoming fibers originating in other motor and sensory regions. As its name implies, the Purkinje cell layer contains the cell bodies of the **Purkinje cells**, which

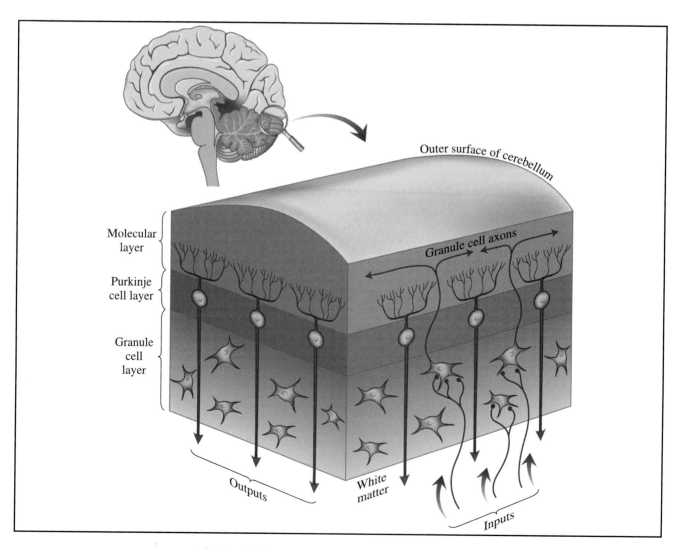

Figure 19.7.

The positions of granule cells and Purkinje cells in the cortex of the cerebellum.

are the output neurons of the cerebellum. The outermost molecular layer contains the dendrites of the Purkinje cells and the axons of the granule cells, which make excitatory synaptic contact with Purkinje cell dendrites. In addition to these layers, the cerebellum also includes the deep cerebellar nuclei (see Chapter 9).

During development, the immature neurons slated to become Purkinje cells arise in the ventricular zone, at the dorsal margin of the nascent fourth ventricle of the brain. In this regard, Purkinje cell development follows the general plan for neurogenesis, shown in Figure 19.4. The first neurons born in the cerebellar ventricular zone are the neurons destined to make up the deep nuclei of the cerebellum. These deep nuclei neurons migrate from the ventricular zone and form a separate layer, shown in Figure 19.8A. As the Purkinje cells arise in the ventricular zone, they must migrate through the layer containing the neurons of the deep nuclei in order

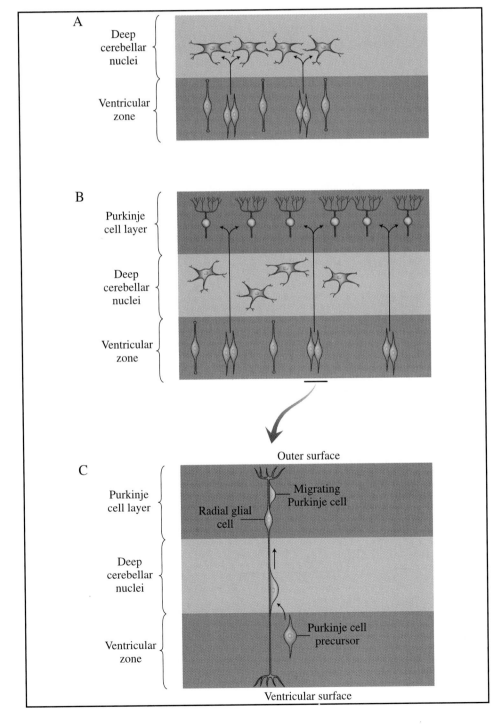

Figure 19.8.

The development of cerebellar Purkinje cells. **A.** At early stages, neurons of the deep cerebellar nuclei are born and migrate out of the ventricular zone. **B.** The Purkinje cells are born at a later stage and must migrate past the neurons of the deep cerebellar nuclei to reach their appropriate position. **C.** The migration of Purkinje cell precursors takes place along long, thin glial cells, called radial glial cells.

to take up their appropriate positions (see Fig. 19.8B). The immature Purkinje cells make this trip along a cellular highway consisting of a special class of glial cells that form early during development. These glial cells are called **radial glial cells** because they have a single, thin process that extends radially from the ventricular surface to the outermost surface of the developing cerebellum.

Granule Cell Migration in the Cerebellum

The granule cells are the last type of cerebellar neuron to be generated during development. Their genesis represents an exception to the general rule that neurons are generated within the ventricular zone. Instead, the granule cells arise at the *outer* surface of the developing cerebellum, in a layer of neuronal precursor cells called the **external granule layer**. This layer is produced by the proliferation of cells within the neural tube at the posterior margin of the cerebellum. As the cells divide, they spread out in an anterior direction over the outer surface of the cerebellum in the manner shown in Figure 19.9A. The immature neurons produced within the external granule layer are destined to become the granule cells in the deepest of the three layers of the cerebellar cortex. Thus, these cells must migrate from the outer surface where they arise, through the Purkinje cell layer, to reach their adult positions (see Fig. 19.9B).

Figure 19.10 shows the stages in the development and migration of a granule cell. An immature granule neuron extends two processes parallel to the surface of

Figure 19.9.

Cerebellar granule cells originate in the external granule layer. **A.** The part of the neural tube just posterior to the developing cerebellum spreads out anteriorly over the surface of the cerebellar region. **B.** The granule cell precursors divide in the external granule cell layers, producing immature granule cells that must migrate through the Purkinje cell layer to reach the appropriate position.

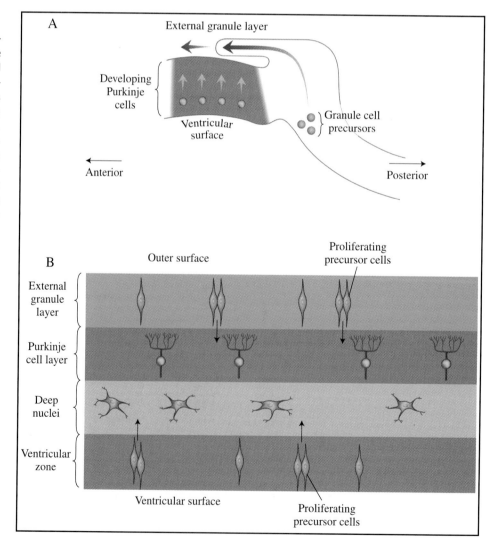

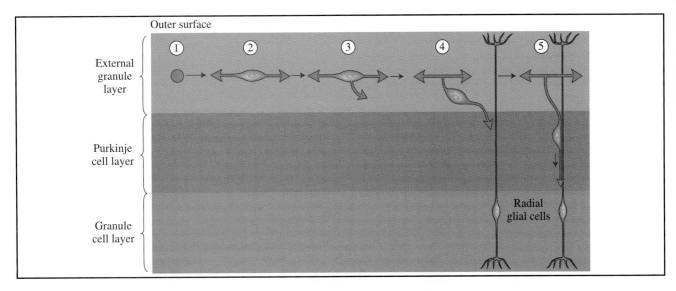

Figure 19.10.

Stages in the migration of a cerebellar granule cell. The migration occurs along the radial glial cells.

the cerebellum. These processes will become the axon projection of the mature granule cell within the molecular layer of the adult cerebellum (see Fig. 19.7). Next, the cell extends a third process perpendicular to the cerebellar surface. The growing third process contacts a radial glial cell and follows the glial cell deeper into the cerebellum. The cell body of the granule cell then begins to migrate along this third process, following the glial cell path toward the deeper parts of the cerebellum. Thus, as with the Purkinje cell, the migration of the granule cell is guided by the fibers of the radial glial cells, although the direction of movement is inward rather than outward.

The granule cell maintains close contact with the radial glial cell during its migration, entwining itself around the glial cell process as it moves along. This close contact of the two cells is accomplished via complementary cell-surface molecules—one on the glial cell membrane and one on the granule cell membrane—that interact strongly with one another. Because they keep the cells together, these molecules are called **cell adhesion molecules**.

Many different types of adhesion molecules are expressed by different cell types throughout the tissues of the body, including the nervous system. The cell adhesion molecule in the granule cells is a membrane glycoprotein called **astrotactin**. A **glycoprotein** is a membrane protein with molecules of sugar attached at various points on the extracellular part of the molecule. The sugar molecules extend into the extracellular space and are thought to provide a unique molecular surface that can be recognized by appropriate receptor molecules on target cells. The match between the two molecules in the extracellular space promotes adhesion between the two cells expressing the molecules. The matching cell adhesion molecule on the radial glial cell that interacts with astrotactin has not been identified.

The importance of a proper binding partner for cell adhesion molecules in neuronal migration is indicated by a neurological mutation in mice called *reeler*. In *reeler* mice, neurons fail to migrate correctly during development of the brain, and layered structures such as the cerebellum and cerebral cortex do not form properly. The mutated gene in the *reeler* mouse encodes a protein called **reelin**, which is a signaling or adhesion molecule, or both, found in the extracellular matrix. Reelin helps guide migrating neurons to their proper positions during the early stages of brain development. The role of the extracellular matrix in neuronal guidance is discussed in more detail in the next section.

PROCESS OUTGROWTH

After a neuron has migrated to its final position within the nervous system, it must create the processes (dendrites and axons) by which it connects to other neurons and receives and sends information. Collectively, dendrites and axons are called **neurites**. Neurites often must travel long distances to reach their targets. Consider the neurons involved in the patellar stretch reflex, for example. The motor neuron must grow an axon that connects with muscle fibers of the quadriceps muscle. To do so, the axon must travel through the ventral root of the spinal cord and navigate correctly past numerous branch points in the growing nerve before finding its synaptic target in the leg. The distance covered by the axon of the sensory neuron of the stretch receptor—from the dorsal root ganglion to the quadriceps muscle via the same nerve branches as the motor axon—is also very long. In addition, the sensory neuron must send a branch of its axon into the spinal cord, where it must seek out and contact the dendrites of the quadriceps motor neurons. In this section we will examine the mechanisms that allow growing neural processes to find their way to the proper targets.

The Growth Cone

How do growing neurites navigate to find the proper path?

At the leading edge of a growing neurite is a specialized structure called the **growth cone**, which is illustrated in Figure 19.11. Neurites may simultaneously have several growing branches, each with a growth cone at its tip. The growth cone is actively mobile, extending amoeboid fingers called **filopodia** (singular: **filopodium**) that interact with the immediate environment and propel the growth cone forward. The movement of the filopodia is driven by filaments of actin, which are connected to the plasma membrane and to molecules of myosin associated with the cytoskeleton. As the filopodia at the advancing front of the growth cone extend in the direction of movement, actin filaments are assembled at the leading edge to enable further movement. The filopodia at the trailing edge retract to allow the entire growth cone to move forward. The actin networks of the retracted filopodia are disassembled and reused to construct new motile lattices at the advancing front of the growth cone. The flattened region between filopodia, called the **lamellipodium** (see Fig. 19.11), also contains actin filaments. When an extended filopodium adheres to the substrate over which the neurite is growing, the lamellipodium moves forward to meet the tip of the filopodium. New filopodia then extend from the leading edge, and the whole process is repeated. As a result, the growth cone inches forward over an adherent substrate.

As the growth cone moves forward, the backbone of the neurite is continually laid down along the path covered by the growth cone. This backbone consists of filamentous **microtubules**, which are constructed of the protein **tubulin**. Membrane is added to the growing tip of the neurite by the fusion of vesicles, which are transported from the cell body of the neuron along the microtubules of the advancing neurite (see Fig. 19.11B). In addition to providing membrane to the growth cone, these transport vesicles supply various membrane proteins, including ion channels, cell adhesion molecules, and membrane receptors for external chemical signals.

If the growth cone is to be able to move, it must adhere to the surrounding cells and extracellular matrix—that is, it must have traction. Adhesion is carried out by cell adhesion molecules similar to those that underlie the cell-to-cell interactions

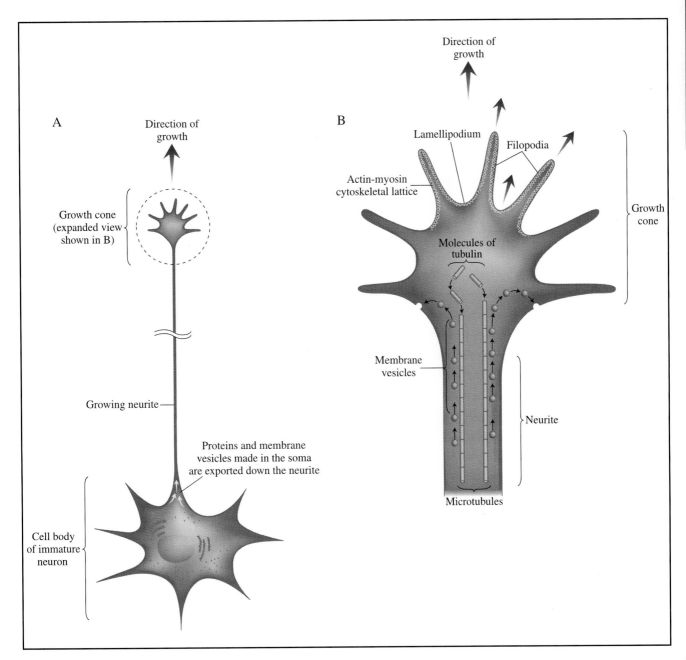

Figure 19.11.

The structure of a growth cone. **A.** An immature neuron gives rise to a neurite, which extends toward its target region to either receive or transmit synaptic signals. The growth cone is located at the end of the neurite. Protein molecules and membrane vesicles are manufactured in the cell body and exported to the growth cone down the interior of the growing neurite. **B.** A close-up view of the growth cone. Movement of the growth cone is mediated by a cytoskeletal lattice containing two motor proteins, actin and myosin. As the neurite extends behind the moving growth cone, the microtubule backbone of the neurite is constructed from molecules of tubulin. Membrane is added to the growth cone by the fusion of vesicles that move along the microtubules.

in neuronal migration. Although a wide variety of different cell adhesion molecules exist, a given neuron expresses only a particular subset during neurite outgrowth. Thus, neurons might be able to interact with and grow on some substrates but not others, depending on whether the substrate incorporates adhesion molecules that are complementary to the neuron's cell-surface molecules. In Figure 19.12, for example, neuron A has adhesion molecules that can interact with substrate molecule

Figure 19.12.

Cellular path finding during neurite outgrowth depends on the ability of cellular adhesion molecules of the growing neurite to combine with substrate adhesion molecules. Neuron B (*red*) can adhere to substrate molecule Y (*red dots*); neuron A (*green*) can adhere to substrate molecule X (*green dots*).

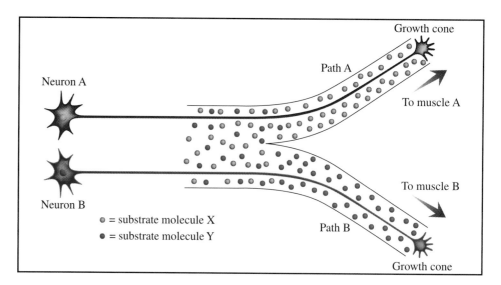

X but not substrate molecule Y; neuron B has different adhesion molecules that can bind to Y but not X. If a path consists of cells or extracellular matrix structures that have both molecules X and Y, then the neurites of both neurons can grow along that path. If the path diverges, with molecule X found only on one path and molecule Y only on the other, then the growth cones of the two neurons will also diverge and follow the paths to which they can adhere. If the two paths represent branches of a peripheral nerve leading to two separate muscles, this type of mechanism could allow motor and sensory neurons targeted for one of the muscles to separate from the neurons targeted for the other muscle.

Families of Cell Adhesion Molecules

What roles do cell adhesion molecules play in neural development?

The specific adhesion of neurite growth cones to particular pathways can be mediated via cell-to-cell interactions (as with the migration of cerebellar neurons along radial glial cells) or via interactions between the growth cone and the extracellular matrix. The **extracellular matrix** is a ubiquitous external material found in most all tissues. It is secreted by the cells that make up the tissue and in some cases by specialized cells such as fibroblasts. The two main classes of macromolecules that provide the structural backbone of the extracellular matrix are **collagen**, which is a protein, and **glycosaminoglycans**, which are large polysaccharide molecules that often combine with proteins to form **proteoglycans**. The extracellular matrix also contains glycoprotein molecules, which are the binding partners for adhesion molecules in the membranes of growing nerve fibers. Two important glycoproteins of the extracellular matrix are **fibronectin** and **laminin**, both of which promote the adhesion of cells to the matrix. Another glycoprotein found in the extracellular matrix is **tenascin**, which can either inhibit or promote neurite attachment and growth, depending on the type of neural cell. In addition, collagen is recognized by some types of cell-surface adhesion molecules.

The molecular makeup of the extracellular matrix is not constant in all parts of the developing organism. By varying the polysaccharide composition and the glycoprotein content of the extracellular matrix, the cells that secrete the matrix can bestow a distinct chemical "flavor" on the matrix in various tissues through which peripheral nerves migrate. Within the developing nervous system itself, different parts of the brain and spinal cord express different extracellular adhesion molecules. The chemical composition of the extracellular environment can promote or retard the growth of neurites from different subsets of neurons and thus help guide neurites to their proper targets.

On the external surface of the plasma membrane are **cellular adhesion molecules**, which enable cells to adhere to one another or to the extracellular matrix. Four families of cellular adhesion molecules have been identified: the **integrins**, the **cadherins**, the **selectins**, and the **immunoglobulin superfamily**. Each family consists of a number of related proteins. Integrins, for example, are formed by the combination of two protein subunits, an alpha-subunit and a beta-subunit (Fig. 19.13). Several types of both alpha- and beta-subunits exist and can associate in various combinations to produce over 20 different kinds of integrins. Each type of integrin binds a particular set of complementary adhesion molecules in the extracellular matrix, including fibronectin and laminin. This is shown schematically for different integrins in Figure 19.13.

The immunoglobulin superfamily of cellular adhesion molecules includes molecules such as **N-CAM** (*n*euronal *c*ell *a*dhesion *m*olecule) and **Ng-CAM** (*n*euronal-*g*lial *c*ell *a*dhesion *m*olecule). These molecules are involved in cell-to-cell adhesive interactions, rather than cell-to-extracellular matrix interactions. The immunoglobulin superfamily receives its name because the extracellular part of the molecule contains several repeated amino acid sequences that are structurally similar to immunoglobulin molecules of the immune system. The adhesion molecules of the immunoglobulin class are thought to bind to molecules of the same type on

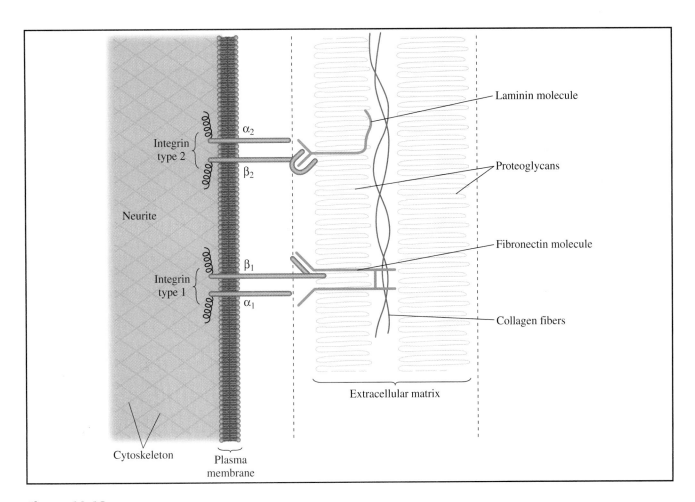

Figure 19.13.

The interaction between cellular adhesion molecules and adhesion molecules of the extracellular matrix. Two types of integrin molecules are shown. One type binds to laminin molecules, and the other type binds to fibronectin molecules.

neighboring cells, as shown in Figure 19.14. Thus, an N-CAM molecule binds to another N-CAM molecule on a neighboring cell, an Ng-CAM molecule binds to another Ng-CAM molecule, and so on. The adhesion molecules of the immunoglobulin family also include extracellular regions that resemble part of the fibronectin molecule of the extracellular matrix. This raises the possibility that N-CAM and Ng-CAM also may bind via their fibronectin-like region to integrins (which normally interact with extracellular matrix components) on neighboring cells.

During neuronal determination, sets of genes specific for each neuronal subtype (see, for example, Fig. 19.5), including genes for selected subtypes of cellular adhesion molecules, are expressed. Thus, the growing neurites of each neuronal class are endowed with specific adhesion molecules, which in turn determine the pathways that the neurite can follow as it grows. These cellular adhesion molecules are an important determinant of the migratory path taken by a newly born neuron and of the sites to which its axons and dendrites ultimately project. Thus, genetic programming is important in determining the pattern of neural migration and neurite projection during development.

In addition to their roles as structural elements that adhere cells to each other and to the extracellular matrix, cellular adhesion molecules also may send and receive cellular signals, based on their interactions with complementary adhesion molecules. These signals can affect further gene expression and help determine final neuronal phenotype. Thus, some of the environmental factors that affect

Figure 19.14.

Cell adhesion by cell-to-cell contact. Two types of cell adhesion molecules, neuronal cell adhesion molecule (N-CAM) and neuronal-glial cell adhesion molecule (Ng-CAM), are shown, each of which binds exclusively to partner molecules of the same type on other cells.

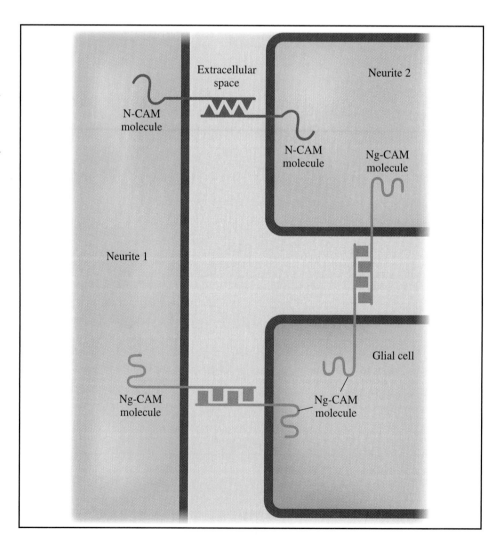

neuronal differentiation involve interactions between cellular adhesion molecules and the extracellular environment contacted by the cell and its neurites.

Neurite Guidance

Our discussion to this point has emphasized the role of molecular interactions that arise from direct contact between adhesion molecules on the surface of neurites and adhesion molecules in the extracellular environment. In addition to these contact-mediated growth cues, movements of growth cones are guided by molecules that are released into the extracellular space and diffuse some distance from their source to the growth cone. These signal molecules either attract growth cones, causing them to turn toward the source of the signal, or repel growth cones, causing them to turn away from the source. Molecules that attract are called **chemoattractants**, while those that repel are called **chemorepellents**. As a group, chemoattractant and chemorepellent molecules are known as **chemotropic molecules**. Cells that release these chemotropic signals can serve as guideposts or beacons to aid the navigation of nearby growth cones.

A particular chemotropic substance might attract growth cones of one type of neuron, have no effect on growth cones of a second type, and repel growth cones of a third class of neuron. The functional effect of a chemotropic molecule depends on the cellular action triggered by the receptor for the molecule in the receiving neurite. Figure 19.15 provides an example of the differential effect of a chemotropic molecule called **semaphorin III** on the growth of neurites of different sensory neurons. The growing neurites of group Ia sensory neurons (mechanoreceptor neurons, including the stretch receptor neurons of stretch reflexes) are insensitive

What is the influence of chemotropic molecules on neurite growth?

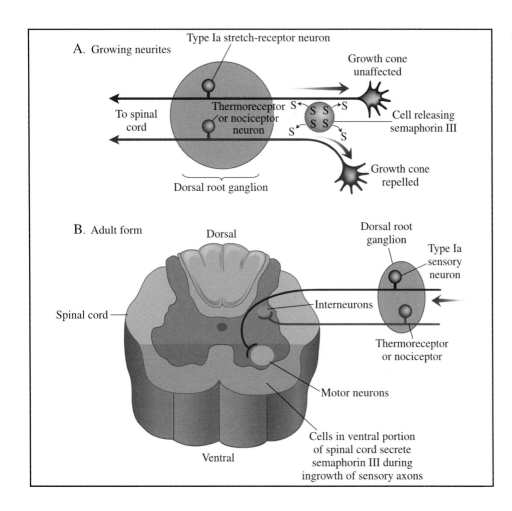

Figure 19.15.

An example of axonal guidance by a chemotropic molecule, semaphorin III. **A.** Growing neurites of thermoreceptor and nociceptor neurons (*red*) are repelled by semaphorin (*S*) and turn away from a cell that secretes the signal molecule. Neurites of group Ia sensory neurons (*green*) are insensitive to semaphorin III and continue to grow straight past the semaphorin-secreting cell. **B.** In the developing spinal cord, cells in the ventral part of the spinal cord secrete semaphorin III at the stage when sensory neurites are growing into the spinal cord. The thermoreceptor and nociceptor neurites are repelled and stay in the dorsal part of the spinal cord, where they synapse onto interneurons. The group Ia sensory neurites continue to grow into the ventral part of the spinal cord and form synapses with motor neurons.

to the semaphorin protein because they lack the membrane receptors that detect semaphorin in the extracellular space. Therefore, growth cones of group Ia neurons pass by semaphore-releasing cells without altering their direction of growth (see Fig. 19.15A). In contrast, semaphorin III repels the neurites of thermoreceptor or nociceptor neurons, which possess semaphorin receptors. As the growth cones of thermoreceptors or nociceptors approach a cell releasing semaphorin III, they change direction, taking the neurite on a path away from the guidepost cell (see Fig. 19.15A).

In the developing spinal cord, the differential effect of semaphorin III on the two types of sensory neurons may help to arrange the projection patterns of the sensory axons, as shown in Figure 19.15B. The stretch receptor axons project directly to the motor neurons of the ventral part of the gray matter in the spinal cord, where they make direct excitatory synaptic connections that underlie the stretch reflex. Nociceptor and thermoreceptor neurons, on the other hand, synapse onto interneurons located in the dorsal part of the gray matter of the spinal cord. At the stage of embryonic development when the axons of the sensory neurons are growing into the spinal cord, cells in the ventral part of the spinal cord secrete semaphorin III. The presence of semaphorin III in the ventral part of the spinal cord repels the growth cones of thermoreceptors and nociceptors but allows the insensitive growth cones of stretch receptor neurons to continue to their motor neuron targets in the ventral part of the gray matter. Although additional cues undoubtedly help direct sensory neurons to their appropriate synaptic targets, semaphorin III helps produce the adult pattern by keeping thermoreceptor and nociceptor growth cones in the dorsal part of the spinal cord.

Semaphorin III is a member of a family of related proteins (the semaphorins) that act as chemotropic signals for the developing nervous system. Another family of chemotropic proteins, the **netrins**, also act as either attractants or repellents, depending on the nature of the receiving growth cone. Little is known about the membrane receptor molecules in the growth cones that detect chemotropic molecules. Chemotropic molecules (and contact-mediated adhesion molecules) affect the direction of growth cone movement by differentially promoting either extension or retraction of filopodia near the location where a signal molecule binds to its membrane receptor. A repellent promotes retraction of filopodia, whereas an attractant promotes extension. Both repellents and attractants affect the assembly and disassembly of the actin filaments responsible for filopodial and lamellipodial movements. The coupling between the activated chemotropic receptors and the actin filaments probably involves intracellular second messengers, including calcium ions and protein kinases, but the exact scheme has not been fully elucidated.

Neurotrophic Factors

What are neurotrophins?

Soluble proteins secreted into the extracellular space during development have additional effects on growing neurons, beyond the steering of growth cones. Certain classes of secreted proteins, called **neurotrophins**, are required for the initiation of neurite outgrowth and even for the survival of neurons. As a result, they are often referred to as **growth factors**. Neurotrophins are secreted by target tissues and detected by specific receptor molecules located on the membranes of the neurons that will ultimately innervate the target.

The first neurotrophin to be discovered is **nerve growth factor** (NGF). If a small piece of dorsal root ganglion or a sympathetic ganglion is placed in a culture dish in a nutrient medium (Fig. 19.16), the neurons in the explanted ganglion attempt to grow neurites. The neurites are feeble, however, and do not extend far from the

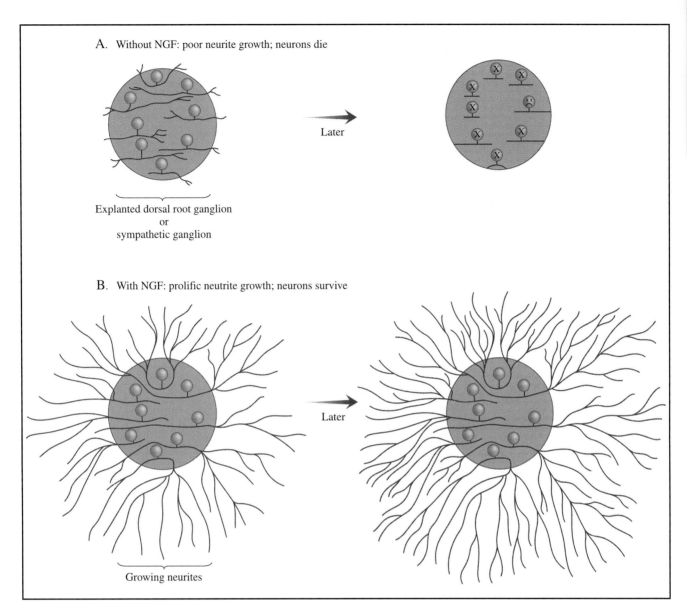

A. Without NGF: poor neurite growth; neurons die

Later

Explanted dorsal root ganglion
or
sympathetic ganglion

B. With NGF: prolific neutrite growth; neurons survive

Later

Growing neurites

Figure 19.16.

Nerve growth factor (NGF) promotes the survival of neurons in cell culture and stimulates neurite outgrowth. **A.** In the absence of NGF, cultured neurons fail to grow neurites and die. **B.** When NGF is added to the culture medium, the neurons survive and grow extensive neurites.

piece of ganglion. Eventually, the neurons in the ganglion die, even though the nutrients in the artificial external medium are sufficient to support the continued survival of other cell types. If NGF is included in the nutrient medium, however, the majority of the neurons in the ganglion survive, and neurite outgrowth is strongly stimulated (see Fig. 19.16B).

In addition to promoting neurite outgrowth and neuronal survival, NGF acts as a chemotropic signal for growth cones. If NGF is provided by a localized source placed to one side of the ganglion, rather than distributed uniformly throughout the medium, the growing neurites orient themselves toward the NGF source. If the source is moved, the growing neurites turn to follow it. NGF is secreted by a variety of target tissues that are normally innervated by sensory neurons of the dorsal root ganglia and by sympathetic neurons. Consequently, NGF may serve multiple roles in stimulating neurite growth, directing incoming growth cones, and promoting the survival of neurons that reach the correct destination.

The early nervous system overproduces neurons. Many more neurons are produced during neurogenesis than are found in the adult nervous system. The missing cells die via a form of cellular suicide called **programmed cell death**, in which "suicide genes" are activated. The products of these genes are proteins that enzymatically attack the cell's vital machinery (including the cellular DNA itself). The developing embryo generates many more neurons than needed, and many of the immature neurons commit suicide. The reason for this overproduction of neurons is uncertain, but it may relate to the difficulty of the wiring task faced by the nervous system. To ensure that sufficient numbers of neurons of each subtype reach their correct targets and form appropriate synaptic connections, perhaps an overabundance of immature neurons is necessary. However, the neurons that die are not only those whose growth cones went astray and failed to reach the proper destination. A substantial number of neurons among the population whose axons contact appropriate target cells often die as well.

Programmed cell death may be the default state for neurons, and neurotrophins like NGF, produced in the target tissue, prevent activation of the programmed death sequence. If the target secretes only enough neurotrophin to support the "correct" number of incoming neurons, the excess cells will die. Experimentally, it is possible to rescue the excess neurons by injecting NGF into embryos, resulting in a higher-than-normal number of neurons in sensory and sympathetic ganglia. Conversely, it is also possible to cause an abnormally high rate of cell death—and reduced numbers of ganglionic neurons—by injecting antibodies that inactivate NGF. These findings demonstrate that neurotrophins do indeed influence neuronal death and survival during development.

Brain-derived neurotrophic factor (BDNF) and **neurotrophin-3 (NT-3)** are two other neurotrophins that are closely related to NGF. NGF, BDNF, and NT-3 have similar amino acid sequences and are encoded by three distinct genes that probably evolved from a common ancestral gene. Therefore, these three neurotrophins are referred to as the NGF family. Different types of neurons have different sensitivities to the three members of the NGF family. For example, group Ia sensory neurons that innervate the muscle spindles are sensitive to NT-3, while nociceptor neurons that innervate the skin are sensitive to NGF. BDNF also promotes the survival of certain classes of sensory neurons. For sympathetic ganglia, however, only NGF is effective, and neither NT-3 nor BDNF supports the survival of sympathetic neurons in culture.

Other neurotrophic proteins, such as **ciliary neurotrophic factor (CNTF)**, are not related to the NGF family. In some cases, growth factors that were first discovered to affect the growth of non-neuronal cells also act as neurotrophins. For instance, **fibroblast growth factor (FGF)** not only induces the proliferation of fibroblasts but also promotes the survival of neurons in both the central and peripheral nervous systems. Like the NGF family, CNTF and FGF differentially affect various neuronal subtypes in different parts of the nervous system.

Nonprotein substances can act as neurotrophic factors as well. **Steroid hormones** affect neuronal growth and differentiation in various parts of the nervous system. Although **corticosteroid hormones** are primarily involved in adrenal gland function, they also affect the development of adrenal chromaffin cells from sympathetic neuron precursors. **Sex steroid hormones** affect sexual differentiation in a variety of tissues, including the parts of the nervous system concerned with the sex organs or sexual behavior. Finally, in insects, steroid hormones (for example, **ecdysone**) play a role in metamorphosis from larval to adult forms. In this process, muscles and motor neurons that are used in the larva but not in the adult die as a result of increased steroid levels during metamorphosis.

Neurotrophin Receptors

Neurotrophin molecules interact with specific receptor molecules that are tuned to detect particular neurotrophins. When the neurotrophin binds to the receptor, the activated receptor molecule in turn sets in motion a series of intracellular events, leading to the complex changes in gene expression required to alter neuronal differentiation and survival. For the NGF family of growth factors, the receptor molecules are members of a family of related transmembrane proteins called **tyrosine receptor kinases** (abbreviated **trk**, which is pronounced "track"). NGF binds to a specific trk called **trkA**, BDNF binds to a different receptor called **trkB**, and NT-3 to **trkC**. The type of trk expressed in a neuron determines the neurotrophins to which the cell will respond during development. Expression of trks may be regulated by genetic and environmental factors and can vary during the course of development, thereby contributing to the specification of neuronal subtype during differentiation.

The binding of NGF to the trkA receptor is shown schematically in Figure 19.17. NGF consists of two identical protein subunits that combine to form a **dimer** (such a dimer formed from two identical subunits is called a **homodimer**). Each NGF subunit binds separately to a single trkA receptor molecule, which brings the two trkA molecules into close proximity. The trkA receptor is a transmembrane molecule, with an extracellular portion that binds NGF and an intracellular portion that generates intracellular signals when the receptor is occupied. The intracellular part of trkA includes a **tyrosine protein kinase** domain that enzymatically attaches phosphate derived from adenosine triphosphate (ATP) onto tyrosine residues in other protein molecules. In the case of the pair of trkA receptors brought together by the binding of NGF, each of the kinase domains phosphorylates the other trkA receptor of the pair (see Fig. 19.17). Phosphorylation activates the trkA receptor and initiates signal cascades that culminate in diverse responses, such as neurite outgrowth and suppression of programmed cell death. The only NGF-dependent step in the activation of the receptor is the formation of the receptor dimer, which allows the two receptor partners of the dimer to phosphorylate and activate each other.

Signal Paths from NGF Receptors to Gene Expression

As might be expected from the diversity of cellular responses evoked by NGF, the activated trkA receptor affects a variety of intracellular signaling mechanisms. The known signaling pathways for trkA are summarized in Figure 19.18. The three major signal systems are indicated by the three branches emanating from the activated receptor at the top of the diagram. The best-understood pathway is that initiated by the G-protein **Ras**. A series of intermediary proteins intervene between the trkA receptor and Ras. The first intermediary is phosphorylated by trkA to start the signal sequence; the last intermediary activates Ras by replacing guanosine diphosphate (GDP) with guanosine triphosphate (GTP), as with other G-proteins. Ras belongs to a different class of G-proteins than the heterotrimeric G-proteins we encountered in sensory systems, however. Heterotrimeric G-proteins are combinations of three different protein subunits. G-proteins like Ras, on the other hand, consist of a single, smaller subunit and hence are called **small G-proteins**. Heterotrimeric G-proteins interact directly with activated receptors, which then catalyze the replacement of GDP by GTP on the alpha-subunit and the dissociation of the activated alpha-subunit from the beta- and gamma-subunits (see, for example, the description of the rhodopsin-transducin interaction in Chapter 15). In contrast, Ras and other small G-proteins are activated by **GTP exchange factors**,

Figure 19.17.

A schematic diagram of the interaction of nerve growth factor (NGF) with its receptor molecule. **A**. NGF consists of two identical protein subunits, each of which binds to a molecule of the NGF receptor, trkA. **B**. An intracellular portion (*purple*) of the trkA receptor molecule acts as a tyrosine kinase enzyme. The kinase attaches phosphate groups to tyrosine in proteins, including trkA itself. NGF binding brings two trkA receptors into close proximity, and the receptor molecules phosphorylate each other (*arrows*). The phosphorylated receptor is activated and then can trigger other signal cascades.

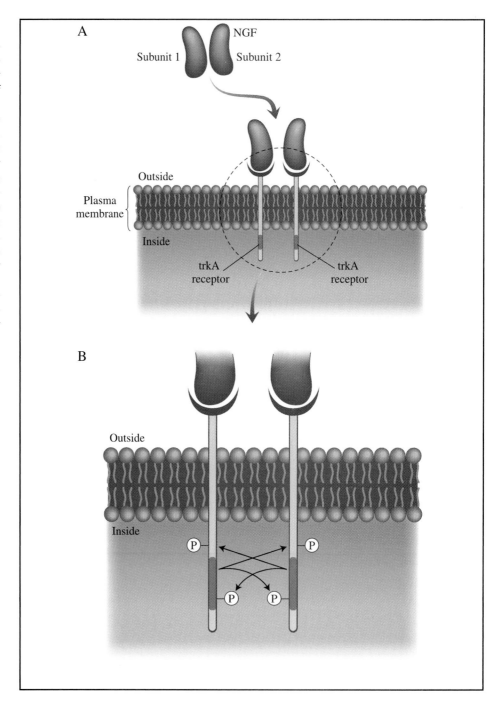

which are proteins that are not receptors. In the case of Ras activation by trkA receptors, the GTP exchange factor is the third of a series of three intermediary proteins that are recruited in sequence to carry the signal from the receptor to the G-protein.

The primary target of the Ras-dependent NGF signal cascade is gene expression in the nucleus of the neuron. Ras, like trkA, is a plasma membrane protein, and its activation is signaled to the cell nucleus via diffusible messengers. As shown in Figure 19.18, the first step in this stage of NGF signaling is the activation of a protein kinase called **Raf** by Ras. Raf triggers a cascade of kinase activation that involves a series of distinct protein kinase subtypes, each of which phosphorylates and activates the next kinase in the sequence. The final step is thought to be the activation

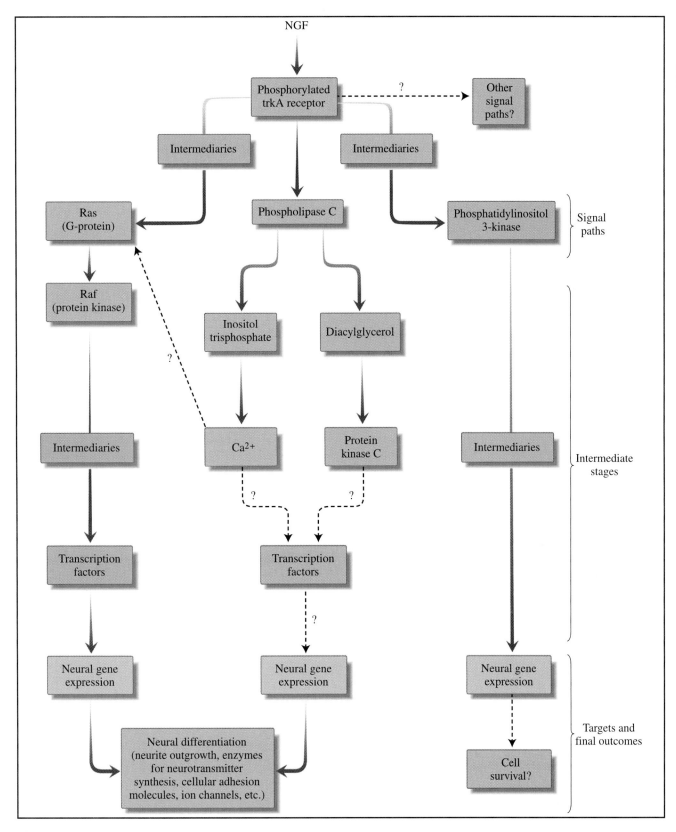

Figure 19.18.

Three signal cascades triggered by the activated trkA receptor. See text for a full description. NGF = nerve growth factor.

of **mitogen-activated protein kinase** (**MAPK**), which penetrates into the nucleus and phosphorylates transcription factors that control gene expression. The phosphorylated transcription factors bind to the regulatory regions on the DNA that initiate the transcription of a set of genes called **immediate early genes**. The proteins produced from the immediate early genes are transcription factors that in turn induce expression of a variety of neural genes required for neuronal differentiation (see Fig. 19.18).

The other two pathways leading from trkA receptors to neural gene expression (see Fig. 19.18) are not as thoroughly characterized as the Ras-initiated pathway. One involves direct interaction between the trkA receptor and an enzyme called **phospholipase C**. Phosphorylated trkA receptors activate the enzyme, which acts on phospholipid molecules in the plasma membrane to release the intracellular messenger molecules **inositol trisphosphate** and **diacylglycerol**. These dual messengers operate in parallel—inositol trisphosphate increases the intracellular calcium concentration, while diacylglycerol activates a protein kinase called **protein kinase C**. Both calcium and protein kinase C can alter gene expression by indirectly affecting transcription factors. The third pathway, shown in Figure 19.18, involves the activation by trkA of another protein kinase, **phosphatidylinositol 3-kinase**, which targets genes that suppress cell death and promote cell survival.

The intracellular signaling systems activated by NGF are complicated, as expected for the intricate task of activating a wide variety of genes in the proper sequence to produce a functional neuron. Our discussion has focused on only one type of neurotrophin receptor, the trkA receptor. The other members of the trk receptor family also activate multiple signal paths. Other neurotrophic factors, such as CNTF, activate non-trk receptors that generate equally complex internal signals leading from the receptor to the genome. Unraveling these molecular signals will keep molecular neurobiologists busy for many years to come.

BOX 1

IN THE CLINIC

Damage to the adult nervous system is usually irreversible, partly because adult neurons are incapable of undergoing cell division, and so neurons lost to disease or accident cannot be replaced. For this reason, there is currently great interest in neurotrophic factors such as brain-derived neurotrophic factor as a means to induce growth and regeneration of damaged neural pathways. Knowledge of neuronal growth factors and their cellular actions is of potentially great benefit to the restoration of neural function. Nevertheless, molecular studies on the development of the nervous system teach us that successful restoration of function requires more than just the generation of new neurons and the induction of neurite outgrowth. During development, neurites travel great distances in the nervous system and connect with diverse targets, and successful neural function requires that these connections must be reproduced after damage to the intervening tissue. Successful navigation of growing neurites requires a variety of signposts and beacons that guide the neurites along the correct path. Unfortunately, many of these molecular guides are expressed only transiently during embryonic development and are absent in adults. Restoration of a functional neural circuit, then, requires recapitulation of a complex developmental sequence.

SYNAPSE FORMATION

At this point, we have examined some of the mechanisms by which nerve cells are generated and then grow axons to appropriate targets, sometimes over long distances. Once the axon reaches the target, it must form synaptic connections. In this section we will examine the stages involved in forming a synapse at the contact point between the ingrowing axon and the target cell. As an example, we will consider the neuromuscular junction. Recall from Chapter 5 that the synaptic terminals of motor neurons release the neurotransmitter acetylcholine (ACh) at the vertebrate neuromuscular junction. ACh depolarizes the muscle cell by binding to and opening ACh receptors, which are nonspecific cation channels in the membrane of the muscle cell. The ACh receptors are clustered at the end-plate of the muscle cell, just opposite the site of ACh release from the motor nerve terminal. We will now examine how this specialized synaptic contact arises during embryonic development, as the motor neuron axons grow out from the developing spinal cord and contact the embryonic muscle.

What mechanisms lead to the formation of a synapse?

Stages of Synapse Formation at the Neuromuscular Junction

Figure 19.19 presents an overview of the important stages in the development of the mammalian neuromuscular junction. When the growth cones of motor neurons reach the muscle, the muscle cells are still in a primitive form. Even at this early stage, the muscle cells produce ACh receptors, but the receptors are inserted throughout the membrane instead of being concentrated at the end-plate region. When an advancing growth cone contacts a muscle cell, forward movement and filopodial extensions halt, and the tip of the neurite begins to convert from a growth cone to a synaptic terminal. The recognition signal that triggers this conversion from motile machinery to synaptic machinery has not been identified, but it presumably involves interactions between cell adhesion molecules like those that guide movements during neurite outgrowth.

At this developmental stage, more than one neuronal growth cone contacts each muscle cell, and each growth cone begins to form a functional synaptic connection. As development proceeds, the multiple synaptic contacts from different motor neurons are eliminated, leaving the mature muscle cell with only a single synaptic contact from one motor neuron. Overproduction of synapses is commonly observed during the initial stages of synapse formation throughout the nervous system. Eventually, the excess synapses are eliminated through a combination of programmed cell death and axon branch pruning, in which the surviving neurons retract some of their branches and contact fewer postsynaptic target cells. The immature neurons evidently compete for a limited number of postsynaptic target sites (one per muscle cell in the case of the neuromuscular junction). The mechanism by which the outcome of this competition is decided is not understood.

As the synaptic connection between the motor neuron and the muscle cell consolidates, ACh receptors cluster at a high density in the membrane of the postsynaptic muscle cell at the point of contact (see Fig. 19.19). At the same time, the number of ACh receptors in the nonsynaptic portions of the muscle cell begins to decline. The clustering of receptors at the end-plate occurs for two reasons: newly synthesized receptor molecules are inserted preferentially at the nerve contact, and previously synthesized receptors migrate to the end-plate. In the adult muscle, very few ACh receptors are found outside the end-plate region, and the receptor density at the point of nerve contact is very high. When the terminal of the incoming motor neuron contacts the muscle cell, the rate at which new ACh receptors

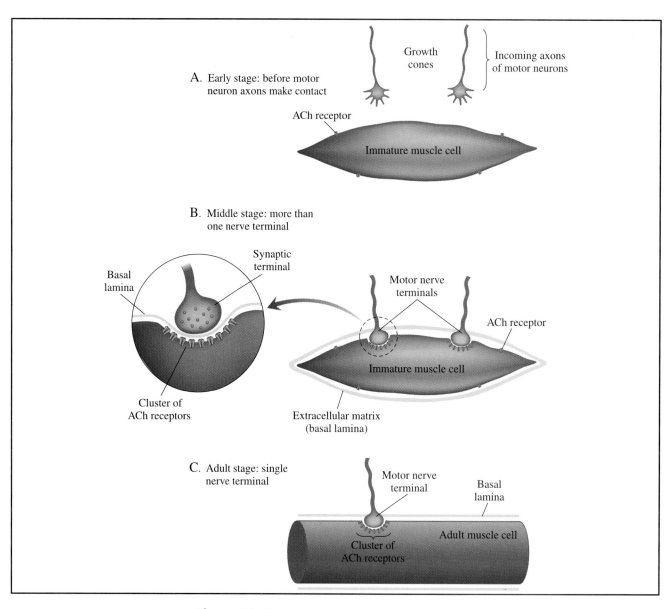

A. Early stage: before motor neuron axons make contact

Growth cones

Incoming axons of motor neurons

ACh receptor

Immature muscle cell

B. Middle stage: more than one nerve terminal

Basal lamina

Synaptic terminal

Motor nerve terminals

ACh receptor

Immature muscle cell

Cluster of ACh receptors

Extracellular matrix (basal lamina)

C. Adult stage: single nerve terminal

Motor nerve terminal

Basal lamina

Cluster of ACh receptors

Adult muscle cell

Figure 19.19.

The stages of synapse formation at the neuromuscular junction. **A.** The growth cones of motor neurons enter the immature muscle. **B.** The growth cones stop when they encounter muscle cells and begin to transform into synaptic terminals. The contact of the nerve terminal induces clustering of acetylcholine (ACh) receptors in the muscle cell at the site of contact. Muscle cells typically receive inputs from more than one synaptic terminal at this stage. **C.** The adult muscle cell receives only a single synaptic input, and the ACh receptors are present almost exclusively at the end-plate region of the muscle cell.

are synthesized increases in the muscle cell, providing the large numbers of receptor molecules needed to achieve the high density in the adult end-plate.

The muscle cell also secretes acetylcholinesterase (the degradative enzyme responsible for terminating the action of released ACh; see Chapter 5) into the developing synaptic cleft. The acetylcholinesterase molecules bind to the extracellular matrix in the cleft, which keeps the enzyme anchored in the proper spot in the extracellular space. The extracellular matrix encasing the muscle cell and synaptic terminal is known as the **basal lamina**, and at the synaptic cleft it contains components that are produced and secreted by both the muscle cell and the motor neuron terminal.

Cell-Cell Communication at the Neuromuscular Junction: Receptor Clustering

The ability of the nerve contact to induce changes in the muscle cell, including increased synthesis and clustering of ACh receptors, implies that some signal is sent from the nerve to the postsynaptic muscle cell. We will consider receptor clustering first, before describing the stimulation of receptor synthesis.

The clustering of receptors is triggered by a protein called **agrin**, which is manufactured by the motor neuron and secreted into the synaptic cleft, where it is incorporated into the basal lamina. As shown in Figure 19.20, agrin interacts with a special receptor molecule called **dystroglycan**, located in the membrane of the postsynaptic muscle cell. Dystroglycan is a transmembrane glycoprotein that connects on the intracellular face of the membrane to the cytoskeleton of the muscle cell, via a linking protein called **dystrophin**. The dystroglycan-dystrophin complex

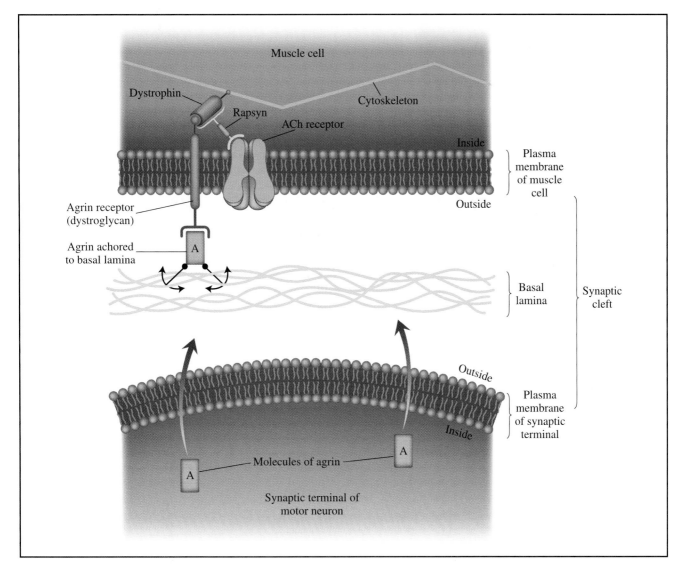

Figure 19.20.

The extracellular protein agrin anchors acetylcholine (ACh) receptors at the end-plate. Agrin is secreted by the motor nerve terminal and incorporated into the extracellular matrix in the synaptic cleft. The coupling to the ACh receptor molecule is accomplished via a series of three linking proteins: dystroglycan, dystrophin, and rapsyn. Dystrophin is also connected to the cytoskeleton of the muscle cell.

also serves as a binding site for another linking protein, **rapsyn**, which also binds to ACh receptors (see Fig. 19.20). Thus, this interconnected set of proteins tethers the ACh receptors to the cytoskeleton of the muscle cell on the one hand and to the basal lamina in the synaptic cleft on the other. Because the anchored ACh receptors can no longer move away from the end-plate, receptors accumulate at the end-plate as more and more are captured at the critical site. In addition, evidence suggests that agrin triggers phosphorylation of the ACh receptor by activating a tyrosine kinase in the muscle cell. The role played by this phosphorylation of the ACh receptor remains unclear, however.

Cell-Cell Communication at the Neuromuscular Junction: Receptor Synthesis

We will now turn to the increased synthesis of ACh receptors in the muscle cell induced by contact with the motor nerve. Muscle cells (**myocytes**) are long, thin cells that extend for the entire length of the muscle. Myocytes arise during development through the fusion of many, smaller precursor cells (**myoblasts**). Thus, a muscle cell contains many nuclei, one for each of the myoblasts that fused to produce the muscle cell (Fig. 19.21). Each nucleus contains DNA and the machinery for gene regulation and gene transcription; thus, each nucleus can produce messenger RNA (mRNA) and direct protein synthesis. At early developmental stages, after the formation of myocytes but before nerve contact, all of the nuclei produce mRNA coding for the subunits of the ACh receptor (albeit at a low rate). During this period, ACh receptors are distributed uniformly throughout the surface of the muscle cell.

When the synaptic terminals of the motor neurons begin to form on the muscle, two changes, which are summarized in Figure 19.21, take place. First, the onset of nerve-triggered electrical activity in the muscle cell globally *inhibits* the production of mRNA for ACh receptors in the myocyte. Second, a trophic factor released from the nerve terminals *stimulates* the production of mRNA for ACh receptors in nuclei near the point of contact, locally overriding the global inhibitory effect of electrical activity.

The global inhibitory effect arises as a by-product of the initiation of normal synaptic transmission at the forming neuromuscular junctions. As synaptic terminals form, the agrin-anchoring mechanism causes preexisting ACh receptors to cluster at the points of nerve contact. As receptors accumulate, ACh released from the newly formed nerve terminal in response to action potential activity in the motor neuron depolarizes the muscle fiber, stimulating action potentials in the muscle cell. The onset of electrical activity of the muscle inhibits the further production of ACh receptor mRNA in the chain of nuclei throughout the muscle cell (see Fig. 19.21C).

The synthesis of ACh receptors is stimulated locally in nuclei near the developing neuromuscular junction by a protein called **ARIA** (*acetylcholine receptor inducing activity*), which is released from the synaptic terminal. ARIA combines with a postsynaptic trk and activates tyrosine phosphorylation of other intracellular signaling molecules, in a manner analogous to the action of NGF described earlier. In this case, the trk activation initiates a signal cascade that culminates in the expression of ACh receptor genes. The signal evidently has only a limited spatial spread within the muscle cell, because the activation of ACh receptor synthesis remains spatially restricted to the point of nerve contact (see Fig. 19.21C). The combination of the electrically mediated inhibition of ACh receptor synthesis in nuclei outside the end-plate and ARIA-stimulated synthesis of ACh receptors at the end-plate ensures that newly made receptor molecules are inserted into the plasma membrane where they will be needed—at the developing end-plate region.

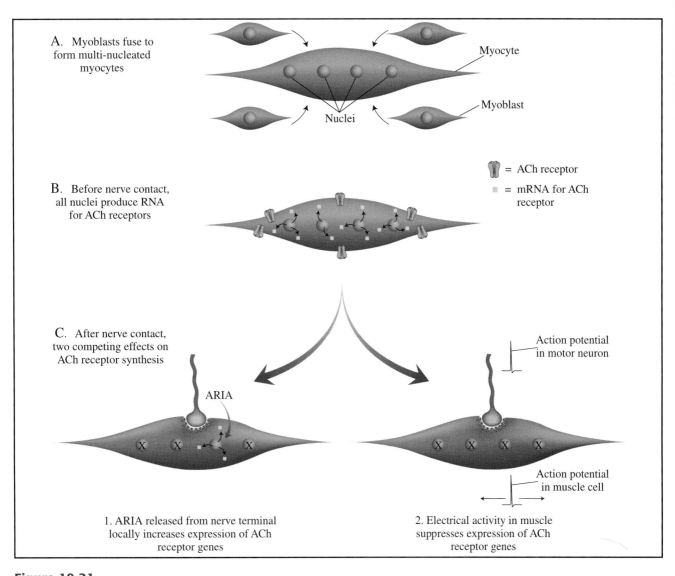

A. Myoblasts fuse to form multi-nucleated myocytes

Myocyte

Myoblast

Nuclei

= ACh receptor

= mRNA for ACh receptor

B. Before nerve contact, all nuclei produce RNA for ACh receptors

C. After nerve contact, two competing effects on ACh receptor synthesis

ARIA

Action potential in motor neuron

Action potential in muscle cell

1. ARIA released from nerve terminal locally increases expression of ACh receptor genes

2. Electrical activity in muscle suppresses expression of ACh receptor genes

Figure 19.21.

The stages in the modulation of acetylcholine (ACh) receptor synthesis in the muscle cell by the motor neuron synaptic terminal. **A.** Muscle cells (myocytes) form by the fusion of precursor cells (myoblasts). **B.** In the fused myocytes, all nuclei produce messenger RNA (mRNA) for ACh receptor proteins. **C.** Contact with the nerve influences the production of mRNA for ACh receptor in two ways. Action potentials (induced in the muscle cell by the activity of the motor neuron) inhibit the expression of the ACh receptor genes (*right diagram*). The trophic substance ARIA (acetylcholine receptor inducing activity), which is released from the synaptic terminal of the motor neuron, activates an intracellular signal cascade that locally stimulates the production of mRNA for ACh receptor subunits in nuclei near the point of nerve contact (*left diagram*).

Cell-Cell Communication at the Neuromuscular Junction: Muscle-to-Nerve Signaling

So far, we have concentrated on signal molecules—agrin and ARIA—that are released by the presynaptic nerve terminal and act on the postsynaptic muscle cell. For effective synapse formation, however, signals also must be generated by the muscle that affects the ingrowing motor axons. For example, a "stop sign" must exist that halts the motor neuron growth cone at the muscle cell and induces formation of a neuromuscular synapse. One candidate for this molecular stop sign is a special form of laminin, **s-laminin**, which is manufactured by the muscle cell and secreted into the developing synaptic cleft. In the extracellular space, the secreted s-laminin incorporates into the basal lamina in the synaptic cleft. Like other cell adhesion molecules, s-laminin promotes adhesion of the motor neuron's neurite to the extracellular matrix. In addition, s-laminin inhibits neurite outgrowth, even in the presence of other adhesion molecules that stimulate outgrowth. S-laminin effectively freezes the growth cone at the point of contact with the muscle fiber, even though the surrounding environment supports growth (a necessity, because the growth must traverse that surrounding environment in order to reach its contact point with the muscle).

Once agrin and s-laminin become part of the basal lamina in the synaptic cleft, neither the nerve terminal nor the muscle cell is required to maintain the signal activity of the extracellular matrix. This fact was demonstrated in experiments like those shown in Figure 19.22. In adult frog muscle, it is possible to destroy both the

Figure 19.22.

The extracellular matrix (the basal lamina) is important for the clustering of postsynaptic acetylcholine (ACh) receptors and for localization of the synaptic terminal of the motor neuron. **A.** In the adult form of the neuromuscular junction (*upper diagram*), the basal lamina (*yellow*) forms a sheath around each muscle fiber. The basal lamina within the synaptic cleft (*pink*) incorporates special molecular components that mediate the clustering of ACh receptors and localize the nerve terminal to the correct spot. If the nerve is cut and the muscle is crushed, both the motor nerve in the muscle and the muscle cells will degenerate, leaving an empty sheath of basal lamina. **B.** The nerve is allowed to regrow, but regeneration of the muscle cells is prevented. The growth cones of the regenerating axons return and form new synaptic terminals at the old location of the end-plate, even though the muscle cell is absent and the target position is marked only by the basal lamina. **C.** The muscle cells are allowed to regenerate, but regeneration of the nerve is prevented. The muscle cells refill the basal lamina sheaths, and ACh receptors cluster at the site of the previous synaptic terminal, which is now absent.

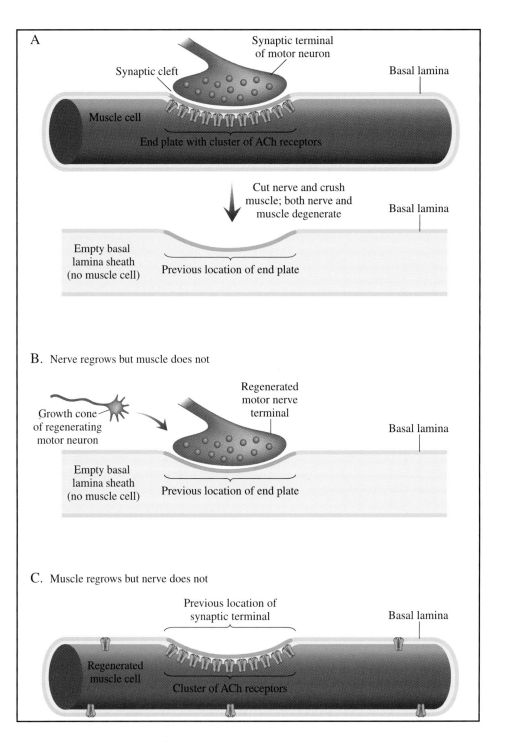

nerve and the muscle cells and then allow the muscle cells, the nerve axons, or both to regenerate. The basal lamina remains intact when the cells are destroyed, leaving behind an empty sheath of extracellular matrix (see Fig. 19.22A). When the nerve is allowed to regrow but regeneration of the muscle cells is prevented, the incoming motor axons stop growing and form presynaptic terminals at the synaptic locations that were previously occupied by the destroyed terminals, even though the muscle cell is now absent (see Fig. 19.22B). The re-formation of the synaptic terminal at the old location reflects the fact that s-laminin—previously incorporated into the basal lamina at the synaptic cleft by the now-defunct muscle cell—remains in place. When the muscle, but not the nerve, is allowed to regenerate, the new muscle cells refill the previous basal lamina. ACh receptors accumulate at the old synaptic site, even though the nerve is no longer present, because agrin remains in the basal lamina at the previous synaptic cleft and is still able to tether ACh receptors. These experiments underscore the importance of the extracellular matrix in synapse formation.

SUMMARY

The nervous system develops from embryonic ectodermal cells, which are induced to form the neural plate during the process of gastrulation. Neural induction is stimulated by a part of the mesoderm, the notochord, which lies beneath the dorsal portion of the ectoderm that will become the nervous system. As development proceeds, the cells of the neural plate proliferate and form a groove along the midline of the embryo (the neural groove); the edges of the neural groove then fuse to create the neural tube. The margins of the neural groove left behind during fusion form the neural crest, which generates the cells of the peripheral nervous system. The neural tube becomes the spinal cord and brain. Neurons are produced by the division of precursor cells located at the innermost edge of the neural tube, the ventricular zone. The newly born neurons then migrate to assume their final positions within the growing three-dimensional structure of the brain and spinal cord. Neurons born in the neural crest also migrate to the adult positions of the peripheral ganglia within the body.

As neurons of a particular type mature, neuronal genes are activated in sequence, specifying the characteristics of that cell type in increasingly finer detail. An important aspect of cell type specification is the determination of the classes of cell adhesion molecules expressed by the immature neuron. Cell adhesion molecules are used for cell-to-cell recognition and cell-substrate interactions during migration and during the growth of axons and dendrites (collectively called neurites). The tip of a growing neurite forms a growth cone, a motile structure responsible for moving the extending neurite along the proper path, guided by molecular guideposts found on cells and in the extracellular matrix. In addition to cell adhesion molecules, chemotropic molecules act as diffusible messengers that either attract or repel growth cones.

Neurotrophic factors are secreted by various neural and non-neural cells and influence the survival and growth of neurons. The best-studied example of a neurotrophin is the protein NGF. NGF is detected by specific neurotrophin receptor molecules in the membrane of the receptive neuron. The NGF receptor is a member of a family of receptors called trks. The activated receptor is a kinase that phosphorylates tyrosine residues on a variety of cellular target proteins. The phosphorylated target proteins serve as internal signals that initiate a series of events leading to the expression of genes appropriate for growth and for the development of neuronal characteristics.

SUMMARY

The formation of a synapse involves signals that are sent and received by both the presynaptic cell and the postsynaptic cell. At the neuromuscular junction, the contact of the growth cone with the immature muscle cell induces clustering of ACh receptors in the muscle cell membrane at the point of nerve contact. In addition, nerve contact increases the rate at which the muscle cell synthesizes ACh receptors. These effects are mediated via two molecular signal proteins, agrin and ARIA, that are secreted by the nerve terminal into the developing synaptic cleft. The muscle cell secretes a special form of an extracellular matrix molecule called s-laminin into the cleft, which acts as a stop signal for motor neuron growth cones.

REVIEW QUESTIONS

1. Identify the Spemann organizer and describe its role in development.
2. Briefly describe suppressor and inducer mechanisms for neural development and give specific examples of molecular mechanisms.
3. Identify the following: notochord, neural plate, neural tube, neural crest.
4. Describe the steps in the development of Purkinje cells in the cerebellar cortex.
5. What mechanisms underlie the motility of growth cones?
6. List the four families of cellular adhesion molecules.
7. What are the main molecular components of the extracellular matrix?
8. Provide an example of a chemotropic molecule that affects the direction of neurite growth.
9. Describe how NGF activates its receptor.
10. Identify the role of each of the following in synapse formation at the neuromuscular junction: agrin, ARIA, s-laminin, dystrophin, dystroglycan, rapsyn.

INTERNET ASSIGNMENT   CHAPTER 19

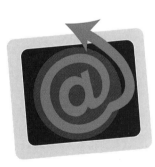

Growth cones are the motile ends of growing neurites. Find images, movies, and other information about growth cones and how they move. In the images you find, identify the filopodia and lamellipodia.

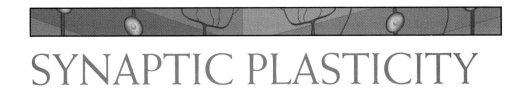

SYNAPTIC PLASTICITY

Animals alter their behavior based on experience. Even animals with simple nervous systems can learn to associate previously neutral sensory stimuli with biologically significant events, learning to avoid situations signifying danger and to approach stimuli associated with reward. These behavioral changes are the external manifestations of underlying changes in the neural systems that control the behavior. Thus, the nervous system is capable of changing the strength of synaptic connections—perhaps even breaking and making synaptic contacts among neurons—based on past experi-

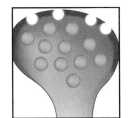

ence. The outcome of this learning process lasts for a long time (decades in some cases).

How does the nervous system modify itself to produce learning and memory? Few answers to this question have been found, partly because the basic circuit underlying a particular behavior must be understood before it is possible to identify the changes in the circuit accompanying learning. This understanding has been reached in very few instances, and then only for simple types of behaviors such as reflexes. We normally envision reflexes as being fixed patterns of behavior, determined by the fixed wiring of simple combinations of neurons. In many cases, however, reflexes are adaptable on the basis of experience and show changes attributable to learning and memory. We will discuss two examples of modifiable reflexes later in this chapter.

In the first part of this chapter, we will describe some simpler changes that occur in the strength of synaptic connections among neurons. In several cases, cellular mechanisms have been discovered that underlie time-dependent changes in the strength of synaptic connections among neurons. Although these synaptic modifications cannot account for all aspects of learning and memory, they do suggest ways that changes in synaptic efficacy can be accomplished in the nervous system.

SHORT-TERM CHANGES IN SYNAPTIC STRENGTH

Synaptic Enhancement

What are the differences between the different forms of short-term synaptic plasticity: facilitation, augmentation, and potentiation?

Neurons tend to fire action potentials in bursts. When a series of action potentials closely spaced in time arrive at a single synaptic terminal, the postsynaptic effects of each successive action potential will add together, producing temporal summation (see Chapter 8). In some cases, each action potential in the series releases the same amount of neurotransmitter, which produces linear summation of the postsynaptic potentials (see Fig. 20.1A). More often, however, the amount of neurotransmitter released by each action potential changes progressively during a burst of presynaptic action potentials. Thus, presynaptic action potentials leave an aftereffect that alters the release of neurotransmitter in response to subsequent action potentials. If the aftereffect *increases* the amount of neurotransmitter released by successive action potentials, it is referred to as **synaptic enhancement** (see Fig. 20.1B). Conversely, if the aftereffect *depresses* the release by subsequent action potentials, it is referred to as **synaptic depression** (see Fig. 20.1C).

Neurobiologists distinguish among different types of activity-dependent changes in synaptic efficacy, based on how long the effect persists and how many presynaptic action potentials are required to elicit the effect. The most rapid type of synaptic enhancement, called **synaptic facilitation**, can be observed after a single action potential, but the enhancement lasts only tens or hundreds of milliseconds. Figure 20.2A shows the rapid time course of facilitation, which decays within a second or less.

In a longer-lasting form of synaptic enhancement, called **synaptic augmentation**, the amount of neurotransmitter released by a single test action potential is increased for a period of several seconds. Augmentation does not occur after a single action potential or even a train of several action potentials. Instead, augmentation requires that the presynaptic neuron fire several hundred action potentials within a few seconds, as shown in Figure 20.2B.

If a presynaptic neuron continues to fire action potentials at a high rate for a minute or more, an even longer-lasting form of synaptic enhancement, called **potentiation**, is sometimes observed. Potentiation persists for several minutes after the train of action potentials (see Fig. 20.2C). This type of enhancement was first described at the neuromuscular junction, where prolonged trains of action potentials cause a sustained contraction of the muscle called **tetanus** (see Chapter 7). By analogy, a sustained burst of action potentials fired at a high rate in any neuron (not just in motor neurons) is also called a tetanus. For this reason, potentiation following a sustained, high-frequency burst of action potentials is sometimes referred to as **post-tetanic potentiation**.

All the forms of short-term synaptic enhancement—facilitation, augmentation, and potentiation—are thought to be triggered by the buildup of intracellular calcium inside the presynaptic terminal during action potential activity. Recall from

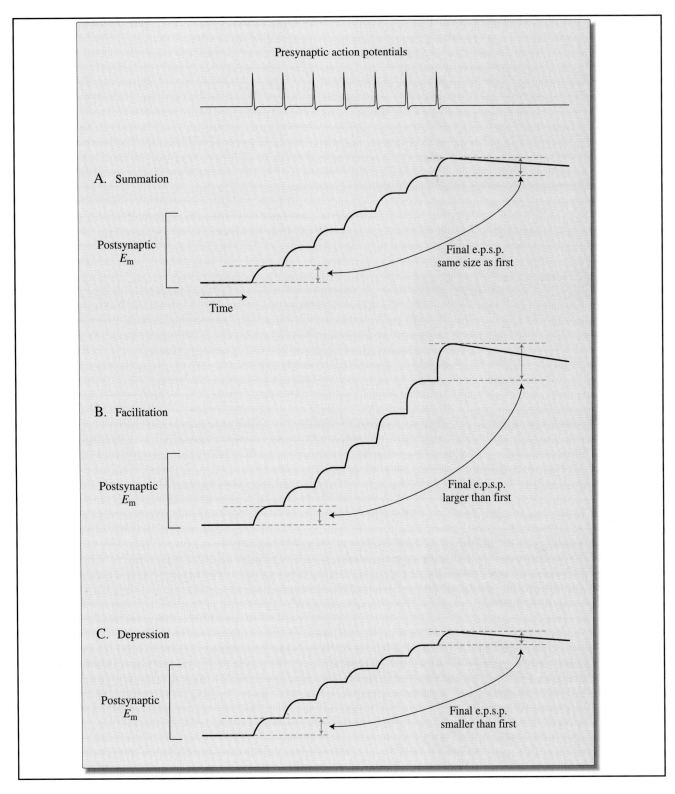

Figure 20.1.

Postsynaptic responses to a burst of presynaptic action potentials, which are shown in the *top trace.* **A.** Each excitatory postsynaptic potential (e.p.s.p.) has the same amplitude, and the postsynaptic response shows simple temporal summation. **B.** In synaptic facilitation, the postsynaptic responses become progressively larger during the burst of presynaptic action potentials. **C.** In synaptic depression, the postsynaptic responses become progressively smaller during the burst of presynaptic action potentials.

Figure 20.2.

Three different forms of synaptic enhancement. Each graph plots the amplitude of the excitatory postsynaptic potential (e.p.s.p.) elicited in a postsynaptic neuron by a single presynaptic action potential. At the time indicated by the *bar* below each graph, a burst of presynaptic action potentials was given to activate synaptic enhancement. The amplitude of the e.p.s.p. is expressed as percentage of the pre-enhancement baseline amplitude. **A**. Facilitation is triggered by a small number of action potentials and lasts for a second or less. **B**. Augmentation is triggered by a longer burst of action potentials and lasts for a few seconds. **C**. Potentiation lasts several minutes after a prolonged burst of presynaptic action potentials.

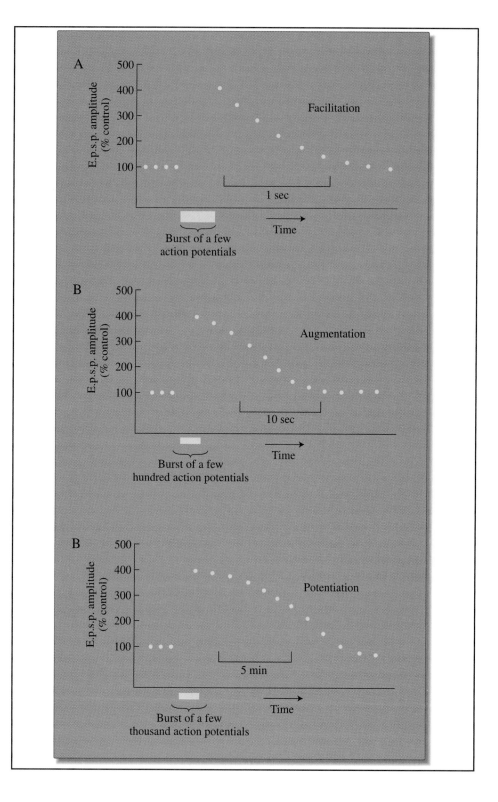

Chapter 5 that neurotransmitter release from the synaptic terminal is initiated by the influx of calcium ions through voltage-dependent calcium channels. The calcium ions that enter the terminal during an action potential are removed by calcium pumps, which restore the intracellular calcium concentration to its normal low level. If a second action potential arrives while some calcium remains from a prior action potential, the calcium ions that enter during the second spike add to the residual calcium, causing calcium ions to accumulate inside the terminal. The time course of removal of this calcium buildup correlates well with the time course of enhanced transmitter release during facilitation, augmentation, and potentiation.

Figure 20.3 shows a schematic diagram of this "residual calcium" model of synaptic enhancement. Calcium ions that enter during an action potential directly trigger the fusion of synaptic vesicles with the plasma membrane. In addition, calcium ions initiate biochemical events that potentiate the release of transmitter during subsequent action potentials. Although the identity of these biochemical events remains unknown, their activity persists—and neurotransmitter release is enhanced—as long as the calcium level remains elevated after a series of action potentials.

The synaptic enhancement just described tends to make synapses more effective if the presynaptic neuron has recently undergone intense activity. Thus, if a postsynaptic neuron receives inputs from a variety of presynaptic cells, the presynaptic cells that have recently fired most intensely will have the greatest weight in determining the activity of the postsynaptic cell. The synaptic influence changes on a scale of seconds or minutes, depending on the level of activity in the presynaptic cell. As a result, neurons within a neural circuit "pay attention to" the presynaptic cells that have been most active in the recent past and thus are most involved in whatever aspect of behavior the organism is engaged in at the moment.

Synaptic Depression

Although enhancement of synaptic efficacy during sustained activity may be desirable in some circumstances, it may be detrimental in other situations. For example, in sensory systems, the nervous system is often more interested in changes in stimulus conditions and less interested in the constant aspects of the environment. Thus, presynaptic inputs that have been most active in the recent past may receive *less* weight in determining the response of postsynaptic cells. This goal can be

What mechanisms can cause short-term depression of neurotransmitter release?

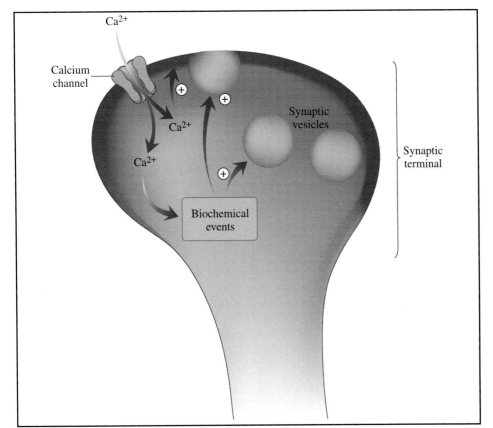

Figure 20.3.

Calcium ions accumulate inside the presynaptic terminal during a burst of action potentials. The depolarization produced by the action potential opens voltage-dependent calcium channels, allowing calcium to enter the terminal. In addition to directly stimulating vesicle fusion, the accumulation of calcium activates biochemical events that potentiate the fusion of synaptic vesicles triggered by subsequent action potentials.

achieved by synaptic depression (see Fig. 20.1), in which the amount of neuro-transmitter released by a single action potential decreases with time during sustained firing. In this way, the greatest amount of transmitter release—and hence the greatest postsynaptic response—will occur at the onset of a burst of action potentials.

Three possible mechanisms for synaptic depression are illustrated in Figure 20.4. In many synaptic terminals, especially in the central nervous system, only a limited pool of synaptic vesicles is available for rapid release during action potential activity. During a series of presynaptic action potentials, this vesicle pool may be depleted faster than it can be replenished, causing the amount of released neurotransmitter to decline with time (see Fig. 20.4A). Other possible mechanisms for synaptic depression are based on the accumulation of calcium ions within the presynaptic terminal, as described for synaptic enhancement. In synaptic depression, the targets for accumulated calcium are different, however, as shown in Figure 20.4B. Accumulation of calcium ions can cause voltage-dependent calcium channels to close, as described for calcium channels in cardiac-muscle cells in Chapter 11. Calcium-dependent inactivation of calcium channels reduces the amount of calcium entering during an action potential, which reduces the amount of neurotransmitter released. Intracellular calcium ions also open calcium-activated potassium channels (see Chapter 4). When calcium accumulates inside the presynaptic terminal, calcium-activated potassium channels hyperpolarize the terminal and promote rapid repolarization following an action potential. These actions also reduce the amount of calcium entry during an action potential and decrease the amount of neurotransmitter released.

Feedback mechanisms also are thought to play a role in synaptic depression (see Fig. 20.4C). The neurotransmitter released by previous action potentials feeds back, either directly or indirectly, onto the releasing terminal and influences the release of transmitter by subsequent action potentials. Indirect feedback can occur via presynaptic inhibition (see Chapter 6). Direct feedback occurs via **autoreceptors** in the plasma membrane of the presynaptic terminal. Autoreceptors are activated by neurotransmitter released from the synaptic terminal on which they are located. Because they are usually located in parts of the synaptic terminal at a distance from the synaptic cleft (see Fig. 20.4C), autoreceptors are activated only when enough neurotransmitter is released to spill out of the synaptic cleft and reach the surrounding parts of the extracellular space. Autoreceptors are usually members of the G-protein–coupled family of receptors, linked indirectly to ion channels via intracellular second messengers. In some cases, the activated autoreceptors reduce neurotransmitter release by closing calcium channels, which reduces the amount of calcium entering during a presynaptic action potential. In other cases, they are linked to the opening of potassium channels, which hyperpolarizes the terminal and speeds repolarization during a presynaptic action potential.

LONG-TERM CHANGES IN SYNAPTIC STRENGTH

Long-Term Potentiation

What is LTP?

Short-term changes in synaptic strength produce an activity-dependent increase or decrease in the presynaptic release of neurotransmitters on a time scale of seconds to minutes after a burst of activity. In addition, neuronal activity can lead to longer-term aftereffects that alter the release of neurotransmitters on a time scale of hours or days. Such long-lasting changes require cellular mechanisms different from those that underlie short-term synaptic enhancement and depression. In this section, we will examine a particularly well-studied example of these long-term

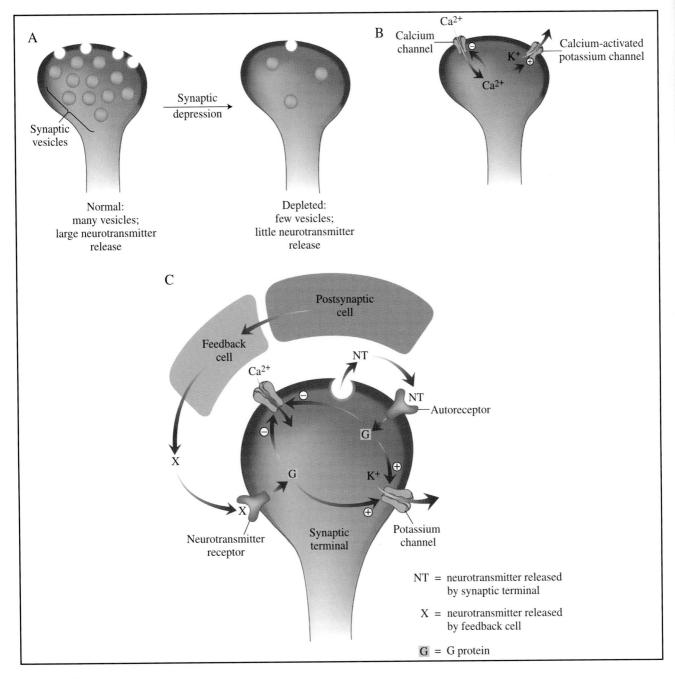

Figure 20.4.

Three mechanisms for synaptic depression. **A**. After repetitive presynaptic action potentials, the pool of releasable synaptic vesicles can become depleted, leaving fewer vesicles available to respond to subsequent action potentials. **B**. Accumulation of calcium ions inside the terminal can inactivate calcium channels (*negative sign*) or activate calcium-sensitive potassium channels (*plus sign*). **C**. The neurotransmitter molecules (*NT*) released by a synaptic terminal bind to autoreceptors on the surface of the terminal. The activated autoreceptors then activate G-proteins (*G*), leading to the closure of voltage-dependent calcium channels (*negative sign*) or the opening of potassium channels (*plus sign*). In addition, the postsynaptic cell contacted by the synaptic terminal can feed back either directly or indirectly and release a different neurotransmitter (*X*), which alters the opening of calcium or potassium channels.

changes: **long-term potentiation** (abbreviated **LTP**). As the name implies, LTP involves a long-lasting enhancement of synaptic strength. Although LTP occurs at a variety of sites in the nervous system, we will concentrate on LTP in synaptic connections in a brain region called the **hippocampus**.

We choose the hippocampus for our discussion because behavioral evidence suggests that this brain structure is involved in the formation of new memories—a finding that has motivated neurobiologists to focus a great deal of experimental attention on synaptic plasticity in the hippocampus. If the hippocampus is destroyed surgically or by disease, short-term memory (memory lasting a few seconds—like the memory we use to recall a phone number we have just looked up) is unimpaired. Likewise, long-term memory (memory lasting years) of events that occurred before the destruction remains unaffected. The ability to place new information into long-term memory is severely impaired, however, which suggests that the hippocampus is involved in a form of intermediate-term memory used to transfer information from short-term to long-term storage. The process by which this transfer takes place remains obscure.

Synaptic Organization of the Hippocampus

The location of the hippocampus is illustrated in Figure 20.5. The hippocampus is a tapered, C-shaped structure tucked under the lower lip of the neocortex. The hippocampus is a simplified type of cerebral cortex called **archicortex**, to distinguish it from the more complex and phylogenetically newer neocortex. The two major parts of the hippocampus are the **dentate gyrus** and the **CA fields** (*CA* is an abbreviation for "cornu ammonis," or "Ammon's horn"). The neurons of the CA fields are pyramidal neurons, shaped like the pyramidal neurons in neocortical areas, whose cell bodies form a single layer. The neurons in the dentate gyrus also form a single layer, but they have rounded cell bodies and are called **granule cells**.

The synaptic connections in the hippocampus related to LTP are shown in Figure 20.6. Incoming axons from neurons in the **entorhinal cortex** enter the hippo-

BOX 1

IN THE CLINIC

Information about the organization of human memory and the differentiation of the different types of memory has come from studies of human neurological patients with defects in particular aspects of memory. For example, memory for motor tasks can be intact even though memory for faces, objects, and places is severely impaired. A role for the hippocampus in human memory was suggested by instances of bilateral damage to the hippocampus in neurological patients. A particularly well-studied case is an individual known in the literature by his initials, H. M., whose hippocampus and associated medial portions of the temporal lobe were surgically removed from both sides in an operation to treat epilepsy. Unfortunately, after the operation H. M. was unable to remember new information for more than a brief time, although his memory for events before the operation was virtually intact. The analysis of H. M.'s deficits gave rise to the idea that the neurons of the hippocampus are involved in some way in the translation of short-term memories into long-term memories. Because of these observations and related experiments on animals, neurobiologists have focused much research on understanding the mechanisms of synaptic plasticity in the hippocampus.

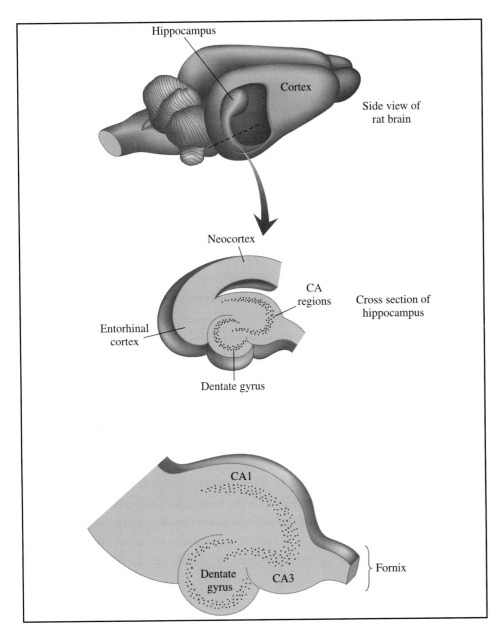

Hippocampus

Cortex

Side view of
rat brain

Neocortex

CA
regions

Cross section of
hippocampus

Entorhinal
cortex

Dentate gyrus

CA1

Dentate
gyrus

CA3

Fornix

Figure 20.5.

The location of the hippocampus in the rat brain. The *upper drawing* shows the location of the hippocampus, and the *lower drawings* show cross sections in the plane indicated in the upper drawing.

campus via a fiber tract, the **perforant path**, and make excitatory synaptic contact onto granule cells in the dentate gyrus. The granule cells in turn send axons (**mossy fibers**) to **subregion CA3** of the CA fields, where they make excitatory synapses onto pyramidal cells. The CA3 pyramidal cells send axons out of the hippocampus via the **fornix**, a large fiber bundle connecting the hippocampus to other brain regions (including the contralateral hippocampus). In addition, the axons of the CA3 cells branch and make excitatory connections with pyramidal cells of **region CA1** of the CA fields. The axon branches of the CA3 neurons extending to region CA1 are called **Schaffer collaterals**. All of the excitatory synapses within the hippocampus release the neurotransmitter glutamate, which is an important point to keep in mind when we discuss proposed mechanisms of LTP.

Long-Term Potentiation Is Associative

All three excitatory synaptic pathways within the hippocampus exhibit post-tetanic potentiation. A burst of high-frequency activity in the presynaptic axons enhances subsequent postsynaptic excitatory responses. Instead of lasting min-

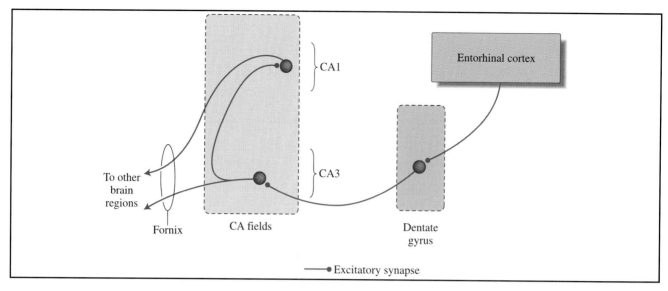

CA1

Entorhinal cortex

CA3

To other
brain
regions

Fornix

CA fields

Dentate
gyrus

Excitatory synapse

Figure 20.6.

The excitatory synaptic circuitry within the hippocampus.

utes, however, the enhanced postsynaptic response persists for as long as a week or more. This long persistence makes LTP interesting as an event that produces enduring changes in synaptic effectiveness. Another property makes LTP even more interesting: the potentiation is *heterosynaptic* and *associative*. That is, activity in one synapse can affect subsequent responses evoked by another synapse (heterosynaptic interaction), provided the two synapses are active at approximately the same time (associative requirement). This aspect of LTP is shown schematically in Figure 20.7. Not only is synaptic transmission enhanced after strong stimulation in the synapses that received the strong stimulation, but also it is enhanced in synapses that were only weakly stimulated, as long as the weak stimulation was closely temporally associated with the strong stimulus. In other words, weakly stimulated synapses that are active contemporaneously with strong stimulation of the postsynaptic cell become potentiated. Further, the potentiation does not produce a general increase in all synaptic inputs after strong stimulation, regardless of whether the synapses were silent or active during the strong stimulus. To become potentiated, synapses must be activated (albeit weakly) nearly simultaneously with the strongly activated synapses. Synapses that are silent during strong stimulation are not potentiated (see Fig. 20.7).

Mechanism of Long-Term Potentiation

How does strong synaptic activation of a neuron trigger LTP?

Although much progress has been made toward a molecular understanding of LTP, the underlying mechanisms have not been established unequivocally. In this section, we will describe some current theories of LTP that incorporate key features of the phenomenon. It is likely that synaptic strength increases during LTP for multiple reasons, each of which may play a greater or lesser role at synapses in particular parts of the nervous system.

Strong synaptic stimulation produces substantial depolarization of the postsynaptic neuron, and *depolarization of the postsynaptic neuron initiates LTP*. Figure 20.8 illustrates an experiment that demonstrates the importance of postsynaptic depolarization in LTP. If the postsynaptic neuron is depolarized by injecting positive current into the cell through a microelectrode, LTP is triggered in the synaptic responses to presynaptic cells that were active during the artificial depolarization.

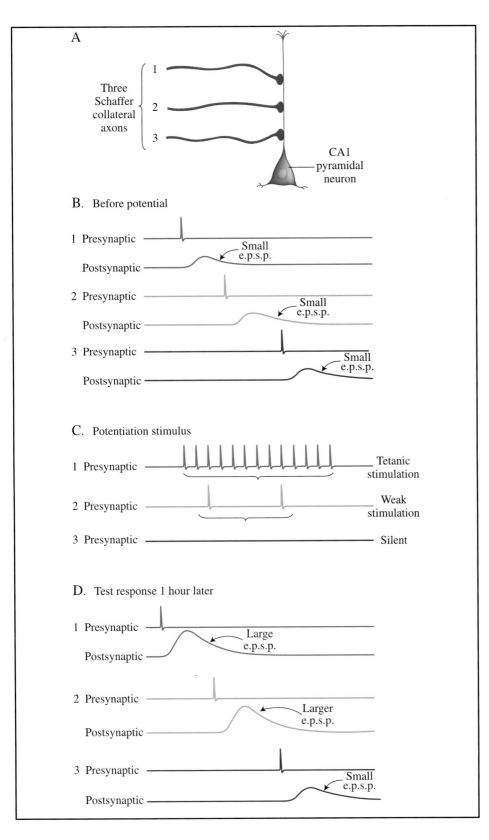

A

Three
Schaffer
collateral
axons
{
1
2
3

CA1
pyramidal
neuron

B. Before potential

1 Presynaptic

Postsynaptic
Small
e.p.s.p.

2 Presynaptic

Postsynaptic
Small
e.p.s.p.

3 Presynaptic

Postsynaptic
Small
e.p.s.p.

C. Potentiation stimulus

1 Presynaptic
Tetanic
stimulation

2 Presynaptic
Weak
stimulation

3 Presynaptic
Silent

D. Test response 1 hour later

1 Presynaptic

Postsynaptic
Large
e.p.s.p.

2 Presynaptic

Postsynaptic
Larger
e.p.s.p.

3 Presynaptic

Postsynaptic
Small
e.p.s.p.

Figure 20.7.

Long-term potentiation of excitatory synapses in the hippocampus. **A**. A schematic
diagram of a pyramidal neuron in subregion CA3, receiving excitatory synapses from
three Schaffer collateral axons. The axons are labeled 1,
2, and 3, and each one can be
separately stimulated to fire
an action potential. **B**. Prior to
potentiation, each input synapse produces a similar excitatory postsynaptic potential
(e.p.s.p.) (traces labeled *postsynaptic*). Each of the three inputs (numbered 1 to 3 on the
left side of the traces) is stimulated separately to fire a
single presynaptic action potential (traces labeled *presynaptic*). **C**. A rapid burst of
action potentials is triggered
in input 1, while input 2 fires
at a low rate and input 3
remains inactive. Although
postsynaptic traces are not
shown for reasons of simplicity, the burst of action potentials in input 1 would produce
summated e.p.s.p.'s and substantial depolarization of the
postsynaptic cell. **D**. One hour
after the potentiating burst of
action potentials, the postsynaptic responses to single
action potentials in the three
input fibers are tested. The
e.p.s.p.'s elicited by input 1
and input 2 are larger, while
the response to input 3 remains the same as before
potentiation.

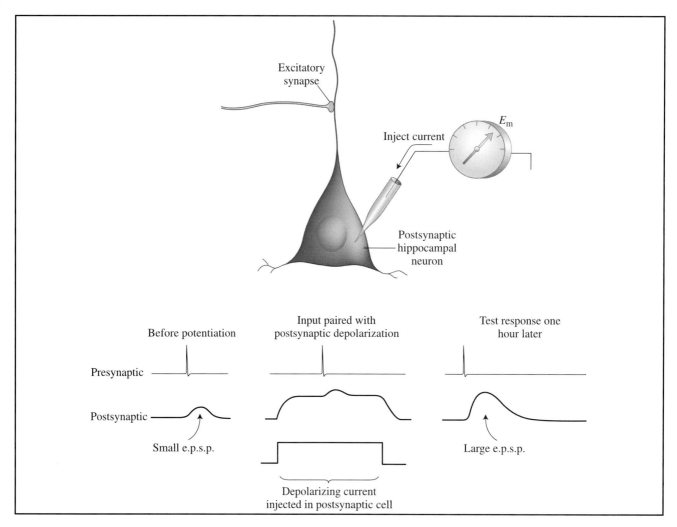

Figure 20.8.

Long-term potentiation in a single input can be triggered by postsynaptic depolarization. A single excitatory input is stimulated to fire a single action potential (traces labeled *Presynaptic*). Before potentiation, a small excitatory postsynaptic potential (e.p.s.p.) is recorded in the postsynaptic cell. After the stimulation of the input is paired with depolarizing current injected into the postsynaptic cell (*middle set of traces*), the postsynaptic response is enhanced (*right set of traces*).

Thus, postsynaptic depolarization is sufficient to initiate LTP, even without tetanic stimulation of the presynaptic inputs. Under normal circumstances, however, the requisite large postsynaptic depolarization occurs only when multiple synaptic inputs are stimulated repetitively, which explains why tetanic stimulation of the input fibers is normally required to elicit LTP.

How does depolarization of the postsynaptic cell affect subsequent synaptic responses, and why does the potentiation affect only those synapses that are active during the depolarization? To answer these questions, we must first examine the anatomical arrangement of the excitatory synapses in the hippocampus and the properties of the postsynaptic receptor molecules that detect glutamate released by the presynaptic terminals. As with many other excitatory synapses in the central nervous system, the synaptic terminals contact the dendrites of hippocampal neurons at short, hair-like protuberances called **dendritic spines**. At high magnification, each spine is seen to consist of a knob-like swelling connected via a thin neck of cytoplasm to the main branch of the dendrite, as shown

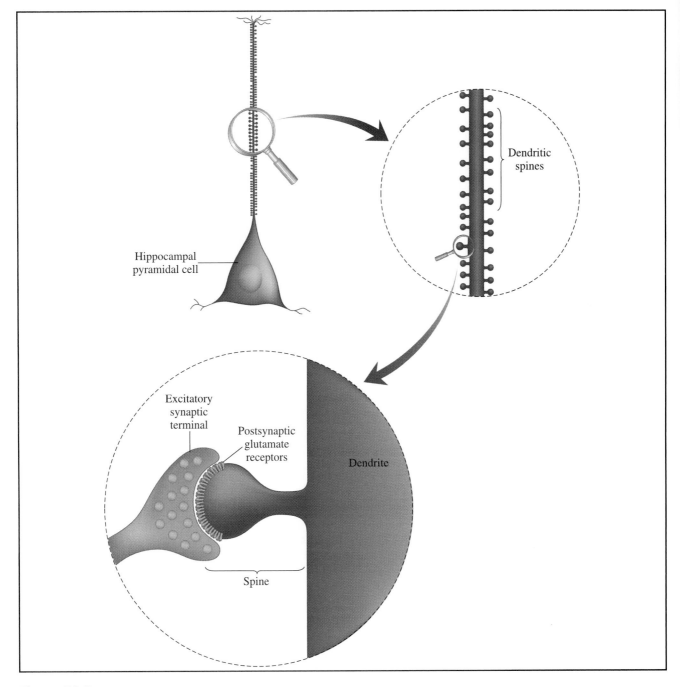

Figure 20.9.

Excitatory synaptic terminals on hippocampal pyramidal cells connect to spike-like protrusions of the dendrites, called dendritic spines.

schematically in Figure 20.9. The thinness of the connecting neck allows each spine to behave as a separate intracellular compartment, within which biochemical events can occur in isolation from the rest of the cell. Thus, internal signals can be generated in one spine without spreading to and affecting other spines on the dendrite. Each spine receives input from a single excitatory synaptic terminal. The combination of one terminal and one spine forms a functional synaptic unit that can be modulated separately from the other units on the dendrite of a single neuron. This structural organization may play a central role in the ability of LTP to selectively enhance transmission at active synapses, leaving inactive synapses unaffected.

The excitatory neurotransmitter released from the synaptic terminals onto the dendritic spines of hippocampal neurons is glutamate. Glutamate binds to and opens ligand-gated ion channels (glutamate receptors) in the postsynaptic membrane of the dendritic spine. The resulting change in ionic permeability produces the excitatory postsynaptic potential (e.p.s.p.) in the postsynaptic cell. In hippocampal neurons, two different types of postsynaptic glutamate receptors, known as **NMDA receptors** and **non-NMDA receptors**, are located in the membrane of the dendritic spine at the contact point with the presynaptic terminal. NMDA (N-methyl-d-aspartate) is an artificial glutamate analog that can activate NMDA receptors but not non-NMDA receptors. The non-NMDA receptors are sensitive to a different glutamate analog, AMPA (α-amino-3-hydroxy-5-methyl isoxazole proprionic acid), and are therefore called **AMPA receptors**.

Both NMDA receptors and AMPA receptors are activated by glutamate released into the synaptic cleft by presynaptic action potentials. Although both receptor types are nonspecific cation channels, AMPA receptors do not have an appreciable permeability for calcium ions. NMDA receptors, on the other hand, permit an influx of calcium ions when the channel is open. Thus, AMPA receptors increase the postsynaptic permeability to potassium and sodium ions, like the nicotinic acetylcholine-activated channels at the neuromuscular junction (see Chapter 5). The NMDA receptors increase the postsynaptic permeability to calcium, as well as potassium and sodium.

Another important difference between the two receptor types is that AMPA receptors open when glutamate binds, regardless of the membrane potential, whereas NMDA receptors require both binding of glutamate and depolarization to open. The voltage dependence of the NMDA receptors does not arise from an inherent voltage sensor in the channel, like the voltage-sensitive gates of the sodium and potassium channels that underlie the action potential (see Chapter 4). Instead, the NMDA receptors fail to conduct inward current at negative membrane potentials because external magnesium ions block the channels. Magnesium, a divalent cation, enters the channel when the membrane potential is strongly negative. Unlike calcium, magnesium does not go through the open NMDA channel but plugs up the pore. Upon depolarization, the electrical gradient across the membrane is reduced, and magnesium is less likely to enter and block the open channel.

The behavior of the NMDA and AMPA glutamate receptors is summarized in Figure 20.10. In the absence of strong excitatory synaptic activity, the postsynaptic membrane potential remains at its usual negative level. Under these conditions (see Fig. 20.10A), glutamate released from a single presynaptic terminal opens AMPA receptors but not the NMDA receptors, which require both glutamate and depolarization to conduct inward current. As a result, a small e.p.s.p. arises that is governed by the AMPA receptors acting alone. This small postsynaptic depolarization is insufficient to reach the range of membrane potential required to open the NMDA channels.

If multiple synaptic terminals are active simultaneously, the summated e.p.s.p.'s depolarize the postsynaptic cell to a greater extent. This larger depolarization allows both NMDA and AMPA receptors to open when glutamate is released from the presynaptic terminal. *The open NMDA receptor channels allow calcium influx, which is the actual trigger for LTP.* Because each spine is separated from its neighbors, the internal calcium concentration increases only in the spines whose terminals are releasing glutamate at the time of depolarization. The synapse at a neighboring spine whose terminal is not active will not become potentiated because no glutamate is available there to occupy the NMDA receptors. Thus, synaptic inputs that are active during a period of depolarization (which would normally correspond to a period of intense excitatory synaptic activity) will become potentiated, while silent inputs will not.

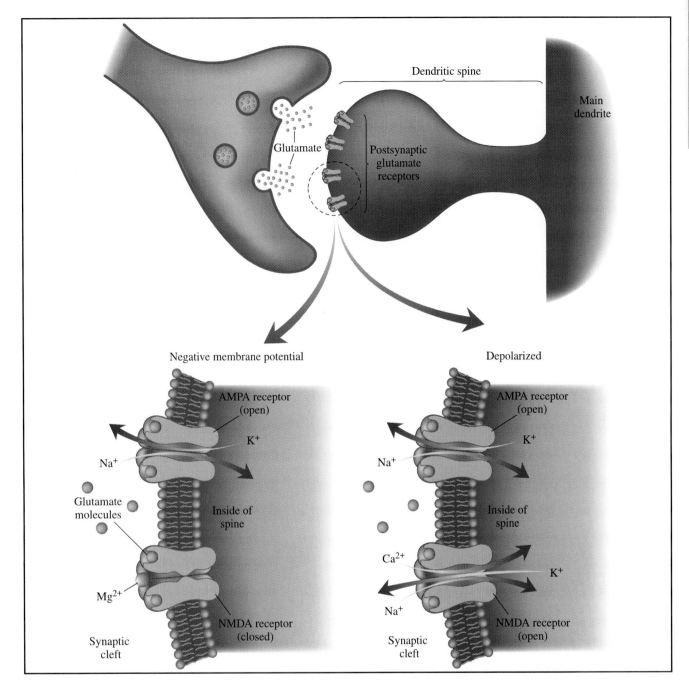

Figure 20.10.

The postsynaptic membrane of the dendritic spine contains two types of glutamate receptors: NMDA receptors and AMPA receptors. Both receptors require the binding of the neurotransmitter glutamate in order to open (*bottom diagrams*); NMDA receptors also require depolarization of the postsynaptic cell in order to open, because the channel is blocked by external magnesium ions at negative membrane potentials. Both types of glutamate receptors allow sodium and potassium ions to move through the open channel, but the NMDA receptor also admits calcium ions.

Long-Term Potentiation May Involve Presynaptic and Postsynaptic Changes

How the increase in internal calcium in the dendritic spine causes LTP of the synapse is less clear, despite intense research activity in recent years. The size of an e.p.s.p. can be increased in two ways: by increasing the amount of neurotransmitter released by a presynaptic action potential (presynaptic mechanisms) or by increasing the postsynaptic sensitivity to a fixed amount of released neurotransmitter (postsynaptic mechanisms). Examples of presynaptic mechanisms are provided by the various forms of short-term synaptic enhancement described earlier in this chapter. A possible postsynaptic mechanism is an increase in the density of functional glutamate receptors in the postsynaptic membrane of the dendritic spine. Evidence suggests that both presynaptic and postsynaptic factors can contribute to LTP in the hippocampus, although there is disagreement about the relative importance of these factors.

If LTP is, at least in part, attributable to an increase in neurotransmitter release, then the question immediately arises of how an increase in calcium in the *postsynaptic* cell triggers a change in neurotransmitter release in the *presynaptic* cell. Clearly, such a mechanism requires that a **retrograde signal** must be transmitted from the dendritic spine to the synaptic terminal. Although the identity of this retrograde signal remains unknown, one proposed signaling scheme is illustrated in Figure 20.11. Among the cellular targets for elevated calcium in the dendritic spine is **nitric oxide synthase**, which is an enzyme that produces **nitric oxide** (chemical structure = NO) from the amino acid arginine. NO is a small, membrane-permeant molecule that can readily diffuse from the dendritic spine into the presynaptic terminal. NO is known to be a cellular messenger that activates intracellular signaling molecules, including guanylyl cyclase. In this scheme, ele-

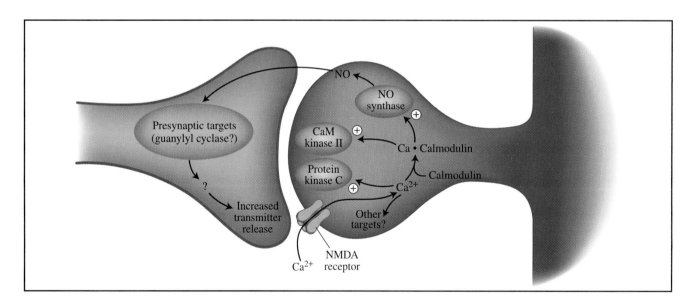

Figure 20.11.

Elevated intracellular calcium levels activate several cellular signals in dendritic spines. Calcium influx through NMDA receptors increases the concentration of intracellular calcium, which binds to calmodulin. Calcium/calmodulin then activates two enzymes: nitric oxide (NO) synthase and calcium/calmodulin-dependent protein kinase II (CaM kinase II). Calcium also activates protein kinase C. NO synthase produces NO from arginine, and the membrane permeant messenger is thought to diffuse to the presynaptic terminal. NO then interacts with cellular signaling pathways, possibly including guanylyl cyclase, to potentiate transmitter release.

vated calcium levels in the postsynaptic cell activate NO synthase. The released NO diffuses to the presynaptic terminal, where it activates an unknown biochemical cascade leading to enhanced neurotransmitter release.

Retrograde signaling need not involve a diffusible messenger like NO, however. At the neuromuscular synapse, signals are sent in both directions through molecules incorporated into the extracellular matrix in the synaptic cleft (see Chapter 19). A similar signal mechanism could be used to communicate from a dendritic spine to the corresponding presynaptic terminal during LTP. For instance, an increased density of postsynaptic glutamate receptors (a postsynaptic mechanism) might alter the availability of an extracellular molecule that in turn affects the number of neurotransmitter release sites (active zones) in the presynaptic terminal (a presynaptic mechanism).

Several possible mechanisms for enhanced postsynaptic sensitivity to glutamate have been suggested. Figure 20.11 illustrates some other cellular targets for calcium in the dendritic spine, including two different kinases: **protein kinase C (PKC)** and **calcium/calmodulin-dependent kinase II (CaM kinase II)**. When activated by elevated calcium levels, these enzymes phosphorylate specific target proteins in the postsynaptic cell. As we saw with neuronal growth factors in Chapter 19, phosphorylation is a cellular signal often used to activate or inactivate various kinds of proteins. In the case of LTP, the targets for phosphorylation by calcium-dependent kinases have not been established. Phosphorylation may increase the number of functional postsynaptic glutamate receptors, either because phosphorylation allows the channels to open in response to glutamate or because phosphorylation allows channels to attach to the cytoskeleton, anchoring them at the appropriate position in the postsynaptic membrane.

Increased glutamate sensitivity also might arise from an insertion of additional AMPA receptors into the postsynaptic membrane. The number of AMPA receptors in the membrane represents a balance between the fusion and retrieval of intracellular vesicles whose membranes contain AMPA receptors (see Fig. 20.11). Elevated calcium levels might favor insertion over retrieval and thus increase the number of AMPA receptors available to respond to glutamate released from the presynaptic terminal.

LTP also can be produced in the nervous system by mechanisms that do not involve postsynaptic NMDA receptors. Even within portions of the hippocampus, LTP can arise in other ways. For example, LTP occurs at the synaptic connection between granule cells of the dentate gyrus and pyramidal cells of area CA3 (see Fig. 20.6), but the postsynaptic response at this synapse does not involve NMDA receptors. Thus, alternative ways to initiate LTP, besides the depolarization-dependent influx of calcium through NMDA receptors, must exist. Because synaptic plasticity plays such an important role in the alteration of behavior based on experience, it should not be surprising that multiple mechanisms have evolved to accomplish this task.

Long-Term Depression of Synaptic Strength

In our discussion of short-term changes in synaptic strength, we saw that synaptic efficacy can either decrease or increase as a result of presynaptic activity. The same is true for longer-term changes in synaptic strength. **Long-term depression (LTD)**, lasting hours or weeks, is also observed at synaptic connections in a variety of brain regions. The stimulation conditions that elicit LTD differ somewhat at various synapses. In some cases, such as in the cerebellum, LTD is heterosynaptic and associative—that is, it requires the temporal pairing of two different synaptic inputs. In other cases, LTD is homosynaptic—that is, it is based on activity in one set of synapses without requiring co-activation of a different set of synapses.

How does LTD differ from LTP?

481

The excitatory synapses in the hippocampus demonstrate LTD as well as LTP. If a synaptic input is activated at a low rate for a few minutes without strong activity in other synapses, the size of the e.p.s.p. elicited by that synaptic input diminishes and remains at this lower level for many hours. In this regard, LTD can be considered the opposite of LTP. In LTP, the effectiveness of a weakly stimulated synaptic input is enhanced when it is paired with strong activation of other pathways. In LTD, the effectiveness of a weakly stimulated synapse becomes reduced if its activation occurs in the absence of strong stimulation in other synaptic inputs. If LTP is induced at a particular synapse, it can subsequently be reversed by LTD. This fact suggests that LTD represents an erasure mechanism for LTP in the hippocampus: unless activation of a synaptic input is *consistently* strongly activated or paired with strong activation of other inputs, potentiation of that input is reversed by LTD.

Even less is known about the mechanism of LTD in the hippocampus than the mechanism of LTP. Evidence suggests that LTD may involve the activation of protein phosphatases, which are enzymes that remove phosphate groups from previously phosphorylated proteins. Given that phosphorylation has been proposed as a mediator of at least some aspects of LTP, the activation of dephosphorylating enzymes seems to be an attractive mechanism for reversing potentiation.

MODIFICATION OF SYNAPTIC STRENGTH IN REFLEX CIRCUITS

We have frequently used reflexes as examples of neuronal signals and their interactions. The simplicity of reflex circuits allows us to readily appreciate the underlying principles of circuit organization. Even these simple neuronal circuits are capable of modification based on experience, however. In this section, we will consider some examples of learned changes in reflexes. In these examples, we will see that learning is accompanied by changes in the effectiveness of synaptic connections that are similar to those we encountered when considering short-term alterations in synaptic efficacy.

Habituation

What synaptic changes underlie habituation of a reflex?

Our first example of simple learning in a reflex circuit is reflex habituation. If a stimulus is presented repeatedly, it typically becomes progressively less effective in eliciting a reflexive response. This reduction of response strength with repetition of a stimulus is called **habituation**. It allows the nervous system to disregard constant stimuli and accentuate changing conditions. The best-studied example of habituation of a reflex is a type of withdrawal reflex in the sea hare, *Aplysia californica*. Like other gastropod molluscs, *Aplysia* has a relatively simple nervous system and a correspondingly simple repertoire of behaviors. This simplicity facilitates the task of sorting out the neural circuitry responsible for particular aspects of behavior and thus makes it feasible to discern the changes in circuitry that underlie behavioral changes.

The overall body structure of *Aplysia* is shown in Figure 20.12. The animal's respiratory organ, the gill, resides within a fleshy pouch on the dorsal surface. Under normal circumstances, the lips of the pouch remain slightly open to allow entry of sea water, which is expelled toward the rear of the animal through a spout called the siphon. In this way, a steady flow of water moves over the gill. If the extended siphon is touched, the siphon and gill are reflexively withdrawn into the pouch, and the pouch closes. This defensive reflex protects the more vulnerable, fleshy parts of the animal from predators. With time, the withdrawn body parts resume their normal positions. If another tactile stimulus is then applied to the siphon,

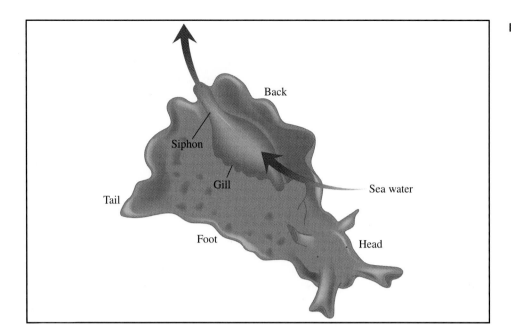

Figure 20.12.
The sea hare, *Aplysia californica*. When the siphon is
touched, the siphon and gill
are reflexively retracted within
a protective pocket on the animal's back.

Siphon

Back

Gill

Tail

Sea water

Foot

Head

withdrawal occurs more slowly and is less complete. After a series of touch stimuli, the reflex habituates, and the gill no longer withdraws when the siphon is touched.

The circuitry of the gill withdrawal reflex and the neuronal changes that produce habituation of the withdrawal reflex are summarized in Figure 20.13A. Touch-sensitive sensory neurons make excitatory synaptic connections directly onto the motor neurons that control the gill muscles. In addition, the sensory neurons make excitatory synaptic contact with interneurons, which then make excitatory connections with the gill motor neurons. Thus, there are both direct and indirect synaptic paths from the sensory neurons to the gill motor neurons.

In the unhabituated state, each action potential in a sensory neuron produces a large e.p.s.p. in the motor neurons (see Fig. 20.13B) and the interneurons. The interneurons also produce a strong e.p.s.p. in the motor neurons. Through these direct and indirect synaptic connections, a burst of action potentials in the touch-sensitive sensory neuron produces a prolonged, high-frequency discharge in the motor neurons and a rapid, complete withdrawal of the gill.

If the tactile stimulus is presented repeatedly, the e.p.s.p.'s produced by the sensory neurons in the motor neurons and interneurons become progressively smaller, as shown in Figure 20.13B. In addition, the synaptic connection between the interneurons and the motor neurons also becomes weaker. The overall result is that fewer action potentials are evoked in the gill motor neurons in response to touch of the siphon, and so the strength of the reflexive withdrawal declines. Thus, habituation of the withdrawal reflex is produced by synaptic depression in the excitatory synapses of the underlying neuronal circuit. The mechanism of the depression is thought to involve an inactivation of calcium channels in the presynaptic terminals and a reduction in the pool of synaptic vesicles available for release at each synaptic active zone. Both of these mechanisms are among those we discussed earlier in this chapter in our discussion of short-term synaptic depression.

Sensitization

Experience can also strengthen a reflex. For example, exposure to a painful or noxious stimulus produces a generalized increase in the vigor of withdrawal reflexes, a phenomenon called **sensitization**. A noxious stimulus may signify that the organism has entered a hostile environment, and therefore the potentiation of de-

What synaptic changes
underlie sensitization of a
reflex?

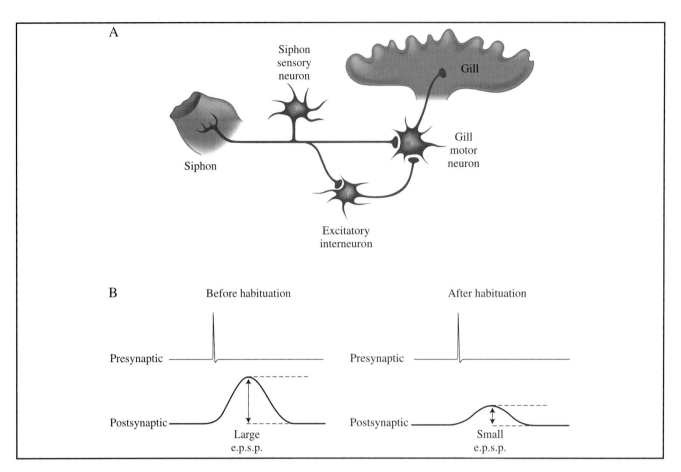

Figure 20.13.

The neural circuit for the gill withdrawal reflex in *Aplysia*. **A**. Touch-sensitive sensory neurons that innervate the siphon project both directly and indirectly via interneurons to the motor neurons of the gill muscles. **B**. Habituation of the withdrawal reflex is produced by synaptic depression in the excitatory synapses of the neural circuit. e.p.s.p. = excitatory postsynaptic potential.

fensive withdrawal reflexes is adaptive. The sensitizing stimulus can occur outside the sensory realm of the reflexes that are potentiated. For instance, a pinch applied to an animal's tail potentiates withdrawal reflexes of the foot and gill. This global action differs from habituation, in which the change in reflex strength is specific to the stimulus that elicits the reflex. Therefore, we would expect the synaptic mechanisms of sensitization to differ from those of habituation.

Facilitation of Neurotransmitter Release Underlies Sensitization

To examine the cellular mechanisms of sensitization, we return to the gill withdrawal reflex of *Aplysia californica*. After an electrical shock (which a human would perceive as painful) is applied to the tail of the animal, touching the siphon elicits faster and stronger gill withdrawal than usual. In other words, the gill withdrawal reflex exhibits sensitization in response to a noxious stimulus.

To account for sensitization, we must expand the circuit for the withdrawal reflex to include inputs originating from the sensory neurons of the tail, as shown in Figure 20.14A. The sensory neurons from the tail indirectly excite a class of interneurons, called **facilitatory interneurons**, which make synaptic contact with the presynaptic terminals of the excitatory synapses in the gill withdrawal circuit.

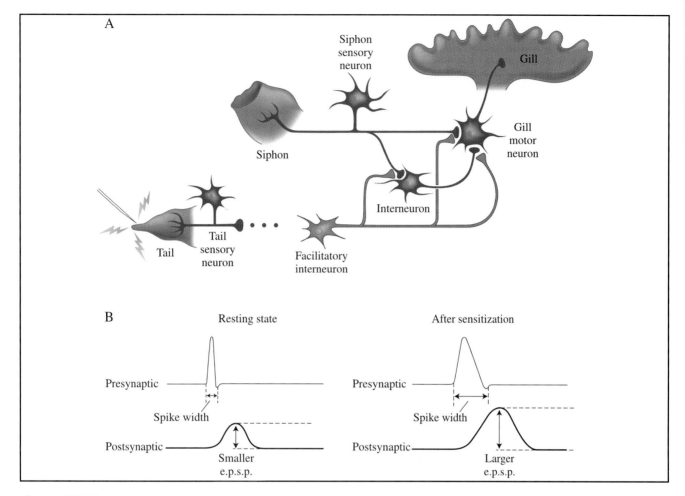

Figure 20.14.

The neural basis of sensitization of the gill withdrawal reflex in *Aplysia californica*. **A.** The excitatory synapses in the gill withdrawal circuit receive presynaptic inputs from a facilitatory interneuron. The facilitatory interneuron is activated by noxious stimuli applied to the tail of the animal. **B.** Sensitization produces larger excitatory postsynaptic potentials (e.p.s.p.) in the withdrawal circuit, reflecting the longer duration of the presynaptic action potential after sensitization.

Activation of the facilitatory interneurons does not produce a typical inhibitory postsynaptic potential (i.p.s.p.) or e.p.s.p. in the postsynaptic target but instead enhances the release of neurotransmitter in response to presynaptic action potentials at the synapses of the withdrawal circuit. After stimulation of the facilitatory interneuron, each action potential in the siphon sensory neuron produces a larger-than-normal e.p.s.p. in its postsynaptic targets, the motor neurons and interneurons (see Fig. 20.14B). The same is true for the excitatory synapses from the interneurons onto the motor neurons. As a result, excitation of the motor neurons is greater, and the reflex response is stronger. The enhanced postsynaptic response reflects an increased release of neurotransmitter at the excitatory synapses in the withdrawal circuit.

The facilitatory interneuron enhances neurotransmitter release by increasing the duration of the action potential (see Fig. 20.14B). The repolarizing phase of the action potential is produced by the opening of potassium channels (see Chapter 4), and slowing of repolarization implies reduced potassium permeability. Figure 20.15 summarizes the mechanism underlying the increase in action potential duration. The facilitatory interneurons release the neurotransmitter serotonin onto the

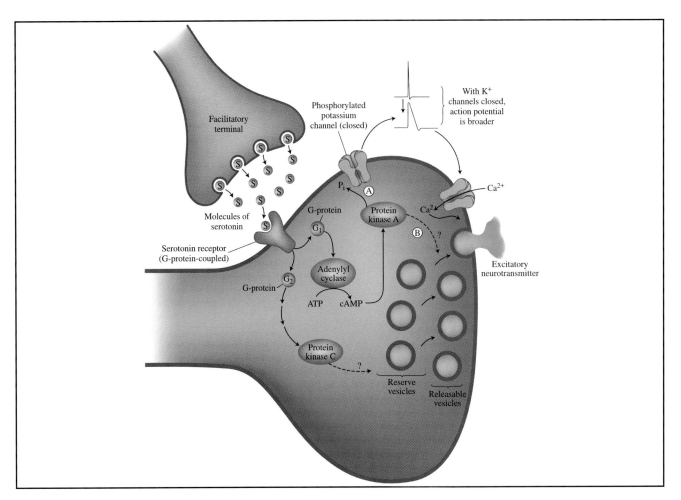

Figure 20.15.

A model for presynaptic changes associated with sensitization of the gill withdrawal reflex in *Aplysia*. The synaptic terminals of the facilitatory interneuron release the neurotransmitter serotonin (*S*), which combines with serotonin receptors in the membrane of the excitatory synaptic terminals of the gill withdrawal circuit. The activated receptor stimulates two G-proteins: one increases intracellular cyclic AMP (*cAMP*) via adenylyl cyclase, and a second activates protein kinase C. Cyclic AMP stimulates protein kinase A, which in turn phosphorylates and closes potassium channels. Reduced potassium permeability broadens the presynaptic action potential and enhances calcium influx through voltage-dependent calcium channels. In addition, protein kinase A and possibly protein kinase C may promote the movement of synaptic vesicles from reserve pools to releasable pools, thereby potentiating transmitter release. ATP = adenosine triphosphate; P_i = inorganic phosphate.

synaptic terminals of the siphon sensory neuron (other neurotransmitters also are used by the interneurons, but we will focus on serotonin). Serotonin activates receptors that stimulate G-proteins in the synaptic terminal. One type of G-protein stimulated by serotonin activates the enzyme adenylyl cyclase, which produces cyclic adenosine monophosphate (cyclic AMP) from adenosine triphosphate (ATP), thereby increasing the concentration of cyclic AMP inside the synaptic terminal. This rise in cyclic AMP enhances neurotransmitter release in two ways.

First, increased cyclic AMP enhances the influx of calcium ions into the terminal (pathway A in Fig. 20.15) by prolonging the presynaptic action potential. This effect of cyclic AMP is mediated by protein kinase A (the cyclic AMP–stimulated protein kinase), which phosphorylates potassium channels. The phosphorylated channels do not open during depolarization, which slows the repolarization of the action potential and allows voltage-activated calcium channels to remain open for a longer time. Thus, a single action potential releases a greater amount of neurotransmitter.

Second, the number of synaptic vesicles available to be released by a presynaptic action potential increases in response to cyclic AMP. This effect may be generated by the movement of vesicles from a reserve group to the active zones, where they can fuse with the plasma membrane in response to calcium influx (pathway B in Fig. 20.15). The molecular mechanism of this second action of cyclic AMP remains unknown.

Evidence suggests that PKC may be involved in the enhancement of neurotransmitter release during sensitization. During sensitization, serotonin receptors indirectly activate PKC via a pathway initiated by a different subclass of G-proteins (see Fig. 20.15). Activation of PKC closes potassium channels and broadens action potentials, which potentiates calcium influx as described earlier. In addition, PKC may increase the pool of releasable synaptic vesicles at active zones.

The Transition from Short-Term to Long-Term Habituation and Sensitization

The cellular mechanisms described in previous sections produce habituation and sensitization lasting a few minutes. If we expose an animal to repeated bouts of habituation or sensitization, however, we can produce changes in the strength of the reflex lasting for days or weeks. What factors account for the transition from short-term to long-term changes in reflex excitability after repetitive experience? Although not all of the molecular answers to this question have been established, RNA synthesis and protein synthesis are required for long-term sensitization of the gill withdrawal reflex. Short-term sensitization is unaffected by inhibition of RNA and protein synthesis, as expected from the fact that the scheme shown in Figure 20.15 for short-term sensitization depends on already-existing proteins within the synaptic terminal. The requirement for new RNA and new protein shifts the focus from the presynaptic terminal, where the short-term changes occur, to the cell body of the neuron, where RNA transcription and protein synthesis take place. Thus, some signal is transmitted from the synaptic terminal to the cell nucleus after repetitive bouts of sensitization, producing long-term changes in synaptic strength.

Long-term synaptic facilitation in the gill withdrawal circuit can be triggered by elevation of intracellular cyclic AMP levels, which is the cellular signal involved in at least part of short-term sensitization (see Fig. 20.15). This finding suggests that cyclic AMP–dependent gene transcription factors may turn on genes involved in long-term facilitation in the sensory neuron. Such cyclic AMP–dependent transcription factors are known to play important roles in other situations in the regulation of neuronal gene expression. The current theory is that protein kinase A, which is activated in the synaptic terminal during sensitization, finds its way to the cell body of the neuron, where it phosphorylates and activates transcription factor proteins. The transcription factors then bind to the regulatory regions of the genes that encode the proteins necessary for maintaining the facilitated state of the synaptic terminals. These proteins have not yet been identified, although some may be transcription factors that in turn either activate or suppress other genes.

One theory holds that this cascade of gene regulation ultimately reduces the amount of the regulatory subunit of protein kinase A. Like many other signaling proteins (for example, heterotrimeric G-proteins), protein kinase A consists of multiple protein subunits. Two different subunits make up protein kinase A: a **catalytic subunit**, which is the kinase enzyme that phosphorylates target proteins, and

What mechanisms produce a long-term shift in the strength of a synaptic connection during sensitization?

a **regulatory subunit**, which binds to and inhibits the catalytic subunit. (Actually, two copies of each subunit constitute a complete protein kinase molecule.) If the amount of regulatory subunit in the cell is insufficient to bind all of the catalytic subunits, protein kinase A will be continually activated, even at basal levels of cyclic AMP. This continuous activation would produce a persistently facilitated synapse. During long-term sensitization, the amount of regulatory subunit is thought to be reduced by selective proteolysis, which suggests that long-term sensitization involves genes encoding proteins that promote proteolysis.

Although these changes in cyclic AMP signaling may be partly responsible for long-term changes in synaptic efficacy, other mechanisms also may play a role. Anatomical experiments suggest that some of the long-term synaptic changes produced by repetitive habituation and repetitive sensitization reflect changes in the *number* of synaptic connections between the sensory neurons and the motor neurons in the reflex circuit. Correlated with the development of long-term sensitization, the sensory neuron makes more synaptic connections with the motor neuron. A larger number of synaptic connections produce greater spatial summation and thus larger excitatory postsynaptic potentials. Conversely, after long-term habituation, the number of synapses declines below normal levels. No changes in the number of synapses are observed during short-term habituation or sensitization.

The synaptic connectivity pattern among neurons is plastic, not fixed. Evidence from imaging studies demonstrates that synaptic connections are added and subtracted on a continual basis in the mammalian nervous system, as well as in the *Aplysia californica* withdrawal reflex. Thus, long-term changes in synaptic strength may partly reflect increasing or decreasing numbers of synaptic contacts among neurons, based on the recent history of neuronal activity in a circuit.

REFLEX PLASTICITY IN THE PRIMATE CENTRAL NERVOUS SYSTEM

Learning in the Vestibulo-Ocular Reflex

What modifications are observed in the VOR on the basis of experience?

Changes in reflex circuits based on experience are not restricted to marine mollusks, like *Aplysia californica*. Even in the human brain, such reflexive learning occurs. A well-studied example is the **vestibulo-ocular reflex** (VOR), which was a major focus of our discussions of sensorimotor integration (see Chapter 10). The VOR prevents the image of the visual world on the retina from moving during passive or active movements of the head. To compensate for visual motion during head movements, the VOR moves the eyes within their sockets. The sensory information for the reflex derives from the motion sensors of the vestibular apparatus, in the semicircular canals of the inner ear. Within the brain, only a single relay interneuron (in the vestibular nuclei, just beneath the cerebellum) intervenes between the vestibular ganglion cells and the motor neurons of the eye muscles (see Fig. 20.16).

One important consideration is that the VOR is an **open loop reflex** (see Chapter 10), operating without the benefit of immediate sensory feedback. As a result, the strength of synaptic interactions in the reflex circuit must be precisely "calibrated" to produce the amount of eye movement necessary to prevent image motion on the retina at each velocity of head rotation. The performance of the VOR is constantly monitored, and the calibration of the reflex is updated appropriately to maintain a match between head motion and eye motion. Thus, the strength of synaptic connections in the VOR is based on experience and represents a form of learning. As we have seen, synaptic strength can be modified on a short- or long-term basis by simple cellular learning mechanisms. In this section, we will examine the modifiability of the VOR from this perspective.

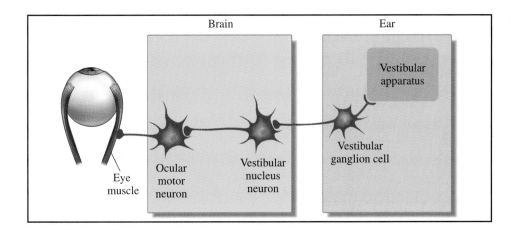

Figure 20.16.

The basic circuit for the vestibulo-ocular reflex in the primate brain.

Learning in the VOR can be demonstrated in experiments in which an observer wears eyeglasses that magnify the visual world, creating a mismatch between the eye movements produced by the VOR and the amount of movement required to keep the image in place on the retina. Without the magnifying eyeglasses, a rotation of the head to the right at 10°/sec requires movement of the eyes to the left at 10°/sec to keep the image of the world at the same position on the retina. With the magnifying spectacles, however, the image projected onto the retina is larger than normal. As a result, rotation of the head at 10°/sec produces movement of the image on the retina at *greater* than 10°/sec. When the VOR produces the previously correct eye movements at 10°/sec, the motion of the eyes is insufficient to correct the slippage of the image on the retina, and the visual world appears to move to the left as the head rotates to the right. With time, however, the output of the VOR increases until the image once again stabilizes on the retina as the head rotates. This change in the VOR is a form of learning.

We can express the relation between the input (head rotation) and the output (eye rotation) of the VOR in terms of the gain of the reflex. The gain is simply the output velocity divided by the input velocity (both expressed in degrees per second). Under normal conditions, the correct gain would be 1.0, corresponding to equal head and eye rotation velocities. With magnifying eyeglasses, however, the required gain is greater than 1.0; with demagnifying glasses, the required gain is less than 1.0. When the magnification of the visual world is altered experimentally, the observed gain of the VOR changes with time to closely match the required value. This change of gain of the reflex is what we mean by VOR learning. In the absence of counterexperience, the modified gain of the VOR is retained indefinitely; thus, it represents a long-term change in synaptic processing.

The Cerebellum in VOR Learning

The cerebellum is involved in the modification of motor behavior based on sensory information about the outcome of the behavior (see Chapter 9). In keeping with this general role, the cerebellum plays an important role in adjusting the gain of the VOR to minimize image motion during head rotation. If the cerebellar cortex is removed surgically, the normal VOR is not affected very much (as expected from the circuit diagram shown in Fig. 20.16). Without the cerebellum, however, VOR learning is abolished, and the gain of the reflex cannot be modified based on experience.

It is not necessary to destroy all of the cerebellar cortex to prevent VOR learning. Like other parts of the brain, the cerebellum is regionally specialized for specific types of sensory and motor systems. The portion concerned with vestibular sensory information and eye movements is the **floccular complex** (which consists

How does the cerebellum affect learning in the VOR?

of the **flocculus**—a lobe at the most lateral part of the cerebellum on each side of the brain—and the **ventral paraflocculus**). Removal of the floccular complex is sufficient to abolish VOR plasticity. If the floccular complex is destroyed *after* the VOR has been modified, the modifications are mostly retained. However, if the normal optical conditions are restored (for example, magnifying eyeglasses are removed) after destruction of the floccular complex, the normal VOR cannot be restored. Thus, the cerebellum is required to acquire modifications of the VOR; once acquired, the altered VOR gain is retained in portions of the VOR circuitry outside the cerebellum.

Connections Between the Cerebellum and the VOR Circuitry

Figure 20.17 summarizes the synaptic connections between the cerebellum and the VOR circuitry. The arrangement follows the general plan for cerebellar circuits presented in Chapter 9: the sensory inputs project in parallel to the cerebellar cortex and to the deep cerebellar nuclei. In the case of the VOR, the floccular complex is the relevant part of the cerebellar cortex, and the vestibular nucleus is the relevant deep cerebellar nucleus. The output cells of the cortex, the **Purkinje cells**, project back to the vestibular nucleus, where they make inhibitory synaptic connections.

The VOR utilizes two sources of sensory information: vestibular inputs provide information about head rotation, and inputs from the visual system provide information about direction and velocity of image motion on the retina. The vestibular inputs inform the cerebellar cortex about head motion and supply the excitatory drive for the basic circuitry of the VOR (see Fig. 20.16). The visual inputs provide an error signal that indicates how successfully eye movements stabilize the image on the retina. A third input to the cerebellum is a feedback signal from the motor neurons of

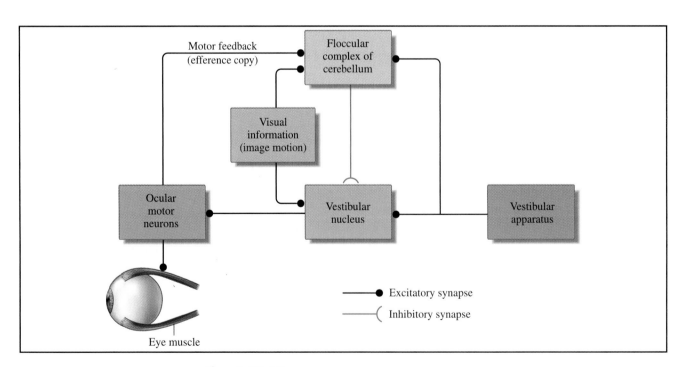

Figure 20.17.

The floccular complex of the cerebellum influences synaptic transfer in the vestibular nucleus during the vestibulo-ocular reflex. The cerebellum receives excitatory inputs from the vestibular system and visual system, which also provide excitatory inputs to the vestibular nucleus. Feedback from the motor output of the ocular motor neurons also reaches the cerebellum.

the ocular muscles (see Fig. 20.17). This type of motor feedback signal, called **efference copy**, gives information about the output signal being sent to the eye muscles. The three signals to the cerebellum permit a comparison among head rotation velocity, image slippage on the retina, and strength of excitatory drive to the eye muscles.

Although the diagram in Figure 20.17 is specific for the VOR, the same general plan of signal connections is used for other sensory-motor combinations in other portions of the cerebellum. Consequently, the calculation of a correction signal, like that thought to be carried out for the VOR, may be carried out in other parts of the cerebellum for various motor systems.

Synaptic Circuitry Within the Cerebellar Cortex

Figure 20.18 summarizes the synaptic connections among the neurons of the floccular complex, a pattern that is repeated throughout the cerebellar cortex. Two types of incoming axons are the **climbing fibers** and the **mossy fibers**, which are distinguished on the basis of their distinctive synaptic connections. Climbing fibers synapse exclusively on Purkinje cells, which are the large neurons whose axons provide the sole output from the cerebellum. Mossy fibers make contact with **granule cells**, which are smaller interneurons whose cell bodies are located deeper in the cerebellum than the Purkinje cells. Both climbing fibers and mossy fibers make excitatory synaptic connections onto their target neurons.

Axons of granule cells extend toward the surface of the cerebellum, where they branch into **parallel fibers** that parallel the surface for long distances. The dendrites of the Purkinje cells receive extensive excitatory synaptic input from the parallel fibers. In addition to these excitatory interactions, Purkinje cells and granule cells receive inhibitory inputs from inhibitory interneurons (stellate, basket, and Golgi cells), which receive excitatory inputs from the parallel fibers.

In the floccular complex, mossy fibers provide the vestibular sensory inputs, while visual information arrives via both mossy fibers and climbing fibers. The efference copy feedback from oculomotor neurons is transmitted via mossy fibers. It is not clear whether the different types of incoming information on mossy fibers are segregated to different sets of granule cells.

It is also not known how the synaptic interconnections summarized in Figure 20.18 compare vestibular, visual, and motor inputs to generate an error signal. Purkinje cells of the floccular complex show little change in action potential activity during the VOR under normal conditions, when the gain of the reflex is at its normal value of 1.0. Although ongoing activity of the Purkinje cells provides a tonic level of inhibitory input to the neurons of the vestibular nucleus, the firing rate of the Purkinje cells neither increases nor decreases during the VOR. Thus, the inhibitory input from Purkinje cells to the vestibular relay neurons of the vestibular nucleus does not normally change during the reflex. However, when the VOR gain is lower than normal as a result of training (that is, the gain is less than 1.0), the floccular Purkinje cells increase their firing rate during the VOR. As a result, inhibition of the neurons in the vestibular nucleus is increased during the reflex, diminishing the excitatory drive provided to the oculomotor neurons. Conversely, the firing rate of the Purkinje cells decreases during the VOR when the gain is higher than normal (that is, the gain is greater than 1.0). This decreased activity of Purkinje cells reduces inhibition of the vestibular nucleus neurons during the VOR and causes greater excitatory drive to be transmitted to the oculomotor neurons. The changes in inhibitory action of the Purkinje cells contribute to the changes in excitation from the vestibular nucleus to the oculomotor neurons that underlie the altered gain of the VOR.

Although the altered inhibition provided by Purkinje cells may contribute to the acquisition of the modified reflex during learning, the Purkinje cells cannot account for the retention of the modified gain. Learned changes in VOR gain persist

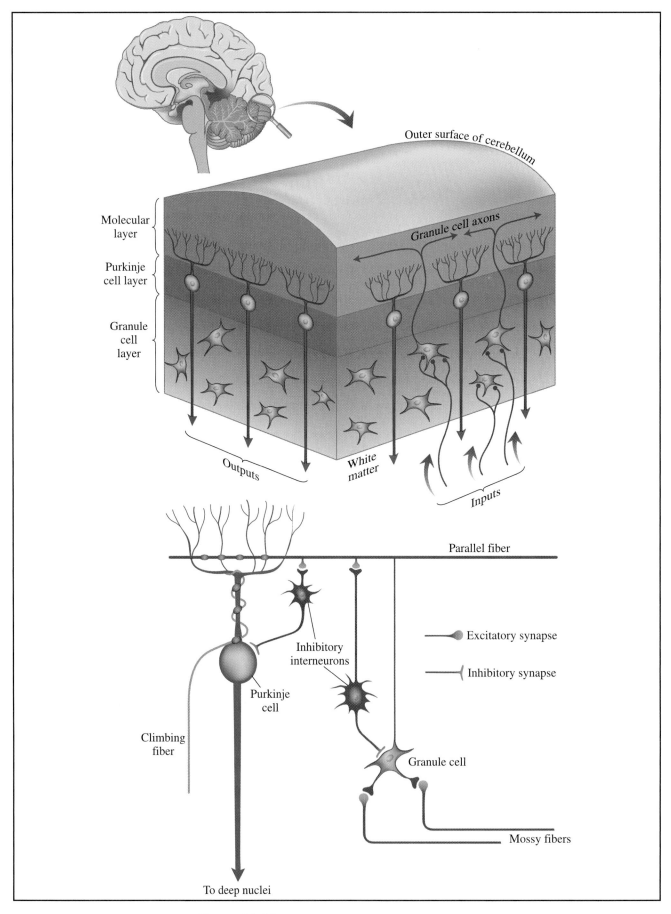

Outer surface of cerebellum

Molecular layer

Purkinje cell layer

Granule cell layer

Granule cell axons

Outputs

White matter

Inputs

Parallel fiber

Inhibitory interneurons

Excitatory synapse

Inhibitory synapse

Purkinje cell

Climbing fiber

Granule cell

Mossy fibers

To deep nuclei

Figure 20.18.

Synaptic interactions in the cerebellum.

when the floccular complex is destroyed and the inhibitory input from the Purkinje cells to the vestibular nucleus is removed. Thus, changes in synaptic efficacy within the basic VOR circuitry must be at least partly responsible for the long-term storage of learned changes in reflex strength.

Long-Term Depression in Purkinje Cells

The long-term changes in synaptic strength in the VOR are reminiscent of LTP and LTD, which were discussed earlier in this chapter. Considerable attention has been directed toward understanding LTD in the excitatory synaptic connections of the parallel fibers with cerebellar Purkinje cells. Activation of the climbing-fiber input to a Purkinje cell produces a long-term decrease in the synaptic effect of parallel-fiber inputs in that same cell that are active at the same time. Thus, concurrent activation of climbing fibers produces an associative depression of parallel-fiber synapses. A single action potential in a climbing fiber produces a large e.p.s.p. and an increase in intracellular calcium in a Purkinje cell, and these responses trigger the depression of the active parallel-fiber synapses in a manner thought to be similar to associative LTP. This LTD mechanism may allow an interaction between signals derived from motion of the visual image (climbing fibers) and signals derived from vestibular inputs (a portion of the parallel-fiber inputs). In turn, altered activity of Purkinje cells during modification of the VOR may result from these synaptic interactions. Because destruction of the cerebellar cortex fails to abolish previously learned changes in the VOR, however, other synaptic sites outside the cerebellum must be involved in the storage of the learned changes.

The circuit diagram shown in Figure 20.17 suggests that the vestibular nucleus might be another site where all of the relevant sensory and motor information is represented. LTP and LTD of synaptic responses in neurons of the vestibular nucleus could produce the changes in synaptic strength required to alter the overall gain of the VOR. The cerebellar output to the vestibular nucleus might then be necessary in some way to set up the long-term changes in synaptic efficacy within the vestibular nucleus. At present, no evidence is available regarding the plasticity of the synaptic connections within the vestibular nucleus.

Although the VOR is one of the simplest reflex circuits in the primate central nervous system, the state of knowledge of its mechanisms of plasticity is primitive compared with the knowledge of reflex plasticity in *Aplysia californica*, for example. Until the sites of long-term alteration in synaptic strength in the VOR are established, it is impossible to identify the cellular and molecular mechanisms that give rise to and sustain the learned modifications of the VOR. As research on neural plasticity proceeds, it will be interesting to see if the molecular changes underlying synaptic plasticity in simple systems such as *Aplysia* also take place in mammalian models of learning and memory, such as the hippocampus and the VOR.

SUMMARY

Synaptic connections among neurons change in strength over time, giving rise to both short-term and long-term changes in the behavior of the organism. This is true for both complex neural circuits and simple reflexes.

Activity-dependent changes in synaptic effectiveness within a single synaptic terminal are the simplest type of synaptic plasticity. An action potential in a presynaptic terminal leaves behind an aftereffect that alters the amount of neurotransmitter released by subsequent action potentials. This aftereffect can either enhance or depress the subsequent release of neurotransmitter. Short-term enhancement mechanisms include the following processes: facilitation, which is triggered by a small number of presynaptic action potentials and lasts for a few hundred milliseconds or less; augmen-

SUMMARY

tation, which lasts for several seconds and is triggered after action potentials are fired at a high rate for a few seconds; and potentiation, which is triggered by still-longer periods of high-frequency firing and lasts for minutes. Short-term enhancement is triggered by a buildup of calcium ions inside the presynaptic terminal during bursts of action potentials. Short-term depression of neurotransmitter release also can occur after a burst of presynaptic action potentials. Multiple mechanisms of depression have been identified, including calcium-dependent inactivation or activation of ion channels, depletion of releasable synaptic vesicles, and activation of autoreceptors on the synaptic terminal by neurotransmitter released from the same terminal.

Long-term changes in synaptic strength last for days or weeks, rather than minutes. LTP has been studied extensively in the hippocampus, a brain region thought to be involved in the formation of memories. LTP occurs when a synaptic input is activated simultaneously with strong depolarization of the postsynaptic cell, which normally occurs only during a period of strong synaptic activation. Thus, LTP requires the association between the activation of an input and the postsynaptic state of the receiving neuron. The potentiated synaptic input then produces a larger-than-normal excitatory postsynaptic potential, an effect that lingers for days or weeks. LTP is thought to be triggered by the influx of calcium ions through postsynaptic glutamate receptors, called NMDA receptors, that require both glutamate and postsynaptic depolarization to open. The increase in postsynaptic calcium triggers cellular messengers that enhance future transmission via both presynaptic and postsynaptic changes. These changes are localized to the activated synapse. Some synapses in the central nervous system also show LTD, but the conditions for triggering LTD are less clearly established.

Cellular mechanisms of learning in simple reflexes have been studied extensively using withdrawal reflexes in a marine mollusk, *Aplysia californica*. Habituation of a reflex refers to the progressive decline in vigor of the reflexive response with repeated presentations of the eliciting stimulus. In the withdrawal reflex, habituation results from synaptic depression in the excitatory synapses in the reflex circuit. Sensitization refers to the enhancement of a reflex following contact with a noxious stimulus. Sensitization of the withdrawal reflex in *Aplysia* occurs when facilitatory interneurons are stimulated by the noxious stimulus. These interneurons release the neurotransmitter serotonin, which acts via G-protein–coupled receptors to increase the concentration of the second messenger, cyclic AMP, inside the excitatory synaptic terminals of the withdrawal reflex circuit. Cyclic AMP induces phosphorylation of potassium channels, which then become inactivated. With fewer potassium channels available to contribute to repolarization, presynaptic action potentials repolarize more slowly, allowing greater calcium influx during an action potential. The increased calcium influx triggers greater neurotransmitter release at the excitatory synapses, producing a stronger withdrawal response.

Reflexive learning is also observed in the primate central nervous system. For example, learning occurs in the VOR, which moves the eyes to keep the visual image stable on the retina when the head rotates. The strength of the motor output to the eye muscles is adjusted based on experience, to adjust for any inaccuracies in maintaining a stabilized retinal image during head motion. This reflex learning reflects changes in the strength of synaptic connections in the VOR circuit. The cerebellum is required for learning in the VOR.

1. Describe the role of intracellular calcium in short-term synaptic enhancement.

2. List three different mechanisms for short-term synaptic depression.

3. Identify the following: dentate gyrus, CA fields, perforant path, Schaffer collaterals.

4. What do we mean when we say that LTP is an *associative* form of synaptic plasticity?

5. What are the important functional differences between the two types of glutamate receptors found in the postsynaptic dendritic spines of hippocampal pyramidal neurons?

6. Describe the role of calcium in the induction of LTP in the hippocampus.

7. Compare and contrast LTP and LTD.

8. Draw the neural circuit for the siphon withdrawal circuit in *Aplysia californica*, and describe the changes that occur during short-term habituation of the reflex.

9. Describe the mechanism of short-term sensitization of the withdrawal reflex in *Aplysia californica*. Include molecular mechanisms where possible.

10. How is the transition from short-term to long-term sensitization thought to occur in the withdrawal reflex in *Aplysia californica*?

11. Discuss the implications of the fact that the VOR is an open loop reflex. What is meant by the "gain" of the reflex?

12. Draw the synaptic interactions among the neurons of the cerebellar cortex and their incoming fibers, and specify the incoming fiber types that carry vestibular, visual, and efference copy information.

13. Describe the changes in the firing rate of Purkinje cells in the floccular complex during the VOR under the following conditions: gain of reflex of 1.0, gain of reflex less than 1.0, gain of reflex more than 1.0.

INTERNET ASSIGNMENT   CHAPTER 20

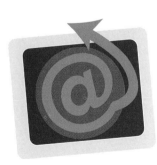

1 Use the anatomical resources you have found on the Internet to view the location of the hippocampus in mammalian brains.

2 Cyclic AMP plays an important role in the long-term modification of reflexes in *Aplysia*. Evidence from *Drosophila* mutants also suggests a role for cyclic AMP and its signaling partners in learning. Use PubMed to investigate fruit fly mutants that affect learning and memory and describe the role of cyclic AMP in those mutations.

LANGUAGE AND COGNITION

In mammals, the evolutionary trend toward an increasingly important forebrain is manifested predominantly in the progressively larger proportion of the forebrain accounted for by the neocortex. For example, the large size of the neocortex is one of the principal distinguishing features of the human brain. Significant parts of this large neocortex are devoted to the control of motor behavior (see Chapter 9) or to the processing of specific sensory information, es-

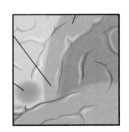

pecially visual information (see Chapter 16). However, the primary sensory and primary motor areas together account for only about 20% of the human cortex. The remaining areas, sometimes referred to as the **association cortex**, are involved in further perceptual processing of sensory information, in motor planning, and in cognition. **Cognition** is a collective term for the complex functions of the brain having to do with language and thought. This chapter examines the role of different parts of the cortex in language and cognition.

LANGUAGE

Lateralization of Language Function

The two halves of the cerebrum are not functionally identical. For example, the somatosensory and motor systems in each cerebral hemisphere are concerned with the contralateral half of the body. Thus, the left cerebral hemisphere receives sensory inputs from and sends motor commands to the right side of the body, while the right cerebral cortex handles the left side of the body (see Chapters 9 and 14). Although this scheme implies an approximately equal division of labor between the two cerebral hemispheres, the two halves of the motor cortex in the human brain are not equally adept at fine-motor control of the hand. Over 90% of people are right-handed, which means that the motor control circuits in the left cerebral cortex are capable of finer control of the hand and fingers than are the circuits in the right hemisphere. In right-handers, fine-motor control is **lateralized** to the left hemisphere, which is referred to as the **dominant hemisphere** for hand control.

Language function is also lateralized in the human brain. In almost all right-handers, the dominant hemisphere for language function is the left hemisphere. As a result, lesions of the relevant parts of the left cortex selectively disrupt the production or comprehension of language, whereas lesions in the corresponding parts of the right hemisphere do not affect language. The left hemisphere is also dominant for language in more than half of left-handed people, in whom the right motor cortex handles fine-motor control. In the remaining left-handers, the right hemisphere is dominant for language. Overall, then, linguistic abilities are localized to the left hemisphere in over 95% of the human population.

Although the left hemisphere is dominant for language in most people, the right hemisphere dominates in other cognitive abilities. For example, musical abilities, such as the ability to sing a melody, are localized to the nondominant hemisphere (typically, the right hemisphere). Spatial abilities, such as the perception of geometrical relationships among objects, are also localized to the nondominant hemisphere.

Hemispheric dominance for language emerges slowly during childhood, and plasticity in the choice of dominant hemisphere persists for some time. As a consequence, a lesion in the left hemisphere of a right-handed child may have no lasting effect on language, although a comparable lesion produced by disease or accident in the adult brain would have devastating effects on language abilities. In the child's brain, the normally nondominant right hemisphere remains capable of taking over the linguistic functions.

Split-Brain Patients Reveal Lateralization of Language Function

Lateralization of cortical function, including language, has been studied extensively in "split-brain" patients whose corpus callosum has been cut surgically in an effort to control severe epilepsy. The corpus callosum is a large fiber bundle—the largest in the brain, in fact—containing axons that connect the two cerebral hemispheres (Fig. 21.1A). Transecting the corpus callosum eliminates most communication between the two halves of the neocortex, and as a result, each cerebral hemisphere behaves independently of the other.

Under normal circumstances, split-brain patients are indistinguishable from normal individuals. However, specially designed experimental conditions reveal differences in the capabilities of the two separated hemispheres, as illustrated in Figure 21.1. Recall that each half of the visual field projects to the thalamus and

What is hemispheric dominance?

Figure 21.1.

Lateralization of language function is revealed in a split-brain patient. The corpus callosum connecting the two cerebral hemispheres has been cut, eliminating communication between the two halves of the cortex. A visual stimulus is presented in either the right or the left visual field sufficiently briefly that the subject cannot move his or her eyes during presentation of the stimulus. **A**. A picture of a fork is presented in the right visual field, which projects to the left visual cortex. The visual information can be relayed to the language system in the left hemisphere, and the patient can verbally identify the stimulus. **B**. A picture of a fork is presented in the left visual field, which projects to the right visual cortex. The visual information cannot be relayed through the corpus callosum to the language system in the left cortex, and the patient cannot verbally identify the stimulus. The left hand can correctly pick out the stimulus object, however, because it is controlled by the right motor cortex.

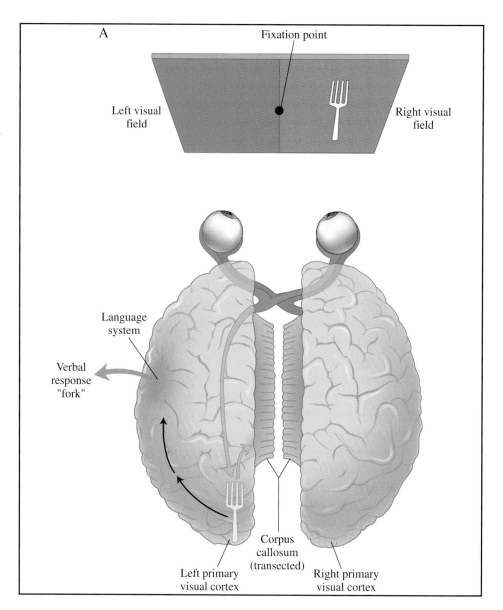

primary visual cortex in the opposite cerebral hemisphere (see Chapter 16, Fig. 16.2). Normally, the visual information in each hemisphere is relayed through the corpus callosum to the opposite hemisphere, but this pathway is no longer available in split-brain individuals. In the absence of the corpus callosum, a visual stimulus briefly presented in the right half of the visual field is seen only by the visual cortex in the left hemisphere (see Fig. 21.1A). Because language is localized to the left hemisphere in most people, the visual information is available for transmission to language areas in the same hemisphere, and the split-brain patient is able to verbally identify an object seen in the right visual field.

If the visual stimulus is briefly presented in the left visual field, split-brain subjects can no longer identify the object verbally. As shown in Figure 21.1B, the visual information is restricted to the right visual cortex under these conditions and cannot be transmitted to the verbally competent left hemisphere in the absence of the corpus callosum. Although the right cortex is mute, it is able to identify the stimulus by nonverbal means. For example, the left hand—which is controlled by the right cortex—can correctly select the stimulus object from a group of other objects, even though the subject is still unable to say what the object is. Similarly, a split-brain patient is unable to verbally identify an object placed in the left hand,

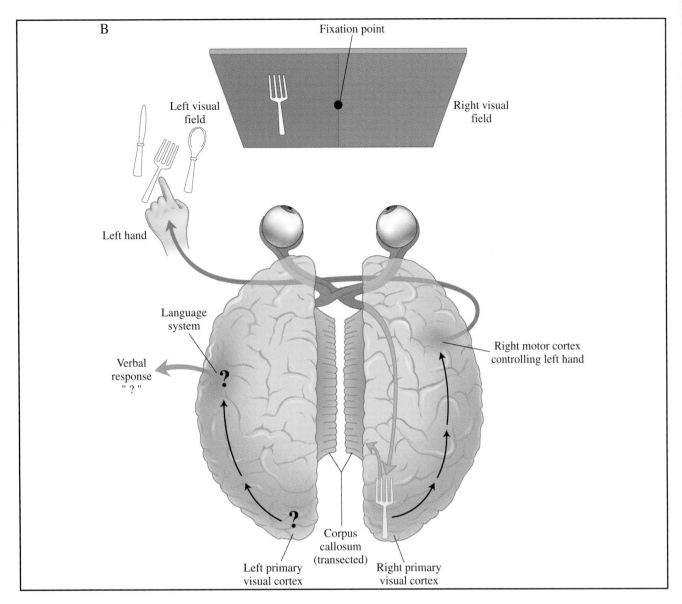

Figure 21.1.

(continued)

because somatosensory information from the left hand projects to the right somatosensory cortex and thus is unavailable to the language areas of the left hemisphere.

Cortical Areas Involved in Language

Language is a uniquely human characteristic. Thus, experimental studies of animal brains cannot provide information regarding language function in the neocortex. Instead, knowledge about the brain regions involved in language has come largely from studies of neurological patients whose brains were damaged by disease, accident, or surgical trauma. (However, see "In the Clinic" for a description of noninvasive techniques used to study the normal human brain during the performance of cognitive tasks.) **Aphasia** is a disorder of the ability to understand or produce spoken language. Although neurologists recognize several different types of aphasia, the two major types are **Broca's aphasia** and **Wernicke's aphasia**, which are

What features distinguish receptive and expressive aphasia?

named for the nineteenth-century neurologists who first described the syndromes and localized the site of the corresponding cortical lesions.

Patients with Broca's aphasia can understand spoken language but produce speech only haltingly. Because Broca's aphasia represents a defect in speech production, it is also referred to as **expressive aphasia**. The corresponding cortical lesion is found in **Broca's area**, which is located in the lateral portion of the frontal cortex of the dominant hemisphere—usually the left hemisphere. As shown in Figure 21.2, Broca's area overlaps part of the premotor cortex, just anterior to the portion of the primary motor cortex that controls the muscles of the mouth and tongue. Although these muscles are responsible for producing speech, Broca's aphasia is not a simple motor defect resulting from paralysis of the relevant muscles. In fact individual words are pronounced normally, but the smooth flow of words into normal speech is disrupted. This type of deficit is consistent with the general role of the premotor cortex in programming complex sequences of movements (see Chapter 9). Thus, Broca's aphasia involves problems translating verbal thought into the required motor movements of the speech apparatus. In addition to deficits of spoken language, patients with Broca's aphasia often have difficulty writing, which suggests that they have a generalized defect of the translation of verbal thought into motor acts.

In Wernicke's aphasia, comprehension of written and oral language is impaired. For this reason, Wernicke's aphasia is also called **receptive aphasia**. Wernicke's aphasia is associated with lesions in the temporal lobe surrounding the primary auditory cortex, which is referred to as **Wernicke's area** (Fig. 21.3). Thus, Wernicke's area is closely associated with the primary sensory cortex for speech perception, just as Broca's area is closely associated with the primary motor cortex for speech muscles. The cortical locations of the lesions are consistent with the principal effects of Broca's and Wernicke's aphasias on the production and understanding of speech, respectively. Patients with Wernicke's aphasia hear normally but are unable to attach meaning to words. In other words, the semantic content of word sounds is lost.

Although Wernicke's aphasia primarily affects comprehension, speech production also may be affected in patients with Wernicke's aphasia. The flow and rhythm of speech production are typically normal, but the correct use of words and grammar may be disrupted, resulting in impairment of meaningful speech. These defi-

Figure 21.2.

The location of Broca's area in the frontal lobe of the left hemisphere of the cerebral cortex. Lesions in this area interfere with the production of spoken language (expressive aphasia).

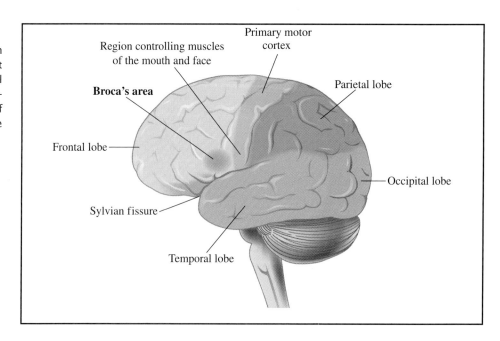

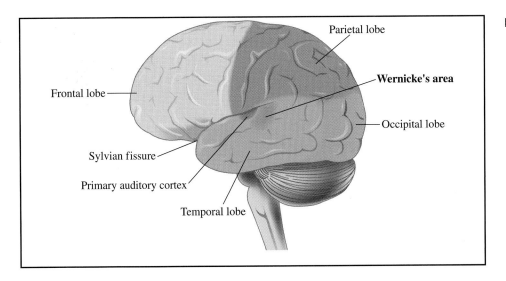

Figure 21.3.

The location of Wernicke's area in the temporal lobe of the left hemisphere of the cerebral cortex. Lesions in this area interfere with the comprehension of spoken language (receptive aphasia).

cits of spoken language associated with damage to Wernicke's area suggest that Wernicke's area communicates with Broca's area during normal speech production.

Evidence for communication between Wernicke's and Broca's areas also is provided by the existence of a third form of aphasia, called **conduction aphasia**. This type of aphasia results from damage to the **arcuate fasciculus**, which is a fiber tract in the cortical white matter that contains axons interconnecting frontal cortex and posterior cortical regions (Fig. 21.4). The arcuate fasciculus includes axons that connect Wernicke's area with Broca's area. Damage to these axons produces speech difficulties, even if both Wernicke's and Broca's areas are intact. Patients with conduction aphasia comprehend spoken language normally, which is consistent with the sparing of Wernicke's area. However, the fluency of speech production is impaired.

Broca's area, Wernicke's area, and the interconnecting arcuate fasciculus surround the perimeter of the large fissure separating the temporal lobe from the rest of the cortex, the **Sylvian fissure** (also called the lateral sulcus). For this reason, the language areas are sometimes referred to as the **perisylvian region**.

In addition to the global forms of aphasia associated with lesions in Wernicke's and Broca's areas, damage to other cortical regions in the dominant hemisphere can produce more restricted forms of language disturbance. For example, an inability

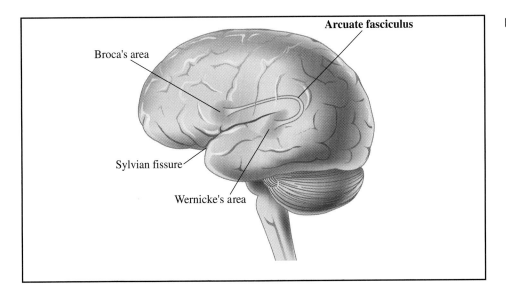

Figure 21.4.

The arcuate fasciculus is an axon bundle that connects neurons of Broca's area and Wernicke's area. Lesions that interrupt the arcuate fasciculus produce conduction aphasia.

to name things (**anomia**) can result from damage to the posterior part of the inferior temporal lobe in the language-dominant hemisphere, near Wernicke's area.

As expected from the strong lateralization of language function to the left hemisphere in most people, lesions in the right hemisphere do not produce the dramatic impairment in language comprehension or production that results from lesions in the perisylvian region of the left hemisphere. However, right cortical lesions do impair other aspects of oral communication. For example, the ability to perceive or to express emotional content (anger, fear, joy, sadness, and so on) in language may be diminished following damage to the perisylvian region in the right hemisphere. Lesions in the right hemisphere may also affect other subtle facets of language, such as irony and humor.

Deficits of Reading and Writing

What parts of the cerebral cortex are involved in reading and writing?

Linguistic communication involves written words, as well as oral and auditory communication. Specific disruption of reading (**alexia**) can result from damage in the **angular gyrus** of the dominant hemisphere, which is located near the border between the temporal, occipital, and parietal lobes (Fig. 21.5). Note that alexia is distinguished from **dyslexia**, which is a congenital disorder of the brain that makes it difficult for children to learn to read. By contrast, alexia arises suddenly as a result of cortical damage produced by accident or disease. Alexia is often combined with **agraphia** (inability to write) as a result of lesions of the angular gyrus. Damage in the frontal lobe, just in front of the region of the primary motor cortex controlling the hand, can also interfere with writing.

Alexia without associated agraphia also can occur after destruction of the left occipital cortex, even though the angular gyrus remains intact. The affected individual is blind in the right visual field but has normal vision in the left visual field, which projects to the intact right occipital cortex. Although words can be seen in the left visual field, comprehension is not possible because the axons that cross from the right to the left visual cortex in the corpus callosum are destroyed by the left occipital lesion. Thus, the visual information remains restricted to the right hemisphere and cannot be transmitted to the language areas of the left hemisphere. In these patients, then, alexia arises from a mechanism that is functionally similar to the visual language deficits observable in split-brain patients (see Fig. 21.1).

Figure 21.5.

The location of the angular gyrus in the posterior portion of the parietal lobe.

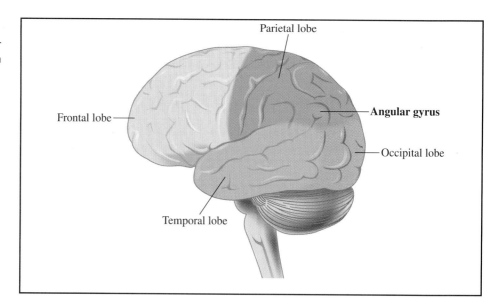

COGNITION

The neocortex is responsible for a variety of higher-level mental functions, in addition to language. As a group, these mental functions are referred to as cognition, which underlies the aspects of behavior we consider to indicate intelligence and rationality. These aspects include such things as recognition of complex objects and their appropriate use, the proper execution of complicated series of motor actions, and the ability to formulate and carry out long-term plans of action. Cognition encompasses a broad range of human abilities, and this section describes selected examples.

As with language, much information about cognitive function in humans has emerged from studies of patients who have had brain damage from surgery, accident, or disease. In the case of nonlanguage forms of cognition, however, additional insight into cortical roles has been obtained from experimental studies of animals, particularly nonhuman primates.

IN THE CLINIC

Much of what is known about cognitive functions of the cortex was learned from studies of neurological patients who had lesions in specific cortical areas caused by head trauma or stroke. Until recently, detailed characterization of the lesion underlying a particular cognitive defect was possible only postmortem, by direct anatomical examination of the brain. The development of noninvasive imaging techniques, commonly used to diagnose neurological problems, now allows lesions of the brain to be visualized in living patients. These techniques include computed tomography (CT), which is a method of constructing three-dimensional images of the body interior based on X-ray absorption, and magnetic resonance imaging (MRI), which uses the magnetic behavior of the nuclei of molecules to construct a three-dimensional representation of internal structures. These techniques provide useful but static information about the structure of the brain.

Dynamic information about changes in neuronal activity during cognitive processes is provided by variants of the imaging techniques, such as positron emission tomography (PET) and functional MRI (fMRI). These techniques can be applied in normal human subjects, allowing neuroscientists to obtain information about normal brain function. In PET, a subject is injected with a radioactive form of a compound, and gamma rays created by positrons emitted by the decaying isotope are used to locate the compound. To obtain information about neuronal activity, a radioactive glucose analog (2-deoxyglucose) is injected, and the glucose analog accumulates in neurons that are firing more frequently and thus have higher metabolic needs.

The technique fMRI detects the increased flow of oxygenated blood to regions that are more active. When neural activity increases at a particular location in the brain, the blood flow in the blood vessels that supply that part of the brain increases. This leads to a corresponding increase in the amount of oxygenated hemoglobin in that part of the brain. The magnetic properties of oxygenated hemoglobin differ from those of hemoglobin without oxygen, and the magnetic resonance signal is therefore different in parts of the brain where activity is higher. Thus, both PET and fMRI can be used to determine which brain regions are more active when a subject is asked to carry out a particular cognitive task, such as reading.

Damage to which parts of
the cortex produce agnosia
and apraxia?

Agnosia

Agnosia is a collective term for the inability to identify objects based on sensory information, even though the primary sensory cortical areas are intact (*agnosia* is derived from Greek words meaning "no recognition"). In general, specific types of agnosia result from lesions in the parietal or temporal lobe, in areas near the primary sensory cortex for the major senses. Agnosias are classified according to the sensory modality that is affected. For instance, tactile agnosia arises from lesions in the parietal cortex near the primary somatosensory cortex. Visual agnosia is caused by lesions near the primary and higher-order visual cortical regions, and auditory agnosia results from damage in the temporal lobe near the primary auditory cortex.

In tactile agnosia (also called **astereognosia**), objects cannot be identified using the sense of touch alone, although the same object can be readily identified if it can be seen. Auditory agnosia refers to the inability to identify nonspeech sounds (for example, a siren, a barking dog, and so on). Because Wernicke's area is also near the primary auditory cortex, cortical lesions that produce auditory agnosia sometimes result in receptive aphasia, as well. Visual agnosia can involve a general impairment of the ability to recognize objects using visual information, but it also can involve more specific deficits in recognizing particular types of objects. For instance, alexia, characterized by the inability to recognize words visually, can be considered a subtype of visual agnosia.

Other subtypes of visual agnosia are also distinguished. One interesting variant is **prosopagnosia** (*prosopon* is Greek for "face"), in which patients are unable to recognize faces of familiar people, including the patient's own face. This highly specific form of agnosia results from lesions in the right hemisphere (that is, the nondominant hemisphere for language). Figure 21.6 shows the location of the region of the right cortex where damage results in prosopagnosia. The lesion in-

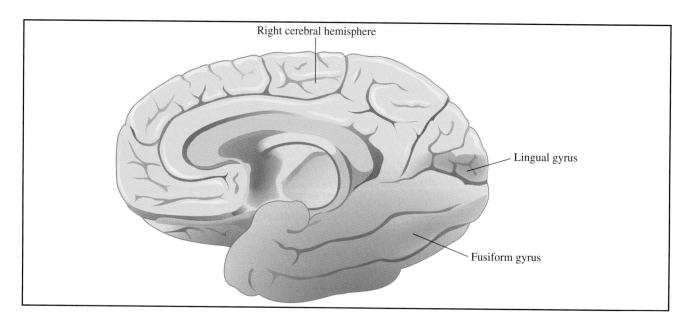

Right cerebral hemisphere

Lingual gyrus

Fusiform gyrus

Figure 21.6.

Lesions in the fusiform gyrus and the lingual gyrus in the right hemisphere interfere with the recognition of familiar faces. The fusiform gyrus is located on the bottom surface of the temporal lobe and is usually mostly hidden from view by the overlying cerebellum. The lingual gyrus is located on the medial surface of the occipital lobe and is also hidden from external view. In the view shown in this figure, all parts of the brain posterior to the thalamus, including the cerebellum, have been cut away to reveal the bottom surface of the temporal lobe.

volves the fusiform gyrus on the bottom surface of the posterior temporal lobe and the lingual gyrus on the medial aspect of the occipital lobe, near the border with the temporal lobe. This general area of cortex is a portion of the **inferotemporal cortex**. Electrical recordings from the inferotemporal cortex of monkey brains reveal that some neurons are activated specifically when pictures of faces are presented. This observation is also consistent with a role for this cortical region in face recognition.

Damage to the parietal lobe of the nondominant (right) hemisphere sometimes results in another form of agnosia, called **contralateral neglect syndrome**, in which the patient ignores the contralateral half of the body. Affected individuals fail to dress, wash, or even acknowledge the existence of the side of the body contralateral to the lesion. If shown the arm or leg from the neglected side, patients with neglect syndrome may claim that the limb belongs to someone else.

In contrast to prosopagnosia and contralateral neglect syndrome, other agnosias arise from lesions in the dominant hemisphere for language. Agnosias that involve an inability to verbally name or describe objects typically are a result of damage in the left hemisphere. For instance, **color agnosia** is a form of visual agnosia that arises from lesions in higher-order visual cortical areas in the left occipital cortex (see Chapter 16). In this disorder, color vision is intact, but patients are unable to name colors.

Apraxia

In addition to the perceptual disturbances observed in agnosias, damage to the cortex also can produce deficits in carrying out motor tasks. Lesions in a variety of cortical areas can lead to different forms of **apraxia**, which refers to a difficulty in programming complex series of movements, without paralysis, sensory defects, or problems performing simple tasks. Many everyday acts, such as getting dressed, require specific motor programs to be carried out in a particular order. In some apraxic patients, cortical damage interferes with the ability to execute the motor programs in the correct order. Although each motor program (for example, putting on socks, putting on shoes, tying shoelaces) is intact, the order of execution is incorrect (for example, tying the laces, then attempting to put on the shoes). In Chapter 9, we learned that the premotor cortex and supplementary motor area in the frontal lobes are important to the performance of complex movements. However, apraxias of various types commonly result from lesions in the parietal/temporal association areas, which suggests that the more posterior cortical regions are involved in planning a series of actions whose individual programs are formulated in the frontal cortex.

In some cases, apraxia is associated with aphasia. For example, lesions in the **supramarginal gyrus** at the border between the temporal lobe and the parietal lobe (Fig. 21.7) can produce both conduction aphasia (see above) and apraxia in which patients cannot properly follow verbal commands to carry out motor actions. As with conduction aphasia, the lesion probably produces apraxia by destroying axons that carry commands from the temporal and parietal areas to the motor areas of the frontal cortex.

Although lesions in discrete sites in the neocortex can produce defects in specific aspects of language or cognition, it should be emphasized that there is not a single "center" for a particular complex function. Successful comprehension or production of language, for example, requires the concerted action of a variety of cortical circuits spread through parietal, temporal, and frontal cortex. Each region of the cortex is interconnected with a variety of other areas, and the neurons at a particular site may participate in numerous, related functions. Functional imaging of the activity of human brains during the performance of mental tasks reveals that

Figure 21.7.

The location of the supramarginal gyrus, at the border between the parietal and temporal lobes.

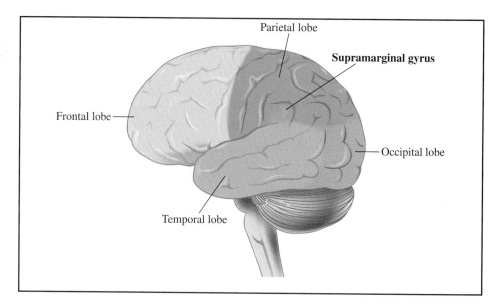

wide-ranging areas of the cortex become active during specific functions and that a given area shows an increase in neural activity during more than one type of task. Also, lesions produced by an accident or a stroke are likely to damage not just the neurons of the outer layers of the cortex at that location but also the underlying axons of the white matter. The white matter may contain axons that originate in and terminate in distant parts of the cortex serving other cognitive functions. Therefore the fiber bundles that carry axons providing interconnections among the cortical areas are also important in cognitive functions, and a lesion in these fiber bundles can produce defects as severe as those associated with damage to the cortex itself.

Cortical Lesions Affect Emotion and Personality

What changes in personality accompany damage to the frontal lobes?

In addition to the effects on cognition and language discussed previously, cortical damage in the human brain can affect emotional behavior and produce changes in an individual's overall personality. As described in Chapter 12, neocortical structures form part of the limbic system, including the cingulate gyrus and the orbitofrontal cortex. Because of their extensive interconnections with noncortical limbic system structures, these cortical areas are involved in emotional behavior and the conscious perception of emotions. Figure 21.8 shows the location of the orbitofrontal cortex, which lies along the bottom surface of the frontal lobes (just above the orbits of the eyes, from which it receives its name). Because cutting fiber bundles that connect the orbitofrontal cortex with the rest of the brain reduces aggressiveness and has a calming effect in experimental animals, similar surgical lesions ("frontal lobotomy") were used to control disturbed emotional behavior in human mental patients. With the advent of drug treatments for mental illness, such psychosurgical treatments have become largely obsolete.

Disconnection of the orbitofrontal cortex has additional effects beyond its calming effect, however. Lobotomized patients commonly fail to make or carry through on long-term plans (that is, they lack "drive" or "initiative"). Damage to the anterior parts of the frontal lobes may also promote impulsive, irresponsible behavior, and social behavior may be disrupted. For example, individuals with frontal lobe damage may lack the ability to edit their verbal output in socially acceptable ways and may use excessive profanity. Thus, association cortex in the frontal lobes appears to be involved in significant ways in determining an individual's personality.

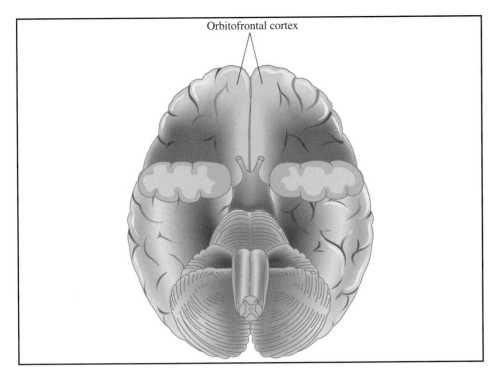

Figure 21.8.
The location of the orbito-frontal cortex (*orange*) on the bottom surface of the frontal lobes. The anterior poles of both temporal lobes have been removed to reveal the underlying parts of the frontal lobes.

Dementia and the Loss of Cognitive Abilities

With increasing age, a significant proportion of the population experiences a loss of mental abilities. In severe cases, progressive and global loss of language, memory, and perceptual abilities leads ultimately to incapacitation and death. The most prevalent form of serious age-related dementia is **Alzheimer's disease**, which is produced by the progressive death of neurons in a wide range of brain regions, including the neocortex.

Alzheimer's disease is characterized by two types of abnormal structures that ac-cumulate in areas where neurons are dying: **neuritic plaques** and **neurofibrillary tangles**. Neuritic plaques are extracellular accumulations of protein, consisting pre-dominantly of β-**amyloid protein** (abbreviated **Aβ**). Neurofibrillary tangles are ab-normal intracellular aggregates of a microtubule-associated protein, called **tau**.

The current theory of plaque formation is illustrated in Figure 21.9. Aβ is a pep-tide fragment derived from selective proteolysis of a protein called **amyloid precur-sor protein**, which is a normal component of neuronal membranes. The function of the precursor protein in normal neurons remains unknown. Aβ is derived largely from the extracellular portion of amyloid precursor protein, and the proteolytic fragment is released into the extracellular space when the precursor is cleaved by proteases. In the extracellular space, Aβ peptides adhere to each other to form a cluster of tangled fibrils (see Fig. 21.9), which then form the nucleus of the plaque.

Aβ is produced normally in the brain, but most of it remains soluble in the extracellular space and does not precipitate to form plaques. Although some plaques are found in brains from aged individuals who did not suffer from demen-tia, many more plaques are present in the brains of patients with Alzheimer's dis-ease, suggesting that a larger proportion of the normally released Aβ precipitates into plaques. Why Aβ precipitates into plaques in dementia is not yet completely understood. Different forms of Aβ exist, depending on exactly which peptide fragment is cut out of amyloid precursor protein by proteases. Some of these forms of Aβ are more soluble than others, and mutations in the precursor protein that favor the insoluble forms underlie certain inherited forms of dementia, in

Abnormal accumulations of what proteins are associated with Alzheimer's disease?

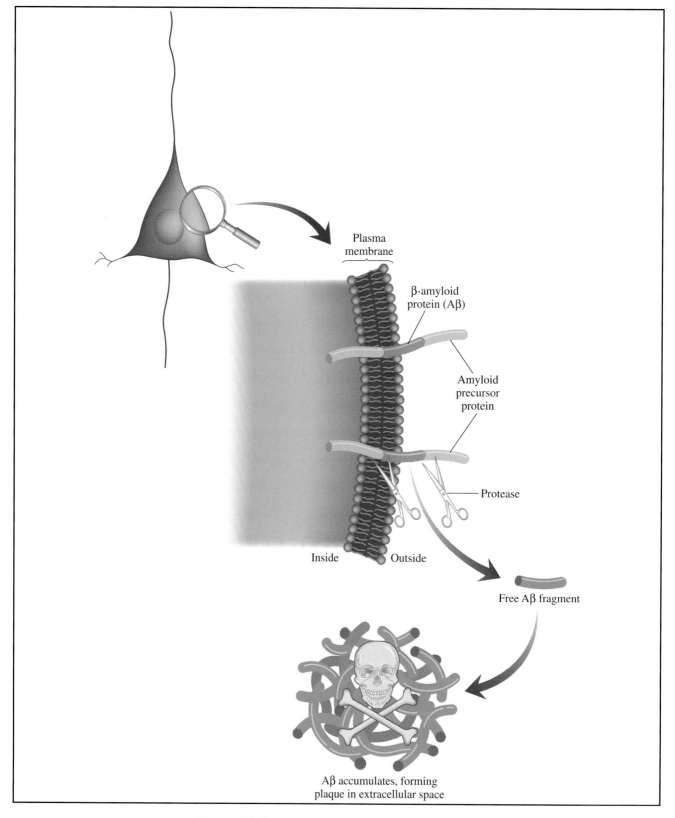

Plasma membrane

β-amyloid protein (Aβ)

Amyloid precursor protein

Protease

Inside   Outside

Free Aβ fragment

Aβ accumulates, forming
plaque in extracellular space

Figure 21.9.

The formation of neuritic plaques in the extracellular space in brains affected by Alzheimer's disease. Amyloid precursor protein is a protein normally found in the plasma membrane of brain neurons. β-Amyloid protein (Aβ) is a peptide fragment embedded within the precursor protein. Aβ is released by proteolysis and accumulates in the extracellular space, forming large clusters called plaques. The plaques are toxic to surrounding neurons.

which symptoms of Alzheimer's disease develop severely and at unusually early ages. Thus, the production of insoluble Aβ and the subsequent plaque formation are thought to trigger neuronal death in some manner. The mechanism by which plaques induce neuronal death is also unknown. The Aβ peptide itself may be toxic to surrounding neurons. Also, an inflammatory response to the abnormal protein deposit may cause damage to nearby tissue, leading to the death of neurons in the vicinity of the plaque.

Neurofibrillary tangles are bundles of filaments formed inside neurons by insoluble accumulations of the neuronal protein tau, as described in Figure 21.10. Tau is normally a component of microtubules, which form the backbone of neurites (see Fig. 19.11). Microtubules consist of the protein tubulin, and tau interacts with tubulin to stabilize the microtubules. Although the tau protein includes a number

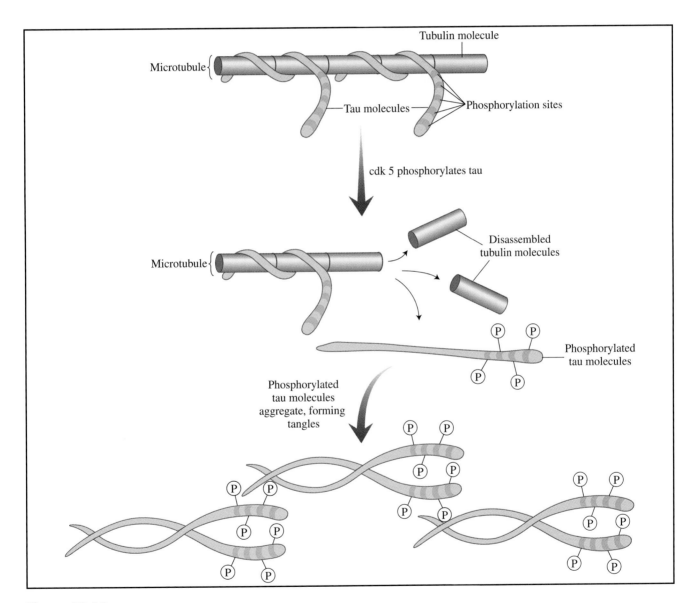

Figure 21.10.

The formation of neurofibrillary tangles within neurons in Alzheimer's disease. Neurons normally contain the microtubule-associated protein tau, which stabilizes the assembly of tubulin molecules into microtubules. To carry out this function, tau must not be phosphorylated. In Alzheimer's disease, tau becomes phosphorylated by cyclin-dependent kinase 5 (cdk5), and the phosphorylated tau dissociates from microtubules, which then disintegrate. Phosphorylated tau molecules bind to each other and form insoluble tangles that accumulate within affected neurons.

of sites that can potentially be phosphorylated by kinase enzymes, tau can interact with microtubules only when these sites are not phosphorylated. In the normal brain, tau exists largely in the dephosphorylated state. In the brain affected by Alzheimer's disease, however, tau becomes highly phosphorylated, causing it to dissociate from microtubules and interact with other phosphorylated tau molecules. As a result, microtubules disintegrate and the abnormal filaments making up the tangles form in the neurites and cell bodies of affected neurons.

Neuroscientists do not yet know why tau becomes unusually phosphorylated in Alzheimer's disease. A kinase called **cyclin-dependent kinase 5 (cdk5)** is thought to carry out the phosphorylation of tau, but how this kinase becomes activated in the disease is not firmly established. Like many other kinases, cdk5 consists of both catalytic and regulatory subunits. Evidence suggests that an abnormal form of the regulatory subunit of cdk5 is found in neurons of patients with Alzheimer's disease, and the abnormal regulatory subunit causes the kinase to become overactive and to hyperphosphorylate tau. The resulting loss of microtubules disrupts the neuronal cytoskeleton and prevents the normal transport of materials from the cell body to the neurites, which may lead to the death of the affected neurons.

SUMMARY

The majority of the neocortex consists of association cortex, which is a collective term for cortical regions that are not directly linked to arriving sensory information or outgoing motor commands. In the human brain, various parts of the association cortex are concerned with complex functions, such as language and thought. These functions are not equally distributed in the two cerebral hemispheres of the brain. Instead, the brain commonly exhibits lateralization of function, in which one hemisphere or the other is dominant for a particular cognitive task. For example, language is localized to the left cortical hemisphere in the great majority of the human population, whereas complicated spatial abilities are localized to the right cortical hemisphere. Lateralization of function is particularly clearly demonstrated in split-brain patients, in whom the corpus callosum, the major fiber tract connecting the two cortical hemispheres, has been cut.

Aphasia is a neurological disorder characterized by a difficulty in understanding or producing spoken language. The two major types of aphasia are Broca's aphasia (or expressive aphasia) and Wernicke's aphasia (or receptive aphasia). Broca's aphasia results from damage in the lateral portion of the frontal lobe, anterior to the portion of primary motor cortex concerned with the muscles of the mouth and tongue. Patients with Broca's aphasia have difficulty producing speech, although comprehension is unaffected. Patients with Wernicke's aphasia cannot understand speech because of a lesion in the temporal lobe near the primary auditory cortex. Damage to the axon tract connecting Broca's area in the frontal cortex and Wernicke's area in the temporal cortex—the arcuate fasciculus— also can produce aphasia. Alexia (inability to read) and agraphia (inability to write) are often associated with damage to the angular gyrus, near the border between the temporal, parietal, and occipital lobes of the dominant hemisphere for language.

Agnosia refers to the inability to identify objects based on sensory information, without damage to the primary sensory cortex. Selective forms of agnosia are associated with each major sensory modality. Failure to recognize specific subtypes of stimuli can also result from cortical damage. For example, an inability to recognize familiar faces (prosopagnosia) results from lesions in the inferotemporal cortex in the nondominant cortical hemisphere (usually the right hemisphere). Cortical lesions also affect the ability to carry out complex series of movements, a disorder called apraxia. Lesions in parietal and temporal association areas often result in a type of apraxia, such as an inability to put on clothing in the proper order.

Global loss of mental abilities (dementia) is frequently observed with aging. The most common form of dementia is Alzheimer's disease, which results from the progressive death of neurons in many brain regions, including the neocortex. Alzheimer's disease is characterized by accumulations of protein in the extracellular space (neuritic plaques) and inside neurons (neurofibrillary tangles). Plaques are formed by aggregations of a peptide called β-amyloid protein, which is a proteolytic fragment of a normal neuronal membrane protein called amyloid precursor protein. Neurofibrillary tangles are aggregates of a microtubule-associated protein, tau, which normally stabilizes microtubules in neurons.

REVIEW QUESTIONS

1. A right-handed patient shows impaired comprehension of speech. In which lobe of the cortex would the underlying lesion most likely be located?

2. Describe the symptoms expected for a lesion in Broca's area. Where is Broca's area located?

3. Why would a lesion in the arcuate fasciculus affect language function, even if the lesion does not destroy any of the cortical gray matter?

4. A split-brain patient is shown an object only in the left half of the visual field and asked to verbally identify the object. Would the patient be able to identify the object? Why or why not?

5. The left hemisphere of the brain is dominant for all cognitive abilities. Do you agree or disagree with this statement? Explain your answer.

6. Define each of the following: apraxia, agnosia, contralateral neglect.

7. Locate each of the following in the human brain: orbitofrontal cortex, angular gyrus, inferotemporal cortex.

8. What is a neuritic plaque, and how is it formed?

9. What protein forms neurofibrillary tangles, and what is its normal function in neurons?

INTERNET ASSIGNMENT   CHAPTER 21

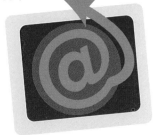

1 Locate the following language areas in the human brain, using on-line images and brain atlases: Broca's, Wernicke's, supramarginal gyrus, and arcuate fasciculus.

2 Functional MRI (fMRI) is being used to study a variety of brain functions in normal human subjects. Use the Internet to investigate how fMRI works. Then, find fMRI images related to language function.

DERIVATIONS OF THE NERNST AND GOLDMAN EQUATIONS

Nernst Equation

The Nernst equation is used extensively in the discussion of resting membrane potential and action potentials in this book. The derivation presented here is necessarily mathematical and requires some knowledge of differential and integral calculus to understand thoroughly. However, I have tried to explain the meaning of each step in words; this approach is intended to allow those without the necessary background to follow the logic qualitatively.

This derivation of the Nernst equation uses equations for the movement of ions down concentration and electrical gradients to arrive at a quantitative description of the equilibrium condition. The starting point is the realization that at equilibrium there will be no net movement of the ion across the membrane. That is, in the presence of both concentrational and electrical gradients, the rate of movement of the ion down the concentration gradient is equal and opposite to the rate of movement of the ion down the electrical gradient. For a charged substance (an ion), movement across the membrane constitutes a transmembrane electrical current, I. Thus, at equilibrium

$$I_C = -I_E \tag{A.1}$$

or

$$I_C + I_E = 0 \tag{A.2}$$

where I_C and I_E are the currents due to the concentrational and electrical gradients, respectively.

Concentrational Flux

Consider first the current due to the concentration gradient, which will be given by

$$I_C = A\Phi_C ZF \tag{A.3}$$

In words, Equation A.3 states that the current through the membrane of area A will be equal to the flux, Φ_C, of the ion down the concentration gradient (number of ions per second per unit area of membrane) multiplied by Z (the valence of the ion) and F (Faraday's constant; 96,500 coulombs per mole of univalent ion). The factor ZF translates the flux of ions into flux of charge and hence into an electrical current. The flux Φ_C for a given ion (call the ion Y, for example) will depend on the concentration gradient of Y across the membrane (that is, $[Y]_{in} - [Y]_{out}$) and on the membrane permeability to Y, p_Y. Quantitatively, this relation is given by

$$\Phi_C = p_Y([Y]_{in} - [Y]_{out}) \tag{A.4}$$

Note that p_Y has units of velocity (cm/sec), so Φ_C has units of molecules/sec/cm^2 (remember that $[Y]$ has units of molecules/cm^3). The permeability coefficient, p_Y, is in turn given by

$$p_Y = D_Y/a \tag{A.5}$$

where D_Y is the diffusion constant for Y within the membrane and a is the thickness of the membrane. D_Y can be expanded to yield

$$D_Y = uRT \qquad (A.6)$$

where u is the mobility of the ion within the membrane and RT (the gas constant times the absolute temperature) is the thermal energy available to drive ion movement. Substituting Equation A.6 in A.5 and the result in Equation A.4 yields

$$\Phi_C a = uRT([Y]_{in} - [Y]_{out}) \qquad (A.7)$$

Equation A.7 gives us the flux through a membrane of thickness a, but we would like a more general expression that gives us the flux through any arbitrary plane in the presence of a concentration gradient. To arrive at this expression, consider the situation digrammed in Figure A.1, which shows a segment of membrane separating two compartments. The dimension perpendicular to the membrane is called x, and the membrane extends from 0 to a (thickness = a). In this situation, Equation A.7 can be expressed in the form of an integral equation:

$$\Phi_C \left(\int_0^a dx \right) = uRT \left(\int_0^a dC \right) \qquad (A.8)$$

Here, C stands for the concentration of the ion; therefore, in reference to Figure A.1, C_a is $[Y]_{in}$ and C_0 is $[Y]_{out}$. Differentiating both sides of Equation A.8 yields

$$\Phi_C dx = uRT \, dC \qquad (A.9)$$

which can be arranged to give the more general form of Equation A.7 that we desire:

$$\Phi_C = uRT \left(\frac{dC}{dx} \right) \qquad (A.10)$$

Equation A.10 can be substituted into Equation A.3 to give the ionic current due to the concentration gradient.

Current Due to Electrical Gradient

Return now to the current driven by the electrical gradient, which can be expressed

$$I_E = A\Phi_E ZF \qquad (A.11)$$

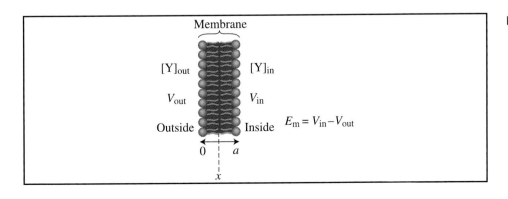

Figure A.1

Segment of membrane separating two compartments.

The flux, Φ_E, of a charged particle through a plane at position x in the presence of a voltage gradient dV/dx will be

$$\Phi_E = uZFC\left(\frac{dV}{dx}\right) \tag{A.12}$$

Again, u is the mobility of the ion, and C is the concentration of the ion at position x. The factor ZFC is then the concentration of charge at the location of the plane; this factor is necessary because the voltage gradient dV/dx acts on charge and ZFC gives the "concentration" of charge at position $= x$. Equation A.12 is analogous to Equation A.10, except that the voltage gradient rather than the concentration gradient is of interest.

Total Current at Equilibrium

Equations A.12, A.11, A.10, and A.3 can be combined into the form of Equation A.2 to give

$$uAZF\left(RT\frac{dC}{dx} + ZFC\frac{dV}{dx}\right) = 0 \tag{A.13}$$

This expression requires that

$$RT\left(\frac{dC}{dx}\right) = -ZFC\left(\frac{dV}{dx}\right) \tag{A.14}$$

Equation A.14 can be rearranged to give a differential equation that can be solved for the equilibrium voltage gradient:

$$\left(-\frac{RT}{ZF}\right)\left(\frac{dC}{C}\right) = dV \tag{A.15}$$

This equation can be solved for V by integrating across the membrane. Using the nomenclature of Figure A.1, the integrals are

$$-\frac{RT}{ZF}\int_{[Y]_{out}}^{[Y]_{in}} \frac{dC}{C} = \int_{V_{out}}^{V_{in}} dV \tag{A.16}$$

The solution to these definite integrals is

$$-\frac{RT}{ZF}(\ln[Y]_{in} - \ln[Y]_{out}) = V_{in} - V_{out} \tag{A.17}$$

or

$$\frac{RT}{ZF}\ln\left(\frac{[Y]_{out}}{[Y]_{in}}\right) = V_{in} - V_{out} = E_M \tag{A.18}$$

Equation A.18 is the Nernst equation.

GOLDMAN EQUATION

The Goldman equation, or constant-field equation, is important for understanding the factors that govern the steady-state membrane potential. As discussed in Chapter 3, the Goldman equation describes the nonequilibrium membrane potential reached when two or more ions with unequal equilibrium potentials are free to move across the membrane. The basic strategy in this derivation is to use the flux equations derived in the previous section to solve separately for the ionic current carried by each permeant ion and then to set the sum of all ionic currents equal to zero. The derivation is somewhat more complex than that of the Nernst equation, and it requires some knowledge of differential and integral calculus to follow in detail. Nevertheless, it should be possible for those without the necessary mathematics to follow the logic of the steps and thus to gain some insight into the physical mechanisms described by the equation.

When several ions are moving across the membrane simultaneously, a steady value of membrane potential will be reached when the sum of the ionic currents carried by the individual ions is zero; that is, for permeant ions A, B, and C

$$I_A + I_B + I_C = 0 \tag{A.19}$$

The first step in arriving at a value of membrane potential that satisfies this condition is to solve for the net ionic flux, Φ, for each ion separately. The total flux for a particular ion will be the sum of the flux due to the concentration gradient and the flux due to the electrical gradient:

$$\Phi_T = \Phi_C + \Phi_V \tag{A.20}$$

The expressions for Φ_C and Φ_V are given by Equations A.10 and A.12. Thus, Equation A.20 becomes

$$\Phi_T = uRT(dC/dx) + uZFC(dV/dx) \tag{A.21}$$

If it is assumed that the electric field across the membrane is constant (this is the constant-field assumption from which the equation draws its alternative name) and that the thickness of the membrane is a, then

$$dV/dx = V/a \tag{A.22}$$

In that case, Equation A.21 can be written

$$\frac{\Phi_T}{uRT} = \frac{dC}{dx} + \frac{ZFV}{RTa}C \tag{A.23}$$

This expression is a differential equation of the form

$$Q = \frac{dC}{dx} + P(x)C$$

which has a solution

$$C\exp\left(\int P(x)dx\right) = \int Q\exp\left(\int P(x)dx\right)dx + \text{constant} \tag{A.24}$$

In this instance, $Q = \Phi_T/(uRT)$ and $P(x) = (ZFV)/RTa)$. Making these substitutions and integrating Equation A.24 across the membrane of the thickness a (that is, from 0 to a) gives

$$C\exp\left(\frac{ZFV}{RTa}\right)\Big|_0^a = \frac{\Phi_T}{uRT}\int_0^a \exp\left(\frac{ZFVx}{RTa}\right)dx \tag{A.25}$$

515

This expression becomes

$$C_a \exp\left(\frac{ZFV}{RT}\right) - C_0 = \frac{\Phi_T}{uRT}\left[\exp\left(\frac{ZFVx}{RTa}\right)\bigg/\left(\frac{ZFV}{RTa}\right)\right]_0^a$$

or

$$C_a \exp\left(\frac{ZFV}{RT}\right) - C_0 = \frac{\Phi_T}{uRT}\frac{RTa}{ZFV}\left[\exp\left(\frac{ZFVa}{RTa}\right) - \exp\left(\frac{ZFV \cdot 0}{RTa}\right)\right]$$

Rearranging and combining terms yields

$$C_a \exp\left(\frac{ZFV}{RT}\right) - C_0 = \frac{\Phi_T a}{uZFV}\left[\exp\left(\frac{ZFV}{RT}\right) - 1\right]$$

This expression can be solved for Φ_T to yield

$$\Phi_T = \frac{uZFV}{a}\left[\frac{C_a \exp(ZFV/RT) - C_0}{\exp(ZFV/RT) - 1}\right] \tag{A.26}$$

Now, C_a and C_0 are the concentrations of the ion just within the membrane. These concentrations are related to the concentrations in the fluids inside and outside the cell by $C_a = \beta C_{in}$ and $C_0 = \beta C_{out}$, where β is the oil-water partition coefficient for the ion in question. Substituting these parameters in Equation A.26 gives

$$\Phi_T = \frac{\beta uZFV}{a}\left[\frac{C_{in} \exp(ZFV/RT) - C_{out}}{\exp(ZFV/RT) - 1}\right] \tag{A.27}$$

The permeability constant, p_i, for a particular ion is given by $p_i = \beta uRT/a$, or $p_i/RT = \beta u/a$. Making this substitution in Equation A.27 gives

$$\Phi_T = \frac{p_i ZFV}{RT}\left[\frac{C_{in} \exp(ZFV/RT) - C_{out}}{\exp(ZFV/RT) - 1}\right] \tag{A.28}$$

The flux, Φ_T, for an ion can be converted to a flow of electrical current, as required in Equation A.19, by multiplying by ZF (the number of coulombs per mole of ion); therefore

$$I = \frac{p_i Z^2 F^2 V}{RT}\left[\frac{C_{in} \exp(ZFV/RT) - C_{out}}{\exp(ZFV/RT) - 1}\right] \tag{A.29}$$

This expression is needed for each ion in Equation A.19. For instance, if the three permeant ions are Na, K, and Cl with permeabilities p_{Na}, p_K, and p_{Cl}, then Equation A.19 becomes (keeping in mind that the valence of chloride is -1)

$$\frac{F^2 V}{RT}\left[\frac{p_K([K]_{in}e^{FV/RT} - [K]_{out}) + p_{Na}([Na]_{in}e^{FV/RT} - [Na]_{out})}{\exp(FV/RT) - 1} + \frac{p_{Cl}([Cl]_{in}e^{-FV/RT} - [Cl]_{out})}{\exp(-FV/RT) - 1}\right] = 0$$

Multiplying through by $-\exp(FV/RT)/-\exp(FV/RT)$ and rearranging yields

$$\frac{F^2 V}{RT(\exp(FV/RT) - 1)}[(p_K[K]_{in} + p_{Na}[Na]_{in} + p_{Cl}[Cl]_{out})e^{FV/RT} - (p_K[K]_{out}$$
$$+ p_{Na}[Na]_{out} + p_{Cl}[Cl]_{in})] = 0$$

This expression requires that

$$(p_K[K]_{in} + p_{Na}[Na]_{in} + p_{Cl}[Cl]_{out})e^{FV/RT} - (p_K[K]_{out} + p_{Na}[Na]_{out} + p_{Cl}[Cl]_{in}) = 0$$

or

$$e^{FV/RT} = \frac{(p_K[K]_{out} + p_{Na}[Na]_{out} + p_{Cl}[Cl]_{in})}{(p_K[K]_{in} + p_{Na}[Na]_{in} + p_{Cl}[Cl]_{out})}$$

Taking the natural logarithm of both sides and solving for V yields the usual form of the Goldman equation

$$V = \frac{RT}{F} \ln\left(\frac{p_K[K]_{out} + p_{Na}[Na]_{out} + p_{Cl}[Cl]_{in}}{[p_K[K]_{in} + p_{Na}[Na]_{in} + p_{Cl}[Cl]_{out}}\right)$$

ELECTRICAL PROPERTIES OF CELLS

Electrical signals are fundamental to the function of the nervous system. The electrical properties of cells are important in determining how electrical signals spread along the plasma membrane. This Advanced Topic explores the electrical characteristics of cell membranes as electrical conductors and insulators. These passive electrical properties arise from the physical properties of the membrane and from the ion channels in the membrane.

The Cell Membrane as an Electrical Capacitor

An electrical capacitor is a charge-storing device that consists of two conducting plates separated by an insulating barrier. Because the lipid bilayer of the plasma membrane forms an insulating barrier separating the electrically conductive salt solutions of the intracellular fluid (ICF) and extracellular fluid (ECF), the plasma membrane behaves as a capacitor. When a capacitor is hooked up to a battery as shown in Figure B.1, the voltage of the battery causes electrons to leave one conducting plate and to accumulate on the other plate. This charge separation continues until the resulting voltage gradient across the capacitor equals the voltage of the battery. The amount of charge, q, stored on the capacitor at that time will be given by $q = CV$, where V is the voltage across the capacitor and C is the **capacitance** of the capacitor. Capacitance is directly proportional to the area of the plates (bigger plates can store more charge) and inversely proportional to the distance separating the two plates. Capacitance also depends on the characteristics of the insulating material between the plates, which is the lipid of the plasma membrane in cells.

The unit of capacitance is the farad (F): a 1-F capacitor can store 1 coulomb of charge when hooked up to a 1-volt battery. Biological membranes have a capacitance of approximately 10^{-6} F (that is, 1 microfarad, or μF) per square centimeter of membrane area. From this value of membrane capacitance, the thickness of the insulating lipid portion of the membrane can be estimated using the following relation:

$$x = \frac{\varepsilon_0 \kappa}{C} \tag{B.1}$$

In this equation, x is the distance between the conducting plates (that is, the ICF and the ECF), C is the capacitance of the plasma membrane (1 μF/cm^2), ε_0 is the permittivity constant (8.85×10^{-8} μF/cm), and κ is the dielectric constant of the insulating material separating the two conducting plates ($\kappa = 5$ for membrane lipid). The calculated membrane thickness is approximately 4.5 nm, which is similar to the membrane thickness of approximately 7.5 nm estimated with electron microscopy. The thickness estimated from capacitance is smaller because it is determined by the insulating portion of the membrane, whereas the total membrane thickness, including associated proteins, is observed through the electron microscope.

Electrical Response of the Cell Membrane to Injected Current

Many electrical signals in nerve cells arise when ion channels open in the plasma membrane, allowing a flow of electrical current, carried by ions, to move across the membrane and alter the membrane potential of the cell. This situation can be mimicked experimentally by placing a microelectrode inside a cell and injecting charge into the cell through the microelectrode. Figure B.2 shows the response of a cell to

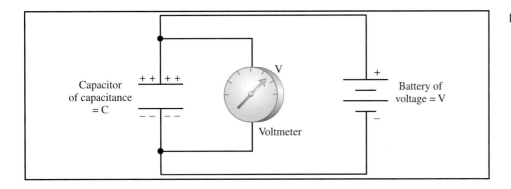

Figure B.1.

When a battery is connected to a capacitor, charge accumulates on the capacitor until the voltage across the capacitor equals the voltage of the battery.

injected current, considering only the capacitance of the cell membrane. If a constant current, I, is injected into the cell, then the charge, q, is added to the membrane capacitor at a constant rate ($I = dq/dt$). Because $q = CV$ for a capacitor, we obtain the following result:

$$I = C\frac{dV}{dt} = \text{constant} \qquad (B.2)$$

In other words, dV/dt is a constant, and voltage changes linearly (that is, at a constant rate) during injection of constant current.

The response of the cell to injected current is different, however, if we take into account the presence of ion channels in the cell membrane. Ion channels provide a path for injected charge to move across the membrane, instead of being added to the charge on the membrane capacitor. The electrical analog of the current path provided by the ion channels is an electrical resistor. Figure B.3 illustrates the effect of adding a resistive path for current flow in the cell membrane, in parallel with the capacitance of the cell membrane. In a spherical cell, the injected current has equal access to all parts of the cell membrane at the same time. Therefore, we can combine all of the resistors and all of the capacitors for each patch of cell membrane, resulting in the analogous electrical circuit shown in Figure B.3, consisting of the combined, parallel resistance R and the combined parallel capacitance C. The injected current now consists of two components: i_C, the component that flows onto the capacitor, and i_R, the component that flows through the membrane resistor, R. The capacitative current is given by Equation B.2, and the resistive current is given by Ohm's law: $i_R = V/R$. Hence, the total current is

$$I = \frac{V}{R} + C\frac{dV}{dt} \qquad (B.3)$$

Solving Equation B.3 for V yields

$$V = IR(1 - e^{-t/RC}) \qquad (B.4)$$

Thus, voltage rises exponentially during injection of a constant current, I. The product, RC, is the exponential time constant of the rise in voltage, which is abbreviated τ. The asymptotic value of the voltage is IR, which is the voltage expected when all of the current is flowing through the membrane resistance. Initially, all of the injected charge flows onto the membrane capacitor, but as charge accumulates, more and more charge flows instead through the resistor, until finally all of the current flows through the resistive path. When the injection of current stops, the accumulated charge on the capacitor discharges through the parallel resistance, R. This decay of voltage is also exponential, with the same time constant, τ, given by RC.

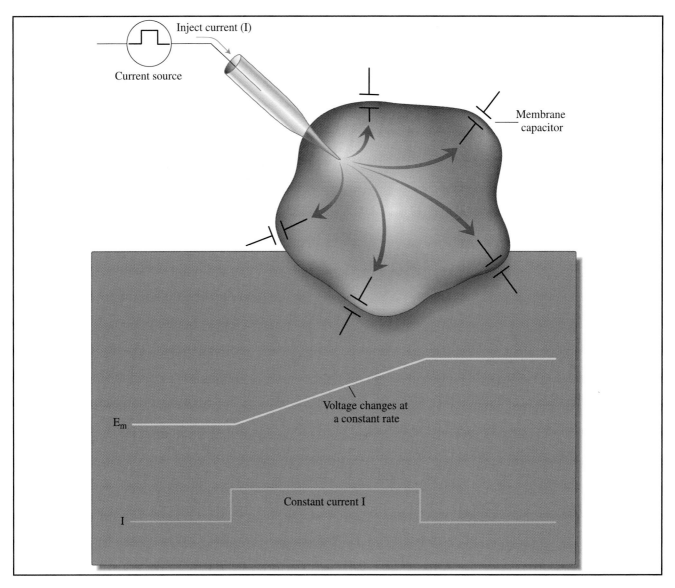

Figure B.2.

The rise of voltage during injection of constant current in a cell. Only the contribution of the membrane capacitance is considered, and the effect of membrane resistance is neglected. During the constant current, I, charge is injected at a constant rate, and as a result, the voltage on the membrane capacitor rises linearly.

The Response to Current Injection in a Cylindrical Cell

In a spherical cell, as in Figure B.3, the injected current flows equally to the resistors and capacitors in all parts of the membrane at the same time. However, neurons typically give rise to many long, thin neurites that extend long distances to make contact with other cells. Current injected in the cell body of the neuron, for example, must flow along the interior of a neurite to reach the portion of the cell membrane located in the neurite at a distance from the cell body. In this situation, then, current does not have equal access to all parts of the membrane.

Figure B.4 illustrates the analogous electrical circuit for a long cylindrical cell. To reach the parallel resistor and capacitor at progressively more distant portions of the cell membrane, current injected at one end of the cell must flow through the resistance provided by the interior of the cell. This resistance can be quite large for

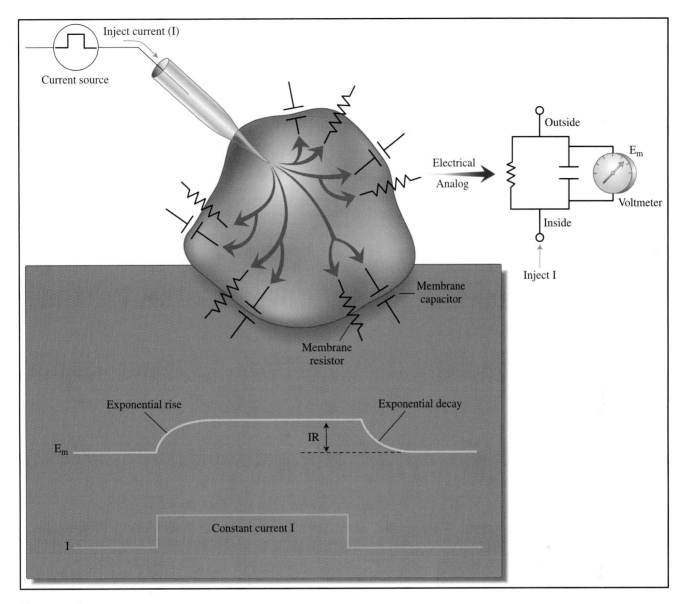

Figure B.3.

The rise of voltage during injection of constant current into a spherical cell, considering both the capacitance and the resistance of the cell membrane. The membrane capacitors represent the insulating portion of the cell membrane, and the membrane resistors represent open ion channels that allow charge to move across the membrane. At the onset of the injected current, all of the injected charge initially flows onto the membrane capacitance. As the voltage on the capacitor builds up, progressively more of the current flows through the resistance. Finally, all of the current flows through the membrane resistance, and the asymptotic voltage is governed by Ohm's law ($V = IR$). Both the rise of the voltage at the onset of the current and the fall of the voltage when the current is turned off follow an exponential time course.

cylindrical neurites of neurons. The resistance of a cylindrical conductor is given by

$$R = \frac{r4l}{\pi d^2} \qquad (B.5)$$

where r is the specific resistance of the conducting material, l is the length of the cylinder, and d is the diameter of the cylinder. For the cytoplasm of a neurite, r is

Figure B.4.

The equivalent electrical circuit for a long cylindrical cell. A constant current is injected at one end of the cell. At each position along the cell, current divides into a membrane component, i_m, flowing onto the membrane resistance and capacitance at that point, and a longitudinal component, i_l, that flows through the resistance of the cell interior to more distant portions of the membrane. The amount of current remaining at each position along the cell is indicated by the thickness of the *arrows*.

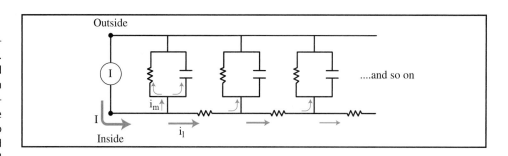

approximately 100 Ω cm, which is about 10^7 times worse than copper wire. Thus, a neurite 1 μm in diameter would have an internal resistance of approximately 1.3×10^6 Ω per μm of length.

The current at the site of injection divides into two components. Some of the current (designated i_m, for membrane current) flows onto the parallel membrane resistance and capacitance at the injection site. The remainder of the current (indicated by i_l, for longitudinal current) flows through the internal resistance of the neurite. At the next portion of the neurite, the current again divides into membrane and longitudinal components. Thus, the amount of current declines with distance along the neurite. In addition, current entering the parallel RC circuit at each position changes with time, because the voltage on the capacitance at each local position builds up as described previously for the spherical cell. As a result, the change in membrane voltage produced by the injection of current in the cylindrical cell varies as a function of both time and distance from the injection site.

Analysis of the electrical circuit shown in Figure B.4 leads to the following equation for membrane voltage:

$$V + \tau\frac{\partial V}{\partial t} = \lambda^2 \frac{\partial^2 V}{\partial x^2}, \text{ where } \tau = r_m c_m \text{ and } \lambda = \sqrt{\frac{r_m}{r_i}} \qquad (B.6)$$

In this second-order, partial differential equation, r_m and c_m are the resistance and the capacitance of the amount of membrane in a 1-cm length of the cylindrical cell, and r_i is the internal resistance of a 1-cm length of the cylindrical cell. For an infinitely long cylindrical cell, the solution of Equation B.6 is the cable equation:

$$V(x,t) = V_{\substack{x=0 \\ t=\infty}} \frac{1}{2}\left\{e^{-X}\left[1 - erf\left(\frac{X}{2\sqrt{T}} - \sqrt{T}\right)\right] - e^{X}\left[1 - erf\left(\frac{X}{2\sqrt{T}} + \sqrt{T}\right)\right]\right\} \quad (B.7)$$

In this equation, $X = x/\lambda$ and $T = t/\tau$. That is, both distance and time are normalized with respect to λ and τ, which are defined in Equation B.6. As in the exponential equation governing the rise of voltage during current injection in a spherical cell, τ is the time constant of the cylindrical cell. The constant factor, λ, is called the **length constant** of the cylindrical cell.

The function *erf* in Equation B.7 is the error function, which is defined as

$$erf(z) = \frac{1}{\sqrt{\pi}}\int_{-z}^{+z} e^{-y^2} \, dy \qquad (B.8)$$

The error function, $erf(z)$, is the integral under a Gaussian probability distribution from $-z$ to $+z$, as illustrated graphically in Figure B.5. Note that as z increases from 0, the integral of the Gaussian function first increases rapidly, then progressively more slowly. The rise of $erf(T)$ with increasing T is shown in Figure B.5B, compared on the same time scale with an exponential rise. When $t = \tau$ (that is, when $T = 1$),

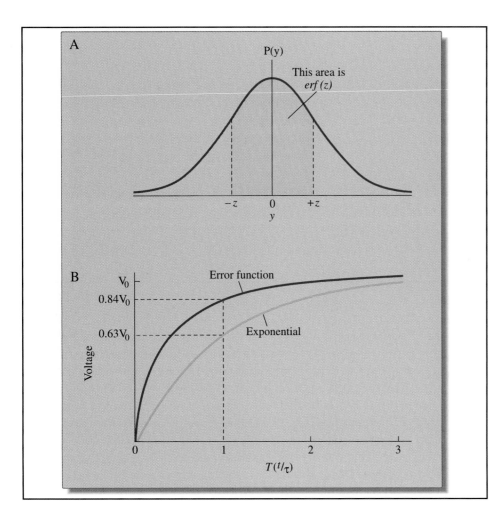

Figure B.5.

The error function represents the area under a Gaussian curve. **A**. The bell-shaped curve represents a Gaussian function. The error function (*erf*) of a variable, *z*, is the integral of the Gaussian function from −*z* to +*z*. **B**. The time course of the rise of voltage with time after the onset of a constant current. The error function rises more steeply than an exponential function. Time is normalized with respect to the time constant, τ, in both cases. When $t = \tau$ (that is, $T = 1$), the error function has reached 0.84 of its final value, V_0, but the exponential function has reached 0.63 of its final value.

the exponential function rises to 0.63 (that is, $1 - 1/e$) of its final, asymptotic value, whereas the error function rises to 0.84 of its asymptotic value.

Although Equation B.7 may seem daunting, it reduces to simpler relations under certain circumstances. For example, the steady-state decay of voltage with distance from the injection site (that is, $V(x)$ at $t = \infty$) can be obtained by recognizing that dV/dt eventually becomes zero a long time after the onset of current injection. Thus, when $dV/dt = 0$, Equation B.6 becomes

$$V = \lambda^2 \frac{d^2V}{dx^2} \tag{B.9}$$

which has an exponential solution:

$$V(x) = V_0 e^{-x/\lambda} \tag{B.10}$$

In this equation, V_0 is the steady-state voltage at the injection site at $t = \infty$. Thus, in the steady state, voltage declines exponentially with distance from the injection site, and the spatial decay is governed by the length constant, λ. Figure B.6 summarizes the decline of voltage along a cylindrical neurite. At a distance λ (that is, one length constant) from the injection site, the steady-state voltage declines to $1/e$ (that is 0.37) of the voltage at the injection site.

Another special case is the rise of voltage with time at the site of current injection (that is, $V(t)$ at $x = 0$). With $x = 0$, Equation B.7 reduces to

$$V(t) = V_0 erf(\sqrt{T}) \tag{B.11}$$

Figure B.6.

The steady-state decay of voltage with distance when a constant current is injected at $X = 0$ in an infinitely long cylindrical cell. Distance is normalized with respect to the length constant, λ. At $x = \lambda$ (that is, $X = 1$), steady-state voltage is 37% of the steady-state voltage at the site of current injection, V_0.

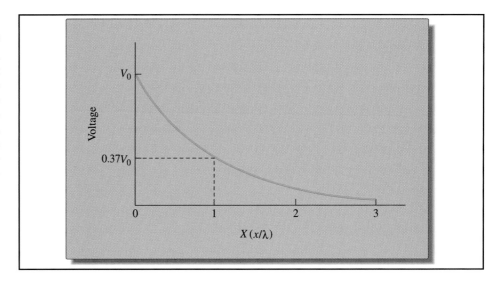

In other words, voltage at the injection site rises with a time course given by the error function, as shown in Figure B.7. At a distance $x = \lambda$ from the injection site, the asymptotic voltage at $t = \infty$ is $0.37V_0$, as described above, and the time course of the rise is given by the cable equation (Equation B.7) with $X = 1$. This time course is also shown in Figure B.7. Note that unlike the rapid rise at $x = 0$, the voltage at $x = \lambda$ rises with a pronounced delay, which represents the time for the injected current to begin to reach the part of the membrane distant from the injection site. Because of the appreciable internal resistance to current flow, injected charge will flow first onto the membrane capacitance at the injection site and then in the intervening portions of the membrane, before reaching more distant parts of the membrane. Thus, the rise of voltage is not only smaller but also slower at progressively greater distances from the point where current is injected into a cylindrical cell.

In the nervous system, the passive cable properties of neurites have functional significance for the influence exerted by a particular synaptic input on action potential firing in a postsynaptic neuron. A synaptic input located on a dendrite at a distance from the cell body of the neuron would produce a smaller, slower change in membrane potential in the cell body than would a synaptic input located near the cell body. Thus, nearby synaptic inputs have greater influence on the activity of postsynaptic cells.

Figure B.7.

The rise of voltage with time after the onset of current injection at two locations along an infinitely long cylindrical cell. Time is normalized with respect to the time constant, τ. At the site of injection ($x = 0$), the voltage rises according to the error function. At a distance of λ from the injection site ($x = \lambda$), the voltage rises with an S-shaped delay to its final value, which is 37% of the steady-state voltage at the site of current injection, V_0.

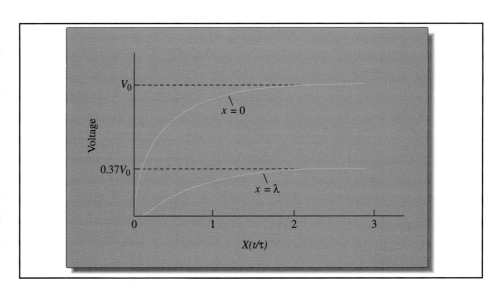

ANALYSIS OF ION CHANNEL GATING

The properties of voltage-sensitive sodium and potassium channels underlying the action potential were described in Chapter 4. This Advanced Topic provides a more quantitative description of these ion channels and their dependence on membrane voltage. The experimental evidence for the role of voltage-dependent ion channels in the action potential was obtained in voltage-clamp experiments performed by Alan L. Hodgkin and Andrew F. Huxley in the period from 1949 to 1952. We begin with the Hodgkin-Huxley model of the nerve action potential and then discuss the behavior of individual voltage-dependent ion channels.

Voltage-Clamp Analysis

In the voltage-clamp technique, membrane voltage is held at a constant value, or "clamped." The time course of the flow of membrane current at the clamped membrane voltage provides an index of the underlying changes in membrane ionic conductance. The voltage-clamp procedure is diagrammed in Figure C.1. Two long, thin wires are threaded longitudinally down the interior of an isolated segment of a squid giant axon, which can be up to 1 mm in diameter. One wire measures the membrane potential, and the other wire passes current into the axon from the output of the voltage-clamp amplifier. The measured membrane potential is connected to one input of the amplifier, and the other input is connected to an external voltage source, the command voltage. The command voltage determines the clamped membrane potential that will be maintained by the voltage-clamp amplifier.

The voltage-clamp amplifier feeds a current into the axon that is proportional to the difference between the command voltage and the measured membrane potential, $E_C - E_m$. If that difference is zero (that is, if $E_m = E_C$), the amplifier puts out no current, and E_m will remain stable. If E_m does not equal E_C, the amplifier will pass current that drives the membrane potential toward the command voltage. For example, if E_m is –70 mV and E_C is –60 mV, then $E_C - E_m$ is a positive number, and the amplifier injects positive charge into the axon and depolarizes the axon. Depolarization continues until the membrane potential equals the command potential of –60 mV.

A current monitor in the output line of the amplifier allows us to measure the amount of current passed by the amplifier to keep the membrane voltage equal to the command voltage. How does this measured current provide information about changes in ionic current and, therefore, changes in ionic conductance of the membrane?

First, we will examine the membrane current and membrane potential without the voltage clamp, using the principles discussed in Chapter 3. Figure C.2 shows the changes in transmembrane ionic current and membrane potential in response to a stepwise increase in g_{Na}, with g_K remaining constant. Under resting conditions, the steady-state membrane potential lies between E_{Na} and E_K, at the membrane voltage at which the inward sodium current exactly balances the outward potassium current (that is, the total membrane current is zero: $i_{Na} + i_K = 0$). When g_{Na} increases, the steady state is perturbed, and i_{Na} increases, as well. The increase in sodium influx causes E_m to become more positive, and the cell depolarizes. Depolarization enhances potassium current, however, because depolarization increases the electrical driving force for potassium to exit. The membrane potential will reach a new steady state, at which both i_{Na} and i_K are larger than their initial values but once again exactly balance one another (see Fig. C.2).

Consider now what happens if the same change in g_{Na} occurs under voltage-clamp conditions, as shown in Figure C.3. The voltage-clamp apparatus now introduces an addition source of current, i_{clamp}. If we set the command voltage, E_C,

Figure C.1.

A schematic diagram of a voltage-clamp apparatus. Two electrodes are inserted into a giant axon, one to measure the membrane potential, E_m, and the other to inject current into the axon to alter the membrane potential. The voltage clamp amplifier injects current that is proportional to the difference between E_m and a command voltage, E_C, which is under experimental control.

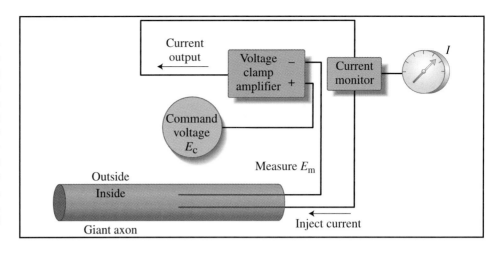

equal to the normal steady-state membrane potential, the current injected by the voltage-clamp apparatus will be zero, because $E_C = E_m$. When g_{Na} increases and the rise in sodium influx begins to depolarize the cell, the voltage-clamp circuit detects the depolarization and injects negative current to counter the increased sodium current (see the trace labeled i_{clamp} in Fig. C.3). The voltage clamp continues to inject this holding current to maintain E_m at its usual resting value as long as g_{Na} remains elevated. The injected current, i_{clamp}, is equal in magnitude to the change in sodium current resulting from the increase in sodium conductance. Unlike the situation without voltage clamp (see Fig. C.2), i_K does not change under voltage clamp because neither E_m nor g_K changed. Thus, the current injected by the voltage clamp

Figure C.2.

Ionic currents flowing in response to a stepwise change in g_{Na}. In the absence of voltage clamp, both i_{Na} and i_K increase in response to the increase in g_{Na}, and a new steady-state membrane potential is reached at a more depolarized level.

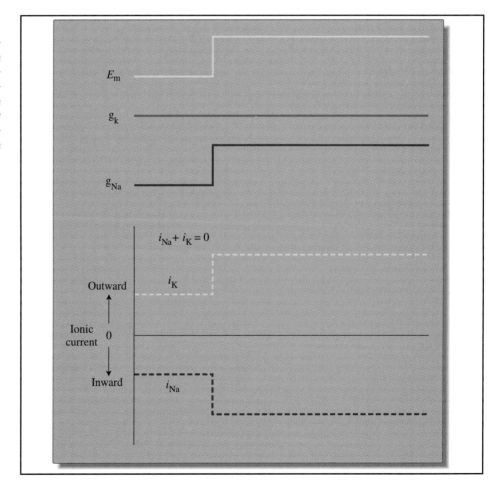

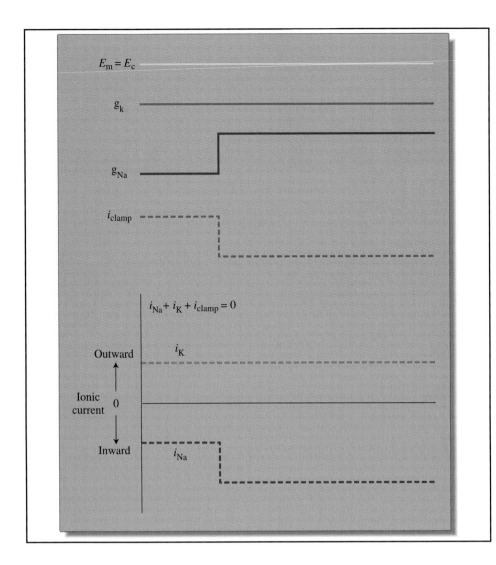

Figure C.3.

Ionic currents flowing in response to a stepwise change in g_{Na}. With voltage clamp, the membrane potential remains constant because the voltage-clamp apparatus injects current (i_{clamp}) that compensates for the increased sodium current. Potassium current remains constant because neither g_K nor E_m changes.

gives a direct measure of the change in ionic current resulting from a change in membrane conductance to an ion.

The measured change in membrane current is related to the underlying change in membrane conductance, using the ionic form of Ohm's law (see Chapter 3). For example, for sodium ions,

$$i_{Na} = g_{Na}(E_m - E_{Na}) \tag{C.1}$$

We can obtain g_{Na} from the measured i_{Na} according to the relation

$$g_{Na} = i_{Na}/(E_m - E_{Na}) \tag{C.2}$$

In this calculation, E_m is set by the voltage clamp, and E_{Na} can be calculated from the Nernst equation, using the internal and external sodium concentrations for the particular experimental situation.

The Gated Ion Channel Model

Membrane Potential and Peak Ionic Conductance

As described in Chapter 4, the voltage-clamp procedure can be used to obtain information about the time course of the voltage-dependent sodium and potassium conductances underlying the action potential (see Figs. 4.16 and 4.17). Hodgkin and Huxley used the voltage clamp to study the voltage dependence of the sodium and potassium channels. They found that the peak magnitude of the conductance change produced by a depolarizing voltage-clamp step depended on the size of the step, as shown in Figure C.4. For example, a voltage step to –50 mV barely increased g_{Na}, but a step to –30 mV produced a large increase in g_{Na}.

Hodgkin and Huxley suggested a simple model that could account for the voltage sensitivity of the sodium and potassium conductances. Their model assumes that many individual ion channels, each having a small ionic conductance, determine the behavior of the whole membrane as measured with the voltage-clamp procedure. Each channel has two conducting states: an open state in which ions are free to cross through the pore, and a closed state in which the pore is blocked. Changing the membrane potential alters the probability that a channel enters the open, conducting state. Depolarization enhances the probability that a channel opens and hence increases the total membrane conductance to that ion.

If the conducting state of the channel depends on transmembrane voltage, an electrical charge associated with the channel is required to provide sensitivity to the voltage. This electrical charge is called the **gating charge** of the channel, because it imparts the voltage dependence of channel gating. The S-shaped relationship between ionic conductance and membrane potential shown in Figure C.4 is expected from basic physical principles for the movement of charged particles under the influence of an electric field, as is presumed to occur for the gating charge of voltage-sensitive sodium and potassium channels. The distribution of charged particles within the membrane is related to the transmembrane electric field according to the Boltzmann relation:

$$P_0 = \frac{1}{1 + e^{\left(\frac{W - z \varepsilon E_m}{kT}\right)}} \tag{C.3}$$

Figure C.4.

The voltage dependence of peak sodium conductance (**A**) and potassium conductance (**B**) as a function of the amplitude of a maintained voltage step.

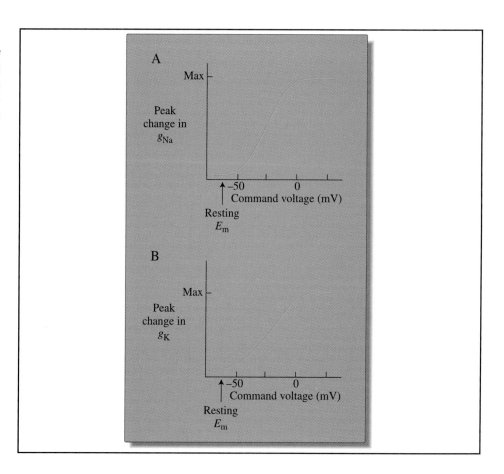

where P_o is the proportion of positively charged gating particles on the outside of the membrane, z is the valence of the gating charge, ε is the electronic charge, E_m is membrane potential, k is Boltzmann's constant, T is the absolute temperature, and W is a voltage-independent term giving the offset of the relation along the voltage axis. The steepness of the rise in P_o with depolarization depends on the valence, z, of the gating charge; the larger z becomes, the steeper the rise of P_o (and, hence, conductance) is with depolarization. The sodium and potassium conductances are steeply dependent on membrane potential, which implies that the gating charge has a large valence. For example, from Hodgkin and Huxley's experiments, the effective valence of the gating charge for the sodium channel is ~6 (that is, $z \approx 6$ in Equation C.3). We now know that the gating charge of the voltage-dependent sodium channel consists of several positively charged amino acids found in transmembrane segment 4 in each of the four domains that make up the channel (see Fig. 4.12). The large number of these charged amino acid residues probably accounts for the high effective valence of the gating charge and the steepness of the voltage dependence of sodium conductance.

Kinetics of the Change in Ionic Conductance Following a Step Depolarization

Upon depolarization, sodium channel activation, sodium channel inactivation, and the opening of voltage-dependent potassium channels take place on different time scales. These differences in the time course of channel gating are important for generating the action potential (see Chapter 4). Hodgkin and Huxley assumed that the rate of change of the membrane conductance to both sodium and potassium following a step depolarization was governed by the rate of redistribution of gating charges in the channels.

For example, consider the kinetics of sodium channel opening following a step depolarization. In the Hodgkin-Huxley theory, channel opening is assumed to be triggered by the movement of gating charges from the inner to the outer surface of the membrane, as shown schematically in Figure C.5. At the normal negative resting membrane potential, the positive charges on the S4 segments of the channel are largely located near the intracellular face of the membrane (see Fig. C.5A), and the channel is closed. Upon depolarization, gating charges are less attracted to the cell interior, and the S4 segments begin to relocate within the electric field across the membrane (see Fig. C.5B). With sufficient depolarization, the charges eventually redistribute so that they are near the outer face of the membrane (see Fig. C.5C). The channel then opens.

If m is the proportion of gating charges near the outer surface of the membrane, then $1 - m$ is the proportion of charges near the inner surface. The movement of gating charges between these two states can be described by the following first-order kinetic model:

$$m \underset{\beta_m}{\overset{\alpha_m}{\longleftrightarrow}} (1-m) \tag{C.4}$$

The rate constant, α_m, represents the rate at which gating charges move from the inner to the outer face of the membrane, and β_m is the rate of reverse movement. A change in membrane voltage instantly alters the rate constants α_m and β_m. For instance, a step depolarization would increase α_m and decrease β_m, leading to a net increase in m and a corresponding decrease in $1 - m$.

The equation governing the rate at which the charges redistribute following a change in membrane potential is

$$dm/dt = \alpha_m(1-m) - \beta_m m \tag{C.5}$$

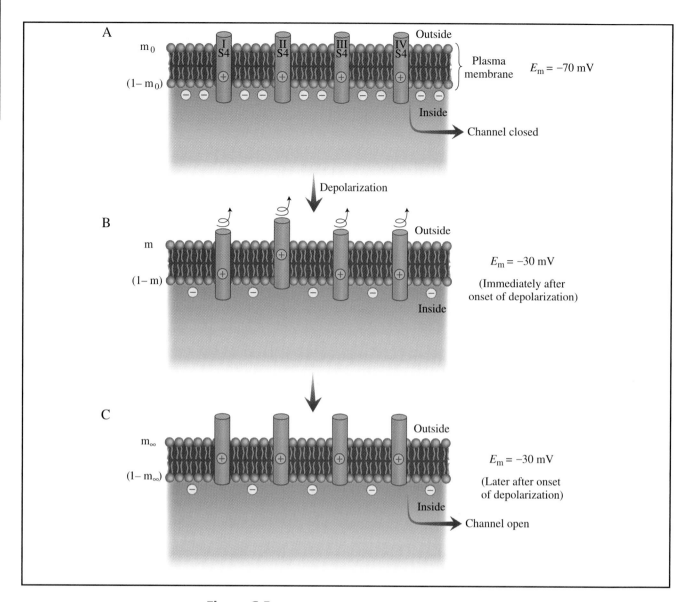

Figure C.5.

The change in distribution of the gating charges of a voltage-dependent sodium channel upon depolarization. The positively charged amino acids in transmembrane segment S4 of each domain of the sodium channel are indicated by the *plus sign*. The four domains are indicated by Roman numerals I through IV. Only the S4 domains are shown for simplicity. **A.** At the normal negative resting potential, the positive charges are located nearer the intracellular face of the membrane, and the sodium channel is closed. **B.** Upon depolarization, the positive charges are less attracted to the cell interior, and the S4 segments begin to alter their position in the membrane. **C.** With time, all four of the S4 segments take on a position nearer the outer surface of the membrane, and the channel opens.

The solution of Equation C.5 is an exponential function:

$$m(t) = m_\infty - (m_\infty - m_0)e^{-(\alpha_m + \beta_m)t} \tag{C.6}$$

Following a change in membrane potential, *m* will change exponentially from its initial value (m_0) to its final value (m_∞) at a rate governed by the rate constants for movement of the gating charges at the new value of membrane potential.

Figure C.6 illustrates the exponential rise of *m* with time after a depolarization. If the movement of a single S4 segment were sufficient to cause the channel to open,

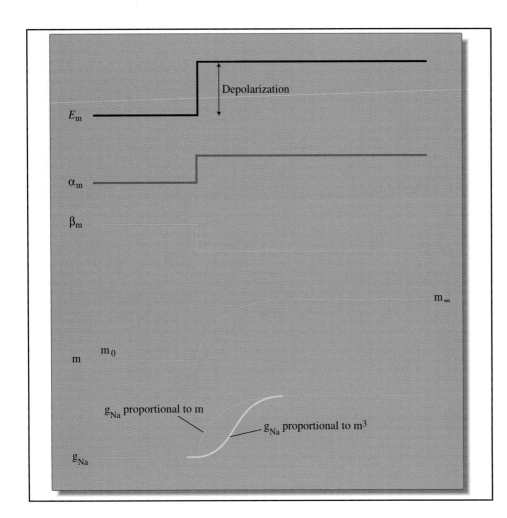

Figure C.6.

The effect of a step change in membrane potential (*top trace*) on sodium channel activation. Depolarization alters the rate constants for movement of the gating charges across the membrane, α_m and β_m. The changes in rate constants induce a change in the proportion of gating charges on the outer face of the membrane (*m*), where they stimulate channel opening. If movement of a single gating charge could activate the channel, g_{Na} would follow the time course of the change in *m* (*orange trace*). The actual change in g_{Na} is proportional to *m* raised to the third power (*yellow trace*).

the number of open channels—and hence g_{Na}—would be proportional to *m*, the fraction of gating charges on the outer face of the membrane. In this case, g_{Na} would also rise exponentially after a depolarization. However, Hodgkin and Huxley found that the rise of g_{Na} after a depolarization actually rose along an S-shaped time course (see Fig. C.6). The nonexponential time course of g_{Na} suggests that more than one gating charge must move within a single channel to cause the channel to open. The probability that a single S4 segment within a channel will move to the outer position is simply proportional to *m*. The joint probability that all of the S4 segments will move for a given channel is given by the product of the probabilities that each single S4 segment will alter its position. Thus, the probability that all S4 segments in the four domains will take on the position required for channel opening is proportional to m^4. The actual rise of g_{Na} following a voltage-clamp step in Hodgkin and Huxley's experiments was proportional to m^3, which is close to the relation expected if all of the charged S4 segments within a single sodium channel must respond to depolarization before the channel can enter the open state.

A similar analysis was carried out for the change in potassium conductance following a step depolarization. The gating charges for the potassium channel redistributed after a change in membrane potential according to a relation equivalent to Equation C.5:

$$dn/dt = \alpha_n(1-n) - \beta_n n \qquad (C.7)$$

By analogy with the sodium channel, n is the proportion of potassium channel gating charges on the outer face of the membrane, $1 - n$ is the proportion on the inner face of the membrane, and α_n and β_n are the rate constants for particle transition from one face to the other. Equation C.7 has a solution equivalent to Equation C.6:

$$n(t) = n_\infty - (n_\infty - n_0)e^{-(\alpha_n + \beta_n)t} \qquad (C.8)$$

In this instance, n_0 and n_∞ are the initial and final values of n. The rise in potassium conductance following a step depolarization was found to be proportional to n^4, which suggests that all four charged S4 segments in the potassium channel redistribute across the membrane to trigger opening of the potassium channel in response to depolarization.

A major difference between the potassium and the sodium channels is that the rate constants, α_n and β_n, are smaller for potassium channels. That is, the sodium channel gating charges are more mobile than their potassium channel counterparts and are able to move more rapidly in response to depolarization. As a result, the sodium channel opens more rapidly after depolarization—a crucial part of the action potential mechanism.

Sodium Channel Inactivation

The change in g_{Na} during sustained depolarization is transient. That is, the sodium channel first activates, then inactivates in response to depolarization. To study the voltage dependence of inactivation, Hodgkin and Huxley performed experiments like that shown in Figure C.7A. A test depolarization was preceded by a prepulse whose amplitude was varied. Depolarizing prepulses reduced the amplitude of the response to the test depolarization by closing inactivation gates, whereas hyperpolarizing prepulses increased the size of the test response by opening inactivation gates that were closed. This effect of prepulses allowed Hodgkin and Huxley to establish the voltage dependence of the inactivation gate on membrane potential, which is shown in Figure C.7B.

The time course of sodium channel inactivation was studied by varying the duration of the prepulse, as shown in Figure C.8. The relation between the size of the test response and the duration of the prepulse (see Fig. C.8B) revealed that inactivation proceeds exponentially during a depolarizing prepulse. By analogy with the sodium channel activation parameter, m, Hodgkin and Huxley described the time course of inactivation with the following exponential equation:

$$h(t) = h_\infty - (h_\infty - h_0)e^{-(\alpha_h + \beta_h)t} \qquad (C.9)$$

The gating parameter, h, governs the opening of the inactivation gate of the sodium channel, just as the parameter m governs the opening of the activation gate. In this case, however, h decreases with depolarization, instead of increasing with depolarization, to reflect the fact that the inactivation gate closes upon depolarization. Thus, upon depolarization, h declines exponentially from its original value (h_0) to its final value (h_∞), at a rate governed by the rate constants, α_h and β_h, for movement of the inactivation gating charge through the membrane. As expected from the discussion in Chapter 4, the closing of the inactivation gate is slower than the opening of the activation gate, implying that the inactivation gating charge is less mobile (that is, the rate constants are smaller).

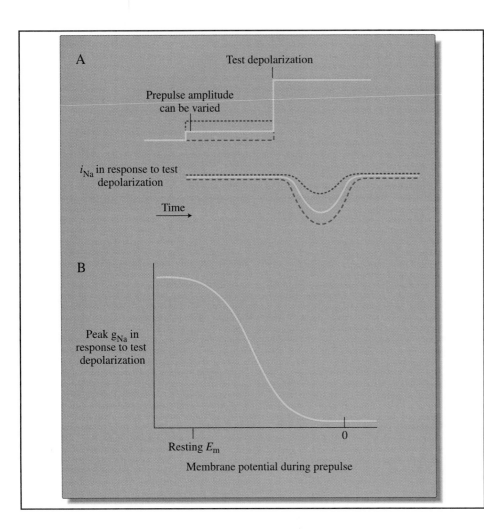

Figure C.7.

The procedure for measuring the voltage dependence of sodium channel inactivation. **A**. A test depolarization is preceded by a prepulse whose amplitude is varied. The subsequent response to the test depolarization provides an indication of how much sodium channel inactivation was produced by the prepulse. **B**. The relation between amplitude of an inactivating prepulse and the peak sodium conductance in response to a subsequent test depolarization. This relation illustrates the voltage dependence of sodium channel inactivation.

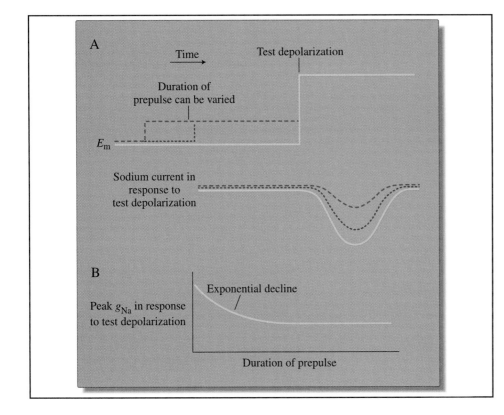

Figure C.8.

The procedure for measuring the time course of sodium channel inactivation. **A**. A test depolarization is preceded by a depolarizing prepulse of varying duration. **B**. The relation between the duration of the prepulse and the peak sodium conductance in response to the test depolarization provides an estimate of the time course of sodium channel inactivation during the prepulse. The decline of the response to the test depolarization follows an exponential time course.

The Temporal Behavior of Sodium and Potassium Conductance

The behavior of the gating parameters m, n, and h provides a quantitative description of the change in sodium and potassium conductance following a depolarizing voltage step under voltage clamp. The sodium conductance is given by

$$g_{Na} = \bar{g}_{Na} m^3 h \qquad (C.10)$$

The potassium conductance is given by

$$g_K = \bar{g}_K n^4 \qquad (C.11)$$

where $\bar{g}_{Na}$ and $\bar{g}_K$ are the maximal sodium and potassium conductances, and m, n, and h are given by Equations C.6, C.8, and C.9, respectively. Thus, following a depolarization, the sodium conductance rises in proportion to the third power of the activation parameter, m, and falls in direct proportion to the decline in the inactivation parameter, h. Figure C.9A summarizes the responses of each gating parameter separately and the product $m^3 h$, which governs the time course of the sodium conductance in response to depolarization. The potassium conductance rises as the fourth power of its activation parameter, n, and does not inactivate, as shown in Figure C.9B.

Figure C.9.

The time courses of sodium conductance and potassium conductance following a step depolarization. **A**. Sodium conductance reflects the time course of both inactivation (h) and activation (m). In the case of activation, channel opening is proportional to the third power of m. The rise and fall of sodium conductance is proportional to $m^3 h$. **B**. The rise of potassium conductance is proportional to the fourth power of the activation parameter, n.

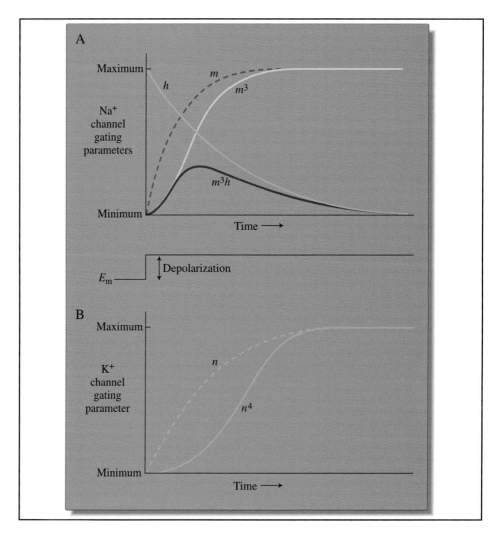

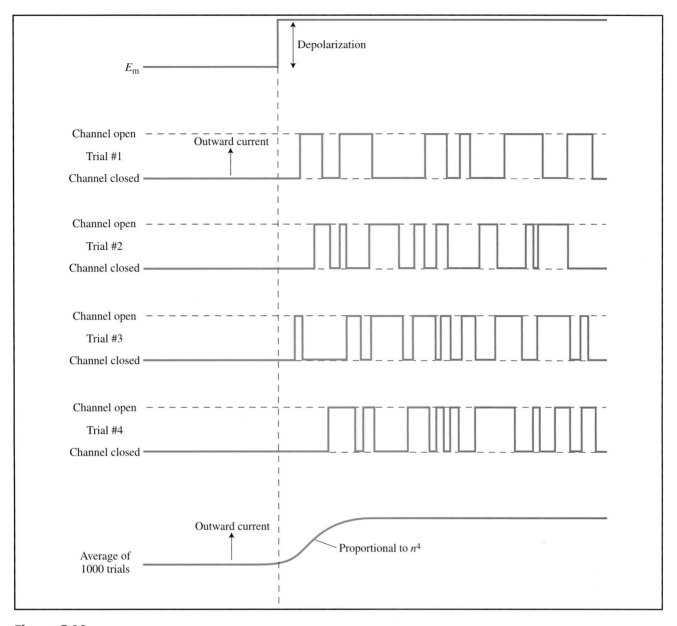

Figure C.10.

The gating of a single voltage-dependent potassium channel in response to a depolarizing voltage step. Channel openings (upward deflections) in response to four sample depolarizations are illustrated. The average response to a series of 1000 trials is shown in the *bottom trace.*

Gating of Single Ion Channels

Voltage Dependence of Potassium Channel Gating

The underlying model for voltage-dependent gating of ion channels assumes that the channels undergo abrupt transitions from closed to open states and that the transition from one state to the other occurs at a rate that depends on the transmembrane voltage. We now consider how individual channels would behave under this model. Figure C.10 illustrates the response of a single voltage-dependent potassium channel after a depolarizing voltage step. After depolarization, the probability that the channel enters the open state is higher than it is when the membrane potential is more negative. This increase in open probability arises because depolarization increases the rate constant, α_n, for movement of gating charges into the position favoring channel opening. Simultaneously, depolarization decreases the rate constant, β_n, for movement of the gating charges in the opposite direction, which results in channel closing. When the channel opens, a steady current (i_S) flows through the channel, determined by the single-channel conductance, g_S, and the electrical driving force ($E_m - E_K$):

$$i_S = g_S(E_m - E_K) \tag{C.12}$$

If the depolarizing stimulus is repeated many times, the response of the channel to each stimulus trial is unique. In some trials, the channel opens rapidly after depolarization, and in other trials the first opening occurs with a longer delay after the voltage stimulus. Thus, at each instant the channel behaves randomly, and entry into the open state is not deterministic. Although at each instant the channel may randomly open or close, the probability that the channel is open rises in proportion to n^4. As a result, the average of a large number of trials (bottom trace, Fig. C.10) provides a smoothly rising response identical to the overall potassium current recorded after a single depolarization in a cell containing a large number of channels.

Open Duration of Voltage-Dependent Potassium Channels

The time that the potassium channel spends in the open state is also random. In the Hodgkin-Huxley model, the channel opens when all four gating charges have moved to the outer face of the membrane, as illustrated schematically in Figure C.11A. Therefore, at the instant the channel opens, all of the charges must be in the "open" position. If any one of the charges redistributes to the "closed" position, the channel closes (see Fig. C.11A). The rate constant for this backward transition (that is, the transition from n to $1 - n$ in the Hodgkin-Huxley formulation) is β_n, and the equation for the rate of change of n is

$$dn/dt = -\beta_n n \tag{C.13}$$

In this case, n refers to the gating charges of the open channel, and thus there is no forward movement from $1 - n$ to n (see Equation C.7). The solution of Equation C.13 is a decaying exponential function:

$$n(t) = n_0 e^{-\beta_n t} \tag{C.14}$$

Equation C.14 provides the probability that a single gating charge remains in the "open" position at time $= t$, given that the channel was open at time $= 0$. The time course of this probability is an exponential decay, with time constant $1/\beta_n$ (see Fig. C.11B). Because the movement of any of the four gating charges induces channel closure, the rate of channel closing will be four times β_n. As a result, the probability that the channel remains open, given that it was open at time $= 0$, is given by:

$$\text{probability (open)} = e^{-4\beta_n t} \tag{C.15}$$

As shown in Figure C.11B, the probability that the channel remains open decays more rapidly than the probability that a single charge remains in the open position. The exponential time constant of decay of open probability is thus $1/4\beta_n$.

If the durations of a large number of individual channel openings are measured, the frequency distribution of observed open durations coincides with the

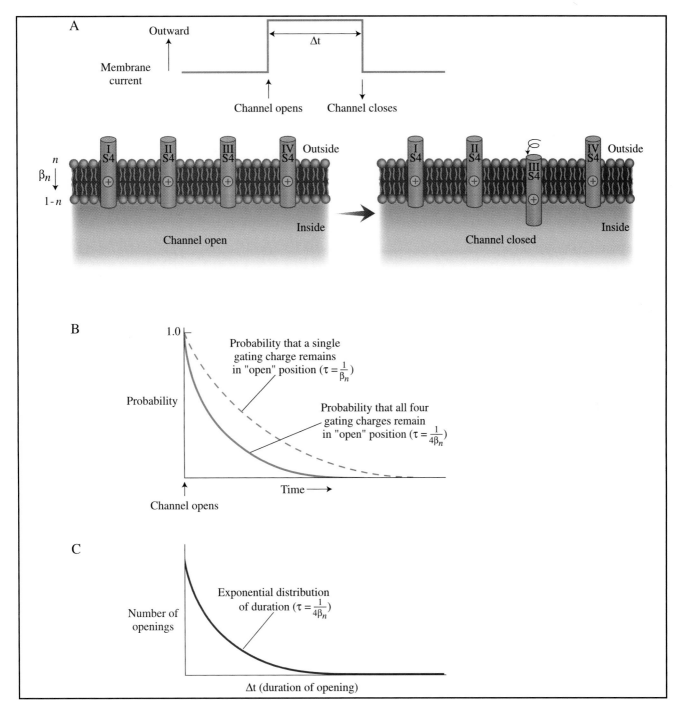

Figure C.11.

The open duration of a single voltage-dependent potassium channel. **A.** The opening of the channel requires that all four gating charges in the four subunits that make up the channel must move to the "open" position near the outer surface of the membrane. If any one of the gating charges relaxes to the inner surface of the membrane, the channel closes. **B.** The probability that a single gating charge moves to the "closed" position is governed by the rate constant, β_n. The probability that the channel remains open declines exponentially with a time constant equal to $1/4\beta_n$. **C.** The frequency distribution of open duration is exponential, also with a time constant of $1/4\beta_n$.

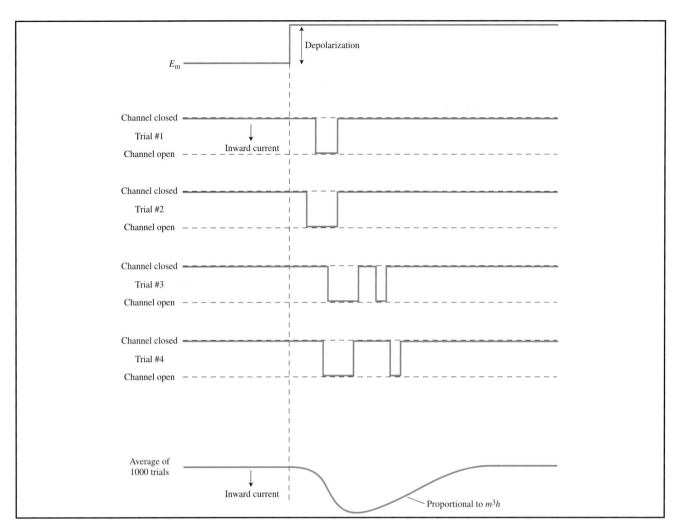

Figure C.12.

The gating of a single voltage-dependent sodium channel in response to a depolarizing voltage step. Channel openings (downward deflections) in response to four sample depolarizations are shown. The *bottom trace* shows the average response to a series of 1000 trials.

probability distribution given by Equation C.15. The expected distribution of open durations for the potassium channel is shown in Figure C.11C. For an exponential distribution, the average open duration is simply the exponential time constant, τ, which is $1/4\beta_n$.

Voltage Dependence of Sodium Channel Gating

Single sodium channels also exhibit voltage dependence of the probability of channel opening. As shown in Figure C.12, the probability that the channel enters the open state is increased by depolarization. However, as expected from the delayed closing of the inactivation gate, the probability of opening declines again during maintained depolarization. On each individual trial, the pattern of channel opening is random after depolarization. However, the average of a large number of trials reveals the time course of open probability, which is proportional to the product of m^3 and h, the activation and inactivation gating parameters in the Hodgkin-Huxley model of voltage-dependent channel gating (see bottom trace in Fig. C.12).

Glossary

A band	A darker band at the middle of a sarcomere of a striated muscle fiber, corresponding to the length of the thick filaments.
absolute refractory period	The period of time after an action potential during which a second action potential cannot be triggered. This period corresponds to the time when sodium channel inactivation gates remain closed after repolarization.
acetylcholine (ACh)	A neurotransmitter in both the central and peripheral nervous system, formed by the combination of acetate and choline, a reaction catalyzed by the synthetic enzyme choline acetyltransferase.
acetylcholinesterase	The degradative enzyme for acetylcholine, which cleaves the ester bond and releases acetate and choline.
ACh receptor	The receptor molecule that detects the presence of acetylcholine in the extracellular space and initiates the postsynaptic response to the neurotransmitter. See muscarinic ACh receptor and nicotinic ACh receptor.
actin	A motor protein. Actin forms the backbone of the thin filaments of striated muscle cells and is also involved in other cellular motions, such as the movement of growth cones.
action potential	The long-distance signal of the nervous system. Action potentials are triggered in excitable cells in response to depolarization that exceeds the threshold potential.
active zone	The subregion of a presynaptic terminal where synaptic vesicles fuse with the plasma membrane, releasing their neurotransmitter content into the synaptic cleft.
adenohypophysis	The anterior portion of the pituitary gland, containing secretory cells that release 7 different hormones into the blood stream, under control of release factors secreted by hypothalamic neurons.
adenylyl cyclase	The synthetic enzyme that converts ATP into cyclic AMP.
ADP	Adenosine diphosphate. ADP results from hydrolysis of ATP by ATPase or kinase enzymes, with the concomitant release of the terminal phosphate group of ATP.
Adrenaline	An alternative term for epinephrine.
afferent pathway	A pathway carrying incoming sensory information into the nervous system.
afterhyperpolarization	A period after an action potential during which the membrane potential is more negative than usual.
agnosia	A collective term for the inability to identify objects based on sensory information, even though the primary sensory cortex is intact.
alpha motor neurons	Large motor neurons that innervate the extrafusal muscle fibers of skeletal muscles.
Alzheimer's disease	The most common type of age-related, progressive dementia, produced by death of neurons in a variety of brain regions. The disease is characterized by two pathological features in the brain: neuritic plaques and neurofibrillary tangles.
amacrine cell	A neuron type found in the retina. Amacrine cells are lateral interneurons that receive input from bipolar cells and make synapses onto the synaptic terminals of bipolar cells and onto the dendrites of ganglion cells.

539

AMPA receptor A subtype of glutamate receptor. AMPA receptors are ligand-gated ion channels that open when glutamate binds and allow cations to enter the postsynaptic cell.

angiotensin A neuroactive hormone involved in the regulation of blood osmolarity and water balance, and in drinking behavior.

angular gyrus A gyrus located at the border between the temporal, parietal, and occipital lobes of the cerebral cortex. Lesions in the angular gyrus of the language-dominant hemisphere interfere with reading and writing.

anion A negatively charged ion.

anterolateral system The sensory projection system carrying pain and temperature information through the lateral sensory tract of the spinal cord to the brainstem, thalamus, and somatosensory cortex.

aphagia Absence of feeding.

aphasia A disorder of understanding or production of spoken language.

apraxia A deficit in programming complex series of movements, without paralysis, sensory defects, or difficulty performing simple movements.

archicortex A simple form of cortex having only a single layer of cells, as opposed to the multiple cell layers found in the neocortex. The hippocampus is an example of archicortex.

arcuate fasciculus A fiber tract in the cortical white matter containing axons that interconnect Wernicke's and Broca's areas. Damage in this fiber tract produces a form of aphasia called conduction aphasia.

area MT A portion of the middle temporal cortex (MT) involved in the detection of visual motion. Also called area V5.

area V1 Another name for the primary visual cortex, or striate cortex, located in the occipital lobe.

ATP Adenosine triphosphate. The high-energy phosphate compound that is the primary source of energy for a variety of energy-requiring cellular processes. ATP also provides the donor phosphate group for phosphorylation of protein molecules by kinase enzymes. The second messenger, cyclic AMP, is synthesized from ATP by the enzyme adenylyl cyclase.

atria (singular: atrium) The upper chambers of the mammalian heart that receive blood returning from the venous circulation (right atrium) or from the lungs (left atrium).

atrioventricular (AV) node A specialized group of muscle cells located near the center of the heart, between the atria and ventricles. Action potentials spread from the atria to the ventricles through the cells of the AV node, which have a slow conduction speed. Contraction of the ventricles is therefore delayed with respect to the contraction of the atria.

autonomic nervous system One of the major subdivisions of the nervous system, containing neurons that provide involuntary control of heart muscle, smooth muscle, and glands. The autonomic nervous system consists of the sympathetic and parasympathetic divisions.

axon The neurite that carries action potentials leaving the cell body of a neuron and distributes the signal to postsynaptic target cells.

basal ganglia	An interconnected group of three forebrain nuclei involved in motor control. The three nuclei are the caudate nucleus, the putamen, and the globus pallidus.
basilar membrane	A membrane within the cochlea that vibrates in response to sound stimuli. The sensory structure of the ear (the organ of Corti) rides on top of the basilar membrane.
beta-adrenergic receptor	A G protein-coupled receptor activated by the neurotransmitter norepinephrine. For example, the sympathetic input to the heart is mediated by beta-adrenergic receptors.
beta-amyloid protein (Aβ)	A peptide fragment that forms the principal component of neuritic plaques in the brains of patients with Alzheimer's disease. Beta-amyloid protein is produced by proteolysis of a normal neuronal membrane protein, amyloid precursor protein.
bipolar cell	A neuron type found in the retina. Bipolar cells are second-order neurons that receive synaptic input from photoreceptors and make synapses on amacrine cells and ganglion cells.
blobs	Groups of neurons within the primary visual cortex, containing color-sensitive cells. The cells within the blobs have high numbers of mitochondria, which are revealed by staining for the mitochondrial enzyme, cytochrome oxidase.
brainstem	A collective term for the midbrain (mesencephalon) and hindbrain (rhombencephalon).
Broca's area	Region of the frontal lobe of the dominant cortical hemisphere for language, where damage produces deficits in production of speech (expressive aphasia). Broca's area is located just anterior to the portion of the primary motor cortex that controls the muscles of the mouth and tongue.
calcium-induced calcium release channel	The ion channel of the sarcoplasmic reticulum that allows calcium ions to flow out of the sarcoplasmic reticulum to trigger contraction of skeletal muscle cells.
cation	A positively charged ion.
caudate nucleus	One of the basal ganglia of the forebrain. Together with the putamen, the caudate nucleus is part of the striatum.
cellular adhesion molecules	Membrane proteins on the external surface of cells that allow cells to adhere to one another or to the extracellular matrix.
center-surround receptive field	A receptive field shape in which a circular central region and a ring-shaped surrounding region have opposing effects on the cell's activity.
central sulcus	The large infolding, or groove, in the dorsal surface of the cerebral cortex, approximately midway between the anterior and posterior poles of the brain.
cerebellum	A major part of the brainstem in mammalian brains, involved in integration of sensory information and motor commands.
cerebral cortex	The outer surface of the cerebrum, containing most of the neurons in the cerebrum.
cerebral ventricles	The fluid-filled canal at the center of the brain.
cerebrospinal fluid (CSF)	The fluid filling the cerebral ventricles and the spinal canal.
cerebrum	A major subdivision of the forebrain. Together, the cerebrum and basal ganglia make up the telencephalon.

C-fibers	Small-diameter, unmyelinated axons of peripheral nerves. C-fibers carry pain and temperature information.
chemoreceptors	Sensory neurons that detect chemical sensory stimuli.
chemotropic molecule	Diffusible extracellular signal molecule that can guide the movements of nearby growth cones. Chemotropic molecules may either repel or attract growth cones.
choline acetyltransferase	The enzyme that synthesizes the neurotransmitter acetylcholine.
cholinergic neuron	A neuron that uses the neurotransmitter acetylcholine.
chromaffin cell	A secretory cell of the adrenal gland that releases norepinephrine and epinephrine into the blood stream.
cingulate gyrus	Part of the limbic system, this outfolding of the cerebral cortex runs front to back, hidden from view within the interhemispheric fissure that separates the two cerebral hemispheres.
cingulum	An axon bundle that contains axons projecting from the cingulate gyrus to the entorhinal cortex in the limbic system.
circadian rhythm	A cyclical change in a physiological or biochemical process having a period of approximately 24 hours.
cochlea	Part of the inner ear that contains the sensory hair cells of the sense of hearing.
cochlear nucleus	A nucleus in the brainstem that receives synaptic input from the spiral ganglion neurons of the cochlea.
collagen	A structural protein that forms the backbone of the extracellular matrix in many tissues.
cones	One of the two major classes of photoreceptors, the other being rods. Cones are less sensitive to light than rods and mediate color vision.
corpus callosum	The large fiber bundle containing axons interconnecting neurons of the two cerebral hemispheres.
corticobulbar system	The motor pathway carrying descending motor commands from the motor cortex to the brainstem.
corticospinal system	The motor pathway carrying axons from the motor cortex to the spinal cord, bypassing the brainstem motor centers.
cranial nerves	Nerves that directly connect the brain to peripheral targets. The human nervous system includes twelve distinct cranial nerves.
cross bridge	A structure visible through the electron microscope, connecting adjacent thick and thin filaments of a myofibril. The cross bridges are formed by myosin molecules that make up the thick filament.
cuneate nucleus	One of the dorsal column nuclei in the brainstem. The cuneate nucleus receives somatosensory inputs from the lateral portions of the dorsal columns of the spinal cord.
cyclic AMP	An intracellular second messenger synthesized by the enzyme adenylyl cyclase from ATP.

cyclic GMP	An intracellular second messenger synthesized by the enzyme guanylyl cyclase from GTP.
decussation	A cross over of axons from one side of the brain to the other.
dendrite	A neurite that receives synaptic inputs from other neurons.
dendritic spine	A short, hair-like projection from dendrite. Excitatory synapses commonly contact dendrites of CNS neurons at dendritic spines.
dentate nucleus	One of the deep nuclei of the cerebellum, in the brainstem.
depolarization	Movement of the membrane potential in the positive direction, from its normal negative level.
diacylglycerol	An intracellular second messenger, formed by the enzyme phospholipase C from membrane lipid.
diencephalon	A subdivision of the forebrain, comprising the thalamus and hypothalamus.
dorsal column nuclei	Nuclei in the brainstem that receive synaptic inputs from somatosensory neurons whose axons are located in the dorsal columns. The dorsal column nuclei are the gracile nucleus and the cuneate nucleus.
dorsal column	A fiber bundle along the dorsal surface of the spinal cord, primarily consisting of branches of primary somatosensory neurons ascending from the spinal cord to the brainstem.
dorsal root ganglion	A ganglion located just outside the spinal cord at each vertebral segment, containing the cell bodies of sensory neurons whose axons enter the spinal cord at that segment.
dorsal root	The fiber bundle containing incoming (afferent) sensory axons entering the spinal cord at each vertebral segment.
efferent pathway	A pathway carrying outgoing motor information from neurons.
emboliform nucleus	One of the deep nuclei of the cerebellum, in the brainstem.
end-plate potential	The postsynaptic electrical response elicited in a skeletal muscle cell by activation of its motor neuron.
end-plate	The synaptic zone of a skeletal muscle cell, where postsynaptic ACh receptors are clustered at high density across from the synaptic terminal of the motor neuron.
entorhinal cortex	A part of the olfactory system and the limbic system. The entorhinal cortex provides input to the hippocampus, and receives synaptic connections from the cingulate gyrus. The entorhinal cortex is an example of paleocortex, having only two cellular layers.
epinephrine	A hormone secreted by adrenal chromaffin cells into the bloodstream. Also used as a neurotransmitter.
equilibrium potential	The value of membrane potential at which a permeant ion is at equilibrium. The equilibrium potential is calculated from the Nernst equation.
excitation-contraction coupling	The process through which an action potential triggers contraction of a muscle cell.

excitatory postsynaptic potential (e.p.s.p.)	A postsynaptic change in membrane potential that promotes firing of an action potential in the postsynaptic cell, by bringing the membrane potential toward the threshold potential.
exteroceptors	Sensory receptors that detect stimuli originating outside the organism. For example, photoreceptors are exteroceptors.
extracellular matrix	An external lattice of proteins and polysaccharides that is secreted by surrounding cells in most tissues.
extrafusal muscle fibers	The muscle cells of a skeletal muscle that generate the contractile force of the muscle and are located outside of muscle spindles.
extraocular muscles	The skeletal muscles that control the movements of the eyes.
fastigial nucleus	One of the deep nuclei of the cerebellum, in the brainstem.
filopodia (singular: filopodium)	Part of a growth cone. Filopodia are finger-like amoeboid structures that interact with the external environment and propel the growth cone forward.
forebrain	The most anterior of the three brain vesicles that arise from the neural tube early in brain development. Also, the adult brain region that arises from the forebrain vesicle. The forebrain consists of the telencephalon and diencephalon.
fornix	A large fiber bundle that contains output axons leaving the hippocampus.
fourth ventricle	The part of the cerebral ventricles located in the hindbrain.
fovea	The part of the retina that receives light from the center of the visual field, at the normal fixation point of the eye.
frontal eye field	Part of the frontal lobe where neurons generate commands that trigger saccades of the eyes.
G protein (GTP-binding protein)	An important class of intracellular signaling molecules that provide the link between activated receptor molecules (such as hormone or neurotransmitter receptors that are not ligand-gated ion channels) and subsequent biochemical events inside target cells. G-proteins are activated when they bind GTP in response to receptor activation.
GABA (gamma aminobutyric acid)	A major inhibitory neurotransmitter in the brain. GABA is synthesized from glutamate by the enzyme glutamic acid decarboxylase.
gamma motor neuron	A special class of motor neurons that innervate the intrafusal muscle fibers within muscle spindles in skeletal muscles.
ganglion (plural: ganglia)	A cluster of neuronal cell bodies, usually located outside the central nervous system in vertebrates. Invertebrate central nervous systems consist of a series of ganglia connected by nerve bundles.
gap junction	A site of electrical connection between two cells, where gap junction channels bridge the gap between the insides of the two cells and allow small molecules such as ions to cross directly from one cell to the other.
GDP	Guanosine diphosphate, which is formed when GTP is hydrolyzed, releasing the terminal phosphate group.
geniculostriate pathway	The visual pathway leading from the lateral geniculate nucleus of the thalamus to the primary visual cortex (striate cortex).

glial cell	A non-neuronal cell in the nervous system that helps regulate the extracellular environment, including uptake of neurotransmitters released from synapses.
globus pallidus	One of the basal ganglia of the forebrain.
glutamate	An amino acid (glutamic acid) used as a neurotransmitter at many excitatory synapses in the central nervous system.
glycosaminoglycans	Large polysaccharide molecules of the extracellular matrix, which often combine with proteins to form proteoglycans.
Golgi tendon organ	A specialized sensory structure that provides an indication of the force applied to a tendon by active contraction of a skeletal muscle.
gracile nucleus	One of the dorsal column nuclei in the brainstem. The gracile nucleus receives somatosensory inputs from the medial portion of the dorsal columns in the spinal cord.
gray matter	A portion of the central nervous system containing predominantly neuronal cell bodies. The relative lack of myelinated axons makes gray matter less opaque than surround areas containing fewer cell bodies and more myelinated fibers (white matter).
growth cone	A motile structure at the leading edge of a growing neurite.
GTP	Guanosine triphosphate. A high energy phosphate compound formed by the combination of guanosine and a chain of three phosphate groups. GTP is an important signaling molecule because it is necessary for activation of G proteins.
guanylyl cyclase	The enzyme that synthesizes the second messenger, cyclic GMP, from GTP.
gyrus (plural: gyri)	An outfolding of the cerebral cortex in brains in which the cortex is highly folded (convoluted), such as the human brain.
habituation	Reduction in the strength of a reflexive response produced by repeated presentation of the eliciting stimulus.
hair cell	A ciliated sensory cell that produces changes in membrane potential in response to movements of the cilia induced by sensory stimuli.
hair follicle receptor	A type of sensory neuron that innervates hair follicles in the skin and is activated when the hair is deflected.
heterologous expression	An experimental technique in which DNA or mRNA for a protein is incorporated into a target cell that does not normally produce the protein.
hindbrain	The most posterior of the three brain vesicles that arise at the anterior end of the neural tube during embryonic development of the brain. Also, the most posterior part of the adult brain, which develops from the hindbrain vesicle, including the pons, medulla, and cerebellum.
hippocampus	A simplified form of cerebral cortex (archicortex) located under the lower lip of the neocortex at the medial border of the temporal lobe. The hippocampus is part of the limbic system and is thought to be involved in certain types of memory.
homeostasis	The maintenance of a relatively constant internal environment despite large changes in external conditions.
horizontal cell	A neuron type found in the retina. Horizontal cells are lateral interneurons that receive synaptic inputs from photoreceptors.

hyperpolarization	A change in membrane potential in the negative direction, making the cell interior more negative.
hypothalamus	A part of the diencephalon involved in a variety of homeostatic functions, in the control of the pituitary, and in motivation and drive. The hypothalamus is a major part of the limbic system.
I band	In a striated muscle cell, the part of the sarcomere corresponding the region occupied only by thin filaments, where thin and thick filaments do not overlap.
immunocytochemistry	An experimental technique in which an antibody specific for a particular protein is used to localize that protein in the cells or tissues.
inferior colliculus	The more posterior of the two colliculi, located on the dorsal surface of the midbrain. The inferior colliculus is a processing center for auditory information ascending from the cochlear nucleus and superior olivary nucleus in the brainstem.
inhibitory postsynaptic potential (i.p.s.p.)	A postsynaptic change in membrane potential that tends to prevent firing of an action potential in the postsynaptic cell, by bringing the membrane potential away from the threshold potential.
initial segment	The initial part of the axon as it leaves the cell body of a neuron. The initial segment is often the point at which action potentials are initiated in response to depolarization.
inositol trisphosphate	An intracellular second messenger, which is produced from membrane lipid by the enzyme phospholipase C.
intermediolateral gray matter	The part of the spinal cord gray matter containing the cell bodies of sympathetic preganglionic neurons.
interneuron	A neuron in the nervous system that receives inputs from other neurons and makes synaptic contact with other neurons.
interoceptors	Sensory receptor cells that detect stimuli arising within the organism. Muscle spindle receptors are an example of interoceptors.
intrafusal muscle fibers	The specialized subset of skeletal muscle cells found within the muscle spindle.
inverse myotatic reflex	The reflex stimulated by activation of sensory neurons of Golgi tendon organs (also called the tendon organ reflex). Activation of this reflex leads to inhibition of the motor neurons for the same muscle, causing a reduction in muscle tension.
ion channel	A membrane protein that forms an aqueous pore through which charged ions can cross the membrane.
isometric contraction	A muscle contraction in which muscle length does not change although muscle tension increases.
isotonic contraction	A muscle contraction in muscle tension remains constant during the contraction.
labyrinth	A collective term for the cochlea, semicircular canals, and otolith organs in the inner ear.
lamellipodium	Part of a growth cone, extending between successive filopodia. When filopodia adhere to the substrate, the lamellopodium fills in the space between the filopodia to bring the growth cone forward in the direction of growth.
lateral column	The lateral white matter of the spinal cord.

lateral geniculate nucleus	The part of the thalamus that receives synaptic inputs from retinal ganglion cells and projects to the primary visual cortex.
lateral inhibition	Inhibition mediated by lateral interneurons, in which sensory stimuli at a particular location on the sensory surface inhibits activity in sensory pathways originating from adjacent regions of the sensory surface.
lateral intraparietal area	A part of the parietal lobe of the cerebral cortex involved in integrating visual stimuli with the control of eye movements.
lateral lemniscus	An axon tract carrying auditory information from the cochlear nucleus and superior olivary nucleus in the brainstem to the inferior colliculus in the midbrain.
lateral line organ	A sensory system found in aquatic vertebrates, containing hair cells that respond to water movement.
lateral sensory tract	Part of the lateral white matter in the spinal cord, containing axons of interneurons that receive inputs from nociceptors and temperature-sensitive sensory neurons.
lateral ventricles	The portion of the cerebral ventricles found in the telencephalon.
leptin	A hormone synthesized by fat cells and thought to be involved in the regulation of feeding behavior.
ligand-gated ion channel	An ion channel in which channel gating is controlled by binding of a chemical signal (the ligand) to a specific binding site on the channel protein. The ACh-gated ion channel of the neuromuscular junction is an example.
limbic system	A brain system involved in the regulation of emotion, motivation, and homeostasis.
Long-term depression (LTD)	A reduction in the strength of a synaptic connection lasting for hours or days.
Long-term potentiation (LTP)	An enhancement of postsynaptic response amplitude lasting hours or days, produced by a burst of presynaptic activity. LTP is commonly studied as a cellular model of learning and memory.
M line	In the sarcomere of a striated muscle cell, the transverse line at the midpoint of the sarcomere. The M line consists of filaments connecting the thick filaments at their midpoint.
mammillothalamic tract	A fiber tract containing axons projecting from the mammillary bodies of the hypothalamus to the thalamus in the limbic system.
marginal zone	The relatively cell free region at the outer edge of the neural tube.
mechanoreceptors	Sensory receptor neurons that respond to mechanical displacement of the sensory surface. Examples are muscle spindle receptors and hair cells.
medial geniculate nucleus	The portion of the thalamus that processes auditory information. The medial geniculate nucleus receives synaptic input from the inferior colliculus and sends axons to the primary auditory cortex.
medial lemniscus	A fiber tract carrying ascending somatosensory information from the dorsal column nuclei of the brainstem to the thalamus in the diencephalon.
medulla oblongata	The most posterior part of the brainstem, at the border between the brain and the spinal cord.

Meissner corpuscle	A rapidly adapting skin mechanoreceptor that is sensitive to touch and pressure.
membrane potential	The electrical voltage difference between the inside and the outside of a cell.
Merkel receptor	A slowly adapting skin mechanoreceptor that signals sustained pressure.
mesencephalon	The midbrain.
midbrain	The middle of the three brain vesicles that arise from the neural tube during embryonic development. In the adult brain, the midbrain consists of brain structures such as the superior colliculus, the inferior colliculus, and parts of the reticular formation.
miniature end-plate potential	A small postsynaptic depolarization at the neuromuscular junction, arising from spontaneous fusion of a single synaptic vesicle in the synaptic terminal.
motor neuron	A neuron that makes synaptic contact with the final target cell, such as a skeletal muscle cell.
motor unit	A single motor neuron and all of the muscle cells that receive synaptic connections from that motor neuron.
muscarinic acetylcholine receptor	A type of G protein-coupled receptor, activated by acetylcholine.
muscle fiber	A muscle cell.
muscle spindle	An encapsulated sensory structure activated by stretch of skeletal muscles.
myelin	The insulating sheath around axons, formed by certain types of glial cells.
myofibril	A bundle of thick and thin filaments that forms an organizational unit within a single muscle cell, which contains several myofibrils.
myosin	The protein that makes up the thick filaments of a myofibril. ATP hydrolysis by myosin provides the energy to drive filament sliding during muscle contraction.
myotatic reflex	The spinal reflex triggered by activation of muscle spindles.
neocortex	A type of cerebral cortex characterized by multiple layers of cells. Most of the cerebral cortex in the human brain consists of neocortex. Examples of neocortex are the primary somatosensory cortex and the primary motor cortex.
Nernst equation	The equation used to calculate the equilibrium potential for a permeant ion.
nerve growth factor	A protein neurotrophin that stimulates neurite outgrowth and influences gene expression in neurons by activating trkA receptors (tyrosine receptor kinase type A).
neural crest	The portion of the neural plate and neural groove containing cells that give rise to the peripheral nervous system. At the neural groove stage, the neural crest occupies the lateral margins of the groove. At the neural tube stage, the neural crest separates from the neural tube.
neural groove	An indentation along the midline of the developing embryo, formed by the proliferation of neuronal precursor cells in the neural plate.
neural plate	The portion of ectoderm overlying the notochord, containing cells that will give rise to the nervous system during further embryonic development.

neural tube	A tubular structure formed by fission of the neural groove from overlying ectoderm. The brain and spinal cord develop from neural tube.
neurite	A collective term for the dendrites and axons of a neuron.
neuritic plaque	A pathological feature found in the brains of patients with Alzheimer's disease. Neuritic plaques are extracellular accumulations of protein, consisting largely of beta-amyloid protein.
neurofibrillary tangle	A pathological feature found in the brains of patients with Alzheimer's disease. Neurofibrillary tangles are abnormal intracellular accumulations of a microtubule-associated protein called tau.
neurogenesis	The stage of neural development when neuronal precursor cells proliferate to produce neurons.
neurohypophysis	The posterior part of the pituitary gland, where nerve terminals of hypothalamic magnocellular neurosecretory cells release the hormones oxytocin and vasopressin.
neuromuscular junction	The synaptic junction between the motor neuron and its postsynaptic skeletal muscle cell.
neuron	A nerve cell.
neurotransmitter	The chemical messenger released from a synaptic terminal to influence a postsynaptic target cell.
neurotrophins	A soluble molecule secreted into the external space that promotes the survival of neurons and stimulates neurite outgrowth.
nicotinic acetylcholine receptor	A type of ligand-gated acetylcholine receptor molecule in which ACh directly binds to the channel protein and opens the channel.
nitric oxide	A small, membrane-permeant molecule that is thought to serve as a cellular signal. Nitric oxide (NO) is formed by the enzyme nitric oxide synthase from the amino acid arginine.
NMDA receptor	A subtype of glutamate receptor. NMDA receptors require glutamate binding and depolarization to allow cations to enter the postsynaptic cell. Open NMDA receptors also allow calcium ions to enter the postsynaptic cell.
nociceptor	A sensory neuron that is activated by stimuli that damage tissue, leading to the sensation of pain.
nodes of Ranvier	Periodic breaks in the myelin sheath, where voltage-dependent sodium channels are clustered and sodium influx occurs to support action potential propagation.
norepinephrine (noradrenaline)	A neurotransmitter released by sympathetic motor neurons and by some neurons in the central nervous system.
notochord	A long, rod-shaped group of cells formed in the mesoderm during gastrulation of the early embryo. The notochord defines the longitudinal axis of the body plan and induces formation of neural tissue in the overlying ectoderm.
nucleus (plural: nuclei)	A cluster of neuronal cell bodies within the central nervous system.
olfactory bulb	The part of the central nervous system that receives synaptic projections from olfactory sensory neurons, via the olfactory nerve.

oligodendrocyte	A type of glial cell that myelinates axons in the central nervous system.
optic chiasm	The cross-over point of the optic nerve, where ganglion cell axons from the temporal and nasal portions of the retina are sorted to ipsilateral or contralateral projections to the lateral geniculate nucleus.
organ of Corti	The sensory structure within the cochlea, where sensory hair cells are located.
osmosis	The movement of water down its concentration gradient.
otolith organ	A sensory structure containing hair cells that detect the organism's orientation with respect to gravity.
oxytocin	A hormone released in the posterior pituitary by hypothalamic neurosecretory neurons.
Pacinian corpuscle	A rapidly adapting skin mechanoreceptor that is sensitive to touch and pressure.
paleocortex	A form of cerebral cortex characterized by two layers of cells, as opposed to the multiple layers of cells found in the neocortex. Entorhinal cortex of the olfactory system is an example of paleocortex.
Papez circuit	The central core of the limbic system, consisting of a loop from the cingulate gyrus, entorhinal cortex, hippocampus, hypothalamus, thalamus, and back to the cingulate gyrus.
parasympathetic division	The acetylcholine-releasing division of the autonomic nervous system.
paravertebral ganglia	The chain of sympathetic ganglia that parallel the spinal column.
Parkinson's disease	A human disease characterized by muscle tremor and difficulty in initiating and sustaining locomotion. The disease results from degeneration of dopamine-releasing neurons of the substantia nigra.
phosphodiesterase	An enzyme that inactivates cyclic nucleotide molecules, such as cyclic AMP or cyclic GMP.
phospholipase C	An enzyme that acts on phospholipid molecules in the plasma membrane to release the intracellular messenger molecules inositol trisphosphate and diacylglycerol. Inositol trisphosphate increases the intracellular calcium concentration, while diacylglycerol activates protein kinase C.
phospholipid	A type of lipid molecule that forms the lipid barrier of cell membranes. A phospholipid molecule includes a hydrophilic portion and a hydrophobic portion.
phosphorylation	Attachment of a phosphate group to specific amino acid residues of a target protein, carried out by a kinase enzyme.
pituitary gland	A master control endocrine gland at the base of the brain. The pituitary gland is controlled in turn by the hypothalamus.
plasma membrane	The external cell membrane separating the interior and the exterior of the cell.
pons	A major subdivision of the hindbrain.
portal vessels	Blood vessels that transport release factors secreted by hypothalamic neurons to the anterior pituitary gland, where they control the release of pituitary hormones.
postcentral gyrus	The gyrus located just posterior to the central sulcus, consisting of the primary somatosensory cortex.

postsynaptic cell	The target cell at a synapse.
post-tetanic potentiation	Synaptic potentiation that follows a sustained, high-frequency burst of presynaptic action potentials.
precentral gyrus	The gyrus located just anterior to the central sulcus, consisting of the primary motor cortex.
premotor cortex	Part of the frontal lobe anterior to the primary motor cortex, containing neurons that encode complex movements.
preoptic area	Part of the telencephalon just anterior and superior to the anterior end of the hypothalamus. The preoptic area is closely associated with the hypothalamus and is usually considered to be part of the hypothalamus.
presynaptic cell	The input cell at a synapse.
prevertebral ganglia	Sympathetic ganglia located in the abdominal cavity.
primary visual cortex	The visual cortical area that receives direct input from the lateral geniculate nucleus. The primary visual cortex (area V1; striate cortex) is located at the posterior pole of the occipital lobe.
process	Another name for a neurite.
proprioceptor	A sensory receptor neuron that detects limb or joint position, muscle length, or muscle tension.
prosencephalon	The forebrain.
protein kinase A	A kinase enzyme that is activated by cyclic AMP. The active kinase phosphorylates target proteins, such as ion channels.
protein kinase C	A kinase enzyme that is activated by an intracellular messenger, diacylglycerol, together with calcium. Diacylglycerol is produced from membrane lipid by the enzyme phospholipase C.
proteoglycans	A constituent of the extracellular matrix, formed by the combination of protein and glycosaminoglycan molecules.
Purkinje cell	The output cells of the cerebellum.
putamen	One of the basal ganglia of the forebrain. Together, the putamen and the caudate nucleus form the striatum.
pyramidal cell	A type of cortical neuron shaped like a pyramid, with a long apical dendrite originating from the narrow end of the cell.
pyramids	The fiber bundles consisting of descending axons from the primary motor cortex.
radial glial cell	A glial cell that extends from the ventricular zone to the marginal zone during early neural development. Migrating neurons leaving the ventricular zone follow the long thin radial glial cells.
raphe nucleus	A nucleus located near the midline of the brainstem, containing (among other neurons) the omnidirectional pause neurons that allow saccades to proceed.
receptive field	The portion of the sensory surface where stimuli affect the activity of a sensory neuron.

receptor potential	The change in membrane potential in a primary sensory receptor neuron in response to a sensory stimulus.
receptor tyrosine kinase (or tyrosine receptor kinase)	A membrane protein whose extracellular portion binds a neurotrophin. The intracellular portion of the molecule includes a tyrosine protein kinase region, which phosphorylates target proteins when the receptor is occupied.
red nucleus	A brainstem motor control nucleus that gives rise to the rubrospinal tract. Activation of the rubrospinal tract promotes limb flexion.
release factor	A substance released into portal vessels by hypothalamic neurosecretory neurons to control release of anterior pituitary hormones.
Renshaw cell	An inhibitory interneuron in the spinal cord that receives excitatory input from a motor neuron and makes inhibitory synapses back onto the same motor neuron.
resting potential	The steady state membrane potential of a neuron in the absence of incoming synaptic or sensory influences.
reticular formation	A diffuse network of neurons in the midbrain and hindbrain, involved in a variety of sensory and motor functions.
reticulospinal tract	A fiber tract consisting of descending axons from neurons in the reticular formation to spinal interneurons and motor neurons.
retina	The multilayered structure at the back of the eye responsible for light reception and processing of visual information. The retina consists of the neural retina, containing the neurons and glial cells, and the retinal pigmented epithelium, which absorbs stray light and supports the outer segments of photoreceptor cells.
retinal (retinaldehyde)	The light-absorbing chromophore group that is chemically attached to the opsin protein to form a visual pigment molecule.
retinal ganglion cell	The output cells of the retina, whose axons form the optic nerve and project to the lateral geniculate nucleus of the thalamus, the accessory optic system, and the suprachiasmatic nucleus of the hypothalamus.
retinohypothalamic tract	The fiber tract consisting of axons of retinal ganglion cells projecting to the suprachiasmatic nucleus of the hypothalamus.
rhodopsin	The visual pigment molecule of rod photoreceptors.
rhombencephalon	The hindbrain.
rods	A subtype of photoreceptor found in the vertebrate retina. Rods are more sensitive to light than cones are responsible for vision under dim illumination.
rubrospinal tract	The fiber tract containing axons descending to the spinal cord from the red nucleus of the brainstem.
Ruffini corpuscle	A slowly adapting skin mechanoreceptor that signals sustained pressure.
saccade	A rapid eye movement used to alter eye position within the orbit, causing a rapid adjustment of the fixation point to different positions in the visual world.
saccule	The horizontally oriented otolith organ of the labyrinth.

saltatory conduction	A form of action potential propagation found in myelinated axons, in which action potentials jump from one node of Ranvier to the next.
sarcomere	The basic repeating unit of striation along the length of myofibrils of striated muscle cells. The sarcomere is defined as extending from one Z line to the next Z line.
sarcoplasmic reticulum	An intracellular store of calcium ions wrapped around the contractile apparatus of myofibrils in striated muscle cells. Calcium released from the sarcoplasmic reticulum triggers contraction.
saxitoxin	A naturally occurring biological toxin that blocks voltage-dependent sodium channels and prevents neurons from firing action potentials.
Schwann cell	A type of glial cell that forms the myelin sheath around axons in the peripheral nervous system.
semicircular canals	The acceleration-sensing, fluid-filled loops that form part of the labyrinth.
sensitization	Enhancement of the strength of a reflexive response produced by the presentation of a noxious stimulus.
sensory adaptation	The reduction in activity of a sensory neuron during sustained application of a sensory stimulus.
sensory neuron	A neuron whose activity is affected by the presence of a particular type of sensory stimulus.
sensory transduction	The conversion of stimulus energy into an electrical signal in a primary sensory receptor neuron.
sinoatrial (SA) node	A specialized group of cardiac muscle cells in the right atrium that normally control the rate of the heart beat.
skeletal muscle	A type of striated muscle responsible for movement of body parts.
SNAP-25	A membrane protein involved in docking and/or fusion of synaptic vesicles at active zones of synaptic terminals.
sodium pump (Na$^+$-K$^+$ ATPase).	A membrane protein that uses energy released by hydrolysis of ATP to actively transport sodium out of the cell and potassium into the cell.
soma	The cell body of a cell, where the nucleus is located.
somatic nervous system	The division of the nervous system that controls the skeletal muscles, as distinguished from the autonomic nervous system.
somatopic map	A form of neural organization in which neighboring regions of a body structure project to or are controlled by neighboring neurons in the brain region that receive sensory inputs from or send motor output to the body structure.
somatosensory system	The sensory system that receives and processes sensory information from the body, including the skin, muscles, and joints.
spatial summation	Summation of postsynaptic responses in a postsynaptic cell from two or more synaptic inputs that are active at about the same time.
spinal canal	The fluid filled space at the center of the spinal cord. The spinal canal is continuous with the ventricles of the brain.

spinal nerve	The mixed motor and sensory nerve connected to the spinal cord at a particular vertebral segment.
spinocerebellar tract	The sensory pathway in the spinal cord carrying ascending axons to the cerebellum.
spiral ganglion	The ganglion in the cochlea containing the cell bodies of sensory neurons that receive inputs from the cochlear hair cells and send axons via the auditory nerve (cranial nerve VIII) to the cochlear nucleus of the brainstem.
stellate cell	A neuron whose dendrites radiate approximately equally in all directions from the soma, producing a starlike pattern.
stem cell	An undifferentiated precursor cell that retains the ability to give rise to a variety of cell types. In the nervous system, stem cells can give rise to various neuron subtypes and to glial cells.
striated muscle cell	A type of muscle cell in which the contractile machinery forms a regular, repeating array, which gives the cell a striped (striated) appearance when viewed through the light microscope.
striatum	A collective term for the caudate nucleus and putamen, which are two of the basal ganglia of the forebrain.
substantia nigra	A midbrain region involved in the control of motor behavior. Loss of dopamine-releasing neurons of the substantia nigra underlies the movement disorder called Parkinson's disease.
sulcus (plural: sulci)	An infolding, or groove, in the cortical surface. A sulcus separates neighboring gyri.
superior colliculus	A brain region on the dorsal surface of the midbrain that is involved in the control of eye movements.
superior olivary nucleus (superior olive)	A nucleus in the brainstem that is involved in the processing of auditory information. The superior olivary nucleus receives inputs from the cochlear nuclei and sends outputs to the inferior colliculus.
supplemental motor area	A higher order cortical motor area located in the medial part of the frontal lobe, just anterior to the primary motor cortex.
suprachiasmatic nucleus	A nucleus of the hypothalamus responsible for synchronizing circadian rhythms in other organs and tissues.
Sylvian fissure	The large sulcus that separates the temporal lobe from the rest of the cerebral cortex. It is also called the lateral sulcus.
sympathetic chains	A series of interconnected sympathetic nuclei (the paravertebral ganglia) that parallel both sides of the vertebral column.
sympathetic division	A division of the autonomic nervous system, containing autonomic motor neurons that release the neurotransmitter norepinephrine. Actions of the sympathetic nervous system typically oppose the actions of the other division of the autonomic nervous system, the parasympathetic division.
synapse	The contact point where a neuron transfers information to a target cell.
synaptic cleft	The extracellular space separating the presynaptic cell and the postsynaptic cell at a synapse.
synaptic vesicle	A small, membrane-bound structure in which neurotransmitter molecules are stored within synaptic terminals.

synaptobrevin	A membrane protein associated with the membrane of synaptic vesicles. Synaptobrevin forms a complex (the SNARE complex) with the plasma membrane proteins syntaxin and SNAP-25 and is thought to play a role in vesicle targeting at the active zone.
synaptotagmin	A membrane protein associated with the membrane of synaptic vesicles that is thought to be responsible for the control of vesicle exocytosis by calcium ions.
syntaxin	A membrane protein involved in docking and/or fusion of synaptic vesicles at active zones of synaptic terminals.
taste bud	A cluster of cells on the surface of the tongue, containing taste receptor cells.
tectorial membrane	A sheet of tissue overlying the organ of Corti in the cochlea. Cilia of outer hair cells are embedded into the surface of the tectorial membrane.
telencephalon	A subdivision of the forebrain, comprising the cerebrum and the basal ganglia.
temporal summation	Summation of successive postsynaptic responses in a postsynaptic cell from two or more action potentials arriving within a brief period in the same synaptic terminal.
tetraethylammonium (TEA)	A drug that blocks potassium channels.
tetrodotoxin	A biological toxin that blocks voltage-dependent sodium channels.
thalamus	One of the two subdivisions of the diencephalon. The thalamus receives and processes sensory information and sends the sensory information to the appropriate regions of the cerebral cortex. The thalamus also plays important roles in motor control.
thermoreceptors	Primary sensory neurons that respond to changes in skin or body temperature.
thick filament	A longitudinal filament found in striated muscle cells, made up of the protein myosin.
thin filament	A longitudinal filament found in striated muscle cells, made up of the protein actin and the associated proteins tropomyosin and troponin.
third ventricle	The part of the brain ventricles that extends from the midbrain through the diencephalon.
threshold (threshold potential)	The value of membrane potential that must be reached in an excitable cell to trigger an action potential.
tonotopic map	The orderly projection of inputs originating from the cochlea to sensory areas in the brain, such that neighboring neurons in the target regions respond to progressively higher frequencies.
transducin	A G protein that is activated by photoactivated rhodopsin during transduction in photoreceptors.
transgenic animal	An animal in which the natural genetic material has been altered by the insertion of exogenous DNA or the deletion of endogenous DNA.
transverse tubules	Invaginations of the plasma membrane in skeletal muscle cells that provide a path for depolarization during the muscle action potential to spread to the cell interior.
trkA, trkB, trkC	Tyrosin receptor kinase molecules that act as receptors for neurotrophin molecules in cells.
tropomyosin	A protein associated with the thin filaments of striated muscle cells. Tropomyosin controls the access of myosin to the myosin binding site of actin.

troponin	A calcium binding molecule associated with the thin filaments of striated muscle cells. Binding of calcium to troponin initiates contraction.
tubulin	A protein molecule that polymerizes to form the backbone of microtubules.
tympanic membrane	The eardrum, which transfers sound pressure waves to the bones of the middle ear.
undershoot	The transient period of increased negativity at the termination of an action potential.
utricle	The vertically oriented otolith organ of the labyrinth.
vasopressin (antidiuretic hormone; ADH)	A hormone released by magnocellular neurosecretory cells of the hypothalamus in the posterior pituitary gland.
ventral column	The white matter on the ventral surface of the spinal cord, containing descending motor axons of the corticospinal tract, the vestibulospinal tract, and the reticulospinal tract.
ventral corticospinal tract	The portion of the ventral column containing descending axons of neurons whose cell bodies are located in the primary motor cortex.
ventral root	The fiber bundle containing outgoing (efferent) motor axons exiting the spinal cord at each vertebral segment.
ventricles	The fluid-filled core of the brain, filled with cerebrospinal fluid.
ventricular zone	The inner layer of the neural tube, next to the fluid-filled ventricle. Dividing precursor cells that give rise to the nervous system are found in the ventricular zone.
vestibular ganglion	A ganglion located just outside the labyrinth of the inner ear, containing the cell bodies of sensory neurons that receive inputs from the hair cells of the semicircular canals.
vestibular nuclei	Nuclei in the brainstem that receive synaptic inputs from sensory neurons of the vestibular ganglion.
vestibulo-ocular reflex	The reflex that induces eye movements in response to head rotation to keep the eyes fixated at a constant point in space.
vestibulospinal tract	A fiber pathway originating in the vestibular nucleus of the brainstem and projecting to the spinal cord. Activation of the vestibulospinal tract promotes limb extension.
voltage-sensitive sodium channel	A sodium channel whose conducting state depends on voltage. Opening of voltage-sensitive sodium channels underlies the depolarizing phase of the action potential.
Wernicke's area	Part of the temporal lobe surrounding the primary auditory cortex. Damage in Wernicke's area produces deficits in understanding spoken language (receptive aphasia).
white matter	Regions of the central nervous system containing few neuronal cell bodies and many myelinated axons. The myelin sheaths are opaque compared to surrounding regions containing mostly neuronal cell bodies (gray matter).
Z line	A crosswise line connecting thin filaments within a myofibril. The sarcomere is defined as extending from one Z line to the next Z line.

Index